Palliative Care in Neurology

Series Editor:

Sid Gilman, M.D., F.R.C.P.
William J. Herdman Professor of Neurology
University of Michigan Medical Center

Contemporary Neurology Series

Palliative Care in Neurology

Edited by

Raymond Voltz, M.D.

Institute of Clinical Neuroimmunology
Department of Neurology and Interdisciplinary Palliative Care Service
Klinikum Grosshadern
D-81366 Munich
Germany

James L. Bernat, M.D.
Neurology Section
Dartmouth Hitchcock Medical Center
One Medical Center Drive
Lebanon NH 03756
USA

Gian Domenico Borasio, M.D., DipPallMed
Interdisciplinary Palliative Care Unit and Department of Neurology
University of Munich
Klinikum Grosshadern
D-81366 Munich
Germany

Ian Maddocks, M.D.
Emeritus Professor
Flinders University of South Australia
215A The Esplanade
Seacliff
South Australia 5049

David Oliver, F.R.C.G.P.
Medical Director
Wisdom Hospice
St William's Way
Rochester
Kent ME1 2NU
UK

Russell K. Portenoy, M.D.
Chairman
Department of Pain Medicine and Palliative Care
Beth Israel Medical Center
First Avenue at 16th Street
New York, N.Y. 10003
USA

OXFORD
UNIVERSITY PRESS

OXFORD

UNIVERSITY PRESS

Great Clarendon Street, Oxford OX2 6DP
Oxford University Press is a department of the University of Oxford.
It furthers the University's objective of excellence in research, scholarship,
and education by publishing worldwide in
Oxford New York

Auckland Bangkok Buenos Aires Cape Town Chennai
Dar es Salaam Delhi Hong Kong Istanbul Karachi Kolkata
Kuala Lumpur Madrid Melbourne Mexico City Mumbai Nairobi
São Paulo Shanghai Taipei Tokyo Toronto

Oxford is a registered trade mark of Oxford University Press
in the UK and in certain other countries

Published in the United States
by Oxford University Press Inc., New York

© Oxford University Press 2004

A catalogue record for this title is available from the British Library
ISBN 0 19 8508433 (Hbk)

10 9 8 7 6 5 4 3 2 1

Typeset by Newgen Imaging Systems (P) Ltd., Chennai, India
Printed and bound in Hong Kong
Produced by Phoenix Offset Ltd/The Hanway Press Ltd

Foreword

This first edition of 'Palliative Care in Neurology' comes at an important time in the evolution of both the fields of neurology and palliative care. For the specialty of neurology, the extraordinary scientific advances that have led to an understanding of the basic and clinical aspects of neurologic disease have opened the door to the availability of a wide range of clinical trials to treat diseases of the nervous system. Many of these new specific treatments are palliative, not curative, and focus on reducing symptoms, improving quality of life, and, in some instances, prolonging life. From Parkinson's disease to multiple sclerosis to the wide range of neurodegenerative diseases, targeted therapies based on new knowledge of the molecular biology of these entities is being translated into therapeutic protocols whose end points are improved quality of life. What had been previously considered untreatable, has become treatable; the unmanageable, manageable. One has only to look at, for example, the treatment of seizures and the evolution of the science of epilepsy to marvel at our ability to control (although not cure) seizure disorders, thus dramatically impacting on the quality of life of seizure victims and their families.

Advances in palliative care parallel those in neurology, where a growing cadre of clinicians in palliative medicine with subspecialty status and a burgeoning research agenda have focused attention on patients with life-threatening illness and the need to improve their quality of life. Although numerous groups have developed varying precepts of palliative care, they all have very similar overarching themes that are best summarized in the 2002 World Health Organization definition of palliative care:

> An approach which improves quality of life for patients and their families facing life threatening illness through the prevention and relief of suffering by means of early identification and impeccable assessment and treatment of pain and other problems, physical, psychosocial and spiritual.

One indicator of the successful evolution of palliative care is evident in several countries including Great Britain, Sweden, Norway, Australia, and Canada, where palliative medicine is a specialty with designated university chairs in palliative medicine and research. In the United States, the American Board of Hospice and Palliative Care Medicine has developed a certifying exam and, to date, over a thousand U.S. physicians have successfully completed this certification and examination process. Palliative medicine is the formal term used to describe this medical specialty—that is, the study and management of patients with active, progressive, life-limiting disease for whom the prognosis is limited and focus of care is quality of life.

Research in palliative care has focused on a wide range of domains that range from symptom assessment and management to understanding psychological, spiritual, and existential factors impacting on patients' quality of life. Research studies have also addressed the multidimensional aspects of the process of dying. Such studies have focused on: the development of methodologies to assess symptoms; pharmacologic approaches for the management of such symptoms; methods to evaluate and compare quality of life with various treatments; ethical and legal aspects of such research and care delivery systems and the legal systems that impact on palliative care; and research into the development of better models of medical decision making and improved communication skills for health-care professionals. Such research has facilitated the role of the palliative care clinician to help patients hear bad news, address serious illness, and find support and knowledge from health-care professionals, who can both lead the way and walk the last mile with the patient.

Palliative care, in short, is an integral part of the continuum of neurologic care from diagnosis to death. Its role is most evident in advanced illness when symptoms are common and complex medical and psychological approaches need to be individualized for each patient.

One can readily see the interface of neurology and palliative care when one looks at the common symptoms of patients with all types of medical and neurologic illness experience in the setting of their advanced disease. Pain, cognitive dysfunction, delirium, anxiety, depression, and psychoses are common symptoms in patients with chronic illness and advanced disease of any type. It is in this area of symptom management that a natural and strong association between palliative care and neurology has formed, as evidenced by the editors of this book, who model an extraordinary partnership with expertise in both fields.

It is hoped that this book will bridge the gap between palliative care experts and neurologists, but with a strong advocacy perspective of the role of the neurologist as a provider of palliative care. This is not to suggest that palliative care experts should assume the role of the neurologist but, rather, should help to educate the neurologist to provide state-of-the-art, evidence-based palliative care to their patients.

Neurologists are providers of palliative care by the very nature of their clinical practice and research. Neurologists commonly care for patients with cerebrovascular disease, stroke, dementia, chronic demyelinating diseases, and chronic neurodegenerative diseases. Most of these diseases are not curative and are associated with disability and dysfunction. In this role neurologists attempt to both prevent neurologic disability and palliate neurologic symptoms. An increasing aging population with an increasing prevalence of dementia, as well as the changing trajectory of dying for patients with multiple sclerosis and amyotrophic lateral sclerosis, Huntington's disease, Parkinson's disease, stroke, and AIDS, point out the increasing need for neurologists to be competent in symptom control and end-of-life care.

For particular symptoms such as the management of pain and delirium, neurologists play a major role because of their special expertise and training. The recent advances in pain management and the availability of evidence-based guidelines for the use of opioid, non-opioid, and adjuvant analgesics in somatic and neuropathic pain states, provides an opportunity for neurologists to undertake sequential trials tailored to individual patients' types of pain. Similarly, in managing delirium, agitation, depression, and anxiety, advances in symptom control research offer an opportunity, through sequential clinical trials, to define the best management approaches to stabilize cognitive dysfunction and/or depression, ideally to enhance cognitive function in the aged population.

The role of neurologists in evaluating patients who are stuporous or in coma, and their role in prognosticating patients' neurologic status, makes it critical for them to be able to communicate difficult and negative information to patients and families in a sensitive, timely, and effective manner. Expanding the communication skills of neurologists is critically important to advance their effectiveness as palliative care physicians. This book offers a practical way forward and marks palliative care in neurology as an evolving discipline of interest among neurologists.

Increasing appreciation of the importance of palliative care for patients with neurologic disorders has been emphasized both by the American Academy of Neurology Ethics and Humanities Committee in its 1996 position statement, which said that it is imperative

...that neurologists understand and learn to apply the principles of palliative care as ... many patients with neurologic disease die after long illnesses during which the neurologist acts as the principal or consulting physician.

Similarly, the World Federation of Neurology has recognized the importance of neurologists expanding their knowledge of palliative care and has supported an international task force.

There is limited data on the specific knowledge base of neurologists in end-of-life care. In a survey of neurologists funded by the American Academy of Neurology in 1996, a sizable gap was identified between established legal, medical, and ethical guidelines for the care of the seriously ill patients with neurologic disease and the beliefs and practices of many neurologists surveyed. For example, although most neurologists supported a patient's right to refuse life-sustaining treatment, many believed that they were killing their patients by supporting such refusals. Thirty-seven per cent of neurologists surveyed thought it was illegal to administer analgesics in doses that risk respiratory depression among terminal ALS patients, and 40% believed that they should obtain legal council when considering stopping life-sustaining treatment. The lack of knowledge of U.S. law and confusion, disagreement, or both concerning medical and ethical guidelines, clearly suggest a need for education in palliative care and end-of-life decision making for neurologists.

A comparable study, using some questions from the U.S. survey, demonstrated a similar sizable gap between established legal, medical, and ethical guidelines in a German population of neurologists. From a survey of practicing neurologists and residency program directors questioned about the role of pain medicine education, 89% of practicing neurologists stated that more pain medicine education was needed for resident training, but only 5% of neurology residencies include a pain clinic rotation and only 29% of residency program directors report having a neurology pain specialist on the faculty. This is particularly important because in this same survey, practicing neurologists reported that 25% of their new patients present with pain as a major complaint.

A recent survey of medical textbooks rated general neurology texts as having minimal to no content on palliative symptom control, ethics, and care of the dying. In contrast, family medicine and geriatrics cover these topics in great detail. These preliminary data, albeit predominantly from the U.S., suggest that there is a lack of educational initiatives focused on palliative care for the practicing neurologist and resident. This creates a barrier to neurologists learning about the practice of palliative care.

There is a growing consensus that education in palliative care needs to be integrated at the undergraduate, graduate, and continuing medical education levels. New initiatives and model programs are underway in medical schools, residency, and faculty development programs. National professional organizations such as the American Academy of Neurology has, along with 17 other subspecialty medical and surgical organizations, signed up to a set of core principles and a consensus statement emphasizing the importance of training neurology residents and practicing neurologists in end-of-life care. To date, the American Academy of Neurology has expanded its courses at its annual meetings in palliative care, pain management, and ethics, and has developed a specific clinical ethics rotation for residents. A series of task forces have worked particularly on palliative care issues that relate uniquely to neurologists. This has included a working group of specialists in amyotrophic lateral sclerosis, who have created end-of-life guidelines and practical assessment tools for neurologists who care for patients with ALS and other neuromuscular diseases. Recent textbooks such as 'Palliative Care in Amyotrophic Lateral Sclerosis', 'Hospice Care for Patients with Advanced Dementia', and 'Palliative Care in Neurology' (Neurologic Clinics series) serve to educate all health-care professionals, but specifically neurologists, to a comprehensive approach for patients with progressive neurologic diseases. These efforts at expanding the knowledge base in the practice of neurology in palliative care are small steps, but still they emphasize the role of the neurologist as a provider of palliative care.

This text is the compendium of information we need and is a comprehensive review of palliative care in neurology. Uniquely, it frames the discipline and defines the role of neurologists in the critical interface of neurologic practice and investigation and palliative care.

Kathleen M. Foley, M.D.

Preface

Palliative care in neurology may be a new topic for a textbook but it comprises an established discipline. In the earliest days of the modern hospice movement, Dame Cicely Saunders addressed palliative care issues in patients dying of brain tumors. In her visionary project, St Christopher's Hospice, patients with amyotrophic lateral sclerosis (ALS) were included from the beginning. Indeed, her concept of a peaceful death in ALS patients represented a turning point in their care.[1]

But despite these accomplishments, physicians, patients, and the public continue to harbor fears and misunderstandings about terminal illnesses and palliative care. Many physicians continue to believe that 'nothing can be done' for such patients because they are inexorably dying, and they remain ignorant of accepted principles and practices of palliative care, as confirmed in the survey of physicians in 1999.[2]

ALS is not the only neurological disease for which the palliative care principles developed by the oncology palliative care community may be applied. Patients with multiple sclerosis (MS) have an increased suicide rate and, in the absence of good palliative care, may request euthanasia and physician-assisted suicide, as Dutch physicians have reported. Surveys of Dutch physicians have shown that 5% of patients with MS and an alarming 20% of patients with ALS die by euthanasia or physician-assisted suicide.[3,4] As a response, palliative care efforts have blossomed in the Netherlands in recent years.

The neurology community has formally embraced palliative care relatively recently. For example, through the influence of one of us (JLB), the American Association of Neurology, in 1996, issued a position statement that 'neurologists have a duty to provide adequate palliative care',[5,6] and the European Neurological Society held a first satellite symposium on this issue.[7] Dr Derek Doyle, one of the founders of academic palliative care, gave the impetus to found an International Working Group on Palliative Care in Neurology, which now is also a Research Group of the World Federation of Neurology. This group has—as a first step in the process of improving the knowledge about palliative care in neurologists—generated the effort to put together this textbook.

This book was written for neurologists and other physicians who wish to continue providing excellent care for neurological patients through the final stage of their disease. Neurologists therefore need to understand both the general principles of palliative medicine and their application to specific diseases of the nervous system. The first section outlines the principles of palliative care; the second summarizes the palliative needs of patients dying from neurological diseases; the third section describes the specific management of the most frequent symptoms encountered in palliative care for neurological patients; and yet another section deals with ethical issues and optimal decision making at the end of life.

In addition to serving as an academic textbook, this book teaches neurologists about palliative care issues. Each chapter begins with a short case highlighting the topic of each chapter, that may also be used for teaching purposes. The book is oriented to the patient's point of view and, in the final chapter, Professor Jaffe discusses his personal experience with far-advanced ALS—no better account of the true meaning of palliative care in neurology can be found elsewhere in the book. Also included are four illustrations by Robert Pope depicting the physical, psychosocial, and spiritual dimensions of chronic illness as he has personally experienced them.

In the near future, palliative care in neurology is likely to shift its focus from diseases such as ALS to areas which have great epidemiological impact, but have not hitherto been strongly associated with palliative care efforts, such as neurovascular disorders and dementias. In the former, despite recent advances in prevention and treatment, incidence and mortality remain high and indeed are likely to increase in the future. The latter group of patients constitutes a formidable challenge, compounded by demographic trends, for interdisciplinary co-operation between neurology, psychiatry, geriatrics, and palliative care. These, and other areas outlined in the book, will require neurologists to expand their knowledge of palliative care and to develop tools and skills that reflect the specific characteristics of the diseases and syndromes with which we are confronted daily. Interdisciplinary and multiprofessional research efforts will establish and enlarge the evidence base for our palliative care interventions and provide us with an increasingly firm basis to better serve the needs of our neurological palliative care patients and their families.

The Editors, January 2003

1. O'Brien T, Kelly M, Saunders C. Motor neurone disease: a hospice perspective. BMJ 1992; 304(6825):471–473.
2. Carver AC, Vickrey BG, Bernat JL, Keran C, Ringel SP, Foley KM. End-of-life care: a survey of US neurologists' attitudes, behavior, and knowledge. Neurology 1999;53:284–293.
3. van der Wal G, Onwuteaka–Philipsen BD. Cases of euthanasia and assisted suicide reported to the public prosecutor in North Holland over 10 years. BMJ 1996;312(7031):612–613.
4. Veldink JH, Wokke JH, van der Wal G, Vianney de Jong JM, van den Berg LH. Euthanasia and physician-assisted suicide among patients with amyotrophic lateral sclerosis in the Netherlands. N Engl J Med 2002;346(21):1638–1644.
5. The American Academy of Neurology, Ethics, and Humanities Subcommittee. Palliative care in neurology. Neurology 1996;46(3):870–872.
6. Bernat JL, Goldstein ML, Viste KM Jr. The neurologist and the dying patient. Neurology 1996;46(3): 598–599.
7. Voltz R, Borasio GD. Palliative therapy in the terminal stage of neurological disease. J Neurol 1997;244(Suppl 4):S2–S10.

Acknowledgements

The editors would like to thank Dr R. Smeding, for her suggestions of increased patient focus within the book, and the Robert Pope Foundation of Hansport, Nova Scotia. We would also like to thank all of our patients, who teach us palliative care daily, and our numerous colleagues who commented on the text. Furthermore, we thank Richard Marley and the editorial staff of Oxford University Press for the enormous support of this project.

Contents

PART 2. NEUROLOGIC OUTCOME AND PALLIATIVE CARE

PART 3. COMMON SYMPTOMS

PART 4. OTHER PROBLEMS WITH ADVANCED ILLNESS

PART 6. GENERAL ASPECTS

Plates

Contributors

JULIA ADDINGTON-HALL
Deputy Head
Department of Palliative Care and Policy
GKT School Of Medicine
King's College London
London, UK

AKIRA AKABAYASHI
Department of Biomedical Ethics
School of Health Science and Nursing
The University of Tokyo
   Graduate School of Medicine
Tokyo, Japan

GOPAL H. BADLANI
Department of Urology
Long Island Jewish Medical Center
New Hyde Park, New York, USA

DERYK BEAL
Division of Haematology/Oncology
The Hospital for Sick Children
Toronto, Canada

JAMES L. BERNAT
Neurology Section
Dartmouth Hitchcock Medical Center
Lebanon, New Hampshire, USA

ALEXANDRE BERNEY
Psychiatry Service
University Hospital
Lausanne, Switzerland

ANNA BLOCKLEY
Department of Neurology
King's College Hospital
London, UK

GIAN DOMENICO BORASIO
Interdisciplinary Palliative Care
   Unit and Department of Neurology
University of Munich
Munich, Germany

MARCO BOSISIO
Psychology Unit
National Cancer Institute
Milan, Italy

ERIC BOUFFET
Division of Haematology/Oncology
The Hospital for Sick Children
Toronto, Canada

AUGUSTO CARACENI
Chief of Neurology Unit and Palliative
   Care Division
National Cancer Institute
Milan, Italy

ALAN CARVER
Department of Palliative Medicine
Mt. Sinai Hospital
New York, New York, USA

DAVID CELLA
Director, Center on Outcomes, Research
   and Education
Evanston Northwestern Healthcare
Professor, Department of Psychiatry
   and Behavioural Sciences
Research Professor, Institute for Health Services
   Research and Policy Studies
Northwestern University Feinberg School
   of Medicine
Chicago, Illinois, USA

WALTER A. CERANSKI
VA Medical Center Nursing Home Care Unit
Phoenix, Arizona, USA

CHRIS CLOUGH
Medical Director
King's College Hospital
London, UK

CARLO A. DEFANTI
Division of Neurology
Ospedale Niguarda Ca'Granda
Milan, Italy

NICHOLAS A. DONINGER
Neuropsychology Fellow
Department of Psychiatry,
The University of Chicago,
Chicago, Illinois, USA

G. FINK
Department of Neurology
Medizinische Fakultät der RWTH
Aachen, Germany

KATHLEEN M. FOLEY
Attending Neurologist
Pain and Palliative Care Service
Department of Neurology
Memorial Sloan-Kettering Cancer Center
New York, New York, USA

MARGARET FOULSUM
Speech Pathology Department
Bethlehem Hospital
Melbourne, Victoria, Australia

FABIO FORMAGLIO
Neuroalgologia
Hopital San Raffaele
Dipartimento di Scienze Neuropsichiche
Milano, Italy

WOLFGANG GRISOLD
Ludwig Boltzmann Institut für
   Neuroonkologie
Kaiser Franz Josef Spital
Wien, Austria

GERHARD F. HAMANN
Department of Neurology
Klinikum Grosshadern
München, Germany

JANET HARDY
Director of Palliative Care
Master Misericordiae Health Services
South Brisbane, Australia

LOUISE HENRY
Senior Dietitian
Royal Marsden Hospital
Sutton
Surrey, UK

SHAROL L. HERR
Mount Carmel Palliative Care Services
Columbus, Ohio, USA

EUGENIA DANIELA HORD
Department of Anesthesia and Critical Care
and
Department of Neurology
Massachusetts General Hospital
Massachusetts, USA

BEN-JOSHUA JAFFEE (DECEASED)

D. KAUB–WITTEMER
Department of Neurology
Klinikum Grosshadern
München, Germany

HEINZ LAHRMANN
Department of Neurology
Kaiser Franz Josef Spital
Wien, Austria

PHYLLIS MCGEE
Division of Haematology/Oncology
The Hospital for Sick Children
Toronto, Canada

A.D. MACLEOD
Nurse Maude Hospice
Christchurch, New Zealand

IAN MADDOCKS
Emeritus Professor
Flinders University of South Australia
South Australia

DONAL MARTIN
Consultant in Palliative Care
Sligo General Hospital
Sligo, Ireland

JEANETTE MEADWAY
Mildmay Mission Hospital
Bethnal Green
London, UK

SEBASTIANO MERCADANTE
Pain Relief and Palliative Care Unit
La Maddalena Cancer Center
Palermo, Italy

WILHELM NACIMIENTO
Klinik für Neurologie
Klinikum Duisburg
Duisburg, Germany

SOHEYL NOACHTAR
Department of Neurology
Klinikum Grosshadern
München, Germany

J. NOTH
Director
Department of Neurology
Medizinische Fakultät der RWTH
Aachen, Germany

DAVID OLIVER
Medical Director
Wisdom Hospice
Rochester
Kent, UK
Honorary Senior Lecturer
Kent Institute of Medicine and Health Sciences
University of Kent
Kent, UK

DAVID OLIVIERE
Director of Education and Training
St. Christopher's Hospice
Sydenham
London, UK

KENDRA PETERSON
Associate Professor
Stanford University Medical Center
Department of Neurology
Stanford, California, USA

RUSSELL K. PORTENOY
Chairman
Department of Pain Medicine and Palliative
  Care
Beth Israel Medical Center
New York, New York, USA

MARIO PROSIEGEL
Medical Director
Neurologisches Krankenhaus München
Tristanstraße
München, Germany

ANGIE ROGERS
Senior Lecturer
Department of Palliative Care and Policy
GKT School Of Medicine
King's College London
Weston Education Centre
London, UK

PAUL ROUSSEAU
Associate Chief of Staff for Geriatrics and
Extended Care
VA Medical Center
Phoenix, Arizona, USA

AMANDA SCOTT
Speech Pathology Department
The Alfred
Prahran, Victoria, Australia

DARSHAN K. SHAH
Consultant Urologist
Akshaya Apollo Hospitals
Dist. Gandhinagar, India

BRIAN TAYLOR SLINGSBY
Department of Biomedical Ethics
School of Public Health
Kyoto University Graduate School of Medicine
Kyoto, Japan

RICHARD SLOAN
Medical Director
Joseph Weld Hospice
Dorchester, Dorset, UK

LEON STERN

FRIEDRICH STIEFEL
Service de Psychiatrie de Liaison
CHUV
Lausanne, Switzerland

NIGEL SYKES
Medical Director
St. Christopher's Hospice
Honorary Senior Lecturer in Palliative
Medicine, King's College
London, UK

ROBERT M. TAYLOR
Mount Carmel Palliative Care Services
Columbus, Ohio, USA

RUDOLF TÖPPER
Neurologische Abteilung
AK Harburg
Hamburg, Germany

LADISLAV VOLICER
Clinical Director GRECC
E.N. Rogers Memorial Veterans Hospital
Bedford, Massachussetts, USA

RAYMOND VOLTZ
Institute of Clinical Neuroimmunology
Department of Neurology and Interdisciplinary
Palliative Care Service
Klinikum Grosshadern
München, Germany

LYNNE I. WAGNER
Clinical Research Scientist, Center on Outcomes,
Research and Education Evanston Northwestern
    Healthcare
Assistant Professor, Department of Psychiatry and
    Behavioral Sciences
Faculty Fellow, Institute for Health Services
    Research and Policy Studies
Northwestern University Feinberg School
    of Medicine
Chicago, Illinois, USA

EDITH WAGNER−SONNTAG
Neurologisches Krankenhaus München
München, Germany

PAUL WALKER
MD Anderson Cancer Center
Department of Symptom Control
and Palliative Care
Houston, Texas, USA

SABINE WEIL
Department of Neurology
Klinikum Grosshadern
München, Germany

HELEN WHITE
Speech and Language Therapist
The Royal Marsden Hospital
Sutton
Surrey, UK

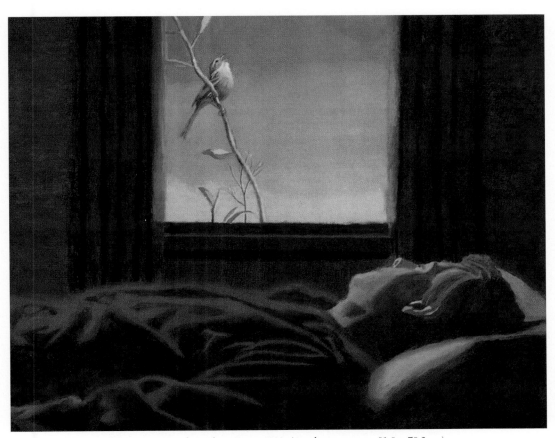

Plate 1 'Sparrow' by Robert Pope, 1989. (Acrylic on canvas, 61.0 × 76.2 cm)

Chapter 1

Palliative Care

David Oliver

Palliative care aims to consider the 'whole patient' within their social support system, allowing the management of symptoms, psychosocial issues, and spiritual issues. The role of palliative care may start from the time of diagnosis or the neurological event and may be combined with other treatment schedules. All health and social care professionals should be involved in the provision of palliative care, usually as members of multidisciplinary teams. There may also be a role for a specialist palliative care team, with specific expertise and training, to support patients and their families and the professional carers involved in the patient's care.

THE PALLIATIVE CARE APPROACH

Palliative care is:

> an approach that improves quality of life of patients and their families facing the problems associated with life-threatening illness, through the prevention and relief of suffering by means of early identification and impeccable assessment and treatment of pain and other problems, physical, psychosocial and spiritual.[1]

The aim of palliative care is to look at the 'whole patient' in the context of their social support system, which is often their family. This holistic approach is crucial in the care of someone with a neurological disease and is relevant from the time of investigation, before the diagnosis has been confirmed, and throughout the progression of the disease.

It is important to stress that palliative care:
- Provides relief from pain and distressing symptoms
- Affirms life and regards dying as a normal process
- Intends neither to hasten or postpone death
- Integrates the psychological and spiritual aspects of patient care
- Offers a support system to help patients live as actively as possible until death
- Offers a support system to help the family cope during the patient's illness and in their own bereavement
- Uses a team approach to address the needs of patients and their families, including bereavement counseling, if indicated
- Will enhance quality of life, and may also positively influence the course of illness
- Is applicable early in the course of the illness.[1]

There have been many debates, especially in the care of cancer patients, about the differing roles of curative and palliative treatment. It has been suggested that curative treatment should be continued until no further benefit can be obtained and at this point palliative care should be instituted. The timing of this sudden switch in the care of the patient can be very variable and may occur very late in the disease process, when death is imminent, and this may deny the patient supportive care, such as the control of symptoms or psychosocial care.

There is now a greater awareness of the need for an integrated approach to the care of a patient with a potentially incurable disease. This may be summarized in Figure 1–1, showing the need to consider:
- Active treatment of the disease, if this is possible
- Active medical treatment of complications of the disease, such as treatment of infection

3

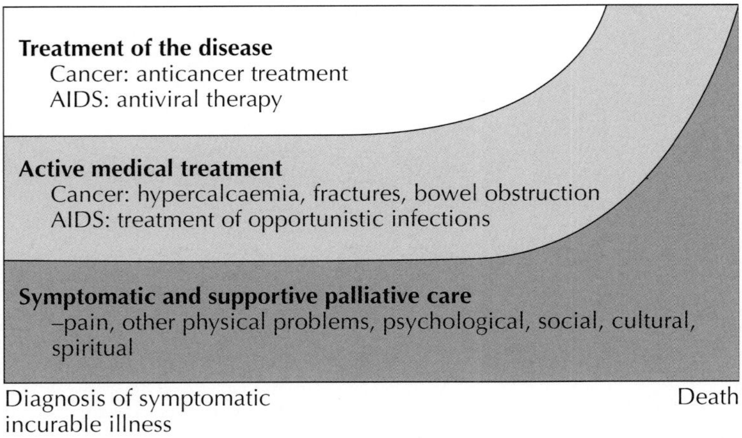

Figure 1–1. Care of a patient with incurable illness. Taken, with permission, from Woodruff, R. (1999). Palliative medicine—symptomatic and supportive care for patients with advanced cancer and AIDS. Third edition. Oxford University Press, Oxford.

- Symptomatic and supportive palliative care—including all aspects of care.[2]

Within neurology there is an increasing appreciation that palliative care is appropriate for patients with certain neurological disorders. The Ethics and Humanities Subcommittee of the American Academy of Neurology has stated that 'neurologists understand, and learn to apply the principles of palliative care'. There are many progressive and incurable neurological diseases where this approach may be appropriate and 'optimal medical care depends on determining the most appropriate means of achieving those goals for each patient'.[3]

However, there is often a reluctance to accept the progressive nature of the disease or the seriousness of the condition (such as after a severe cerebrovascular accident), and patients and their families receive overoptimistic ideas concerning the nature and progression of the disease. Doctors have little training in either the breaking of bad news or palliative care[4] and may find it difficult to provide patients with this information. As a result the care of the patient and family may be less than optimal, symptoms remaining unrelieved and psychosocial concerns never addressed or only partly recognized when near to death, when the possibilities of resolution are limited. In many neurological diseases there is often progressive loss and increasing disability and it is essential that all the following aspects of care are addressed as early as possible:

- Physical aspects, such as the control of symptoms

- Psychological aspects, such as the fears and concerns about the disease
- Social aspects, involving families and those close to the patient
- Spiritual aspects, concerning the meaning of life and the fears for the future

It is very difficult to address the more profound concerns of the patient if communication is limited due to loss of speech. Earlier intervention, when the patient is more easily understood and communication aids are not necessary, allows better interaction and communication.

From the time of diagnosis or the neurological event there is a need to consider the 'whole patient' and to adopt the palliative care approach. This:

aims to promote both the physical and psychosocial well being and is a vital and integral part of all clinical practice, whatever the illness or its stage, informed by a knowledge and practice of palliative care principles.[5]

This approach should be part of the care we give to all patients and comprises:
- Focus on quality of life which includes good symptom control
- Whole person approach taking into account the person's past life experience and current situation
- Care which encompasses both the dying person and those who matter to that person
- Respect for patient autonomy and choice (e.g. over place of death, treatment options)

- Emphasis on open and sensitive communication, which extends to patients, informal carers, and professional colleagues.[5]

This palliative care approach should be part of everyday care, regardless of diagnosis. However, this may not always be the case and there is an increasing need to ensure that the principles are included in the training of all health-care professionals. Many still see their role as the cure and alleviation of disease, whereas in reality the majority of patient care involves the palliation of symptoms and disability. All health-care professionals need to accept the limitations of the care that can be given and to approach patients and their families in a positive, but realistic, way. This particularly applies to the care of people with a serious or progressive neurological disease, who face continual losses as the disease progresses and may require a great deal of help in coping with these losses and the ensuing changes in their lifestyle.

There is evidence of confusion in the care provided by neurologists. A survey of U.S. neurologists showed that there was a lack of clarity regarding the use of morphine. When they were asked about the administration of morphine to a patient with dyspnoea from advanced amyotrophic lateral sclerosis, in a dose which could depress respiration, 26% felt that this was the same as killing the patient and 39% felt that this would constitute euthanasia, even though there are clear guidelines on the use of such medication.[6] There were also strong feelings that not offering intervention, such as tube feeding or assisted ventilation, to a patient who may require this, was the same as killing the patient. The survey showed that there was a need for further education of neurologists, particularly in the techniques of palliative care.[6]

Many people will require more specialized help and rehabilitation. This may be provided by a specialized neurological team, a disability team, or specialist palliative care services. This involves a specialized multidisciplinary team approach, with the many different disciplines working collaboratively together in maximizing the care offered to the patient and family. There may be limitations as to team involvement in the care. For instance in the United States, specialist palliative care services only receive Medicare funding for the last six months of life. However, the need for specialized multidisciplinary care extends throughout

the disease process, perhaps for many years, and it is essential that the same palliative care principles are provided by all the services throughout the patient's care pathway.

SPECIALIST PALLIATIVE CARE

In the United Kingdom, many specialist palliative care providers are involved in the care of people with neurological disease, in particular motor neurone disease (MND)/ amyotrophic lateral sclerosis (ALS). A survey in 1998 showed that at least 75% of inpatient units were involved in the care of patients with MND/ALS.[7] The involvement varied with units providing:

- Care throughout the disease, from the time of diagnosis
- Respite care as the disability progressed
- Terminal care, in the final weeks or days of life

The specialist palliative care services may provide care and support in different ways:

- At home, with the support of the multidisciplinary team, in collaboration with the family physician and community nurses
- In an inpatient palliative care unit or hospice, for symptom control, respite care, or terminal care
- In a day hospice, providing care for the day, allowing respite for carers and the opportunity for multidisciplinary assessment, involvement in rehabilitation and other activities, complementary therapies, and socialization
- In hospital, with a palliative care team providing advice and support to patient and family and the health-care professionals
- Specialist psychosocial care from social workers, counsellors, and psychologists
- Care after the patient's death, with bereavement support and counselling for families

This specialist palliative care follows the patient and the aim should be to provide a seamless service, wherever the patient is at that particular time. The specialist nature of the care is ensured by the close involvement of the multidisciplinary team, including:

- Medical practitioner, in particular a Consultant in Palliative Medicine

- Nursing specialist
- Social worker
- Speech and language therapist
- Occupational therapist
- Physiotherapist
- Chaplain, and others trained in providing spiritual care and support
- Clinical psychologist
- Dietitian
- Pharmacist
- Complementary therapists, providing aromatherapy or massage

All the members of the team should be working primarily within specialist palliative care and have been trained and be receiving ongoing support and training in this area of expertise.

Specialist palliative care aims to look at the positive aspects of a person's life and abilities and to enable patients and their families to remain as active as possible. For many people, including health-care professionals, hospices may be seen negatively, merely in terms of terminal care. However, the services should provide the care that patients require and work with them to make the most of their abilities.

The involvement of specialist palliative care in the care of people with neurological disease varies greatly. There has been appreciable experience in the care of patients with ALS[8–12] and one study found that only 15% of patients had been referred for symptom control although many had uncontrolled symptoms which could benefit from the multidisciplinary assessment of the palliative care team[8].

Although new treatment regimes are being developed in the care of patients with neurological disease there is still a full assessment of the palliative care needs of the patient and family so that palliative care can continue alongside the more active care. This often occurs in the care of patients with cancer, as there are needs for symptom control and psychosocial support while oncological treatments, such as chemotherapy, are continued. There is a need for close collaboration between neurological services and palliative care providers to ensure the patient is offered the maximum number of treatment possibilities.

There is always a need to balance the information given to patients as they may not always be able to cope with the decision. For instance, there is increasing evidence that it is necessary to ensure the best timing for the introduction to the patient of equipment to help with daily living. If information and equipment are presented and discussed too early there may be a negative reaction from the patient who may then not accept them for some time. There may be a conflict in allowing patients full information, when they may find it difficult to cope emotionally with this extra load. However, it is also important that decisions involve patients and their families closely and that health-care professionals do not make a paternalistic decision. This conflict will increase as newer treatment options are developed and there is growing interest in trying to stage the decision-making process, so that the patient and family can make their decisions with the minimum of stress. Palliative care services can be involved in these processes, and the need for accurate and responsible communication is very much part of the role offered by palliative care. Close collaboration is helpful and some neurological centers are suggesting the involvement of palliative care services earlier in the disease progression so that this collaboration can be fostered.

Palliative care aims to help and support the patient and family—not to shorten life. With the control of distress many patients feel more positive and life may even be extended. There may be occasions when the shortening of life may be a foreseeable consequence of treatment, but the *intention* is never to shorten life. On occasions patients may decide against procedures or treatments that could prolong their lives, for instance a feeding gastrostomy or ventilatory support. As long as the patient is able to make this decision clearly (and mental incapacitation rarely affects people with neurological disease), the health-care team should support the patient and family in this decision and help to minimize distress by the provision of good palliative care.[3]

The patient with neurological disease faces many challenges and many losses as the disease progresses. These affect the family and close carers as well, and the health-care professionals involved with the care may also be affected by these losses. Palliative care from a multidisciplinary team, working collaboratively with all the other services involved in the care, helps the patient and family to continue to function as effectively as possible and ensures that the quality of life is as good as possible.

This chapter is based on 'Palliative care' in Palliative Care in Amyotrophic Lateral Sclerosis, edited by D. Oliver, G.D. Borasio, and D. Walsh, Oxford University Press, 2000.

REFERENCES

1. World Health Organization (2002) World Health Organization Definition of Palliative Care *www.who.int/cancer/main.cfm* 2/23/2003.
2. Woodruff R. Palliative Medicine. Symptomatic and Supportive Care for Patients with Advanced Cancer and AIDS, 3rd Ed. Oxford University Press, Oxford, 1999.
3. The American Academy of Neurology, Ethics and Humanities Subcommittee. Palliative care in neurology. Neurology 1996;46:870–872.
4. Borasio GD, Sloan R, Pongratz D. Breaking the news. In: Oliver D, Borasio GD, Walsh D, eds. Palliative Care in Amyotrophic Lateral Sclerosis. Oxford University Press, Oxford, 2000:29–36.
5. National Council for Hospice and Specialist Palliative Care Services. Specialist Palliative Care: A Statement of Definitions. National Council for Hospice and Specialist Palliative Care Services, London, 1995.
6. Carver AC, Vickrey BG, Bernat JL, Keran C, Ringel SP, Foley KM. End-of-life care. A survey of US neurologists' attitudes, behavior, and knowledge. Neurology 1999;53:284–293.
7. Oliver D, Webb S. The involvement of specialist palliative care in the care of people with motor neurone disease. Palliative Medicine 1999;14:47–48.
8. O'Brien T, Kelly M, Saunders C. Motor neurone disease: a hospice perspective. British Medical Journal 1992;304:471–473.
9. Oliver D. The quality of care and symptom control— the effects on the terminal phase of MND/ALS. Journal of Neurological Sciences 1999;139(Suppl.): 134–136.
10. Hicks F, Corcoran G. Should hospices offer respite admissions to patients with motor neurone disease? Palliative Medicine 1993;7:145–150.
11. Neudert C, Oliver D, Wasner M, Borasio GD. The course of the terminal phase in patients with amyotrophic lateral sclerosis. Journal of Neurology 2001;248:612–616.
12. Ganzini L, Johnston WS, Silveira MJ. The final month of life in patients with ALS. Neurology 2002;59: 428–431.

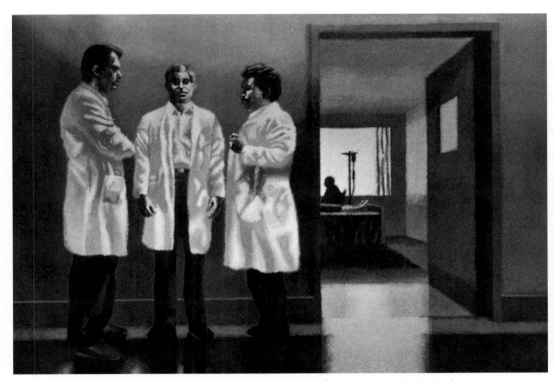

Plate 2 'Conference' by Robert Pope, 1990. (Acrylic on canvas, 61.0 × 91.4 cm)

PART 1

DISORDERS

Chapter 2

Palliative Care in Stroke

Gerhard F. Hamann
Angie Rogers
Julia Addington–Hall

In this chapter we address the palliative care needs of people who are expected to die soon after a severe stroke. We also consider the particular challenges that the care of these patients—and their families—present for neurologists, stroke physicians, nurses, physiotherapists, and others. The use of palliative care in stroke patients has attracted little attention, and consequently there is very little experience on which to draw, particularly when considering the palliative care problems specific for stroke. This chapter focuses, therefore, on identifying those stroke patients particularly likely to have palliative care needs, describing these needs and applying general principles of palliative care to their management.

CASE HISTORY

Mrs Müller was a 64-year-old single woman who had recently retired from her job as a secretary. She

had no children and only one sister and a niece, with whom she was in contact only a few times a year. She had a history of hypertension, hypercholesteremia, and insulin-dependent diabetes mellitus. She lived independently and enjoyed her garden work.

One day she had a sudden onset of vertigo, nausea, and vomiting. Her blood pressure increased to RR 220/120 mmHg. A hypertensive emergency was diagnosed, oral antihypertensive drugs were given, and she was admitted to hospital. Her blood pressure remained elevated for seven days, and the symptoms of vertigo, impaired balance, and nausea persisted. On day seven additional intravenous antihypertensive treatment (Urapidil) was administered. Her blood pressure fell to RR 140/80 mmHg within several hours, and she started to complain of paresthesia in her right arm, followed by a weakness in her right arm and leg. A progressive stroke in the territory of the left middle cerebral artery was suspected and the patient was transferred to an acute stroke unit. On the basis of the neurological examination, which included duplex sonography and a cranial CT scan, a brainstem infarction was diagnosed. She was treated with IV heparin, her blood pressure was kept at a constantly elevated level, and her blood sugar was optimally controlled.

Nevertheless, the paresis of the right as well as of the left side and bilateral dysaesthesia and paresthesia continued to increase, and four days later flaccid tetraplegia and global anesthesia appeared. Her level of consciousness diminished. At this time she was transferred to an intensive care unit (ICU) for artificial ventilation. A cerebellar and spinal stroke was diagnosed on the basis of cranial and cervical MRIs and angiography of the extra- and intracranial vertebral arteries, which showed impaired vertebral blood circulation as a result of reduced blood pressure and subtotal stenosis. The clinical course of the patient deteriorated. As the hospital had a palliative care team, consisting of a consultant physician and two palliative care nurses, they were asked to help with her care two days before her death. They then advised the stroke and ICU team on pain relief medication and sedation.

In neurological terms, the aggressive blood pressure regimen had caused an irreversible secondary deterioration. Aggressive antithrombotic therapy with heparin and artificial blood pressure support did not prevent further deterioration. Revascularization therapy, such as thrombolysis, stenting, or angioplasty, was considered too risky by the neuroradiologist, neurosurgeon, and the vascular neurologist. As the cerebellar, brainstem, and spinal strokes she had experienced had resulted in tetraplegia, deep coma, and loss of brainstem reflexes, the final complication of an obstructive hydrocephalus (occlusion of the fourth ventricle by the swelling of the cerebellar infarcts) was not treated. In accordance with the relatives' wishes, a limitation of the medical therapy was initiated in a conference between the director of the department, the consultant neurologist responsible for the neurointensive care unit, and the colleague responsible for the stroke unit. Antithrombotic therapy was stopped, and artificial ventilation was limited to normoventilation. Pain control with morphine infusion was believed adequate. The next day the patient died without obvious discomfort or pain.

She had been in the hospital for a total of 14 days, initially in the internal ward (seven days), then in the acute stroke unit (three days), and subsequently in intensive care (four days). She had lost the ability to speak after the clinical deterioration on the second day in the acute stroke unit, and had been unconscious for three days when she died.

Case Discussion

The experience of Mrs Müller and her family during her final illness highlights the following points that health professionals interested in providing optimal care for stroke patients at the end of life need to consider.

Sudden onset of disease during health

Most palliative care services to date have focused on patients with cancer, AIDS/HIV, or progressive neurologic conditions such as motor neuron disease. Stroke differs fundamentally from these conditions. An otherwise healthy person, who only has mostly undetected risk factors for vascular diseases, suddenly experiences a stroke. Mrs Müller, for example, progressed in less than two weeks from being a healthy person to a severely disabled patient requiring support for even basic body functions. Her situation, and that of her relatives, dramatically changed within minutes to hours. There was no time to think about the care preferred at the end of life, to complete unfinished business, to gradually assimilate information about the diagnosis, or to adjust to it. They were suddenly faced with an unexpected situation demanding immediate and potentially life-threatening decisions. Those caring for such patients need sensitivity and good communication skills to help patients and families participate in such decision making.

The progressive, unrelenting deterioration

The goal of stroke medicine is to reduce the effect of stroke, enable patients to regain function, and prevent future episodes. Unfortunately, even under optimal conditions and with the use of all technical and human resources, some stroke patients will progressively deteriorate as Mrs Müller did, and will die. This unrelenting course raises feelings of helplessness in physicians, nurses, physiotherapists, and others involved in their care, which can lead to a loss of interest in the patient, avoidance of personal contact with the patient and/or relatives and, in extreme forms, limit even basic interventions for the patient. If this is to be avoided, the whole team involved in the patient's care needs to understand that even with optimal therapy death is unavoidable in some patients, and that while sorrow at the loss of a fellow human being is appropriate, a sense of personal failure is not.

*Severe anxiety associated with
the progressive disease*

Understandably, many people become depressed in the days, weeks, and months following a stroke as they struggle to come to terms with the losses they experience: loss of independence, loss of dignity, loss of life as they knew it. Directing attention to any form of medical therapy that promises to reduce stroke symptoms and to prevent disability is one way health professionals try to offer hope. If these therapies do not influence or only marginally change the clinical course, patients and their families may experience severe anxiety. Such feelings are, of course, well-known to those caring, for example, for terminally ill cancer patients, and palliative care has developed expertise in providing appropriate psychological and spiritual support to patients and families. Anxiety may be particularly high in stroke, however, as patients and families feel caught between the fear of death and the fear of survival with significant disabilities.

*Inability to speak and
communicate*

Following her stroke, Mrs Müller lost control of pharyngeal and laryngeal muscles and consequently was unable to speak. Later she had to be artificially ventilated. This meant that the health-care team had to make decisions about her treatment without knowledge of Mrs Müller's preferences. It was also difficult to assess whether she was comfortable or in pain. Communication problems can be the source of considerable distress to family members, who are denied the opportunity of a final conversation. These problems may be encountered in many stroke patients (e.g. those with aphasia, dysarthria, or consciousness problems). While signs or written communication may be helpful with some patients, they often cannot be used after an acute stroke, since complex neuropsychological symptoms may increase problems of communication.

Inability to swallow

The acute loss of pharyngeal and laryngeal reflex control and muscle activation meant that Mrs Müller could not swallow. We do not know how she experienced this, as she could not communicate. There is anecdotal evidence, however, that the loss of the ability to swallow can be very distressing for patients. After successful rehabilitation, some patients remember the inability to swallow as very threatening and important. This loss put Mrs Müller at risk of secondary medical complications, such as aspiration and subsequent pneumonia, but it also meant she needed to receive artificial hydration and nutrition. In settings in which feeding is not automatic, this can lead to difficult and complex ethical dilemmas about whether to withdraw or withhold nutrition.

*Suspected pain due to the inability to
move and communicate*

Being bedridden without any chance of moving or avoiding less comfortable positions is a major reason for pain and discomfort in stroke patients. Many have a painful shoulder (frozen shoulder syndrome). Regular repositioning, the use of physiotherapeutic concepts such as the Bobath concept, and careful attention to pressure areas are important to avoid decubital ulcers. These measures are labor-intensive and require enough well-trained nursing staff. The maintenance of comfort for Mrs Müller and other patients like her critically depends on the skill of nurses and physiotherapists.

*Integrating family members
into decision making*

Mrs Müller was not close to her sister and niece, who described her as eccentric and reserved. Their conversations never touched on any aspects of how she might like to experience her own death or how she would like to be treated in the case of a life-threatening disease or a hopeless situation. However, the sister remembered that she had not wanted her mother to receive active treatment at the end of life. This elderly lady was diagnosed to have ovarian cancer in the final stages. Chemotherapy and an operation were offered for better symptom control. At that time her mother was undecided, and Mrs Müller advised her not to accept any medical treatment besides pain control medication. She died in the following months. Faced with the final situation of Mrs Müller's loss of consciousness, severe brainstem dysfunction, and tetraplegia, her two relatives urged the physicians to limit medical therapy and to allow the patient to die.

Family and friends often provide the only insight into the values and concerns of the patient once they become unconscious, and are therefore important sources of information for health professionals. Their views will, of course, also be affected by their own experiences, the patient's stroke, and, indeed, their relationship with the patient. They need to know that they are heard by the health professionals, but they may want something else than the patient. This poses a quandary for those caring for the patient.

End of life decision

The health professionals involved in Mrs Müller's care and her relatives agreed that she should not receive any more active treatment and be allowed to die. Such agreement is not always reached, however. Stroke units should have access to palliative care specialists who can help to determine what the patient may have wanted and what the family wants, and to support the multiprofessional team to reach and sustain agreement.

AN INTRODUCTION TO STROKE

Stroke is a heterogeneous group of diseases which includes brain infarction (supratentorial, cerebellar, or brainstem), intracerebral bleeding, subarachnoid hemorrhage, and various rare entities such as vasculitis, dissections, sinus thrombosis, etc. Typical symptoms are paresis (mostly as hemiparesis), hypesthesia, hemianopia, diplopia, visual loss, headache, acute vomiting, aphasia, or loss of consciousness. The etiology of brain infarction includes emboli originating from the heart, aorta, or major brain-supplying vessels, hemodynamic changes due to severe stenosis or occlusions, *in situ* thrombosis of intracranial arteries, and microangiopathy caused by diabetes or hypertension. Basic diagnostic measures are brain CT, cardiac examination including ECG, ultrasound investigations, and lab examination.

There is good evidence for three major therapeutic choices:

1. Stroke unit treatment as a basic therapy including the regulation of imbalanced body hemostasis (blood glucose, temperature, blood pressure, etc.) and avoidance of complications like falls, infections, and decubitus
2. Intravenous thrombolysis in very selected cases within a 3-hour time window following the initial symptoms
3. The immediate administration of aspirin.

The first two therapies result in an improvement in mortality and morbidity of 10%–30%, and aspirin between 1% and 5%.[1] The

long-term prognosis following a stroke is rather poor: about 10%–30% of the patients die within a year, another 20%–25% develop post-stroke dementia, about 40%–50% of all patients experience some kind of disability, and only about 25% survive without any major disability.

EPIDEMIOLOGY

Stroke in General

Prevalence and incidence of stroke vary according to different populations, ethnicity, and age. The Framingham study in the United States estimated the annual age-adjusted incidence of stroke for men to be 6 of 1000 and for women, 4.5 of 1000.[2] Similar rates are reported from the WHO–Monica projects for western Europe. A constant decline of stroke rates in western countries has been accompanied by a steady increase in stroke occurrence in eastern European countries and less developed countries. The Framingham study revealed that about 60% of all strokes are artherothrombotic brain infarctions, 23% cardiac embolism, 7% intracerebral hemorrhage, 7% subarachnoid hemorrhage, and 1.4% of various origins. Age is the major determinant of stroke rate: incidence in 45–54 year-olds is about 0.8 in 1000, rising to 9.4 in 1000 in the age group between 75 and 84 years.[3]

Clinical Deterioration in Stroke

Little is known about the number of stroke patients who experience clinical deterioration. About 30%–50% of all stroke victims show a 'stroke in evolution', with progression after arrival at the hospital.[4] This phenomenon is especially well-known in patients who arrive early, but it does not necessarily lead to a severe life-threatening situation. About 7%–11% of the patients in an acute stroke unit develop severe clinical worsening that requires their transfer to an ICU (for mechanical ventilation, for example). If acute stroke is treated with thrombolysis, clinical deterioration is often related to secondary hemorrhagic transformation[5] or the development of brain swelling with an increase in intracranial pressure.[6]

Various approaches have been used to identify clinically useful parameters to predict severe deterioration in stroke patients. Analyzing data from the National Institute of Neurological Disorders and Stroke (NINDS)– rt–PA study, Frankel and co-workers found a baseline value of more than 17 NIHSS (NIH stroke score) combined with atrial fibrillation to be a negative predictor; an NIHSS of more than 22 points 24 hours after stroke onset had a positive predictive value of 98% for death or severe disability.[7] A patient with this score would be severely disabled with hemiparesis or hemiplegia and additional neurological symptoms such as aphasia, hemianopia, facial paresis, or hemihypesthesia. The evaluation of the European thrombolysis trial (ECASS I) revealed that neurological deterioration was mainly related to cerebral edema and occurred in 37.5% of all patients within 24 hours.[8] Other neurological as well as medical complications, such as seizures, falls, decubital ulcers, or infections (pneumonia or urinary tract infections), may be relevant factors in the secondary deterioration during acute stroke.[9]

Death and Severe Disability in Stroke

Death rates from stroke, like incidence, vary between different countries and according to social and racial determinants, age, and gender. Age-adjusted death rates from the WHO–Monica project show that lowest death rates were found in the United States, Canada, Australia, and Switzerland: 20 of 100,000 females and 40 of 100,000 males die of stroke each year. These rates rise to about 50 of 100,000 for females and 70 of 100,000 for males in Germany, Italy, and most European countries. Eastern European countries have extremely high rates (e.g. Romania with 140 of 100,000 females and 200 of 100,000 males or Bulgaria with 200 of 100,000 females and 300 of 100,000 males).[2] In the United Kingdom about 20% of people who have a stroke will die within one month, 10% in the following year, and another 5% in the next year.[10] Both the death rate and incidence of stroke are declining in western countries (e.g. from 1970 to 1990 stroke incidence declined by 60% in the United States).[2] Better treatment and rehabilitation may account for much of this change, but the natural history of stroke may also be changing.

There are several valid predictors of functional recovery after stroke: age, previous stroke, urinary continence, consciousness at onset, disorientation in time and place, activities of daily living (ADL) score on admission, level of social support, and metabolic rate of glucose outside the infarct area in hypertensive patients.[11]

Although data are available on the incidence and death rate of stroke, there are no data on the number of stroke patients requiring palliative care. One-third of stroke victims can be expected to die within two years of their stroke, but many of these die suddenly. Thus, the number of stroke patients who might benefit from a period of palliative care can only be estimated. A conservative estimate is that 8%– 10% of all stroke patients die after a period of irreversible deterioration, and that these patients and families might benefit from the application of the principles of palliative care or directly from palliative care specialists.

Future Developments

Two conflicting epidemiological trends will influence future developments in stroke:
1. An increase in the elderly population will be accompanied by a rise in stroke incidence and severity
2. Improved lifestyle factors and healthier behavior will work against this trend to reduce the stroke incidence and death rate

Nevertheless, it is likely that both more and more severe strokes will be seen in the following decades. The importance of palliative care in stroke will therefore probably increase.

STROKE SUBTYPES ESPECIALLY REQUIRING PALLIATIVE CARE

Severe Carotid Artery Territory Strokes

MALIGNANT MEDIA INFARCTION

A large middle cerebral artery infarction is likely to develop into a space-occupying situation with the danger of transtentorial herniation. The death rate of patients with this specific type of supratentorial stroke may be as high as 80% when untreated.[12] Decompressive surgery is an option for some, particularly younger patients. For others, medical therapy with artificial ventilation, use of hyperosmolar substances, and adjustment of basic homeostatic body functions (temperature, glucose level, etc.) are required. The rate of fatalities is high. The patients develop mesencephalic and subsequently medullary decerebration caused by transtentorial herniation and herniation at the foramen magnum level. The final result is brain death. At this point there is no need for active pain treatment, but morphine may be required in hopeless situations with progressive herniation to ensure the absence of pain and discomfort. Very old patients and those who do not want intensive care treatment will require palliative care at an earlier stage. Medical therapy may be limited to substituting nutrition, preventing insufficient oxygenation, and reducing any pain and discomfort. The informal caregivers and the family should be actively integrated in the process in order to make the right decisions.

MULTIPLE SUPRATENTORIAL STROKES

Multiple and simultaneously severe supratentorial strokes result in a condition similar to experimental total forebrain ischemia. It is a rare, but devastating condition.[13–15] The acute onset and severe neurological deficits regularly lead to severe disability and have an extremely poor prognosis. Palliative care could play an important role after the initial therapeutic decisions have been made. The limits and strategies are similar to those discussed for patients with malignant media infarction.

Basilar Artery Thrombosis/Severe Brainstem Infarction

The severest form of ischemic stroke is thrombosis of the basilar artery. The blood supply to this brainstem artery is of fundamental importance, since the vegetative centers for breathing, circulation control, and control of almost all basic body functions will be affected. Many patients develop prodromal symptoms before the severe brainstem dysfunction is obvious. Typical prodromal symptoms are vertigo (60%), headache (50%), double vision (33%), paresis (32%), somnolent

states (23%), and dysarthria (23%).[16] These prodromal signs may precede subsequently severe brainstem signs for hours or even days. The prognosis in untreated cases is extremely poor: about 85% of all patients with acute basilar thrombosis will die. The survivors often exhibit severe brainstem dysfunction with long-term disability or even locked-in syndrome.[16]

The state-of-the-art therapy for patients with acute basilar artery thrombosis is local intra-arterial thrombolysis to dissolve the occluding clot. Although the efficacy of this therapy has never been proven in randomized trials, strong empirical evidence urges its use. Neurological intensive care specialists and stroke experts all over the world choose this therapy, since mortality can be reduced to 50%[17] or even less.[18] The collateral flow pattern can determine the prognosis after thrombolysis, and patients with good collateral pathways can have low mortality rates of 17% after successful thrombolysis.[19] Patients with very profound brainstem dysfunction (deep coma with loss of all brainstem reflexes) may not be eligible for intra-arterial thrombolysis if symptoms have been present for longer than 5–10 hours. Therefore, the patients with such long-lasting symptoms and those with unsuccessful thrombolysis continue to have a poor prognosis and should be treated with basic measures to relieve the symptoms. Here, palliative care is very important to ensure that these patients do not suffer from pain or discomfort and to support their family. Death is likely to occur within days.

LOCKED-IN SYNDROME

This is a severe form of brainstem infarction with a decerebration state on the level of the pons. Patients remain tetraplegic but fully awake. They can communicate with eye movements or by closing their eyes; they see and hear and are fully aware of their environment. A recent German essay by a 'locked-in patient' who survived the state and made substantial improvement described this terrifying state as being 'imprisoned in your own body'. The syndrome attracted public interest when a former editor-in-chief of the French journal, Elle, had a brainstem infarction that left him in a locked-in syndrome. Prior to his death he dictated a book (Le Scaphandre et le Papillon (The Butterfly and the Diving Bell), Editions Robert Laffont, S.A., Paris, 1997) using an eye closing–opening alphabet, in which he described the situation of being aware of everything but also dependent for everything.

The prognosis for recovery is poor, but survival after the development of a locked-in-syndrome can last as long as 2 to 18 years.[20] Patients suffering from 'locked-in syndrome' are able to communicate and transfer even very specific thoughts to their environment. Sedation of these patients does not seem justified, since this would reduce their chances of communicating and actively living in their environment. Computerized aids for communicating have been developed. Most recently, very sophisticated tools using the slow cortical potentials (from EEG) to operate communicating devices have been introduced.[21] After training sessions with continuous feedback, the patients achieved 84% correct communicating steps and were able to communicate autonomously.

The key issues involving these long-term survivors are the feasible methods of communication and the emotional and physical stress for the patient's caregivers. The issues these patients raise for palliative care are very different from those raised by stroke patients rendered unconscious by their stroke, for whom the emphasis is on maintaining physical comfort and providing family support. A particularly difficult situation arises when these patients communicate a definite and sustained wish to die. Specialists in palliative care are often experienced in discussing these issues with patients and families, and may be an important resource for the health-care team at such a time.

Severe Intracerebral Hemorrhage

Intracerebral hemorrhages are responsible for 10%–15% of all strokes, especially in far eastern (Chinese and Japanese) populations.[22] Supratentorial hemorrhages exceeding 50 ml of volume have a mortality of around 50%.[22] Most intracerebral hematomas caused by hypertension are found in the basal ganglias, whereas other causes show a preference for lobar occurrence.[23] The situation in severe intracerebral hemorrhage is very similar to that in malignant middle cerebral artery stroke. Evidence-based concepts of treatment are still lacking, although some large trials comparing medical intensive care treatment and surgical hematoma evacuation are currently under

way.[23] Most hospitals try a surgical intervention as a last resort to reduce the hematoma volume and to save the patient from a life-threatening rise in intracranial pressure.[22,23]

Palliative care concepts have to be considered primarily when hemorrhages are extremely large (exceeding 100 ml supratentorially and 50 ml infratentorially), and when there are concomitant severe diseases with expectations of a poor outcome (e.g. severe liver dysfunction with coagulation disorders resulting in a severe intracerebral hemorrhage). Palliative care may also be important for patients without clinical improvement following surgery, or with progressive transtentorial herniation or signs of severe brainstem dysfunction. Patients with severe intracerebral hemorrhages are almost comatose or have severely reduced consciousness functions, communication skills, and awareness of their environment.

SUBARACHNOID HEMORRHAGE (SAH)

Patients with subarachnoid hemorrhage are generally younger than 60 years of age, in contrast to patients with stroke or intracerebral hemorrhage who are usually older and have multiple illnesses.[24] The incidence is around 6 of 100,000 persons, and most of the severe bleedings are caused either by aneurysms (85%) or by arteriovenous malformations (AVMs). The prognosis is determined by the occurrence and the severity of complications following a SAH, mainly due to rebleeding, the development of vasospasms with secondary brain infarction, hydrocephalus aresorptivus, autonomic changes, and the rise in intracranial pressure.[24]

Despite many technical improvements for diagnosis in recent years (e.g. new MRI techniques) or for therapy (such as endovascular aneurysm coiling), the prognosis remains poor. About 50% of the patients with an acute SAH will die and one-third of survivors will remain dependent.[24] This poor prognosis clearly demonstrates the need for specific palliative help for subgroups of patients: those who have an initially severe SAH with deep coma and rapid development of herniation; and those who have aneurysms or AVMs that are so large, difficult to reach, or close to important brain centers that no cure is possible. These patients are treated with a general medical regimen to avoid complications, but they are at extremely high risk of rebleeding and subsequently of dying. Some do well, however; they and their carers therefore have to deal with considerable uncertainty. The age profile of these patients indicates that their families and children may require palliative care expertise as support in the face of life-threatening illnesses and bereavement.

Other Types

It is not possible to describe all possible subtypes of stroke in which palliative care teams may play an important role, since many rare types of stroke may require special handling and information. We therefore refer the reader to the classic handbooks on stroke (see reference[25] for one such handbook). Two special subtypes, however, need to be mentioned: sinus venous thrombosis and vasculitis.

Sinus venous thrombosis is related to coagulation abnormalities and in contrast to most stroke syndromes occurs more frequently in women than men. It is often seen in younger women during pregnancy or the postpartum period. Hereditary coagulation disorders (e.g. activated protein C (APC) resistance) may be found in the patient history. The prognosis for patients suffering from sinus venous thrombosis is rather good; mortality has dropped to about 10% in recent years. Although rare, it affects young women with new babies and thus poses particularly difficult ethical, practical, and emotional problems that are among the most demanding neurologists may ever face. Palliative care may be an important source of support for all concerned in these difficult situations.

Vasculitis is also seen in younger patients. Its severe course can hardly be influenced, so that repeated complications result (such as subarachnoid hemorrhage (SAH), intracerebral hemorrhage (ICH), strokes, or progressive dementia). Palliative aspects are relevant if patients do not respond to the regular immunosuppressive drugs or even radical interventions.

SPECIFIC PROBLEMS

A recent publication on palliative day care in England showed that stroke is, along with HIV/AIDS and motor neuron disease, one of the three second-most important diagnoses after cancer (demanding 90% of all resources) which require palliative care.[26] The stroke literature focuses on diagnosis, treatment, and rehabilitation. There is almost no literature on the needs of patients who are expected to die soon from stroke. A secondary analysis from England by the Regional Study of Care for the Dying involved 237 patients.[27] It showed that 65% were reported by bereaved relatives to have experienced pain in the last year of life, 51% confusion, 57% depressed mood, and 56% urinary incontinence. Pain control was judged as inadequate. A quarter of the relatives felt they had had insufficient choice about treatment. As few other data are available, we will, therefore, draw on our own clinical experience to highlight the specific problems of these patients and their families.

Loss of Consciousness

A variety of stroke syndromes result in primarily disturbed consciousness or severely reduced secondary changes in alertness. Situations with reduced consciousness are severe intracerebral hemorrhage, severe subarachnoid hemorrhage, and basilar thrombosis. Secondarily, many severe strokes may result in an at least temporarily diminished level of consciousness. Important situations include malignant middle cerebral artery infarction, secondary intracranial pressure rise (in supra- and infratentorial strokes), early stroke recurrence (e.g. bilateral infarctions), and thalamic infarctions (small infarcts in the thalamic region with reduced alertness). The reduction in alertness may be considered somnolence in early stages; stupor in more severe stages; and coma in the final, most severe stage of impairment. The degree of coma can be determined by the brainstem responses to external stimuli.

Care must be taken to ensure that unconscious patients receive adequate pain control and good nursing care to prevent distress from such problems as pressure areas or poor mouth care. They may also require artificial hydration and nutrition, although practices vary in different countries. An observational study of care on an acute stroke unit in the United Kingdom reported that these patients seemed to inhabit a 'limbo' land between life and death, and were in danger of 'social death' (i.e. being ignored by clinical staff and being treated as 'non-persons'). This was distressing to relatives, whose own support needs were considerable (but often ignored) when they visited their unresponsive loved ones.[28,29]

Any end-of-life decisions can only be made on the basis of the patient's assumed wishes (which may have been previously stated), the family's views, and the physician's judgement. Other members of the health-care team should also be consulted, as they may have come to know the patient and family well. The institutional ethical committees may also help to reach an ethically and medically justified decision without the fear of legal consequences.

Confusion

Some patients with acute stroke experience a phase of disorientation and confusion. It may be caused by the location of the stroke (e.g. thalamic stroke), a diffuse damage to a postulated integrative system responsible for attentiveness and coherent thoughts,[30] or by accompanying diseases (e.g. blood glucose changes, alcoholic dependency). Confusion impairs the patient's ability to understand medical information and to decide future needs. A further source of confusion is the need to introduce a legal representative of the federal authorities in many countries. Especially longer-lasting confusion or the development of delirium may lead to situations similar to those in patients with communication problems and consciousness disorders.

Loss of Communication Skills

Patients with left side middle cerebral stroke and brainstem infarcts are particularly likely to have communication problems. Prolonged aphasia (difficulties comprehending language and expressing oneself) and dysphasia (difficulty speaking, but with full comprehension) are associated with poor prognosis. Communication with patients and those close to them is likely to be time-consuming and often problematic. It may be hard to find a nonverbal way of communicating, since many patients also have accompanying neuropsychological changes such as apraxia, agnosia, neglect, and problems of visual and spatial orientation. It is important to make every effort to do so, especially since stroke patients and their families are eager for information on stroke, at least in terms of functional recovery. Health professionals tend to avoid giving prognostic information, although patients and families often want this.[31,32] In the Regional Study of Care for the Dying, a population-based, retrospective survey, two-fifths of stroke patients were thought by bereaved relatives to have definitely or probably known that they were dying. Respondents reported stroke patients and their families would have liked improved communication in all care settings.[27] This suggests that a significant proportion of stroke patients would benefit from more open discussion of their prognosis.

Communication is also crucial for monitoring symptoms, both to assess their severity and to achieve patient compliance with treatment. For example, Kehayia and co-workers found significant differences in the use of pain medication in stroke patients with and without aphasia.[33] Aphasic patients received less pain medication and less pro re nata (prn) (as required) medication. If patients have a poor prognosis, an open dialogue between health-care workers and the patient's relatives is essential to establish the patient's previous abilities or quality of life, which is likely to be the key to any decision on the withdrawal or withholding of treatment.[34]

Incontinence

Incontinence is high among stroke survivors. Meta-analysis of studies on the urinary incontinence of stroke patients found that between 32% and 79% of patients were incontinent on admission, 25%–28% on discharge, and 12%–19% had episodes of incontinence some months after discharge. Fecal incontinence has been found in 31%–40% of patients on admission and 18% on discharge, and 7%–9% six months after discharge. Incontinence has been associated with higher mortality and morbidity, and with higher rates of discharge to nursing homes.[35,36] Incontinence may not be related to the stroke itself; but rather be a functional consequence of reduced ability to express oneself and reduced mobility.[37]

Urinary incontinence in stroke patients with a poor prognosis is managed by a catheter, which poses a risk of infection. Poor management of fecal incontinence may compromise the patient's skin and result in increased pain, discomfort, and distress. Fecal incontinence is a very distressing symptom for both patients and their informal carers.[27] Constipation is a common symptom following stroke of all kinds and requires regular monitoring and appropriate medical treatment.

Feeding Problems

Dysphagia (the inability to swallow) is common after hemispheric stroke, and is in itself a predictor of poor outcome and death following stroke:[38] 30% of conscious patients have impaired ability to swallow on the day after their stroke, 16% of survivors after one week, and 2% after one month.[39] Studies that have assessed nutritional status after stroke report malnutrition in 8%–40% of stroke patients.[40] The physical consequences of stroke may result in these patients eating slowly due to facial weakness, poor arm function, and general fatigue. Poor nutritional status has been linked to the development of pressure area sores,[41] and resultant muscular weakness may inhibit rehabilitation.[42]

Patients with persistent dysphagia may need to be fed through a nasogastric (NG) tube, which can be uncomfortable and can often dislodge. Alternatively, they may be given a percutaneous gastrostomy (PG)—a tube that is surgically inserted directly into the stomach. Although this is thought to be better tolerated, there is conflicting evidence about the risks associated with and the outcomes of both NG and PG feeding.[43] A randomized controlled trial of PG and NG feeding found greater mortality and decreased nutritional intake in the NG patients.[43] However, a review of 37 patients who had a PG tube inserted post-stroke found that only 12 patients survived for three months; median survival was 53 days.[42] As it is likely that patients with persistent dysphagia who require enteral feeding have a relatively short prognosis, it is particularly important that doctors communicate openly with these patients and their families.

The question of whether to provide artificial nutrition for patients with a poor prognosis is an important one, and families and friends have strong feelings about this issue.[34] An international trial of different feeding policies for stroke patients is in now progress (International Stroke Trials Collaboration. Food Trial—*http://www.dcn.ed.ac.uk/food.*) Results from this trial are not yet available, but they will provide concrete information on the consequences of feeding stroke patients in terms of recovery. More information will, however, still be needed on the effect of both feeding and hydration in patients with a poor prognosis, including the effect on the mode and 'quality' of dying. There is no objective information on the consequences of decisions to begin or withhold feeding in this group. Again, decisions about whether or not to feed these patients require open and honest communication with families. Palliative care specialists have a particular interest and familiarity with difficult end-of-life decisions. Their input may, therefore, be helpful, particularly if there is disagreement within the medical team or between health professionals and patients or their representatives.

Pain

Stroke patients may suffer pain from a variety of sources. It may be the direct result of the stroke (for example, due to hemiplegia or contracture) or may stem from comorbidities such as arthritis. Up to 72% of stroke patients have a 'shoulder–hand syndrome',[44] in which the patient's upper limb becomes stiff due to reduced movement and, as a result, the hand becomes swollen, blue, hot, and clammy. Between 18%–32% have post-stroke headaches.[45] Additionally 8% of patients have 'central post-stroke pain' (a neuropathic pain syndrome thought to arise from the vascular lesion and characterized by pain in the corresponding body part).[46] This pain is thought to be partially resistant to opioids and remains difficult to treat. Amitriptyline produced a statistical reduction of central post-stroke pain in a small cohort; carbamazepine resulted in some, but nonsignificant, improvement.[47] Lamotrigine, a new antiepileptic drug, has recently been shown to be effective and well tolerated in a trial involving 30 patients with central post-stroke pain.[48]

The expertise of specialist palliative care may be relevant for pain management here. There is a need for better pain control in patients with communication problems. In such cases it is important that analgesia are regularly provided rather than be given 'as required'. Patients who have been taking regular medications for pain prior to their stroke will need to be assessed and assisted in continuing these therapies.

Depression and Anxiety

Post-stroke depression is described as a common problem, although variations in prevalence have been reported. A Scandinavian study included 486 patients aged 55 to 85 years. Major depression was diagnosed in 26% and minor depression in 14% of all patients. Dependency in daily life and pre-stroke depression were found to be the only independent predictors of post-stroke depression.[49] This supports the finding of Gainotti and co-workers[50] that a stroke patient's depressive symptoms were primarily a reaction to the 'devastating consequences of stroke' rather than a consequence of their stroke per se. People dying following a stroke both in the hospital and community were reported to have needed increased psychosocial support, and those in the community who cared for depressed and anxious relatives would have liked more help and support.[27] Depression in stroke patients can be treated with regular antidepressant medication. Thus, post-stroke depression is a common problem, has both organic and psychological causes, and may be relieved with appropriate psychological or medical therapies.

Stroke in Cancer (Thrombogenetic, Neck Dissection)

Some cancer patients may have a stroke as an end-stage complication of cancer. Since 15% of cancer patients have cerebrovascular lesions at autopsy and 50% of these lesions might have been symptomatic,[51] the simultaneous occurrence of both diseases is not a rare event. Different mechanisms have been suggested to explain stroke etiology in cancer patients: metastasis may cause intracerebral hemorrhage, coagulation disorders with hypercoagulability can cause thromboembolic stroke or sinus thrombosis, or leukemic

hypocoagulation may result in intracerebral or subarachnoid hemorrhage. Heparin is thought to be helpful in cancer hypercoagulation. Aggressive therapy with thrombolysis is in most cases contraindicated, since bleeding from the primary tumor or metastasis may result.[52]

A very special case of stroke in cancer is that of head and neck cancer. Patients with, for instance, laryngeal cancer develop compromised carotid arteries, either by the tumor itself growing around the vessels or due to neck dissection with even carotid artery resection[53] or secondary radiation with radiation-induced carotid artery stenosis or occlusion. Non-bacterial thrombotic endocarditis (NBTE) is another special situation in which cancer patients can develop a stroke. This special form of cardiac involvement in cancer is a non-bacterial endocarditis in patients with far-advanced tumors such as adenocarcinomas of the lung (about 10% of autopsies show thrombotic changes), leukemia, lymphomas, and others.

Caregivers

Most non-professional care of people following a stroke is provided by spouses. Various studies have tried to assess the extent of the 'burden' of care on this group. Usually the severity of the stroke and the patient's ability to undertake activities of daily life determines the level of care needed. However, the 'burden' experienced by non-professional carers is also associated with the carer's personal characteristics.[54] Ill health and an overall decrease in the quality of life of informal carers has been reported.[55] Stroke survivors living in the community are underserved by both health and social services and have unmet personal psychosocial needs, both of which increase the load on informal carers.[56,27]

Little attention has been paid to the specific needs of families of stroke patients with a poor prognosis, and who cope with a situation in which a loved one's death is inevitable. In many cases relatives will be involved in the decision making on whether to withdraw or withhold treatment, which may add considerably to their distress and anxiety. Such family members may need help to come to terms with this situation and, following the death of their loved one, may benefit from some form of bereavement support. The dying trajectory seems to have a particular impact on both the needs of families and the support (or lack of it) they receive. Those whose loved one survives for more than five days experience particular stress.[28]

Care in the Last Days of Life

Good supportive nursing care is particularly important for stroke patients at the end of their life. This care should include mouth care to prevent the development of oral candida, a system of turning the patient to avoid sores in pressure areas, and the management of feeding, incontinence, constipation, and pain. Dysphagic patients are especially prone to chest secretions, which can be distressing for both the patient and their family at this time; these can be managed with appropriate suction and medication. Guidelines on Managing the Last Days of Life in Adults (published by the National Council for Hospice and Specialist Palliative Care Services in the United Kingdom[57] and by the American College of Physicians[58]) are relevant to these patients and their adoption may help to improve care.

SUMMARY

The needs of patients expected to die soon after a stroke, and those of their families, have received little attention to date. Few stroke patients in the United Kingdom or elsewhere currently receive care from hospices and specialist palliative care services. The limited available evidence (outlined in this chapter) suggests that palliative care has a greater role to play in stroke than has hitherto been the case. This is not, however, to suggest that all— or, indeed, many—stroke patients who subsequently die should be cared for by hospices or specialist palliative care services. The United Kingdom makes a useful differentiation between the palliative care approach and specialist palliative care. The former is care informed by the principles and practice of palliative care, and it is argued that this should be provided to all patients who need it, regardless of setting, by their current healthcare providers. The latter is provided in specialist settings and/or by specialists in palliative care.

Some stroke patients with particularly complex physical, psychological, or social needs at the end of life may benefit from a hospice and specialist palliative care, and research is urgently needed to establish this. In the meantime, meeting the palliative care needs of stroke patients remains the responsibility of all those who currently care for these patients—at home, in the hospital, and in nursing homes. To do this, they may require education in palliative care and support from such specialists. Providing better care for stroke patients who are expected to die soon will require partnerships between those currently caring for these patients and the growing numbers of doctors and nurses who specialize in palliative care.

REFERENCES

1. Hankey GJ, Warlow CP. Treatment and secondary prevention of stroke: evidence, costs, and effects on individuals and populations. Lancet 1999;354: 1457–1463.
2. Wolf PA, D'Agostino RB. Epidemiology of stroke. In: Barnett HJM, Mohr JP, Stein BM, Yatsu FM, eds. Stroke, Pathophysiology, Diagnosis, and Management, 3rd Ed. Churchill Livingston, New York, Philadelphia, Edinburgh, London, Toronto, Montreal, Sydney, Tokyo, 1998:3–28.
3. Barker WH, Mullooly JP. Stroke in a defined elderly population, 1967–1985—a less lethal and disabling but no less common disease. Stroke 1997;28:284–290.
4. Britton, M, Roden A. Progression of stroke after arrival at hospital. Stroke 1985;16:629–632.
5. Berger C, Fiorelli M, Steiner T, et al. Hemorrhagic transformation of ischemic brain tissue: asymptomatic or symptomatic? Stroke 2001;32:1330–1335.
6. Krieger DW, Demchuk AM, Kasner SE, Jauss M, Hantson L. Early clinical and radiological predictors of fatal brain swelling in ischemic stroke. Stroke 1999;30:287–292.
7. Frankel MR, Morgenstern LB, Kwiatkowski T, et al. Predicting prognosis after stroke: a placebo group analysis from the National Institute of Neurological Disorders and Stroke rt-PA Stroke Trial. Neurology 2000;55:952–959.
8. Davalos A, Toni D, Iweins F, Lesaffre E, Bastianello S, Castello J. Neurological deterioration in acute ischemic stroke: potential predictors and associated factors in the European cooperative acute stroke study (ECASS)I. Stroke 1999;30:2631–2636.
9. Davenport RJ, Dennis MS, Wellwood I, Warlow CP. Complications after acute stroke. Stroke 1996;27: 519–524.
10. Ebrahim S. Clinical Epidemiology of Stroke. Oxford University Press, Oxford, 1990.

11. Kwakkel G, Wagenaar RC, Kollen BJ, Lankhorst GJ. Predicting disability in stroke—a critical review of the literature. Age Ageing 1996;25:479–489.
12. Schwab S, Steiner T, Aschoff A, et al: Early hemicraniectomy in patients with complete middle cerebral artery infarction. Stroke 29:1888–1893, 1998.
13. Bogousslavsky J, Bernasconi A, Kumral E. Acute multiple infarction involving the anterior circulation. Arch Neurol 1996;53:50–57.
14. Catala M, Rancurel G, Raynaud C, Leder S, Kieffer E, Koskas F. Bilateral occlusion of the internal carotid arteries. Analysis of a series of 19 patients. Rev Neurol 1995;151:648–656.
15. Roh JK, Kang DW, Lee SH, Yoon BW, Chang KH. Significance of acute multiple brain infarction on diffusion-weighted imaging. Stroke 2000;31:688–694.
16. Caplan LR. Posterior Circulation Disease. Blackwell Science, Cambridge, Oxford, London, Edinburgh, Carlton, 1996.
17. Hacke W, Zeumer H, Ferbert A, Bruckmann H, del Zoppo GJ. Intra-arterial thrombolytic therapy improves outcome in patients with acute vertebrobasilar occlusive disease. Stroke 1988;19:1216–1222.
18. Berg–Dammer E, Felber SR, Henkes H, Nahser HC, Kühne D. Long-term outcome after local intra-arterial fibrinolysis of basilar artery thrombosis. Cerebrovasc Dis 2000;10:183–188.
19. Cross III DT, Moran CJ, Akins PT, Angtuaco EE, Derdeyn CP, Diringer MN. Collateral circulation and outcome after basilar artery thrombolysis. Am J Neuroradiol 19:1557–1563, 1998.
20. Katz RT, Haig AJ, Clark BB, DiPaolo RJ. Long-term survival, prognosis, and life-care planning for 29 patients with chronic locked-in syndrome. Arch Phys Med Rehabil 1998;73:403–408.
21. Kaiser J, Perelmouter J, Iversen IH, et al. Self-initiation of EEG-based communication in paralysed patients. Clin Neurophysiol 2001;112: 551–554.
22. Kase C, Mohr JP, Caplan LR. Intracerebral hemorrhage. In: Barnett HJM, Mohr JP, Stein BM, Yatsu FM, eds. Stroke, Pathophysiology, Diagnosis, and Management, 3rd Ed. Churchill Livingston, New York, Philadelphia, Edinburgh, London, Toronto, Montreal, Sydney, Tokyo, 1998: 649–700.
23. Fernandes HM, Gregson B, Siddique S, Mendelow AD. Surgery in intracerebral hemorrhage. Stroke 2000;31:2511–2516.
24. Van Gijn J, Rinkel GJE. Subarachnoid hemorrhage: diagnosis, causes and management. Brain 2001;124: 249–278.
25. Barnett HJM, Mohr JP, Stein BM, Yatsu FM, eds. Stroke, Pathophysiology, Diagnosis, and Management, 3rd Ed. Churchill Livingston, New York, Philadelphia, Edinburgh, London, Toronto, Montreal, Sydney, Tokyo, 1998
26. Higginson IJ, Hearn J, Myers K, et al. Palliative day care: what do services do? Palliative Day Care Project Group. Palliat Med 2000;14:277–286.
27. Addington–Hall JM, Lay M, Altmann D, and McCarthy M. Symptom control, and communication with health professionals, and hospital care of stroke patients in the last year of life as reported by surviving family, friends, and offficials. Stroke 1995;26:2242–2248.
28. Rogers A, Addington–Hall JM, Pound P. Investigating the palliative care needs of stroke patients on the acute stroke unit. Abstracts of the Annual Palliative Care Congress, University of Leeds, 15–17 September 1997. Palliat Med 1998;12:481.
29. Rogers A, Addington–Hall JM. 'So I think it's swinging a bit toward not to feed'—decisions not to treat on a stroke unit. Palliative Care Congress, University of Warwick, March 2000. Palliat Med 2000;14: 240–241.
30. Brust JCM. Agitation and delirium. In: Bogousslavsky J, Caplan LR, eds. Stroke Syndromes. Cambridge University Press, Cambridge, Melbourne, 1995: 134–139.
31. Hoffman JE. 'Nothing can be done'—social dimensions of the treatment of stroke patients in the general hospital. Urban Life and Culture 1974;3: 50–70.
32. Becker G, Kaufman S. Managing an uncertain illness trajectory in old age: patients' and physicians' views of stroke. Med Anthropol Q 1995;9:13–18.
33. Kehayia E, Korner–Bitensky N, Singer F, et al. Differences in pain medication use in stroke patients with aphasia and without aphasia. Stroke 1997;28: 1867–1870.
34. British Medical Association. Discussion Document: Withholding and Withdrawing Life-prolonging Medical Treatment: Guidance for Decision Making. BMJ Books, London, 1999.
35. Nakayama H, Jorgensen HS, Pedersen PM, Raaschon HO, Olsen TS. Prevalence and risk factors of incontinence after stroke: the Copenhagen Stroke Study. Stroke 1997;28:58–62.
36. Ween JA, Alexander MP, D'Esposita M, Roberts S. Incontinence after stroke in a rehabilitation setting: outcomes, associations and predictive factors. Neurology 1996;47:659–663.
37. Borrie MJ, Campbell AJ, Caradoe–Davis TH, Spears GFS. Urinary incontinence after stroke: a prospective study. Age Ageing 1986;15:177–181.
38. Gordon C, Laughton Hewer R, Wade DT. Dysphagia in acute stroke. Br Med J 1987;295:411–414.
39. Barer DH. The natural history and functional consequences of dysphagia after hemispheric stroke. J Neurol Neurosurg Psychiatry 1989;52:236–241.
40. Dennis M. Nutrition after stroke. Stroke Review 1998;2:6–10.
41. Finucane TE. Malnutrition, tube feeding and pressure sores: data are incomplete. J Am Geriatr Soc 1995;43:447–451.
42. Wanklyn P, Cox N, Belfield P. Outcome in patients who require a gastrostomy after stroke. Age Ageing 1995;24:510–514.
43. Norton B, McLean KA, Holmes GK. Outcome in patients who require a gastrostomy after stroke. Age Ageing 1996;25:493.
44. Bohannon RW, Larkin PA, Smith MB. Shoulder pain in hemiplegia; statistical relationship to five variables. Arch Phys Med Rehab 1986;67:514–516.
45. Ferro JM, Lelo TP, Oliveira V, et al. A multivariate analysis of headache associated with ischemic stroke. Headache 1995;35:315–319.
46. Vestergaard K, Nielsen J, Andersen G, Arendt–Nielsen, Jensen TS. Sensory abnormalities in consecutive unselected patients with central post-stroke pain. Pain 1995;61:177–186.

47. Leijon G, Boivie J. Central post-stroke pain—a controlled trial of amitriptyline and carbamazepine. Pain 1989;36:27–36.
48. Vestergaard K, Andersen G, Gottrup H, Kristensen BT, Jensen TS. Lamotrigine for central poststroke pain. Neurology 2001;56:184–190.
49. Pohjasvaara T, Leppavuori A, Siira I, Vataja R, Kaste M, Erkinjuntti T. Frequency and clinical determinants of poststroke depression. Stroke 1998;29:2311–2317.
50. Gainotti G, Azzoni A, Razzano C, Lanzillotta M, Marra C, Gasparini F. The post-stroke depression rating scale: a test specifically devised to investigate the affective disorders of stroke patients. J Clin Exp Neuropsychol 1997;19:340–356.
51. Graus, F, Rogers LR, Posner JP. Cerebrovascular complications in patients with cancer. Medicine 1985;64:16–35.
52. Rogers LR. Stroke and neoplasia. In: Welch KMA, Caplan LR, Reis DJ, Siesjö BK, Weir B, eds. Primer on Cerebrovascular Diseases. Academic Press, San Diego, London, Boston, New York, Sydney, Tokyo, Toronto, 1997:313- 314.
53. Maves MD, Bruns MD, Beenan MJ. Carotid artery resection for head and neck cancer. Ann Otol Rhinol Laryngol 1992;101:778–781.
54. Schotte WJM, de Hain RJ, Rijinders P, Limburg Mm Van der Bos GAM. Burden of care after stroke. Stroke 1998;29:1605–1611.
55. Anderson G, Vestergaard K, Ingeman–Nielsen M, Jensen TS. Incidence of post-stroke pain. Pain 1995;61:187–193.
56. Wilkinson PR, Wolfe CDA, Warburton FG, et al. A long-term follow-up of stroke patients. Stroke 1997;28:507–512.
57. National Council for Hospice and Specialist Palliative Care Services. Changing Gear—Guidelines for Managing the Last Days of Life in Adults. The National Council for Hospice and Palliative Care Services, London, 1997.
58. Quill TE, Byock IR. Responding to intractable terminal suffering: the role of terminal sedation and voluntary refusal of food and fluids. American College of Physicians–American Society of Internal Medicine (ACP–ASIM) end-of-life care consensus panel. Ann Int Med 2000;133:561–562.

Chapter 3

Demyelinating Disease

A.D. (Sandy) Macleod
Fabio Formaglio

MULTIPLE SCLEROSIS—BRIEF RESUME
PALLIATIVE MANAGEMENT OF
  NEUROLOGICAL SYMPTOMS
Weakness and Loss of Motor Control
Spasticity
Fatigue
Ataxia and Intentional Tremor
Visual Disturbances
Swallowing Difficulties
Urinary Disorders
Sexual Dysfunction
Bowel Dysfunction
Pain and Paresthesia
Skin Care
Paroxysmal Phenomena

PALLIATIVE MANAGEMENT OF
  PSYCHOBEHAVIORAL AND
  COGNITIVE SYMPTOMS
Grief and Adjustment Reactions
Denial
Autonomy and Individualization
Affective Disorder
Disorders of Emotional Expression
Cognitive Impairments
Psychotic Episodes
Personality Change
Alcohol/Substance Abuse
Sleep Disturbance
THE TERMINAL PHASE

Demyelinating diseases share the common pathologic feature of foci of degeneration, involving the myelin sheath of nervous tissue. Multiple sclerosis (MS) is the commonest demyelinating disease and this chapter will focus on the palliative management of MS.

MS has a variable natural course. Typically, it has an initial relapsing–remitting course followed by progressive deterioration. Neurological deficits tend to accumulate and the burden of illness escalates. In the absence of a known cure—though disease-modifying agents can influence the natural course—a palliative philosophy of care, from the onset, by a multidisciplinary care team, is required. New neurological symptoms may be curtailed by corticosteroid, antispasmodic, analgesic, anticonvulsant, or antidepressant medications, physical therapy, and psychotherapy—all relieve some of the intensity of the acquired deficits. Yet with progression the quality of life risks erosion. Attentive symptom control is

greatly appreciated by the patient and despite the ravages of this cruel disease quality of life can be maintained. Life expectancy is reduced and the final years of life may be undignified because of the burden of symptoms, the profound dependency upon others, and cognitive impairment.

CASE HISTORY

A 37-year-old woman presented with a 17-year history of MS of secondary progressive type. She complained of a new severe burning pain, as well as 'burning bee', in her left hand. She has been restricted to a wheelchair for the last five years by severe lower limb weakness and spasticity, sometimes painful. Spasticity is an obstacle to her physical therapy. Her control of her voiding is compromised by an urgency to micturition, and often she is incontinent. She is severely depressed, and worried about the progression of the disease.

She is afraid of the loss of her residual ability to function. She lost her job 10 years ago, and seven years ago she broke up with her boyfriend. She currently lives alone. Interferon had not arrested the progress of her disease and corticosteroid pulses had not induced significant symptom resolution over the previous few years. Her quality of life had deteriorated and both patient and her carers were tiring of the burden of her care because of the multiplicity and accumulation of symptoms.

MULTIPLE SCLEROSIS—BRIEF RESUME

Multiple sclerosis (MS) is an inflammatory, demyelinating disease of the central nervous system (CNS). The disease is the most common cause of chronic neurological disability among young adults. The etiology of MS is unknown, but there is convincing epidemiological, pathological, and experimental evidence that MS is an autoimmune T-cell mediated inflammatory demyelinating disorder of the CNS, induced by some still unknown environmental factors in genetically susceptible subjects. The pathological lesions consist of discrete areas of inflammation and demyelination (plaques) scattered throughout the CNS. The lesions can disturb conduction of nerve impulses in any CNS pathway and can occur at different sites and at different times. The scattered distribution of MS lesions results in a wide variety of clinical symptoms and signs.[1]

The median age of MS onset is 31 years and the illness is approximately three times as common in women as in men.[1] The natural course of MS is extremely variable. Symptoms may appear, disappear, and reappear; they can gradually worsen or remained unchanged. Approximately 85% of patients start the disease with a relapsing/remitting (RR) course. This form of MS is characterized by episodes (exacerbation or relapses) of neurological dysfunction, persisting for more than 24–48 hours. The recovery from relapses varies among patients and from one attack to the next. The relapses occur at irregular intervals and, over time, the recovery can be incomplete and the patient starts to accumulate disability. 80%–90% of patients with a RR form

of MS convert to a secondary progressive course—a disease pattern of gradual accumulation of irreversible disability, within 20–25 years from onset; the rest have a progressive course from onset, with or without superimposed relapses.[2,3]

Thus, the burden of illness escalates—by 15 years after onset 32%–76% require an aid to ambulate, 65%–75% have left work because of their illness, and 14%–29% are bedridden.[4] Quality of life is progressively eroded. The variable march of MS symptoms is slow, cumulative, and cruel. The median survival from onset is 28 years for men and 33 years for women. The overall life expectancy is seven years less than normal or 75%–85% of expected survival. Mortality increases with disability. Death directly from MS itself is rare; infection is the most common cause of death.[4]

There is no definite cure for MS. The treatment of acute relapse is with corticosteroids administered preferably intravenously for 3–5 days. In recent years, large controlled clinical trials, involving relapsing–remitting MS patients, demonstrated that interferon b-1a, interferon b-1b[5] and glatiramer acetate significantly reduce the frequency of attacks and the accumulation of new demyelinating brain lesions revealed by MRI. Indications for the use of available therapies for MS have changed in a few years, passing from a conservative to a more aggressive attitude. So far, this approach is limited to the early phases of the disease.

However, the mainstay of management is palliative from diagnosis to death. Attempts to relieve the symptoms of neurological relapse and the underlying accumulative deficits is a core clinical task.[6] Invariably, relapses are associated with psychological distress, necessitating an empathic and supportive approach. By reducing the extent of impairment caused by the disease (e.g. fatigue, visual loss, incontinence), the disability may be lessened (e.g. locomotion, reading, personal care) and, likewise, the handicap (immobility, occupation, independence). The sheer number of symptoms of MS and their complex interactions is daunting.[7] The treatment of the effects of the disease (the symptoms and the provision of support) involves a multidisciplinary team which may include, in addition to the family physician and the neurologist, the urologist, psychiatrist, pain specialist, neuro-radiologist, specialist nurse, physical therapist, social worker, occupational therapist, psychologist, speech language therapist, dietician, chaplain, and lay support groups. Involvement of the patient (and their carers) in determining a management strategy is a critical component of the palliative approach to their care. Quality of life needs to be the crucial clinical determinant indicating the extent of medical intervention.

Though a palliative philosophy of care is not likely to be shared by the patient during the early years of disease (for their hope of cure or spontaneous resolution is strong), the natural course of MS dictates this approach for the professional carers. Gradually, the patient's health predicament forces them to move towards their carer's philosophy. Clinical decisions to withhold active life-preserving symptomatic treatments, such as antibiotics, should be by joint agreement and ideally previously rehearsed. The phase of disease at which such decisions need to be made is dependent on disease and patient variables.

J.K. Wolf, a physician and MS sufferer, considered depressive disorder to be the most disabling symptom of MS, spasticity to be the most frequent, bladder symptoms to be the most confusing, and bowel symptoms to be the most humiliating.[8] In clinical practice the most medically intriguing symptoms are often not the symptoms of greatest concern to the patient.

PALLIATIVE MANAGEMENT OF NEUROLOGICAL SYMPTOMS

Weakness and Loss of Motor Control

These symptoms are more prominent in lower limbs; they coalesce with spasticity, fatigue, and ataxia to reduce the patient's mobility. Weight loss, if indicated, can be an important intervention. Crutches and supportive bandaging may improve function, yet enhance muscular disuse. Physical therapy to improve the use of those agonist muscles less involved by the disease may be of benefit.[9]

Spasticity

This is one of the most typical and disabling MS symptoms. It accumulates over time, with the advancing of the disease. The need for symptomatic treatment of spasticity approximately parallels the severity of corticospinal tract involvement. Spasticity increases fatigue and reduces mobility, and may be associated with muscle pain. It prevails on lower limbs, where extensor spasticity can aid weightbearing impaired by strength loss. Thus, it is important to recognize that spasticity overtreatment can impede mobility. In the terminal stage of the disease, spasticity merges with muscle fibrosis and anchylosis, to result in a complete loss of mobility, sometimes in uncomfortable fixed positions. Sleep and rest, and personal care may be deeply impaired.

Spasticity is associated with flexor spasms, or exaggerated avoidance reflexes, triggered by movements or tactile stimuli. Flexor spasms can provoke severe muscle pain and be an obstacle to mobility such as physical activity. Several stressors, such as exposure to cold, severe exertion and muscular stretching, hyperventilation, and a full bladder, may all exacerbate spasticity and precipitate spasms (and are preventable). Spasticity is also worse during fever and urinary tract infections.[9]

Spasticity and flexor spasms can be treated initially with simple preventive measures, such as 'leg warmers' and by supporting the knees, semi-flexed, on pillows. Physical therapy is useful from the beginning of symptoms to prevent muscle contractures and to teach patients to manage the increased muscle tone. However, pharmacotherapy is often necessary (Table 3–1). Oral baclofen, diazepam and other benzodiazepines, dantrolene, and tizanidine are equally effective in MS spasticity and muscle spasm treatment. Comparative studies have not shown drugs with superior profile. Anti-spasticity drugs differ in mechanism of action; therefore they can be alternated and combined. Unfortunately, clinical research on validated score of spasticity and/or gain in quality of life is poor, and does not clearly confirm the clinical impression of efficacy of these drugs.[10]

When the muscle spasm is confined in a few muscle groups, botulinum toxin may be useful. Intrathecal baclofen, delivered in a

Table 3–1. **Anti–spasticity Drugs in Multiple Sclerosis**

Medication	Dosage Range	Potential Side Effects
Baclofen	20–75 mg/day PO 50–200 mcg/day intrathecally	Drowsiness, increased weakness, dizziness, delirium, ataxia, nausea
Tizanidine	4–18 mg/day	Sedation, hypotension, anxiety
Clonazepam	2–6 mg/day PO	Sedation, delirium
Diazepam	5–20 mg/day PO	Sedation, delirium
Dantrolene	100–300 mg/day PO	Sedation, dizziness, diarrhea, hepatitis
Botulinum A toxin	20–100 U muscle	Increased weakness

continuous infusion by implanted pumps, is increasingly recognized as being an effective, but not easy to manage, system to maximize drug efficacy.

Fatigue

A profound sense of physical exhaustion and lack of energy is a constant companion for most MS patients.[11] Generalized fatigue may be enhanced by depression and overexertion, and contributes to the undermining of quality of life and restriction of activity. As in patients with advanced malignancy, fatigue is under-reported, infrequently enquired for, and, for many, is a major disabling symptom. Fatigue may be continuously present or exacerbated by muscular exertion and amplified by heat and humidity. Thus, even if daily activity, such as exercise, may contribute to a sense of health and well-being, care must be taken to control the increase in body heat and to accurately gauge individual exercise tolerance. Temperature management by avoidance of hot environments and rapid changes in ambient temperature, cooling by such simple measures as drinking ice water, a cool bath, or a swim, using a mesh chair which allows good ventilation and lying prone (which prevents temperature elevation locally over the spine) are important measures. Regular rest and sleep are essential. Psychostimulants, such as methylphenidate and pemoline have been trialled and amantadine has been shown to relieve fatigue in one-third to one-half of patients, but its efficacy often wanes quickly. Recently, modafinil has been trialled in a phase II trial with good success.[12] Potassium

blocking agents such as 4-aminopyridine have been used to alleviate temperature sensitivity.[11]

Ataxia and Intentional Tremor

To a degree most MS patients suffer from these symptoms which are provoked by sensory disturbance and damage to the cerebellum and its pathways. Cerebellar dysfunction is associated with poor outcome. Ataxia may be a particularly disabling symptom, reducing manual dexterity and aggravating the risk of falling. Tremor and titubation may be profoundly socially embarrassing symptoms. Physical therapists can teach appropriate movements to compensate for motor disequilibrium. Intentional tremor may be dampened by arm weights that reduce the amplitude of movement. Since anxiety amplifies tremor, benzodiazepines are sometimes useful. Primidone or propranolol may be used if tremor is severe, but generally these treatments are disappointing. There are uncontrolled reports of high-dose isoniazid, associated with pyridoxine to avoid hepatotoxicity or neuropathy, and tetrahydrocannabinols for tremor.[13] In selected cases, thalamic stimulation and surgery may be considered therapeutic options.[14]

Visual Disturbances (Visual Loss, Diplopia, Oscillopsia)

Optic neuritis is one of the most common causes of spontaneous reversible visual loss in young adults. It is the presenting symptom in approximately one-fifth of MS patients, and occurs at some stage in the course of three-quarters of patients. Pendular nystagmus, even if a rare symptom, can be deeply disabling.[15]

Aids for visual impairment and the expertise of those who work with such patients, though often resisted, may be very helpful. Benzodiazepines and baclofen are the mainstay of oscillopsia treatment. High-dose isoniazid has been proved effective in anecdotal reports.

Swallowing Difficulties

Dysphagia tends to be underestimated in MS patients. Dietary advice and education is often warranted. In advanced disease PEG might be considered (see Chapter 16 for details).

Urinary Disorders

Bladder dysfunction develops eventually in 90% of MS patients. Bladder hyperreflexia occurs in approximately two-thirds. Detrusor hyperreflexia results in a sense of urgency, urge incontinence, and increased frequency of micturition. A full bladder, exposure to cold, exercise, hyperventilation, and infection may all aggravate detrusor hyperreflexia. Flaccid bladders are rare. Detrusor hyperreflexia is further complicated by sphincter dyssynergia in half of the patients. This dysfunction results in hesitancy, with interrupted or diminished stream. Obstructive disorder results in gradually increasing residual volumes and, as a consequence, persistent urinary tract infections, stone formation, and bladder 'accidents'.

A urologic evaluation is the first step to determine the urologic dysfunction and appropriate treatment. Patients with spastic bladder should avoid fluid intake before activities where frequent urination is not feasible. Anticholinergic medications, such as oxybutynin, propantheline bromide, and tricyclic antidepressants allow better filling of the bladder but risk retention of urine if sphincter stenosis coexists (Table 3–2). Desmopressin nasal spray or PO and intravesical capsaicin may also assist storage dysfunction. Anti-spasticity drugs (e.g. baclofen, benzodiazepines) and hyoscyamine are preferred in bladder spasms. Bladder massage (or Credè manoeuvre), alpha blockade (e.g. terazosin), and intermittent self-catheterization may help those patients who find it difficult to void. Finally, if all these measures fail, a permanent catheter must be considered.

Bacterial urinary infection is very frequent in MS patients. With a post micturition residual over 50 ml, bacteriuria complications increase three-fold. Preventive techniques

Table 3–2. Medication Used to Treat Bladder Dysfunction

Medication	Indications	Dosage Range	Potential Side Effects
Oxybutynin chloride	Overactive bladder Involuntary bladder contractions	10–20 mg/day PO	Dryness, drowsiness, blurred vision, palpitations
Propantheline bromide	Bladder spasms, cramps	45–90 mg/day	Dry mouth, blurred vision, tachycardia, nausea, constipation
Imipramine and other tryciclic antidepressants	Urinary frequency	10–150 mg/day	Sedation, dizziness, constipation
Desmopressin	Fecal incontinence Urinary frequency	0.2– 0.4 nocte PO/nasal spray	Stuffy nose, abdominal cramps, nausea
Capsaicin (intravesical)	Bladder hyperreflexia		Burning (transient)
Terazosin	Difficulty to void	2–6 mg/day	Hypotension
Hyoscyamine	Bladder spasms	0.75 mg 7/day	Dry mouth, blurred vision, tachycardia, delirium

include regular, frequent urination, with complete bladder emptying, often requiring double voiding or self-catheterization, adequate hydration, acidification of urine, and prophylactic antibiotics (see Chapter 26).

Sexual Dysfunction

In MS patients the preservation of a sexual relationship can be of paramount importance. However, a failure of erection in males and anorgasmy in females frequently intervene. Sildenafil, papaverine, surgical prostheses, and vacuum devices may warrant consideration in the male. However, drugs and techniques requiring dexterity and co-ordination to administer may not be ideal. Psychological counseling and support, irrespective of the cause of the sexual dysfunction, is advisable.

Bowel Dysfunction

Incontinence is an uncommon symptom of MS, however constipation is present in 30%–50%. Immobilization, autonomic dysfunction, anticholinergic medication, and reluctant hydration (for fear of bladder accidents) all contribute to constipation. Anal sphincter dysfunction may cause proctalgia, unexpected leakage, and difficulties emptying. The psychological humiliation caused by these problems may be significant (see Chapter 25).

Pain and Paresthesia

Pain is a frequent symptom in MS, involving about 50%–75% of the patients at some time during the disease course. Pain occurrence and its severity is not related to the length of the disease or severity of the demyelinating lesions. A close relation has been documented between pain and disability and psychological status.[16,17]

In MS, neuropathic pain prevails, triggered by ectopic neuronal activity in the spino–thalamic–cortical pathway, favoured by the demyelination, or by deafferentation of brain centers. In other cases, muscle spasticity or visceral (e.g. bladder) distension may produce nocioceptive painful signals. Not uncommonly, ectopic neural discharge arises from the spinal dorsal column system and presents as tingling, formication, or other non-painful sensation.

Neuropathic pain frequently occurs as burning or throbbing continuous pain in the lower limbs. Paroxysmal pains, as trigeminal neuralgia, Lhermitte's sign, or shooting or burning paroxysmal pain of the limbs, are rarer. Tonic seizures or painful tonic spasms are sudden bursts of spasticity often associated with severe pain, which last seconds or a few minutes and spread from the trunk or limbs, sometimes crossing the midline. Different from flexor spasms, these are unconnected to underlining spasticity. Tonic seizures usually subside spontaneously any time up to a month later. Back and muscle pain are frequent complaints in MS, but pain is usually not severe.

Anticonvulsant drugs are the preferred drugs in paroxysmal neuropathic pains. Carbamazepine and, in recent years, gabapentin and lamotrigine, have been effective in open label trial. Baclofen, mexiletine, and clonazepam are also used in these pains and paresthesia. Long-lasting neuropathic pains may respond better to tryciclic antidepressants. NSAIDs and physical therapy are the main treatment of musculoskeletal pains. Ocular pain in optic neuropathy may require a short course of simple analgesia.

Skin Care

Immobilization and confinement to bed risks decubitus ulceration. Sensory impairments and motor incoordination may increase the likelihood of lacerations and minor injuries. Good nursing care should prevent the development of decubitus ulcerations.

Paroxysmal Phenomena

Brief recurring episodes of paresthesia, numbness, pain, weakness, clumsiness, dystonia, dysarthria, diplopia, visual disturbance, and vertigo are examples of paroxysmal phenomena which may occur during the course of MS. These may respond to anticonvulsants or baclofen. These syndromes may subside within days or months, allowing the withdrawal of medication.

PALLIATIVE MANAGEMENT OF PSYCHOBEHAVIORAL AND COGNITIVE SYMPTOMS

Grief and Adjustment Reactions

The losses incurred during the course of MS are multiple and cumulative. The loss of health, of neurological function, of opportunity, of potential, of independence, of employment, and of vitality occur unpredictably and inevitably. The uncertainties of prognosis, the vicissitudes of hope and denial, the sadness of erupting complications essentially result in a chronic and everlasting adjustment reaction. As one loss may be adjusted to, another loss emerges, and as this process proceeds the failing brain struggles even harder to incorporate and accommodate these losses. Psychotherapeutic interventions need to be supportive, empathic, flexible, and pragmatic. Partners, children, and relatives grieve also, often not in parallel with the patient, for they try to hide their hurt from the hurting patient.

Denial

In the early phases of illness, denying the impact and the sequelae of the disease is a psychological defence mechanism which allows a respite until grieving can proceed. Time for the 'bad news' to sink in and to build up strength to embark upon the work of grief and adjustment is not pathological. In the later stages of MS denial tends to be organically determined, often maladaptive, and creative of major management difficulties such as refusal to comply or even attend therapy or consultations.

Autonomy and Individualization

Physical symptoms of loss of function may result in loss of locomotion, dexterity, and personal care. Ultimately, physical independence may be lost. Being dependent on others—the loss of one's autonomy and independence—may result in devastating psychological injuries including those to self-esteem and dignity. Knowledge about, and experience

of, the illness may empower sufferers to exert influence over their management plans. This necessitates medical and nursing attendants allowing the patient to be a key member of the management team rather than enacting a paternalistic authoritarian medical model of care. However, cognitive decline may eventually reduce the feasibility of such an approach.

Affective Disorder

The lifetime prevalence of a major depression in MS is 40%–60%. Depression in MS is more frequent than in comparable disabling disease and is related to cerebral involvement.[1] The presence of depression is not closely related to the duration of illness or degree of disability or cognitive impairment, but may be more common during relapses or when neurological disability is progressing. Correlation with MRI lesion load has been disappointing. There is little support for genetic predisposition; social factors are of relevance and perceived lack of social support and the degree of social isolation correlate better with the presence of depression than MRI abnormalities.

Disruption of frontal–temporal circuits by MS plaques may be the critical organic risk factor for depression. Depression may herald a relapse, corticosteroids and interferons may induce depression, and complicated grief reaction may predispose to depression. For every individual there is a multitude of risk factors which may accumulate and breech the depressive threshold. Suicide rates are higher than in the normal population: the risk is increased 7.5-fold. The lifetime risk of suicide in MS is 2%.[4,18] Suicide is most likely in the less disabled, young male within five years of diagnosis. In the age of interferon treatment this rate may have even increased due to the depressogenic side effect of interferons.

Despite the frequency and seriousness of major depressive disorder in MS few receive adequate treatment. Tricyclic antidepressants may be effective but drop-out rates because of intolerable side effects are very high. Published trials of sertraline and moclobemide show moderate efficacy and tolerability in MS. Tolerability of agent is the key influence upon pharmaceutical choice. Hence most clinicians use SSRIs first line. Maintenance anti-depressants, possibly lifelong, should be considered in those who clearly benefit and don't wish to risk depressive relapse.[19]

There is a two-fold increase of bipolar mood disorder in MS and mood stabilizers (sodium valproate, lithium carbonate) may be indicated. Corticosteroids at doses of greater than 40 mg prednisone (equivalent), even in short pulses, may induce psychiatric side effects such as depression, mania, and delirium. The therapeutic response of bipolar illness to pharmacotherapy can be adversely affected by coexistent organic disease such as MS.

Disorders of Emotional Expression (Eutonia, Euphoria, Pathological Laughing, Crying, Lability of Mood, Emotional Incontinence)

This may occur in 10%–25%, and is more likely in severely disabled with cognitive impairment. Major depression may coexist, but not invariably. Clinically it is important to differentiate the outward expression of affect from the subjective mood state. Many of these patients may not be sad or miserable; a minor emotional provocation such as a happy or sad moment may result in emotional expressive dyscontrol. This may be indicative of underlying cognitive impairment and not an underlying depression. There is a literature on the use of low-dose antidepressant medications, particularly SSRIs, in this condition and one RTC with amitriptyline. Simple techniques of cognitive and distracting strategies may be helpful, such as a rapid change of content from that provoking the reaction. Though generally self-limiting and brief, the frequency of these reactions may be very high, and increase as does fatigue as a day evolves.[20]

Cognitive Impairments

Though often subtle, cognitive deficits can be detected in 40%–60% of patients and contribute significantly to the burden of disability.[1] Cognitive dysfunction is severe in 21%–33%. Higher cortical function is often normal to a casual observer, or during bedside mental status examination, yet on neuro-psychological testing evidence of subcortical dementia is apparent. Relatives have been shown to report the underlying deficits more accurately than the patient themselves. Slowing of cognitive processing, impaired auditory attention, memory retrieval deficits, executive function deficits (verbal fluency, planning, and organizational difficulties) may be difficult to quantify clinically but hinder daily living even more than gross physical impairment. Language tends to be best preserved.

MS patients with cognitive symptoms are less likely to be employed or engaged in social activities than MS patients without such deficits. Cognitive dysfunctions have potential influence upon issues such as fitness to drive, child custody, jury service, and testamentary capacity and competency. Superimposed depression may amplify cognitive deficits. The natural history of cognitive deficits remains uncertain—they may remain static in the early stages; recovery of cognitive deficit caused by a relapse may or may not occur; there is substantial individual variation; however, in progressive MS, deterioration is likely.

Management involves support and education of the patient and relatives about these deficits, and advice that they are not just behaving poorly. Cognitive retraining and the learning of compensatory strategies such as graded practice on memory tasks and the use of lists and written cues may be of benefit. Parenteral physostigmine can improve memory in MS patients; the cognitive enhancing drugs such as rivastigmine may have possibilities. Corticosteroids and perhaps interferons may induce a remission of cognitive deficits.[21,22]

Psychotic Episodes

These are reported, but uncommon. The threshold for delirium in cognitively impaired MS patients is lower, thus the initial differential diagnosis should always be that of acute delirium.

Personality Change

Though recognized for over a hundred years, the personality changes associated with MS have been little studied. Irritability, apathy, and disinhibition were reported in 35%, 20%, and 13% of MS patients, respectively.[19] The disorders of emotional expression, such as euphoria, may merely be symptoms of frontal lobe/dysexecutive change. Organic disintegration may enhance personality traits previously muted. These changes in behavior are often cause of great concern and management dilemmas for carers and relatives. Strict behavioral interventions may be required, but are not easy to enforce consistently and humanely.

Alcohol/Substance Abuse

Pathological intoxication may occur in the cognitively compromised, however, as a generalization, there is a tendency for alcohol misuse to wane in the presence of neurological impairment, for most recognize that drunkenness merely highlights their neurological deficits. A premorbid pattern of the use of alcohol or substances to cope with adversity augers poorly for the initial phase of adjustment to MS.

Sleep Disturbance

Excessive somnolence and inappropriate daytime sleep can occur in MS but may merely be a reflection of fatigue. Narcolepsy has been reported as associated, and certainly MS patients have reduced sleep efficiency and more awakenings during sleep.

THE TERMINAL PHASE

Fatigue, cachexia, immobilization, cognitive impairment, and weakness all predispose to an enhanced risk of infection. Infection is usually the immediate cause of death.[23,24] The end-of-life phase may be protracted by assertive antibiotic treatment, often at the cost of the quality of remaining life.

REFERENCES

1. McDonald WI, Ron MA. Multiple sclerosis: the disease and its manifestations. Phil Trans R Soc Lond B 1999;54:1615–1622.

2. Lublin FD, Reingold SC, the National Multiple Sclerosis Society (USA) Advisory Committee on Clinical Trials of New Agents in Multiple Sclerosis. Defining the clinical course of multiple sclerosis: results of an international survey. Neurology 1996;46:907–911.

3. Nortvedt MW, Riise T, Myhr K–M, Nyland HI. Quality of life in multiple sclerosis : measuring the disease effects more broadly. Neurology 1999;53:1098–1103.

4. Sadovnick AD, Ebers GC, Wilson RW, Paty DW. Life expectancy in patients attending multiple sclerosis clinics. Neurology 1992;42:991–994.

5. Neilley LK, Goodin DS, Goodkin DE, Hauser SL. Side effect profile of interferon beta-1b in multiple sclerosis: results of an open label trial. Neurology 1996;46:552–554.

6. Clanet MG, Brassat D. The management of multiple sclerosis patients. Current Opinion in Neurology 2000;13:263–270.

7. Thompson AJ. Multiple sclerosis: symptomatic treatment. J Neurol 1996;243:559–565.

8. Wolf JK, Mastering MS. Handbook of Management. Academy Books, Rutland, Vermont, 1996.

9. Mitchell G. Update on multiple sclerosis therapy. Medical Clin North Am 1993;77:231–249.

10. Shakespeare DT, Young CA, Boggild M. Anti-spasticity agents for multiple sclerosis. The Cochrane Library 2000;Issue 4.

11. Krupp LB. Mechanisms, measurement, and management of fatigue in multiple sclerosis. In: Thompson AJ, Polman CH, Hohlfeld R, eds. Multiple Sclerosis: Clinical Challenges and Controversies. Martin Dunitz Ltd., London, 1997:283–294.

12. Rammohan KW, Rosenberg JH, Lynn DJ, Blumenfeld AM, Pollak CP, Nagaraja HN. Efficacy and safety of modafinil (Provigil) for the treatment of fatigue in multiple sclerosis: a two centre phase 2 study. J Neurol Neurosurg Psychiatry 2002;72(2):179–183.

13. Consroe P, Musty R, Rein J, Tillery W, Pertwee R. The perceived effect of smoked cannabis on patients with multiple sclerosis. Eur Neurol 1997;38:44–48.

14. Montgomery EB Jr, Baker KB, Kinkel RB, Barnett G. Chronic thalamic stimulation for the tremor of multiple sclerosis. Neurology 1999;3:625–628.

15. Stark M, Albrecht H, Pollmann W, Straube A, Dieterich M. Drug therapy for acquired pendular nystagmus in multiple sclerosis. J Neurol 1997;244:9–16.

16. Stenager E, Knudsen L, Jense K. Acute and chronic pain syndromes in multiple sclerosis. A 5-year follow-up study. Int J Neurol Sci 1995;16:629–632.

17. Archibald CJ, McGrath PJ, Ritvo PG, et al. Pain prevalence, severity and impact in a clinical sample of multiple sclerosis patients. Pain 1994;58:89–93.

18. Caine ED, Schwid SR. Multiple Sclerosis, depression, and the risk of suicide. Neurology 2002;59:662–663.

19. Diaz–Olavarrieta C, Cummings JL, Velazquez J, Garcia de la Cadena C. Neuropsychiatric manifestations of multiple sclerosis. J Neuropsychiatry Clin Neurosci 1999;11:51–57.

20. Feinstein A, O'Connor P, Gray T, Feinstein K. The effects of anxiety on psychiatric morbidity in patients with multiple sclerosis. Multiple Sclerosis 1999;5:323–326.

21. La Rocca NG, A rehabilitation perspective. In: Rao SM, ed. Neurobehavioral aspects of multiple sclerosis. Oxford University Press, New York, 1990:215–229.
22. Rao SM, Leo GJ, Ellington L, Nauestz T, Bernardin L, Unversagt F. Cognitive dysfunction in multiple sclerosis II. Impact on employment and social functioning. Neurology 1991;41:692–696.
23. Sadovnick AD, Eisen K, Ebers GC, Paty DW. Cause of death in patients attending multiple sclerosis clinics. Neurology 1991;41:1193–1196.
24. Koch–Henriksen N, Bronnum–Hansen H, Stenager E. Underlying cause of death in Danish patients with multiple scleropsis: results from the Danish Multiple Sclerosis Registry. J Neurol, Neurousurg, Psy 1998;65:56–59.

Chapter 4

Neoplasms

Kendra Peterson

INTRODUCTION AND EPIDEMIOLOGY
**COMMON SYMPTOMS OF PRIMARY
 AND METASTATIC BRAIN TUMORS**
Headache
Seizures
Cognitive Dysfunction
Psychological Distress
Immobility
Thromboembolism

**LEPTOMENINGEAL AND SPINAL CORD
 METASTASES**
COMPLICATIONS OF TREATMENT
Radiotherapy
Chemotherapy
Corticosteroids
**COMMUNICATION AND DECISION
 MAKING**
SUMMARY

Although most malignant tumors that affect the nervous system are currently not curable, aggressive multimodality therapies are employed in many instances in an effort to prolong life, and to maintain function and quality of life for as long as possible. Skillful management of a patient with nervous system malignancy includes careful diagnosis and rendering of appropriate treatments; careful attention to symptom management must also be the goal throughout the course of the illness and at the end of life. In addition, the patient must be supported through the transition from hope for cure or prolonged survival, to the acceptance of the terminal illness. Inherent in malignancies that affect the nervous system are changes in cognitive ability, personality, physical function, autonomy, and family and community roles. Family members and other caregivers are profoundly affected by the illness and themselves need support, education, and care. Although the focus of this discussion is the care of patients with incurable, progressive, and malignant nervous system tumors, the remarks are largely applicable to the care of many patients with less malignant tumors and at earlier stages of illness as well.

CASE HISTORY AND DISCUSSION

A 45-year-old man is now at home dying with a malignant brain tumor—glioblastoma multiforme. His wife is his primary caregiver. She has stopped working in order to care for him at home, and has hospice services involved in his care. She describes him foremost as a family man. Throughout his career he always made it home by 6:00 to have dinner with her and their son and rarely missed a soccer game or school performance; he was also the founder of a successful business.

He was diagnosed 12 months ago with a cerebellar tumor and underwent surgical resection and radiation therapy. His tumor recurred in the right frontal lobe five months later, and was treated with additional radiation therapy and experimental chemotherapy. Over the ensuing months he developed changes in personality, exhibited as paranoia, anxiety, and agitation. He became suspicious of his wife's motivations, and began hiding medicines and accusing her of lying to him. His wife and child were distraught by his behavior. He was admitted to the psychiatric ward of a hospital for management of steroid-induced psychosis, secondary to dexamethasone prescribed to control brain swelling. Tumor infiltration likely played a contributing role in his cognitive and behavioral changes. He was discharged from the hospital on antipsychotic medications that calmed his behavior but also slowed his movements and sedated him. He subsequently developed pulmonary embolus, treated with anticoagulants, and focal seizures involving the left upper extremity, treated with anti-convulsant medication. MRI showed extension of the tumor from the cerebellum into the brainstem causing somnolence and difficulty swallowing. He is no longer receiving medical therapies for the brain tumor.

He is now unable to walk though can assist in transfers from the bed to a chair. He is able to interact with his family to a limited degree. He is intermittently awake, and present in the room when the family is having meals, doing homework, or watching television. He does not initiate much conversation with them and answers direct questions briefly. He does not complain of pain. He takes in little food and fluid, although can still swallow medications. His wife has signed a 'do not resuscitate' order. He is not currently able to communicate his understanding of his illness, its prognosis, or his wishes. His wife is exhausted by her efforts to care for him, by her grief resulting from her loss of her partner and his imminent death, by trying to support and care for their young child, and by financial concerns related to loss of his income and her own.

Discussion

This case illustrates some of the commonly encountered symptoms that occur in patients with progressive incurable malignant brain tumors, including cognitive and behavioral changes, progressive functional dependence and immobility, seizures, and thromboembolic disease. It highlights the need for a complex, multi-faceted, and coordinated system of care for these patients, and exemplifies the concerns for advance care planning, financial issues, and caregiver support, all of which have tremendous impact on the total care of patients with brain tumors and their caregivers throughout the course of the illness and at the end of life.

INTRODUCTION AND EPIDEMIOLOGY

The term neoplasm can be used to refer to a wide variety of tumors within the nervous system, with a diverse spectrum of behavior in terms of natural history, response to treatment, and prognosis. On one end of the spectrum are benign tumors such as meningiomas or pituitary adenomas for which surgical resection is often curative. Unfortunately, the more common neoplasms, malignant gliomas and most metastases, are aggressive cancers for which currently available therapies extend survival but are rarely curative. Even low histological-grade, slow-growing tumors eventually end the life of most affected patients, and commonly evolve over time into more aggressive phenotypes.

Primary brain tumors are relatively unusual cancers. Unfortunately, the most common primary brain tumor, glioblastoma multiforme, is also the most malignant. The yearly mortality rate from malignant primary brain tumors is about 5 per 100,000. Metastatic brain tumors occur with much more frequency. They are often diagnosed at an advanced stage of cancer, although occasionally represent a single site of metastasis in a patient with well-controlled systemic disease. Primary and metastatic brain tumors may have similar neurological presentations, although primary brain tumors are more commonly unifocal and therefore predominantly affect a single region of brain function, while metastatic brain tumors are more likely to be multifocal and cause dysfunction at multiple sites or diffusely within the nervous system. The effects of brain metastases may be difficult to distinguish from the dysfunction attributable to systemic disease and metabolic disturbance encountered in patients with widely metastatic systemic cancers.

Systemic cancers also metastasize to other parts of the nervous system, most notably the leptomeninges, causing multifocal nervous system dysfunction, or to the epidural space, resulting in back pain and spinal cord compression. These are typically late manifestations of widely metastatic cancer, although are occasionally the presenting feature of a newly diagnosed malignancy. Involvement of the peripheral nervous system outside of the spine, including the brachial and lumbosacral plexus or peripheral nerves, is also an important contributor to discomfort and dysfunction in patients with cancer but will not be addressed in this chapter.

COMMON SYMPTOMS OF PRIMARY AND METASTATIC BRAIN TUMORS

Headache

Patients with headache are commonly fearful that they may have a brain tumor, and physicians lack the ability to distinguish benign headaches from those related to a brain tumor by the characteristics of the headache alone. The 'classic' headache associated with a brain tumor—a progressive morning headache accompanied by nausea and vomiting—occurs in a minority of patients with brain tumors. More commonly the headache associated with a brain tumor is indistinguishable from tension type headaches, and may have the characteristics of classic migraine in about 5% of patients. The most important distinguishing feature of a headache associated with a brain tumor is its association with other neurological abnormalities, such as seizures, change in personality, focal neurological dysfunction, or change in level of consciousness.[1]

The headache associated with a brain tumor is caused by local or distant traction on pain-sensitive structures within the brain, including the meninges and blood vessels. Its severity often correlates with the degree of intracerebral edema, mass effect, and shift of intracranial structures. Corticosteroid medications are among the most useful agents to relieve the headache associated with a brain tumor. They act by diminishing vasogenic edema surrounding the brain tumor. Any corticosteroid may be useful in this regard, although the synthetic glucocorticoid dexamethasone is often chosen because of its relatively long half-life and limited mineralocorticoid effect. The dose is titrated to maximize headache relief and neurological function, while minimizing the many potential complications of corticosteroid use that will be discussed later in the chapter.

Close to half of patients with brain tumors will have headache as one prominent presenting feature, although in most the headache is relatively easily controlled. For rare patients headache is a severe, persistent, and progressive symptom through the course of the illness and as the tumor progresses. For these patients, the appropriate use of analgesics to control pain and improve quality of life is essential. The World Health Organization analgesic ladder approach to the treatment of pain is as appropriate for patients with headaches as it is for other types of pain.[2] Particular care should be taken for patients with brain tumors to avoid the use of meperidine whose metabolite may lower the seizure threshold. It is also important to monitor for side effects of cognitive disturbance or change in level of consciousness in patients whose brain function may already be somewhat impaired by the disease.

In the final stages of illness, a decline in the level of consciousness and diminished communication may make it difficult to assess a patient's pain and response to treatment. In this setting it is appropriate to interpret physical signs such as rubbing the head and moaning as likely representing pain responses, and to treat accordingly using sublingual, parenteral, or transdermal routes of administration as necessary.

Seizures

Seizures occur in about 20%–40% of patients with brain tumors as a presenting feature, and only about half of patients with brain tumors have a seizure during the course of the illness. Therefore, seizure prophylaxis for patients who have never had seizures is not routinely necessary. An American Academy of Neurology Practice Parameter recommends prophylactic anti-convulsant medications for only one week in the perioperative period following brain tumor resection.[3] This guideline might be modified for patients with large tumors and significant mass effect for whom a seizure causing an elevation of intracranial pressure might be devastating, or for patients with multiple cortical or hemorrhagic tumors in which seizures may be more likely to occur. Patients who drive automobiles or perform other activities in which a seizure might pose a particular risk might also be recommended to receive prophylactic anti-convulsants.

Although not all patients with brain tumors have seizures, it is essential to discuss with the patient and caregivers this possibility in anticipation. Most seizures are brief, self-limited, and rarely harmful in themselves. Patients should be instructed to remove themselves from dangerous situations if they feel the onset of a seizure, which might include feelings of déjà vu, abnormal smells, tastes, epigastric rising, or other unusual sensations. Some seizures have no warning and result in generalized convulsions. Caregivers should be instructed to aid the patient to a place of safety, often on the floor, and that turning the patient on his side may help maintain an open airway. Objects should not be placed in the patient's mouth to prevent him from biting or 'swallowing' his tongue, and in fact this may lead to the caregiver being bitten. It is not always essential to seek emergency medical treatment for every seizure, although a condition of prolonged or recurrent seizures (status epilepticus) is a life-threatening event. Education and guidance about seizures can minimize the impact of seizures on quality of life and avoid unnecessary emergency room visits, while allowing caregivers to recognize the need for medical intervention when prolonged or recurrent seizures occur.

Patients with brain tumors may have generalized convulsions, or may have focal seizures manifested by motor, sensory, visual, or cognitive disturbance, depending on the site of the seizure focus. Whether or not seizures develop probably depends on the site of the tumor within the brain, its rate of growth, and possibly its histology. Once a seizure has occurred it is a common and reasonable practice for a patient with a brain tumor to be treated with anti-convulsant medications for a prolonged period, often until no seizures have occurred for several years. Many patients have no seizures or few seizures during the course of their illness. Rarely, frequent and refractory seizures impose severe limitations on function, autonomy, and safety throughout the course of the illness and at the end of life, and very infrequently are a direct cause of death.

The issue of whether or not a patient with a brain tumor and risk for seizures should continue to drive an automobile is one that takes significant consideration. The inability to drive causes a distressing degree of dependence on many patients. However, the issue of safety for the patient, and for others, is the primary concern. Legal regulations vary from country to country and from state to state within the United States. It is appropriate for physicians to adhere to local regulatory requirements, and in addition to advise patients not to drive if in their judgement driving is unsafe because

of the risk of seizures or impairments in motor or cognitive functioning.

A complete discussion of the use of anti-convulsants is beyond the scope of this chapter, although a few points specific to patients with brain tumors deserve emphasis. First is the reported increased incidence of severe allergic skin reactions—the Stevens–Johnson syndrome—in patients who receive concurrent anti-convulsant medications and cranial irradiation.[4] This has been attributed most frequently to the use of phenytoin, although has been reported with carbamazapine and may occur with other anti-convulsants as well. It is an important consideration guiding the use of anti-convulsants during radiation treatment. Second is the inducement of the hepatic microsomal enzyme system by many of the commonly used anti-convulsants that leads to increased metabolism and lowering of the blood levels of many drugs used in the treatment of patients with brain tumors. This is most significant for corticosteroids and some of the chemotherapeutic agents. Third is the clinical observation that corticosteroids themselves may play a role in reducing seizure activity by decreasing peritumoral edema. Finally is the unwanted effect of many of the anti-convulsants, even at 'therapeutic' serum levels, on the cognitive function of patients whose function may already be limited by the tumor. Careful monitoring of serum drug level, and consideration of alternate anti-convulsants is warranted before attributing all cognitive dysfunction to the direct effects of the tumor.

While seizures usually are not harmful and are rarely a direct cause of death in patients with brain tumor, their presence can be disconcerting to patients and caregivers at the final stage of illness. A supply at home of easily administered sublingual or rectal benzodiazapene or valproic acid often provides a readily available management strategy for seizures that occur in the final stages of illness, and allows a patient to remain in his own home rather than prompting emergency medical intervention.

Cognitive Dysfunction

There is a myriad of reasons for patients with brain tumors to experience cognitive dysfunction. It is essential to distinguish the direct effects of the tumor from other potentially treatable etiologies. Such causes include the effects of radiation or chemotherapy, anti-convulsant toxicity, side effects of corticosteroids, seizures or the postictal state, systemic infection or metabolic derangement, and depression. Cognitive dysfunction is often attributable to multiple causes; optimizing cognitive function therefore depends on evaluating all of the potential contributing factors and intervening where possible.

When the brain tumor is the principle cause of cognitive dysfunction, its specific manifestations are largely related to the location of the tumor within the brain. Patients with dominant hemisphere tumors are more likely to have difficulties with expressive or receptive language function, while those with non-dominant hemisphere tumors may have visuospatial problems, and those with frontal lobe dysfunction disorders of affect and insight.

Cognitive function may improve with treatment of the tumor, correction of metabolic derangement or drug toxicity, and treatment of depression. Methylphenidate may also improve cognitive function and is of most benefit in the management of patients with significant psychomotor retardation.[5] Cognitive dysfunction is an important determinant of health-related quality of life, and it may be an independent predictor of survival for patients with brain tumors.

Eventual cognitive dysfunction is a predictable result of a progressive brain tumor in most patients. The changes may, however, be subtle and occur with insidious progression, or with fluctuating severity depending on the response of the tumor to treatment as well the status of other contributing factors. Careful serial evaluation of cognitive function including bedside testing and formal neuropsychological testing is important to assess the patient's ability to act autonomously and to have decisional capacity in regard to receiving conventional or experimental treatments.

Psychological Distress

Perhaps not surprisingly, psychological distress is a common symptom experienced by patients with brain tumors and their caregivers throughout the course of the illness. Anxiety and depression are commonly encountered as people face a potentially life-ending illness, and experience significant changes in community, occupational, financial, social, and family roles and relationships. Interestingly, these symptoms are not particularly more common than in patients with other chronic neurological diseases.[6] The specific manifestations of psychological distress may relate to location of the tumor within the brain. Patients with frontal lobe tumors are more likely to exhibit abulia or depression, while those with temporolimbic tumors more commonly have mania or panic episodes. Psychological symptoms may also result from medication side effects, most notably the widespread use of corticosteroid and anti-convulsant medications. Psychological symptoms may be difficult to distinguish from the 'organic' symptoms directly resulting from the brain tumor, or from side effects of tumor treatments or adjuvant therapies. Psychological symptoms are best managed with a multimodality approach that includes pharmacological intervention with antidepressants or anxiolytics, individual or family counseling, support groups, and spiritual guidance.

Immobility

Loss of physical mobility and resultant physical dependence is a common symptom of patients with brain tumors. The location of the tumor within the brain is the major determinant to when in the course of the illness this occurs, but it eventually occurs in almost all patients with progressive brain tumors. Corticosteroids may improve physical function to some degree by diminishing peritumoral edema. Immobility renders the patient dependent on assistive devices or other people to ambulate and to carry out essential daily activities. It frequently causes an unwanted degree of dependency, and predisposes the patient to other complications including skin breakdown, venous thromboembolism, painful contractures, and infection.

It is common that aggressive physical therapy is not instituted in patients with progressive brain tumors as they are perceived as having a progressive illness without the potential for benefit. However, physical therapy can play a vital role in optimizing the physical function of a patient with a brain tumor, and patients with brain tumors experience as much functional benefit from rehabilitation programs as do patients with other neurological disease.[7] Physical and occupational therapists can provide ongoing education, equipment, appropriate exercises, and techniques to facilitate an improved quality of life for patients with brain tumors throughout the course of the illness.

Thromboembolism

Venous thromboembolism is diagnosed in about 20% of patients with brain tumors during the course of the illness, and may be present without symptoms and go undiagnosed in an even higher percentage. Patients in the perioperative period and those who are hemiparetic are at particular risk, although this complication may occur even in fully ambulatory patients due to changes in the hemostatic and fibrinolytic systems induced by the tumor itself. Prophylaxis of this complication is therefore appropriate, with the use of pneumatic or gradient compression stockings. Prophylactic anti-coagulation is rarely utilized and not well studied. A high index of suspicion is needed to diagnosis thromboembolic disease. Patients may present with extremity pain or swelling, or chest pain and dyspnea if pulmonary embolism has occurred. A more subtle presentation is mild encephalopathy secondary to hypoxia.

Anti-coagulation with heparin and warfarin is the appropriate treatment for most patients with brain tumors who develop thromboembolic disease, and is not associated with an increased risk for intracranial or intratumoral hemorrhage compared to patients with brain tumors not anti-coagulated.[8] However, complicating factors that might influence the decision to anti-coagulate include the presence of a commonly hemorrhagic brain tumor (eg. metastatic melanoma), chemotherapy-induced thrombocytopenia, or previous gastrointestinal hemorrhage, particularly in a patient on corticosteroid medication. An alternative to anti-coagulation is the use of an inferior vena caval (IVC) filter, but they too have significant associated complications. Recurrent pulmonary embolism may result from the development of collateral circulation, and IVC filter thrombosis and post-phlebitic syndromes are common. An IVC does not relieve the pain, swelling, and dysfunction related to lower extremity thrombosis. Thrombolytic therapies are contraindicated in the treatment of patients with brain tumors. In the terminal phases of illness, it may be appropriate to treat a patient with thromboembolic disease with analgesics and sedatives rather than institute full anti-coagulation.

LEPTOMENINGEAL AND SPINAL CORD METASTASES

Metastasis to the leptomeninges and spinal cord are typically late manifestations of widely metastatic systemic cancers. Rarely are they the initial presentation of a previously undiagnosed cancer, or the only site of disease of a cancer of unknown primary. They are each diagnosed in about 5% of patients with cancer, although may be more common and go undiagnosed in patients who are severely debilitated in the late stages of widely disseminated cancer. Both are thought most commonly to result from hematogenous spread of cancer, though rarely result from direct invasion of the nervous system from a contiguous site of disease. Both require a high index of suspicion to diagnose, as the early symptoms may be subtle. While treatment is not curative, early institution of treatment may provide significant symptom relief and palliation.

Leptomeningeal cancer commonly presents with multifocal, sometimes patchy involvement, of numerous regions of the neuraxis.[9] It commonly presents as basilar meningitis causing multiple cranial neuropathies. Involvement of multiple nerve roots may result in radicular pain, weakness, or sensory loss, usually with diminished deep tendon reflexes. Involvement of the cauda equina may cause urinary or fecal incontinence. Rarely, encephalopathy results from direct cortical invasion, but more commonly is a result of communicating hydrocephalus presumed due to diminished resorption of CSF. Occasional patients have focal cerebral neurological deficits or seizures secondary to direct cortical infiltration.

Diagnosis is made by CSF examination, which commonly shows elevated protein and pleocytosis in addition to malignant cells on cytological examination. Serial CSF examination may be necessary to make a cytological diagnosis. Nearly any cancer may metastasize to the leptomeninges, although lung and breast cancers and lymphoma are among those that do so most commonly.

Treatment of leptomeningeal cancer is not expected to be curative in most cases, although may improve the symptoms and quality of life of an affected patient and may prolong survival, usually in the order of months. Corticosteroids may significantly improve symptoms, especially if neck, back, or radicular pain are prominent symptoms of the disease. Whole-brain radiotherapy is usually employed, as well as radiation therapy to sites of 'bulky' or symptomatic spine disease. Intrathecal chemotherapy, usually administered through a surgically placed intraventricular catheter, is administered once or twice weekly until the CSF normalizes, and then monthly thereafter. Repeated lumbar puncture for administration of chemotherapy may also be performed, and may be warranted if the major site of symptomatic disease is in the lower spine. Methotrexate is commonly used in the treatment of solid cancer metastases, while ara-C (or liposomally packaged ara-C requiring less frequent administration) is used more commonly in the treatment of leptomeningeal lymphoma. Analgesics should be employed as needed if corticosteroids and primary treatments of the tumor are ineffective in relieving pain. Careful attention to bladder and bowel function is important, particularly in patients with cauda equina involvement.

Epidural spinal cord compression most commonly results from direct extension of tumor that has metastasized to the vertebral bodies. It may also result from direct extension through the vertebral foramen from the paraspinal space without bony involvement, especially in the case of lymphoma, and rarely from hematogenous spread to the epidural space without adjacent bony involvement. It is diagnosed most commonly in cancers that frequently metastasize to bone, such as lung, breast, prostate cancers, and multiple myeloma, and in lymphoma. Patients typically present with neck or back pain, often radicular in nature due to involvement of adjacent nerve roots.[10] The pain is often made worse by lying down, coughing, or straining. Patients may experience rapidly progressive neurological dysfunction with extremity weakness, numbness, and sphincter dysfunction, or may exhibit more insidious progression. The mechanism of spinal cord dysfunction is both neurological and vascular, with direct compression of nerves and axons but also vascular compression and congestion resulting in eventual spinal cord ischemia and irreversible infarction.

Corticosteroids should be administered when there is a clinical suspicion of spinal cord compression due to cancer even before a definitive diagnosis is made. Corticosteroids can significantly improve neurological function and outcome by reducing peritumoral spinal cord edema, and may have a dramatic effect in reducing a patient's pain. Corticosteroids may also have a direct oncolytic effect on lymphoma. For patients with severe or rapidly progressive neurological compromise an initial high dose of corticosteroids (such as intravenous dexamethasone 100 mg bolus followed by 24 mg every six hours) is appropriate and may provide prompt relief of symptoms while definitive diagnostic tests are being carried out.[11] The dose of corticosteroid continued after that is determined by the response to corticosteroids as well as the findings on diagnostic studies, with the goal of rapidly reducing the dose once more definitive treatment is instituted.

The diagnosis of spinal cord compression due to cancer is typically confirmed with MRI, although myelogram or contrast CT may be diagnostic in situations when MRI is not available. In patients with known cancer the typical MRI appearance is usually sufficient to make a diagnosis and only in rare instances, if the diagnosis is uncertain, is surgical biopsy necessary. The entire spine should be imaged in order to plan appropriate treatment, as often there are multiple levels of spine involvement.

Radiation therapy is the mainstay of treatment for epidural spinal cord compression. Treatment should be initiated as quickly as possible in order to have the best chance of preserved or improved neurological function. It is common that neurological function will decline slightly and transiently with the first or second fraction of radiotherapy, possibly due to radiation-enhanced cord edema. Rarely, surgical intervention is appropriate, especially for the treatment of known radioresistant tumors, or for patients who experience continued progression of symptoms during the course of radiotherapy. Surgical decompression is most easily performed by removing the posterior vertebral elements. However, in most instances the site of vertebral metastasis is in the vertebral body resulting in anterior spinal cord compression, so posterior decompression does nothing to remove the bulk of the tumor, may lead to spine instability, and is not advised. Consideration is sometimes given to an anterior surgical approach and vertebrectomy, although this more invasive surgical intervention is usually restricted to patients with relatively good overall prognosis, only one site of spinal involvement, and without widely metastatic systemic disease. Chemotherapy does not usually act quickly enough to play a significant role in the treatment of epidural spinal cord compression due to cancer, with the possible exception of lymphoma in which chemotherapy may rapidly and dramatically reduce the size of the tumor.

Corticosteroids and radiotherapy are typically sufficient to relieve the pain associated with epidural spinal cord compression, although analgesics should be employed appropriately if pain is a persistent problem. Aggressive physical therapy, bladder and bowel program, prevention of thromboembolic complications, and exquisite skin care are also essential to maximize the physical function and quality of life of these patients. When epidural spinal cord compression is suspected in the very terminal phase of a patient's illness, at a time when he is already bedridden from other causes, corticosteroids and analgesics alone may be appropriate therapies rather than instituting daily visits for radiation oncology. However, in many instances, aggressive diagnosis and treatment of epidural spinal cord compression effectively reduces pain and improves neurological function and quality of life even in the late stages of a cancer illness.

COMPLICATIONS OF TREATMENT

Radiotherapy

A comprehensive discussion of the effects of radiotherapy on the nervous system is beyond the scope of this chapter and is found elsewhere.[12] A few of the pertinent features will be highlighted. It is important to realize that the effects of radiotherapy are at times difficult to distinguish on clinical and radiographic bases from the effects of progression of the malignancy, but have different implications in terms of clinical course and prognosis. Recognizing the effects of radiotherapy on the nervous system may prevent unneeded antineoplastic treatments, and may themselves be moderated to some degree with appropriate treatments.

The effects of radiotherapy on the brain and nervous system are classically characterized by their timing in relation to radiotherapy. Acute effects occur during radiotherapy and are thought to result from local edema caused by the radiation itself. Cranial irradiation may result in headache, nausea, or worsening of the underlying neurological deficits. Spinal cord irradiation may similarly result in transient worsening of the neurological dysfunction. Fatigue is a common and sometimes debilitating effect of radiotherapy. The acute effects of radiotherapy are typically transient and are often improved with treatment with cortiocosteroid medications.

Early delayed effects of radiotherapy often occur a few weeks to months after completion of radiotherapy. The effects are thought to be the result of demyelination and are often transient. Patients may develop severe somnolence, seen particularly in children who have undergone posterior fossa irradiation, or in worsening of their neurological deficit. Similarly, patients who have received spinal irradiation may have similar transient worsening of their neurological symptoms, sometimes with an associated electric shock-like sensation (Lhermitte's sign) with neck flexion reflecting posterior column dysfunction. These effects are probably spontaneously reversible, although are commonly treated with corticosteroids as well.

The late complications of nervous system irradiation occur months to many years after completion. It may result in frank brain (or rarely spinal cord) necrosis, in global cognitive decline, or in progressive focal neurological decline. Radiation therapy may also cause hypothalamic and pituitary axis dysfunction resulting in hypothyroidism and other hormone imbalance. The pathology of late radiation injury is related to gliosis and microvascular injury. The severity and extent of involvement depend on the volume of tissue irradiated, and on the total radiation dose and daily fraction size. It is also worse in elderly patients or very young children, and possibly in patients with other illnesses that predispose to microvascular injury such as diabetes or hypertension. Brain MRIs may show areas of necrosis that are difficult to distinguish by imaging from recurrent tumor, although MR spectroscopy or PET scan may give a clue to the likely pathological process. MRI may also show periventricular white matter changes, atrophy, and ventriculomegaly, particularly in patients who have received whole brain radiotherapy. The extent of such changes correlates roughly with the extent of cognitive decline that a patient experiences. MRI of the spinal cord is more likely to show atrophy without specific signal abnormalities.

Radiation necrosis in the brain is sometimes appropriately treated with surgical resection of the necrotic mass, both to definitively distinguish it from recurrent tumor and to improve neurological function. More commonly it is managed with corticosteroids, and anti-coagulation or pentoxyphilline have been used in an attempt to improve microvascular blood supply to necrotic tissues. Functional improvements in global cognitive decline may be enhanced with methylphenidate treatment. Rare patients with significant ventriculomegaly out of proportion to global brain atrophy experience gait disorder, cognitive decline, and incontinence that may improve with ventriculoperitoneal shunting.

While the late effects of radiotherapy are rarely the direct cause of a patient's death, they commonly render patients chronically neurologically disabled, and have significant impacts on the ability to perform self-care activities and on occupational, family, and community roles. Adaptation to such changes includes physical, occupational and speech therapy, and sometimes vocational retraining. Tremendous support and counseling may also be required for patients and caregivers to adapt to the chronic changes in roles and relationships that ensue.

Chemotherapy

A discussion of the numerous symptoms that result from the use of chemotherapeutic agents is beyond the scope of this chapter. For the most part, commonly used chemotherapy agents for the treatment of primary brain tumors, including but not limited to nitrosoureas, procarbazine, and temozolomide, do not typically have significant neurological consequences in and of themselves. Any contribution they may have to neurotoxicity in the setting of concurrent nervous system irradiation is not well established. Many chemotherapy agents have well-described neurological consequences reviewed elsewhere.[13] Prominent examples include the leukoencephalopathy seen with high-dose systemic or intrathecal methotrexate, and the cerebellar dysfunction of cytarabine or fluorouracil. Novel strategies for the treatment of brain tumors including angiogenesis inhibition, cell differentiating agents, or gene therapies may result in additional side effects and toxicities that will be more clearly defined in the future.

Corticosteroids

There are numerous unwanted effects resulting from the use of corticosteroid medications.[14] Their frequent substantial benefit in improving neurological dysfunction related to peritumoral edema must be weighed against the potential acute and long-term complications. A detailed discussion of all corticosteroid side effects will not be presented, but a few points particularly relevant to the treatment of patients with nervous system malignancies will be emphasized.

With the exception of lymphoma, corticosteroids generally provide symptomatic treatment without primary effects on the malignant process. It is therefore reasonable to limit the dose of corticosteroid to one that improves function to the greatest degree without causing significant side effects. Although there are several corticosteroid medications to choose from, dexamethasone is most commonly used because of its limited mineralocorticoid effect and relatively long half-life. The dose and schedule is individualized to the patient's needs, but in many instances may be given on a twice-daily schedule.

Common side effects include the Cushingoid appearance and acne production that may be quite troublesome to patients. Most patients develop some degree of proximal myopathy when treated with corticosteroids for more than a few weeks; this is severe and disabling in about 10% of patients.[15] It is more prone to develop on the synthetic fluorinated corticosteroids such as dexamethasone, and decreasing the dose or changing to another agent may improve the condition. It may be less pronounced in patients who receive concurrent phenytoin, possibly due to interactions on drug metabolism or binding.

Cognitive or behavioral changes are common in patients receiving corticosteroids, and may manifest as irritability, euphoria, and, rarely, flagrant psychosis.[16] Cognitive changes may occur at the initiation of steroids or after patients have been on prolonged treatment, and are roughly, although not invariably, dose related. If the patient is otherwise receiving significant benefit from corticosteroid treatment and the symptoms are mild, they are sometimes managed with a small dose of sedative or neuroleptic medication. The symptoms are reversible once the corticosteroid is discontinued. It is essential to distinguish the cognitive changes caused by corticosteroids from the effects of tumor progression, other medications, or metabolic disturbances.

Another potential side effect of corticosteroids is an increased risk for opportunistic infection, in particular *Pneumocystis carinii* pneumonia, which occurs most commonly after prolonged treatment at a time when the corticosteroids are being tapered.[17] Some have advocated prophylactic treatment with trimethoprim sulfa or pentamadine to prevent this complication. Therapy to prevent gastrointestinal hemorrhage is also a common practice, although without good data to support its routine use. Glucose intolerance, osteoporosis, avascular necrosis of joints, and cataracts, are other potential complications of long-term use whose likelihood and severity must be weighed against the benefit of corticosteroids in an individual patient.

In the terminal stages of illness the abrupt withdrawal of steroids could conceivably hasten death by causing adrenal insufficiency or exacerbating cerebral edema. However, this practice commonly occurs at a stage of illness when death is imminent, and patients are comatose and no longer able to take in oral medications, food, or fluids. The usual practice is to discontinue corticosteroids abruptly at that stage, and not to administer them parenterally which would only serve to prolong the dying process. Ideally this issue is discussed with the patient and caregivers long in advance of the terminal stage of illness, and may be included in a written advance directive. If the abrupt withdrawal of corticosteroids results in discomfort, the patient may be appropriately managed with analgesics or sedatives, but the intravenous administration of corticosteroids is rarely appropriate or necessary.

COMMUNICATION AND DECISION MAKING

Most malignant brain tumors and nervous system metastases are incurable. Advance care planning is therefore appropriate early in the course of the disease. In the case of brain tumors, there is a high likelihood of eventual cognitive impairment, pushing the need for this discussion to occur at a point in the illness even earlier than would be appropriate for other patients with serious, potentially life-ending illnesses. Patients need to understand that the time of full intellectual competency is likely to be much more reduced than the time of survival. A written advance directive allows the patient to identify a surrogate decision maker in anticipation of a time when he is no longer able to make his own medical decisions, and articulates and documents his wishes in regard to the use of aggressive medical interventions that have the potential to prolong the dying process.

However, a thoughtful balance must be reached between the patient's hope for prolonged survival and acknowledgement of the disease's likely prognosis. Discussion of prognosis and advance care planning therefore evolves in a continuing conversation that takes place over time. It demands sensitivity and finesse on the part of the physician. Ideally, a physician accompanies and guides a patient and family through the transition from hope for cure or prolonged survival, to acceptance of the terminal nature of the illness, offering life-prolonging therapies when available, and exquisite symptom management throughout the course of the illness.

SUMMARY

The total care of an incurable neoplasm affecting the nervous system is a complex task.

It is best performed by a team of specialized care providers including neuro-oncologists, medical oncologists, radiation oncologists, neurosurgeons, palliative medicine specialists, nurses, neuropsychologists, social workers, and physical and occupational therapists. Hospice providers and spiritual counselors provide particular skilled services to patients nearing the end of life. The role and prominence of each team member evolves during the course of the illness as the disease progresses and the symptoms and needs of the patient change. Family members often provide the bulk of the direct care, and themselves require support, education, counseling, and respite. While there are currently no curative therapies available for most patients with malignant brain tumors and nervous system metastases, careful attention to symptom assessment and management can greatly enhance quality of life throughout the course of the illness and at the end of life.

REFERENCES

1. Forsyth PA, Posner JB. Headaches in patients with brain tumors. Neurology 1993;43:1678–1683.
2. Cancer Pain Relief and Palliative Care. Report of a WHO Expert Committee. World Health Organiztion, Geneva, 1990.
3. Glantz MJ, Cole BF, Forsyth PA, et al. Practice parameter: anti-convulsant prophylaxis in patients with newly diagnosed brain tumors. Report of the Quality Standards Subcommittee of the American Academy of Neurology. Neurology 2000;54:1886–1893.
4. Delattre JY, Safai B, Posner JB. Erythema multiforme and Stevens–Johnson syndrome in patients receiving cranial irradiation and phenytoin. Neurology 1989;38:194–198.
5. Meyers CA, Weitzner MA, Valentine AD, et al. Methylphenidate therapy improves cognition, mood, and function of brain tumor patients. J Clin Oncol 1998;16:2522–2527.
6. Pringle AM, Taylor R, Whittle IR. Anxiety and depression in patients with an intracranial neoplasm before and after tumour surgery. Br J Neurosurg 1999;13:46–51.
7. Huang ME, Cifu DX, Keyser–Marcus L. Functional outcomes in patients with brain tumors after inpatient rehabilitation: comparison with traumatic brain injury. Amer J Phys Med Rehab 2000;79: 327–335.
8. Norris LK, Grossman SA. Treatment of thromboembolic complications in patients with brain tumors. J Neurooncol 1994;22:127–137.
9. Olson ME, Chernick NL, Posner JB. Infiltration of the leptomeninges by systemic cancer. A clinical and pathological study. Arch Neurol 1974;30: 122–137.
10. Gilbert RW, Kim JH, Posner JB. Epidural spinal cord compression from metastatic tumor: Diagnosis and treatment. Ann Neurol 1978;3:40–51.
11. Sorensen PS, Helweg–Larson S, Mourisden H, et al. Effect of high-dose dexamethasone in carcinomatous metastatic spinal cord compression treated with radiotherapy: A randomised trial. Eur J Cancer 1994;30A:22–27.
12. Peterson K, Rottenberg DA. Radiation damage to the brain. In: Vecht ChJ, ed. Handbook of Clinical Neurology. Elsevier Science BV, Amsterdam, 1997: 325–351.
13. Posner JB. Side effects of chemotherapy. In: Reinhardt RW, ed. Neurologic Complications of Cancer. F.A. Davis Company, Philadelphia, 1995: 282–310.
14. Posner JB. Supportive care agents and their complications. In: Reinhardt RW, ed. Neurologic Complications of Cancer. F.A. Davis Company, Philadelphia, 1995:59–66.
15. Dropcho EJ, Soong SJ. Steroid myopathy in patients with primary brain tumors. Neurology 1991;41:1235–1239.
16. Stiefel FC, Breitbart WS, Holland JC. Corticosteroids in cancer: neuropsychiatric complications. Cancer Invest 1989;7:479–491.
17. Henson JW, Jalaj JK, Walker RW, et al. Pneumocystis carinii pneumonia in patients with primary brain tumors. Arch Neurol 1991;48:406–409.

Chapter 5

Parkinson's Disease and Related Disorders

Chris G. Clough
Anna Blockley

Palliative care for Parkinson's disease (PD) is a poorly developed area of care. We do not understand the needs of Parkinson patients close to death and how best to meet these. Although many patients die of other diseases, almost certainly PD itself contributes to terminal decline in others. Despite this lack of knowledge it is possible to define where care can be improved. Knowledge of drug treatment is helpful, as is being aware of the multiplicity of problems of Parkinsonian patients in decline. A multidisciplinary approach is often the best way to address these needs and involvement of the palliative care team should be considered. There is an opportunity for further research to quantify and describe patients' problems close to death to help deliver a better quality of care to end-stage Parkinson patients.

CASE HISTORY 1

Mavis developed PD in her early seventies. She attended for regular neurological follow-up with her husband Peter, who took an obsessive interest in her care, tape recording all conversations with the neurologist so he could review them at a later date. Gradually, Mavis deteriorated, with increasing balance problems and then cognitive decline. The occurrence of hallucinosis led to simplifying her drug regimen, concentrating on levodopa treatment which helped her Parkinsonian symptoms to a degree. When 78 years old she became acutely ill with chest infection leading to admission. As the infection cleared it became clear there had been a serious deterioration in her Parkinsonism. She was fully bedbound, dependent on nursing care, and needed to be roused to consciousness, which revealed the extent of her dementia. She appeared to her nurses and doctors to be in terminal decline with very poor quality of life. She could be fed by nurses but otherwise remained immobile with increasing limb contractures. Peter refused to accept the clinical assessment of the hopelessness of the situation. He arranged for her to go home and to have around-the-clock nursing care.

Six years later she remains bed bound, with extreme contractures of her limbs, mostly appears to be asleep but, if roused, will look around and say a few words which appear to make sense to Peter. She has had numerous crises—bowel obstruction due to constipation, chest infections (presumably secondary to inhalation)—but these have all been aggressively treated at Peter's request. He remains determined that she will make some form of recovery and will not relinquish his hopes despite the evidence that she will not improve and what, to an outsider, appears to be a very low quality of life.

Commentary

This sad case demonstrates a number of important points. It shows the difficulty of trying to predict life span in PD and highlights the problems about cause of death. Patients may survive many years despite loss of many bodily functions and severe dementia. Thus one appreciates the reluctance of palliative care teams with limited resources to commit themselves to the care of PD patients. PD patients will survive if every 'opportunity for death' is aggressively treated. Most of us would not want to survive in Mavis's condition but, as she is not compos mentis, her husband is taking decisions on her behalf, agreeing courses of action, as there was no evidence of an advance directive or living will. Physicians in the United Kingdom can take decisions on behalf of a patient who is not competent, especially if it is clear that a relative is acting against the patient's best interests (N.B. English and European law). However, the reality is that carers and relatives have an important part to play in making decisions about their relative's care and it would be difficult to act counter to those wishes without gaining the support of other professionals and making sure the legal situation is clear to all. Fortunately, Mavis appears peaceful and not distressed.

CASE HISTORY 2

James, who developed PD in his seventies, was a retired hematologist. With drugs, his quality of life remained good for several years. He was a stoic and confronted his loss of independence due to balance problems with good humor. From 77 years onwards, increasing problems emerged—hallucinosis, episodes of confusion, and he had falls and became housebound. Levodopa controlled some of his Parkinsonian stiffness but did little else for his overall quality of life, and the dose was limited because of the risk of aggravating his hallucinosis. Depression emerged and did not respond to drug treatment. He became increasingly frail and reliant on his wife for

support: she was a 'tower of strength'. He was admitted urgently with pneumonia and was given antibiotics. However, he remained bedbound and confused. After repeated discussions with his wife it was clear that his wishes were that, in the emergence of terminal illness, he did not want to be aggressively treated. He was started on a syringe driver with opiates, quickly become sedated and no longer distressed. Intermittently, he would wake to talk to his wife. Nursing care concentrated on keeping him comfortable; L-dopa was continued at low dose to relieve limb stiffness. He quietly 'passed away' two weeks later.

Commentary

Here, the wishes of the patient and his wife were clear. (The physician accepted there was an advance directive.) The physician was able to indicate that aggressive treatment (further antibiotics, physiotherapy) would only attain, at best, a return to his previous life which was no longer acceptable to him. Thus, concentration on control of pain, mental distress, and nursing aspects were the preferred options. The patient's wife was grateful for all the care he received. After his death she did not take up the offer from the neurologist to discuss the decision about the terminal care her husband had, as she was happy all the right decisions had been made. Here, it was clear that a shift in emphasis of management could take place with the agreement of the patient and his wife.

INTRODUCTION

Little has been written about palliative care for PD. It is not that the situation does not arise; more that the approach to PD for those who manage these patients is that they concern themselves with the correct diagnosis, drug treatment, and the multidisciplinary care of what is usually a long-term, progressive disorder.[1] Palliative care specialists, too, have not routinely been involved in the care of PD patients. In the United Kingdom, until recently, hospices and palliative care centers have generally refused referral of PD patients because they are aware of the long duration of the disease and the difficulties in predicting the time of death (see Case History 1). When resources are limited, committing palliative care teams to care for patients over long periods has not been possible. These difficulties highlight that area of care where health services generally perform badly. At the two extremes of care—rehabilitation of acute neurological problems and palliative care—the problems and resources required are more easily identified.

Many health services, along with social service support, fall down in planning and managing the care of progressive disorders such as PD. Additionally, those services, such as they are, along with hospital-based specialists, may not recognize the shift of emphasis and goals when continuing care moves into the palliative care arena. Physicians, patients, and carers alike may find it hard to move from a situation where everybody is doing their utmost to prolong life and quality of life by using all available drug treatment and even neurosurgery. The failure of drug treatment, inappropriateness of surgery, and other critical events (for instance cognitive decline) may indicate that a shift in emphasis is required from an essentially medical approach—'high tech'/pharmacologically led—to one which recognizes that the goal remains qualify of life but in the context of a life span which is considerably shortened by emerging problems of disability, mental decline, or general decline in physical well-being.

PARKINSON'S DISEASE—DIAGNOSIS, TREATMENT, AND COURSE

Parkinsonism is diagnosed when the core symptom of bradykinesia (slowness of movement) occurs with cogwheel rigidity and/or rest tremor.[2] The idiopathic form of the disease—Parkinson's disease—is assumed to be the diagnosis when no cause of symptomatic Parkinsonism is apparent (e.g. neuroleptic-induced Parkinsonism) and there is a positive response to levodopa/dopaminergic therapy (Table 5–1). PD is a progressive neurodegenerative disorder where the brain shows loss of pigmented neurons from the substantia nigra (particularly pars compacta) and the association of a specific intraneuronal inclusion body—the Lewy body.

Table 5–1. **Diagnosis of Parkinson's Disease**

The diagnosis requires bradykinesia plus:
- Tremor (resting)

or

- Rigidity (cogwheel or lead pipe)

Additional features:
- Postural imbalance
- Fixed stooped posture
- Dystonic postures (e.g. striatal hand)H
- Hypomimia (masked faces)
- Shuffling short-step gait (with or without festination)
- Freezing episodes (pdoxical akinesia)
- Seborrhea—scalp scurf
- Constipation
- Bladder symptoms (pseudo prostatism)
- Bulbar symptoms—dysarthria, dysphagia
- Pain
- Cognitive disturbance
- Psychiatric problems—depression, anxiety, hallucinations

It was the discovery of levodopa therapy in the 1960s[3] which revolutionized the treatment of PD (Table 5–2) and led neurologists to consider the disease a pathfinder amongst neurodegenerative disorders. Effective symptomatic treatment led to an overly optimistic view of the outlook for most Parkinsonian patients. It is now clear that not only are there problems of long-term dopaminergic treatment (Table 5–3) but many symptoms of PD are not relieved by PD drug treatment (Table 5–4). Five to ten years following diagnosis many patients are experiencing increasing problems such as drug-induced fluctuations (on–off), dyskinesias, and neuropsychiatric problems.[4] For others the key issue affecting quality of life is depression.

These issues vary enormously from patient to patient; the main predictor of complications being age. Those patients with young onset disease (10% of patients present before age 50) can reasonably expect many years (20–30 years) where the motor component of the disease is controlled by drug treatment and, latterly, by neurosurgical interventions (deep

Table 5–2. **Drugs Used in Parkinson's Disease**

Class	Drug Name	Availability
L-dopa drugs *(Always combine with a decarboxylase inhibitor.)* *Remain the most effective way of reversing PD motor symptoms*	Cocareldopa (Sinemet) Cobenyldopa (Madopar)	Tablets Controlled release capsules and dispersible tablets
Dopamine agents *All (apart from apomorphine) are longer acting than L-dopa but have more side effects (nausea, hypotension, hallucinosis).*	*Ergot derivatives*: Bromocriptine Pergolide Cabergoline Non-ergot: Pramipexole	Tablets
Can be used on their own for new patients and to smooth out L-dopa–induced fluctuations later on.	Ropinirole Apomorphine	Injections (Penject) Infusion
Anticholinergic drugs *Rarely used as can cause confusion.* *May have a role with painful dystonia and to control salivation.*	Benzhexol Bentrophine Orphenadrine	Tablets and intramuscular injections
Other drugs: **Catechol-o-methyl transferase inhibitor**	Entacapone *Used in conjunction with L-dopa to prolong duration of action.* Amantadine hydrochloride *Useful to help control dyskinesias.*	Tablets Capsules
Cholinergic drugs *May have a role to play when cognitive decline occurs.*	Rivastigmine Donepezil	Tablets
Atypical antipyschotics *Used to control confusion when all else fails.*	Clozapine Olanzapine	Tablets

brain stimulation). Older patients (>70 years) are more likely to run into difficulties such as failure to respond to dopa drugs, balance problems, and neuropsychiatric problems. These can considerably limit the impact of drug therapy and necessitate early intervention of a multidisciplinary team (MDT). Where physical and mental decline occur the MDT is particularly important in arranging other support for the patient and carer.

Carers often soldier on without complaint when the problems remain physical (e.g. difficulties with mobility, falls, and impairment of activities of daily living). In contrast, cries for help from carers often occur when patients develop confusion and/or hallucinosis. Though hallucinations can be benign and not need treatment, they also can be very frightening both for the patient and carer. Dementia complicates at least 20% of

Table 5–3. Long-term Problems of Dopaminergic Therapy

Motor

(a) Fluctuations	'Wearing off' phenomenon (end of dose deterioration)
	Random on–off oscillations
	Delayed 'on' response
	Drug-resistant 'off' (dose failure)
	Early morning akinesia
	Freezing
(b) Dyskinesia	Peak dose (choreic)
	'Turning on'
	Diphasic (ballistic)
	'Off period' dystonia
Non motor (off period related)	Pain, akathisia, restless legs
	Sweating, tachycardia, dyspnea
	Depression, panic attacks, hyperventilation, screaming
Neuropsychiatric	Hallucinations
	Delirium and pnoid psychosis
	Hypersexuality
Sleep related	Nightmares
	Vivid dreams
	Fragmented sleep

Table 5–4. Non-motor Complications of Parkinson's Disease

Problem	Symptoms
Cognitive	Dementia, confusion; overlap with diffuse Lewy body disease
Psychological	Depression, anxiety attacks, apathy
Bladder	Frequency, incontinence
Sexual	Erectile failure, psychological impotence, sexual dissatisfaction
Pain	Secondary to dystonia/ dyskinesia, off-period pain, depression
Sleep disturbance	Sleep disruption secondary to nocturia or decreased mobility
Bulbar	Dysphagia, dribbling
Bowel	Constipation, nausea, bloating
Weight loss	Anorexia secondary to depression, dyskinesia, dysphagia
Visual	Hallucinations
Blackouts	Postural hypotension, cardiac, carotid sinus hypersensitivity
Balance	Frequent falls, freezing
Speech	Dysarthria, hypophonia, palilalia, speech initiation failure
Skin	Seborrhoea, scalp scurf, hyperhidrosis

Parkinsonian patients, rising with increasing age of onset of the disease. Most usually, the onset of hallucinations and cognitive decline indicates the onset of diffuse Lewy body disease (also known as dementia with Lewy bodies).[5] Cholinergic drugs (rivastigmine, donepezil) may improve behavior, controlling hallucinosis and memory in this situation, but effects tend to wear off over 12 months.

To summarize, early management of PD with drug treatment can be highly successful but the involvement of the MDT is important for optimal management.

WHY DO PEOPLE WITH PARKINSON'S DISEASE DIE?

It is important to understand the late decline of Parkinsonian patients and the cause of death. Presently, there is little data on the usual cause of death of PD patients; Parkinsonism is rarely cited on death certificates as contributory to death. Though many patients will die of unrelated causes—after all PD is predominantly a disease of the elderly—undoubtedly, PD will be a substantial contributor to death for a large number of patients. With the advent of levodopa, average life expectancy of PD patients has been extended from 7.5 years to an average of 11 years though, as indicated above, there are wide variations as positive response to levodopa is crucial.[6] Expected mortality has fallen from three times normal to about 1.5 times normal.[7]

Typically, a patient will have about five good years; then 10–12 years after diagnosis, increasing problems will occur, managed with frequent drug changes; and then this period is followed by progressive disability with or without mental problems. It will often be the latter that determines whether patients leave their homes to be cared for within residential or nursing establishments. Mortality rises rapidly once this occurs. The cause of death may be due to complications from falls or because the patient has become increasingly bedbound. Thus, bronchopneumonia is often cited as the primary cause of death on death certificates. Some patients develop bulbar problems. Speech problems may be accompanied by swallowing difficulties and hence loss of weight. Dysphagia or cough may indicate inhalation problems which lead to chest infections. Significant dysphagia occurs, on average, 10–11 years after the diagnosis, which is considerably longer than in so-called Parkinson-plus disorders (multi-system atrophy, progressive supranuclear palsy—see following section). Once it occurs, average duration to death is 15–24 months.[8]

Weight loss can be due to poor intake, but can also be caused by excessive dyskinesia and lead to increasing frailty. Excessive dyskinesias can cause death from exhaustion. Troublesome hallucinosis and confusion can be difficult to manage and sedative drugs are often used. Similarly, neuroleptic drugs may be used to control dyskinesia. These drugs almost certainly will aggravate Parkinsonism and, in the late stages, will cause immobility. Thus severe Parkinsonism will cause death through immobility, falls, chest and urinary infections, and exhaustion/weight loss. In this tragic setting the skills of palliative care clinicians become ever more important.

OTHER PARKINSONIAN SYNDROMES

Parkinsonism which does not respond significantly to dopaminergic drugs carries a much worse prognosis and most usually indicates that the underlying disorder is multisystem atrophy (MSA). Unfortunately this group of patients will have an unremitting downward course with life expectancy of 5–8 years.[9] Though the problems will be very similar to those of Parkinsonian patients, they will often have early onset falls and bulbar symptoms. MSA can be accompanied by cerebellar signs, and/or autonomic problems such as early onset erectile dysfunction, bladder disturbance, and postural hypotension.

Hallucination and dementia tend not to be specific features. Management of these cases is aided by early involvement of the MDT but symptomatic drug treatment will often be limited.

Progressive supranuclear palsy (PSP) is another progressive neurodegenerative condition often mistaken for PD.[10] Again it is characterized by early onset falls and near absence of response to dopaminergic drugs. Its particular feature is the occurrence of a severe eye movement disorder starting with impaired voluntary vertical eye gaze and slow saccadic eye movements, progressing to complete plysis of all eye movement and eye lid opening apraxia.

Both MSA and PSP will share with PD common palliative care problems.

SPECIFIC PALLIATIVE CARE PROBLEMS

A change in emphasis in care of PD patients is required when it becomes clear that, despite best medical/surgical care, the patient is becoming ever more disabled or when persistent neuropsychiatric problems or dementia emerge (Table 5–5). The development of this scenario may indicate that the patient is entering a phase of terminal decline. Certainly dementia is a clear marker of a poor prognosis. Experienced clinicians will recognize that the disease is entering the last phase, though the MDT team and relatives may find it hard to accept that future aggressive interventions are not indicated. Frequent discussions with patients, carers, and relatives are required in this setting to enable them to understand the limits of medical interventions. Patients and carers may often press for novel or inappropriate treatments. Every consideration should be given to their suggestions and explanations provided; for instance, drug therapy will not help falls, brain surgery is not indicated where there is dementia. Nevertheless, a number of symptomatic interventions may be possible.

Nursing Needs

Palliative care teams are most likely to become involved when patients become bedbound.

Table 5–5. **Symptom Approach in Parkinson's Disease**

Symptom	Intervention
Balance/gait	Physiotherapy for cueing tricks
Freezing attacks	Occupational therapy assessment of environment
	Metronome, or inward chanting-like singing
	Avoid tasks in sequence
	Wheelchair assessment
	Avoid sticks—cause blocking
	Avoid Zimmer frames—rolators (wheeled frames) are more useful
Delusions/ hallucination/dementia	Withdraw medications that may exacerbate pnoid delusions such as sedatives, anticholinergics
	Remove dopaminergic drugs of least potency such as amantadine and selegeline; remove dopamine agonists before L-dopa; remove L-dopa as a last resort
	Try atypical antipsychotics (clozapine, quetiapine)
	Look for infections that may exacerbate confusion
	Consider the use of cholinesterase inhibitors (e.g. rivastigmine, donepezil)—N.B. carer support
Depression and anxiety	Tricyclics, SSRIs
	Look at social support, increase patient interaction with family, friends, etc.
Troublesome dyskinesia	Reduce overall drug treatments—smaller, more frequent doses of L-dopa
	Continual apomorphine infusion
	Amantadine—possible antidyskinetic effect
	Brain surgery e.g. pallidotomy, deep brain stimulation
Dysphagia	Speech and language therapy/swallow assessment (? need for videofluoroscopy)
	Dietician involvement (? homogenise solids, ? thicken fluids)
	PEG if swallow compromised
Excessive daytime sleepiness and sudden unintended sleep attacks	Decrease sedating drugs
	Decrease dopaminergic medications
	Correct night-time insomnia (good 'sleep hygiene')
	Dopamine agonists for restless legs
	Modafinil
	Is sleep apnea contributing?
Drooling	Anticholinergics e.g. benzhexol, hyoscine patches
	Possible use of oral atropine drops—caution with psychosis
	Possible use of botulinum toxin in the salivary glands
Orthostatic hypotension	Eliminate antihypertensives
	Teach strategies to limit sudden changes in posture
	Increase salt and fluid intake
	Avoid large meals
	Avoid alcohol
	Elevate head of bed

Continued on following page

Table 5–5— *continued*

Symptom	Intervention
	Fludrocortisone
	Midrodine
Pain	Off period—increase dopaminergic medications
	Dystonic—ascertain cause, under- or over-treatment
	Joint—anti-inflammatories
	Painkillers (see text), antidepressants
Urinary incontinence	? Desmopressin for night-time urinary frequency
	? Oxybutinin
	Permanent indwelling urinary catheter/suprapubic catheterization
	Continence advisor
Bowel disturbances	Constipation—avoid bulking agents, use stimulants and osmotics
	Incomplete emptying—consider apomorphine penjects

Nursing needs are the priority in this circumstance e.g. care of skin pressure points, need for comfortable position, bladder and bowel care, oral hygiene, and diet. Social interaction remains important as does maintaining psychological well-being.

Depression

Depression is a common accompaniment of PD. It can occur early as part of the shock of receiving the bad news, but probably is an intrinsic part of the disorder, reflecting a loss of those neurotransmitters (noradrenaline, serotonin) related to good mood maintenance. Studies estimating the frequency of depression have indicated a prevalence of about 50%.[11] However, it is these authors' view that during the disease lifespan most, if not all, patients will develop psychiatric problems. Depression is often part of the terminal decline. It may be manifest by anxiety, mood change, sleep disturbance, or physical decline. A trial of antidepressant is always warranted in this setting. Although there are few comptive trials, selective serotonin re-uptake inhibitors (e.g. paroxetine, citalopram) are probably best as they avoid the potential for anticholinergic side effects from older established tricyclic drugs. Drug treatment may not always be successful in this scenario and it may be worthwhile

re-evaluating the cognitive profile. Apathy can be mistaken for depression and is a significant component of cognitive decline in PD.

Bowel and Bladder

Bowel and bladder involvement is universal in the late stages of the disease. Constipation, due to poor gut motility, is inevitable. Bulk-enhancing laxatives should be avoided; stool-softening agents such as a lactulose or movecol (norgine) should be used, backed up with occasional use of stimulants (senna, sodium picosulphate). This can be a difficult problem, suppositories and enemas may be needed. Manual evacuation can be required and, rarely, patients have needed surgical management with permanent colostomy.

Similarly, bladder problems are not easily solved. Increased urinary frequency and urgency can be helped by anticholinergics (e.g. oxybutynin). In the male, these problems can be mistaken for prostatism. Expert urological assessment may be needed with urodynamics. Surgical management should be avoided as transurethral resection of the prostate can be complicated by permanent incontinence. Anticholinergics will need to be avoided to avoid aggravation of mental problems. Incontinence and urinary retention are not uncommon. Intermittent self-catheterization is rarely feasible. Bedbound patients will often require long-term catheterization to avoid skin and hygiene problems. Suprapubic placement is often best if catheterization is required over long periods.

Skin Care

Skin care can be complicated by specific Parkinsonian dermatological disease—seborrheic dermatitis and scalp scurf. Expert advice may be required and steroid creams and antifungal agents used if skin symptoms impact on quality of life.

Sleep Disturbance

Sleep disturbance is common in PD and increases in frequency and severity with progression of the disease. Restless leg disorder with limb pain relieved by activity is characteristic. Dopamine agonists can help relieve this problem. Rapid eye movement sleep behavioral disorder (RBD) refers to limb or body movements associated with dream mentation. Dreams appear to be acted out and disrupt sleep continuity.[12]

Positioning

Maintaining a comfortable position for Parkinsonian patients, whether in a chair or bed, can be difficult. It is complicated by the flexed posture characteristic of the disease. Thus supportive cushions may be required. Patients, if completely akinetic, will not be able to shift position and will need frequent repositioning. Specially supportive mattresses (air flow, etc.) will help nurses prevent skin sores but do not prevent the need for comfortable repositioning.

Hyperkinesia

In contrast to akinetic patients, there are those with exceptional hyperkinesia (secondary to drug treatment) who are not able to sit/stand/lie in one place without frequent falls. In the worse cases patients will apparently spin uncontrollably on the floor. These patients will often insist on their high doses of dopa drugs, appearing to be addicted to them. Even subtle reductions in overall dose (to their mind)

cause unacceptable reduction in mobility or mood. Advice from a movement disorder specialist is required to decide on a way forward for these patients. Substitution with continuous apomorphine infusion or surgical procedures such as pallidotomy may be needed. Hyperkinetic crises require intervention as patients can die from exhaustion; in this setting the use of powerful neuroleptics (e.g. haloperidol, risperidone) may exceptionally be justified. Usually, though in the terminal stages, drugs have already been reduced because of hallucinations/confusion or have a diminishing effect; most patients are akinetic rigid as in the pre-dopa era.

Contractures

Contractures are common in this situation and are difficult to prevent by physiotherapy. Small doses of L-dopa drugs may be given to try to prevent their occurrence, balancing the beneficial motor effects with the possible deleterious effects on mental state. Botulinum toxin injected into the flexor compartments of arms and legs can reduce tone and enable physiotherapists to stretch limbs into a more normal position. Surgical tenotomies can be helpful in severe cases. The limited aim of such treatment needs to be fully understood by patients and carers. Bedbound patients can progress to tightly contracted hands, arms, and legs. The aim of treatment is usually to improve comfort, limb pain, hygiene (particularly palmar hygiene in contracted hands), and positioning. Functional improvement is not likely at this stage—often the patient is demented and unable to cooperate with any realistic rehabilitation programme.

Pain

Pain for Parkinsonian patients is a difficult problem and especially common in the late stages.[13] Pain related to stiffness and rigidity can be helped by dopaminergic therapy. It can be limb pain related to dystonic spasms, and these can be due to under treatment (N.B. early morning dystonia) or excessive dopaminergic therapy. More diffuse limb and trunkal pain can be difficult to understand. There are likely to be psychiatric features and a trial of antidepressants (e.g. amitriptyline) is always warranted for intrusive pain. Later in the course of the disease, posture and constipation (abdominal pain) may all contribute to pain. Simple painkillers are often used but with limited success. Combination painkillers containing additional codeine-related drugs also have limited success and carry the additional risk of aggravating constipation and mental confusion. The use of opiates for distressed Parkinsonian patients has not been investigated carefully. It would be our view that morphine (via syringe-driver) can be very useful in allaying the pain and distress of Parkinsonian patients in terminal decline. Its use needs to be carefully explained, if possible to the patient, but usually, in this situation, the carer needs to agree on this course of action.

Although some patients may 'improve' with the relief of pain, most will be sensitive to the sedative effects. Not only that but, in order to combat opiate-induced nausea, most syringe drivers also contain neuroleptic-based antiemetics (prochlorperazine, haloperidol) which will aggravate Parkinsonism. The role of domperidone, the preferred antiemetic for Parkinsonian patients (it does not block brain dopamine receptors), has not be assessed in this circumstance. Thus a decision to use a syringe driver containing the usual 'palliative care cocktail' of opiates, antiemetic, and anticholinergic agents needs to be considered carefully as the chances are that bedbound patients will become sedated and immobile, thereby more prone to chest infections, and could proceed to death within days or weeks. Nevertheless, in our view this course of action is justified with the consent of patients and carers when quality of life is extremely poor, all therapeutic options have been exhausted, and it is clear the patient has entered a terminal state.

The aim of treatment with opiates is to control pain and distress. This situation has many similarities with the humane care of terminally ill cancer patients. Similarly, best practice is that these end-of-life decisions are discussed with the patient to preserve their autonomy. There may be an advance directive to take account of. Most usually in this situation, patients are confused, disorientated, and unable to understand these discussions. It is then important to explain the position to the principal carer or relative and have their consent. All such discussions need to be recorded meticulously in the notes, with clear actions agreed.

SUMMARY

The voyage of the Parkinsonian patient is a long one—starting from receipt of the bad news, through the initial years of successful drug therapy, to the later stages of increasing disability and mental problems. More research needs to be directed towards the last years when Parkinsonian patients become ever more difficult to manage and on understanding when the role of the neurologist and team needs to change from aggressive medical management. Palliative care teams need to engage with the management of chronic neurological illness; their skills can support the MDTs in delivering optimum care. They may need to be involved early in the course of the disease and episodically thereafter, and should thus not be identified by the patients and carers as an indication that the stage of terminal decline has been reached.

REFERENCES

1. Parkinson J. An Essay on the Shaking Palsy. Neely and Jones, London Sherwood, 1817.
2. Yahr MD, Clough CG. Parkinson's disease. In: Yhar MD, ed. Houston Merritt Memorial Volume. Raven Press, New York, 1983.
3. Birkmayer W, Hornykiewicz O. Der L-deoxyphenylalanine (=dopa)—effect bei der parkinson—akinese. Weiner Klinische Woochenschrift 1961;73:787–788.
4. Hardie RJ, Lees AJ, Stern GM. On–off fluctuations in Parkinson's disease. Brain 1984;107: 487–506.
5. McKeith I, Galasko D, Kosaka K, et al. Consensus guidelines for the clinical and pathological diagnosis of dementia with Lewy bodies. Neurology 1996;47:1113–1124.
6. Hoehn MM, Yahr MD. Parkinsonism: onset, progression and mortality. Neurology 1967;17:427–442.
7. Shaw KM, Lees AJ, Stern GM. The impact of treatment with levodopa on Parkinson's disease. Quarterly Journal of Medicine 1980;49(195):282–293.
8. Miller J, Wenning GK, Verny M, McKee A, et al. Progression of dysarthria and dysphagia in most mortem-confirmed parkinsonian disorders. Arch Neurol 2001;58:259–264.
9. Quinn N. Multiple system atrophy—the nature of the beast. J Neurol Neurosurg Psychiat 1989;Jun:Suppl 78–79.
10. Steele JC. Progressive supranuclear palsy. Brain 1972;95:693–704.

11. Mindham RHS. J Neurosurg Psychiatry 1970; 33:170–180.
12. Ray Chaudhuri K. The basis for day and nighttime control of symptoms in Parkinson's disease. Eur Neurol 2002;9(suppl 3):40–44.
13. Quinn NP, Lang AE, Koller WC, Marsden CD. Painful Parkinson's disease. Lancet 1986;1:1366–1369.
14. Sawle GV, ed. Movement Disorders in Clinical Practice. Isis Medical Media Ltd, Oxford, 1999.
15. Bajaj NPS, Clough CG. Non motor aspects of idiopathic Parkinson's Disease. 2001 Current Medical Literature—Parkinson's Disease 2001;3:1–6.

Chapter 6

Dementias

Ladislav Volicer

Alzheimer's disease is the most common cause of dementia and progresses in four stages. Management of the patient should include a palliative care approach which includes a decision-making process ahead of time. The use of cardiopulmonary resuscitation (CPR) and tube feeding is seen critically. Also, transfer to an acute medical setting poses serious risks, such as confusion and falls, to the patients. As side effects are rarely reported appropriately, drug treatment must be restricted wherever possible. Also, in life-threatening infections, very often the use of analgesics and antipyretics, maybe with the help of oxygen, may assure comfort without the use of antibiotics. Support for family members must start with diagnosis and continue after the death of the patient with bereavement support for at least one year.

CASE HISTORY

Mr Gray is a 67-year-old gentleman who taught mathematics in a high school. He retired two years ago and spent his time enjoying his hobbies—making model airplanes and gardening. However, recently he has become less interested in his projects and has difficulty remembering which project he is currently working on and what needs to be done in the garden. Last week, Mr Gray got lost when shopping in a neighborhood in which he was born and had to be brought home by the police. His wife, concerned about his condition, insisted that he saw a physician.

Physical examination by Dr Gordon showed that Mr Gray suffered from high blood pressure, controlled by a diuretic and angiotensin-converting-enzyme (ACE) inhibitor, and was otherwise healthy. Elementary cognitive evaluation detected deficits in short-term memory and abstract thinking. Mr Gray was referred for a neuropsychological evaluation and laboratory tests were performed. Laboratory tests were within normal limits and neuropsychological evaluation found deficits in multiple areas of cognitive functioning. Dr Gordon made a diagnosis of probable Alzheimer's disease and invited Mr Gray and his wife to discuss his findings.

CAUSES OF DEMENTIA

Many pathological conditions may lead to development of dementia. Some of these may be reversible, although the number of patients with reversible dementias is rather small. A recent review concluded that most conditions that were considered reversible causes of dementia are not truly reversible because of possible association of treatable disorders with progressive dementias and because the conditions may cause structural changes that do not respond to treatment.[1] Most dementias, especially in older individuals, are caused by degenerative changes in the brain that progress over time and lead to loss of independence of the affected person.

Mr Gray was diagnosed as having probable Alzheimer's disease. That is the most common cause of progressive degenerative dementia. Other frequent forms of progressive dementia are vascular dementia, dementia with Lewy bodies, and fronto-temporal dementia. Although the early symptoms of these dementias may vary, later stages pose similar medical and behavioral problems. In addition, when brains of individuals dying with progressive dementia are examined, very often more than one pathological process that can lead to dementia is present. Thus, clinical management of later stages of dementia is similar regardless of the initial symptoms and diagnosis.

Dr Gordon explained to the Grays that there is currently no treatment available that would stop or reverse the course of Alzheimer's disease. Dr Gordon made it clear that Mr Gray will lose his capacity to make decisions about his finances and medical care as Alzheimer's disease progresses. Therefore, he urged Mr Gray to appoint a proxy who would be able to take over his finances and to discuss which medical treatments he would want in different stages of the disease.

DECISION-MAKING CAPACITY

With the progression of dementia, all individuals eventually lose their decision-making capacity. It is very often at this point that difficult decisions regarding end-of-life care have to be made. These decisions include CPR, transfer from a home or long-term institution to an acute care setting, treatment of systemic infections with antibiotics, and tube feeding. The decisions may be made easier if the patient executed a living will specifying which treatment he would accept. Unfortunately, most living wills are very general, do not provide guidance regarding specific treatment procedures, and do not take into account the slowly progressive nature of

dementing diseases that makes unclear when the living will decisions should be applied. Therefore, in most situations specific decisions have to be made by a patient's proxy. Ideally, this proxy should be appointed by the patient and should have discussed the patient's wishes and philosophy with the patient before he became demented. In this situation, the proxy can decide on the basis of substituted judgement, putting himself into the 'patient's shoes'. Substituted judgement is also promoted by a living will that can be interpreted by the proxy and used to make specific decisions.

STAGES OF PROGRESSIVE DEMENTIAS

Living wills should specify which treatments the patient considers appropriate in each stage of the disease. It is possible to recognize four stages of Alzheimer's disease and other progressive degenerative dementias. In the mild stage, the patient suffers from cognitive impairment and is unable to perform some instrumental activities of daily living, such as shopping or cooking, but is still independent in basic activities of daily living, such as dressing and toileting. In the moderate stage, the patient becomes more confused and apraxic and requires help with basic activities of daily living. He may also engage in unsafe activities when left alone and requires constant supervision. However, he is still able to feed himself and to ambulate independently. When patients become unable to ambulate independently and feed themselves, they progress into the severe stage of dementia. However, they are still able to ambulate with assistance and are able to communicate somewhat with others. In the last, terminal stage of dementia, patients are unable to ambulate even with assistance and lose the ability to communicate with the environment. However, they still perceive pain and may benefit from environmental stimulation because very few, if any, progress into the persistent vegetative state.[2]

Mr Gray decided that he would not want to be resuscitated if he were in the severe stage of dementia but did not want to make any other decisions. However, he appointed his wife as his health-care proxy for making additional decisions. Mr Gray was started on a cholinesterase inhibitor that improved some-what his memory, and continued taking his antihypertensive medications.

During the next two years, Mr Gray's dementia slowly progressed. He developed severe short-term memory deficit and aphasia. One morning, Mrs Gray found her husband on the floor unconscious. She called an ambulance and Mr Gray was brought to a hospital, although he regained consciousness before the ambulance arrived. Physical exam-ination showed blood pressure of 100/60 with significant postural drop. Mrs Gray reported that her husband sometimes lost his balance but never complained of dizziness. The ACE inhibitor was discontinued and Mr Gray became more stable when walking, with blood pressures in the 160/95 range.

MANAGEMENT OF CHRONIC DISEASES

Management of chronic diseases in individuals suffering from progressive dementia should be modified to take account of three factors: patients with advanced dementia have decreased life expectancy, they cannot report side effects of the treatment, and treatment interventions pose more of a burden for them than for cognitively intact individuals.

Decreased life expectancy is related to both age and dementia severity. Mortality rate is increased most in younger demented individuals, being 10 times higher in women and seven times higher in men 65–74 years old, four times higher in women and three times higher in men 75–84 years old, and two times higher in individuals over the age of 85.[3] Four-year survival probability was reported to be 0.85 for cognitively intact, 0.69 for mildly impaired, and 0.51 for severely impaired individuals, and when adjustments were made for the effect of other health and social covariates, severely impaired persons were twice as likely to die as cognitively intact persons.[4] Decreased life expectancy should be taken into considera-tion in management of chronic illnesses that have a long-term effect on mortality in this patient population. Preventive measures, such as restricted diets and screening pro-cedures, may not be appropriate in indivi-duals with progressive dementia.

Because patients cannot report side effects of treatment, pharmacological management of chronic conditions, such as hypertension and diabetes, should be conservative and empha-size prevention of treatment side effects that may lead to serious complications. For instance, dizziness and postural hypotension may lead to a fall and hip fracture, which is much more dangerous for the individual than slightly elevated blood pressure.

Treatment of individuals with advanced progressive dementia should take into con-sideration the burden such treatment imposes and the benefit for the patient. Most medical interventions cause some discomfort for a patient that can be tolerated by somebody who understands the rational for such an intervention. Patients with advanced dementia are unable to comprehend the need for ther-apeutic interventions, do not cooperate with treatment, and may even actively oppose it. Therefore, even routine procedures, such as blood drawing or blood pressure measure-ment, may exacerbate behavioral symptoms of dementia. Thus, the burden of therapeutic interventions in patients with advanced dementia is larger than that in cognitively intact individuals.

With progression of dementia, Mr Gray became incontinent and resisted efforts of his wife to clean him because he did not under-stand what had to be done. He also had delusions that his wife was a stranger and he tried to make her leave his house. Mrs Gray eventually decided to place Mr Gray in a nursing home.

During the admission process, Mrs Gray was asked about advance directives regarding Mr Gray's treatment. She produced the living will but was told that Mr Gray was not yet in the severe stage of dementia and, therefore, his decision about CPR did not apply. After being told about the burdens and benefits of CPR in the institutionalized elderly, Mrs Gray deci-ded that her husband should not be resusci-tated if his heart or breathing stopped.

CARDIOPULMONARY RESUSCITATION (CPR)

CPR performed in a hospital provides immediate survival for 41% of patients and survival to discharge for 13% of them.[5]

However, success is three times less likely in presence of dementia—almost as rare as in metastatic cancer. In addition, many cardiac arrests occur in long-term care institutions caring for demented individuals. The immediate survival of resuscitated nursing home residents is 18.5% with only 3.4% discharged from the hospital alive.[6] If the decreased success rate observed in a hospital population is present also in the nursing home population, only one third of 3.4%, i.e. 1% of demented residents suffering cardiac arrest can be expected to be discharged alive from the hospital.

Potential benefits are, however, diminished by several considerations. CPR is a stressful experience for those who survive, who may experience CPR-related injuries such as broken ribs and often have to be on a respirator. An intensive care unit environment is not conducive to appropriate care for demented individuals who are confused and often develop delirium. Many patients who are discharged alive from the hospital after CPR are much more impaired than they were before the arrest. The experience of CPR is very traumatic for patients and their families, as evidenced by the fact that even residents who have reported no change from pre-arrest status execute frequently a 'Do Not Resuscitate' (DNR) directive preventing repetition of the CPR. Also, other residents of long-term care facilities may be upset by witnessing the CPR procedure.

At the next meeting of the treatment team with Mrs Gray, other options related to medical management of Mr Gray were discussed. These options included transfer of Mr Gray to a hospital for treatment of systemic infections (such as pneumonia), use of tube feeding (if Mr Gray started having difficulties eating), and use of antibiotics in the nursing home for treatment of systemic infections.

PROXY PLANNING FOR MEDICAL CARE

Treatment decisions should be made ahead of the time of crisis at a meeting of proxy and other family members or friends with the treatment team. The treatment team should include the physician or physician extender (e.g. nurse practitioner), a nursing staff representative, and a social worker, who acts as a meeting moderator. Presence of a chaplain is useful for addressing religious and ethical matters. This family conference is a good opportunity to answer all concerns expressed by the proxy and others close to the patient regarding the patient's condition and treatment. During the conference, the treatment team should clarify the patient's prognosis and describe options for management of complications and intercurrent diseases. Risk and benefits of all the management strategies should be clearly explained according to the published evidence. Presence or absence of previous patient's wishes has to be determined at the beginning of the discussion. The discussion may be framed as an opportunity for determining which goals of care are most important—prolongation of life, maintenance of function, or maintenance of comfort.[7]

The decisions regarding treatment limitations are very difficult and the proxies need guidance from the treatment team in this process. Otherwise they may feel overwhelmed and guilty if they decide to forgo some treatment modalities. Recommendations for the proxy should be made not only by the physician but should be developed by the whole treatment team. It should be recognized that nursing staff are moral agents who have to be consulted before treatment decisions are made, because they have to live with the residents and execute these decisions. In reaching consensus, many factors need to be weighed including the patient's decline, the ability of the family to cope, the professional development of the nursing staff, and philosophy of the nursing unit. Consensus is facilitated through trust between the family and staff and by thoughtful consideration of the patient and family readiness.

Mrs Gray reported that Mr Gray did not make any decisions regarding the other treatment options. She felt that at this point the most important goal of care to be maintenance of function, with comfort second, and prolongation of life third. The treatment team recommended to Mrs Gray that Mr Gray should be treated in the nursing home and not transferred to acute care hospital if he developed pneumonia or other life-threatening infections. The team assured Mrs Gray that Mr Gray would be transferred if the transfer was necessary for increased comfort—for instance, if he developed acute abdominal problem that would require surgical treatment or if he suffered a fracture that would require surgical attention. After weighing the risks and benefits for Mr Gray related to a transfer to an acute care setting, Mrs Gray decided that her husband should not be transferred unless it was required for comfort.

TRANSFER TO AN ACUTE MEDICAL SETTING

Transfer of demented individuals to an emergency room or hospital exposes them to serious risks. Even cognitively intact, hospitalized, elderly individuals develop depressed psychophysiological functioning that includes confusion, falling, not eating, and incontinence. These symptoms are often managed by medical interventions, such as psychotropic medications, restraints, nasogastric tubes, and Foley catheters, which expose the patient to possible complications including thrombophlebitis, pulmonary embolus, aspiration pneumonia, urinary tract infection, and septic shock. It was reported that shortly after hospital admission of elderly individuals, functional deterioration occurs in mobility, transfer, toileting, feeding, and grooming, and none of these functions improve significantly by discharge.[8] Risk factors for this functional decline were identified to be decubitus ulcer, cognitive impairment, functional impairment, and low social activity level.[9] Individuals with advanced dementia would exhibit at least three of these risk factors: cognitive impairment, functional impairment, and low social activity level. The functional decline occurred in 63%–83% of individuals exhibiting three or four of the risk factors, and 41%–67% of these individuals either died in the hospital or had to be placed in a nursing home. These data indicate that hospitalization of cognitively impaired individuals exposes them to significant burden that has to be taken into account when such a transfer is considered.

Transfer of long-term care facility residents to an emergency room or hospital for treatment of infections and other conditions may not be optimal for management of these problems. A recent study, which reviewed hospital records of 100 unscheduled transfers to a hospital, found that 36% of emergency room transfers and 40% of hospital admissions were inappropriate.[10] These numbers increased further to 44% of emergency room transfers and 45% of hospital admissions when advance directives were considered. The rate of hospitalization varies widely between different long-term care facilities[11] and could not be predicted by any patient characteristics if all hospitalizations were considered. When only hospitalizations of residents who were not hospitalized during the first six months of their stay were considered, several resident characteristics were associated with hospitalization. These characteristics included severe functional impairment, increased impairment in activities of daily living, decubitus ulcers, feeding tube, and primary diagnosis of congestive heart failure or respiratory disease.[12]

Hospitalization is not necessary for optimal treatment of pneumonia of nursing home residents. Immediate survival is similar in residents receiving treatment and long-term care facility and in the hospital.[13] Similarly, mortality due to pneumonia was similar in two nursing homes despite double the rate of hospitalization in one of them.[11] Longer-term outcomes are actually better in residents treated in a nursing home. It was reported that the six-week mortality rate was 18.7% in non-hospitalized residents and 39.5% in hospitalized residents, despite no significant differences between the hospitalized and non-hospitalized groups before diagnosis.[14] Similarly, a larger proportion of hospitalized individuals had worsening of their functional status or died two months after the episode of pneumonia.[15] This improved outcome in non-hospitalized residents was present only in those who had a lower respiratory rate and was greatest in residents who were independent or mildly dependent at baseline.

The available data indicate that transfer to an emergency room or hospital has significant degree of risks and relatively few benefits for individuals with advanced dementia. Therefore, this management strategy should be used only when it is consistent with overall goals of care and not as a default option.

Another issue that was discussed with Mrs Gray at the meeting with the treatment team was the management of eating difficulties. The team explained to her that although Mr Gray did not have any problem eating at that time, he may start refusing food or have difficulties swallowing food and liquids as the dementia progressed. It was explained to her that the treatment team would always continue feeding Mr Gray using hand feeding and would try to minimize the consequences of dementia by changing the diet composition and texture. The team also explained to Mrs Gray that tube feeding would produce significant discomfort for Mr Gray with little or no benefit. Mrs Gray agreed that use of tube feeding would not be in her husband's best interest.

EATING DIFFICULTIES AND TUBE FEEDING

Eating difficulties develop in all individuals as dementia progresses. They are caused by apraxia that initially prevents patients from using utensils but eventually makes them completely unable to eat unassisted. In addition, patients often develop intermittent food refusal that can be caused by depression, dislike of institutional food, or inability to perceive hunger. With further progression of dementia, patients often develop swallowing difficulties that provoke choking on food and liquids. Choking and food refusal are often exhibited simultaneously. Eating apraxia can be managed by hand feeding, and food refusal often responds to antidepressant treatment or to administration of appetite stimulants. Swallowing difficulties and choking may be minimized by adjustment of diet texture and by replacing thin liquids with thick ones (e.g. yogurt instead of milk).[16] Unfortunately, some practitioners still consider introduction of tube feeding as necessary to assure appropriate nutrition and prevent aspiration.

Two excellent reviews recently summarized available evidence considering the risks and benefits of tube feeding in individuals with advanced dementia.[17,18] Both reviews found no evidence that long-term feeding tubes are beneficial in individuals with advanced dementia. Tube feeding does not prevent aspiration of nasopharyngeal secretions and/or regurgitated gastric contents and does not prevent aspiration pneumonia—indeed, it might actually increase its incidence. Moreover, nasogastric tubes may promote sinus and middle ear infections, and gastrostomy tubes may cause cellulitis, abscesses, necrotizing fasciitis, and myositis. Tube feeding creates

patient discomfort due to the presence of the nasogastric tube and the use of physical restraints to prevent tube removal. In a survey of cognitively intact patients rating discomfort levels of procedures, the nasogastric tube was considered the most uncomfortable procedure, followed by mechanical ventilation, and physical restraints.[19] Tube feeding also deprives the patient of the taste of food, the pleasure of eating, and contact with caregivers during the feeding process.

Feeding tubes may cause many local, pleuropulmonary, abdominal, and other complications.[17] Contaminated feeding solutions may cause gastrointestinal symptoms and bacturiuria. Insertion of a nasogastric tube may provoke a fatal arrhythmia during the procedure and percutaneous endoscopic gastrostomy tube placement may prompt a perioperative death. The common use of restraints and the increased production of urine and stool in patients receiving tube feedings additionally fosters the development of pressure ulcers.. There is no evidence that tube feeding promotes the healing of pressure ulcers, improves the functional status, prevents malnutrition, or increases survival in individuals with advanced dementia.[17] This imbalance of burdens and benefits of tube feeding justifies the recommendation that tube feedings not be used in individuals with advanced dementia—a recommendation supported by secular and religious ethicists.[18]

Even if tube feeding is instituted in a severely demented individual, it may be discontinued. It is possible to convert tube feeding to hand feeding and, in some cases, patients may be able to feed themselves again.[20]

Mr Gray's dementia slowly progressed. He became unable to walk even with assistance and lost the ability to communicate meaningfully with his environment. He was unable to chew food and had to be fed purée food and liquid dietary supplements. Mr Gray also started to choke on thin liquids and had to receive all liquids thickened by addition of yogurt or commercial food thickener. He developed two episodes of aspiration pneumonia that were successfully treated in the nursing home by intramuscular administration of antibiotics. During the next annual meeting of the treatment team with Mrs Gray, the team asked her what she felt was the most important goal of care at this point. Mrs Gray decided that, in view of the progression of dementia into a terminal stage, the main goal of care should be comfort and maintenance of function, and prolongation of life should be no longer considered. The team recommended to Mrs Gray that if Mr Gray again developed pneumonia, the medical treatment should not include antibiotics but should be limited to antipyretics, analgesics, and oxygen. After weighing the risks and benefits of such an approach, Mrs Gray agreed to palliative care only.

ANTIBIOTIC TREATMENT OF LIFE-THREATENING INFECTIONS

Antibiotic therapy is quite effective in treatment of an isolated episode of pneumonia or other systemic infection. In most patients it is possible to limit antibiotic therapy to oral preparations.[21] It is preferable to limit the use of intravenous therapy in cognitively impaired individuals who do not understand the need for intravenous catheters, try to remove them, and have to be often restrained or given psychotropic drugs to allow the treatment to continue. If patient has poor oral intake, it is possible to use intramuscular administration of cephalosporins for treatment of infections.

However, the effectiveness of antibiotic therapy is limited by the recurrent nature of infections in advanced dementia. Antibiotic therapy does not prolong survival in cognitively impaired patients who are in the terminal stage of dementia.[22,23] In addition, antibiotics are not necessary for maintenance of comfort in demented individuals because discomfort increases during the first 3–5 days of an episode of infection similarly in patients treated and not treated with antibiotics, and there is no significant difference in discomfort during the resolution of infection.[24] This indicates that use of analgesics and antipyretics, and of oxygen if necessary, assures comfort without antibiotic administration. Morphine is especially useful in treatment of terminal dyspnea.

Antibiotic use is not without adverse effects. Patients may develop gastrointestinal upset, diarrhea, allergic reactions, hyperkalemia, and agranulocytosis. Diagnostic procedures such as blood drawing and sputum suctioning, which are necessary for rational use of antibiotics, cause discomfort and confusion in demented individuals who do not understand the need for them. In addition, diagnostic procedures fail to indicate the source of infectious episode in 30% of cases.[22] Furthermore, most infections are recurrent in demented individuals, because the underlying causes, such as swallowing difficulties and aspiration, persist. Use of antibiotics in patients with advanced dementia should take into consideration the recurrent nature of infections, the adverse effects produced by antibiotics and the accompanying diagnostic procedures, and the lack of any significant enhancement of patient comfort.

Mr Gray's condition remained stable for another six months. He continued having swallowing difficulties and was sometimes choking on food and liquids. He had several episodes of temperature elevations but they resolved with the use of acetaminophen. One episode resulted in tachypnea but Mr Gray was kept comfortable by morphine and oxygen. Eventually, Mr Gray became unable to open his mouth and swallow. He received comfort care and intensive nursing care, which included maintaining moist oral mucosa and morphine. Mr Gray lapsed into a coma and died peacefully with Mrs Gray at his side. A memorial service was held for Mr Gray at the nursing home, attended by Mrs Gray and nursing home staff. The nursing home social worker continued to contact Mrs Gray from time to time to find out if she needed any help or the attention of a mental health professional.

BEREAVEMENT SUPPORT

Bereavement support is very important for family caregivers of Alzheimer's patients because it provides closure to a long stressful experience of living with slow progressive deterioration of a loved one that can be described as ongoing funeral. Bereavement support should last for at least a year and include three phases: avoidance, confrontation, and re-establishment.[25] The health-care professional has to assess periodically the bereaved caregiver and provide support that is appropriate for the phase that the caregiver is experiencing. This assessment may take the form of open-ended questions that try to detect avoidance or confrontation of feelings.

During the avoidance phase it is important to allow caregivers the necessary time to realize what has happened. Periodically, the staff member should phone the caregivers to let them know that they are available when they are ready to talk about their experience. They should also remind the caregivers about the grieving process and what is to be expected, including the fact that it may take some time for them to realize what has happened.

The confrontation phase may be eased by reminding caregivers that they will have 'good days' and 'bad days', and that this is normal during the grieving process. They should be encouraged to talk with health-care professionals, as well as friends and relatives, about feelings and experiences. The staff member should also encourage caregivers to return to pleasurable activities as soon as they are able to and should link caregivers with community resources, such as bereavement support groups and groups for widows.

During the re-establishment phase, the staff member should continue to encourage caregivers to tell their stories and to identify unresolved aspects of caregiving experience, including feelings of guilt about institutionalization and agreement with treatment limitations. It is also useful to help caregivers develop ways in which memories of their relative can be kept alive (organizing pictures, making contributions in their names) and to help them anticipate difficult times (e.g. anniversaries, holidays) and develop strategies to deal with these times. The staff member may encourage caregivers to identify ways to gain a perspective on their situation (e.g. writing a journal, attending a support group), but has to be always alert to the need for referral to psychological treatment for caregivers who are experiencing sustained depression or anxiety.

SUMMARY

Despite recent advances in neuroscience and psychopharmacology, treatment of individuals suffering from progressive dementias cannot stop or reverse the course of these conditions. Although the death is not caused directly by the dementing process itself, the complications leading to death are inevitable consequences of the diseases. Therefore, an advanced dementia should be considered a terminal illness similar to untreatable cancer, and palliative treatment of medical complications, striving for maximal comfort instead of maximal survival at all costs, is warranted. Such an approach is beneficial not only for patients suffering from dementia but also for their family caregivers.

Management of the patient described in this chapter was 'ideal' in that it did not involve any disagreements about goals of care between the family caregiver and treatment staff. In our experience, in most cases it is possible to reach a consensus regarding goals of care after the benefits and burdens of various interventions are described to family caregivers. However, there are some caregivers who have difficulties realizing that aggressive medical interventions do not provide any long-term benefit and may produce increased discomfort for the patient. A decision to limit treatment based on medical futility is a possibility in such a situation, although in the United States the proxy decision is usually honored.

The author is supported by the USPHS grant P30AG13846 and by the U.S. Department of Veterans Affairs.

REFERENCES

1. Piccini C, Bracco L, Amaducci L. Treatable and reversible dementias: an update. J Neurol Sci 1998;153(2):172–181.
2. Volicer L, Berman SA, Cipolloni PB, Mandell A. Persistent vegetative state in Alzheimer disease—does it exist? Arch Neurol 1997;54(11):1382–1384.
3. Ostbye T, Hill G, Steenhuis R. Mortality in elderly Canadians with and without dementia—a 5-year follow-up. Neurology 1999;53(3):521–526.
4. Kelman HR, Thomas C, Kennedy GJ, Cheng J. Cognitive impairment and mortality in older community residents. AJPH 1994;84(8):1255–1260.
5. Ebell MH, Becker LA, Barry HC, Hagen M. Survival after in-hospital cardiopulmonary resuscitation. A meta-analysis. J Gen Int Med 1998;13(12):805–816.
6. Finucane TE, Harper GM. Attempting resuscitation in nursing homes: policy considerations. J Am Geriatr Soc 1999;47(10):1261–1264.
7. Gillick M, Berkman S, Cullen L. A patient-centered approach to advance medical planning in the nursing home. J Am Geriatr Soc 1999;47:227–230.
8. Hirsch CH, Sommers L, Olsen A, Mullen L, Winograd CH. The natural history of functional morbidity in hospitalized older patients. J Am Geriatr Soc 1990;38(12): 1296–1303.

9. Inouye SK, Wagner DR, Acampora D, et al. A predictive index for functional decline in hospitalized elderly medical patients. J Gen Intern Med 1993;8(12):645–652.

10. Saliba D, Kington R, Buchanan J, et al. Appropriateness of the decision to transfer nursing facility residents to the hospital. J Am Geriatr Soc 2000;48(2):154–163.

11. Thompson RS, Hall NK, Szpiech M. Hospitalization and mortality rates for nursing home-acquired pneumonia. Journal of Family Practice 1999;48:291–293.

12. Fried TR, Mor V. Frailty and hospitalization of long-term stay nursing home residents. J Am Geriatr Soc 1997;45(3): 265–269.

13. Fried TR, Gillick MR, Lipsitz LA. Whether to transfer? Factors associated with hospitalization and outcome of elderly long-term care patients with pneumonia. J Gen Intern Med 1995;10(5):246–250.

14. Thompson RS, Hall NK, Szpiech M, Reisenberg LA. Treatments and outcomes of nursing-home-acquired pneumonia. J Am Board Fam Pract 1997;10(2): 82–87.

15. Fried TR, Gillick MR, Lipsitz LA. Short-term functional outcomes of long-term care residents with pneumonia treated with and without hospital transfer. J Am Geriatr Soc 1997;45(3):302–306.

16. Frisoni GB, Franzoni S, Bellelli G, Morris J, Warden V. Overcoming eating difficulties in the severely demented. In: Volicer L, Hurley A, eds. Hospice Care for Patient with Advanced Progressive Dementia. Springer Publishing Company, New York, 1998:48–67.

17. Finucane TE, Christmas C, Travis K. Tube feeding in patients with advanced dementia: a review of the evidence. JAMA 1999;282(14):1365–1370.

18. Gillick MR. Sounding board—rethinking the role of tube feeding in patients with advanced dementia. N Engl J Med 2000;342(3):206–210.

19. Morrison RS, Ahronheim JC, Morrison GR, et al. Pain and discomfort associated with common hospital procedures and experiences. J Pain Sympt Manag 1998;15(2):91–101.

20. Volicer L, Rheaume Y, Riley ME, Karner J, Glennon M. Discontinuation of tube feeding in patients with dementia of the Alzheimer type. Am J Alzheim Care 1990;5:22–25.

21. Medina–Walpole AM, McCormick WC. Provider practice patterns in nursing home-acquired pneumonia. J Am Geriatr Soc 1998;46(2):187–192.

22. Fabiszewski KJ, Volicer B, Volicer L. Effect of antibiotic treatment on outcome of fevers in institutionalized Alzheimer patients. JAMA 1990;263:3168–3172.

23. Luchins DJ, Hanrahan P, Murphy K. Criteria for enrolling dementia patients in hospice. J Am Geriatr Soc 1997;45(9):1054–1059.

24. Hurley AC, Volicer B, Mahoney MA, Volicer L. Palliative fever management in Alzheimer patients: quality plus fiscal responsibility. Adv Nurs Sci 1993;16:21–32.

25. Liken MA, Collins CE. Grieving: facilitating the process for dementia caregivers. J Psychosoc Nurs 1993;31(1):21–31.

Chapter 7

Infectious Disease

Jeanette Meadway

Two infections are used to illustrate the issues occurring in palliative care of infectious disorders occurring in neurology. The acquired immune deficiency syndrome (AIDS) is caused by the human immune deficiency virus (HIV), whilst CJD is associated with a prion (a protease-resistant protein). Suitable care requires full knowledge of appropriate infection control measures, avoiding those which are unnecessary and present a barrier between carer and patient, often with damaging psychological consequences. The patient may suffer from stigma because of the infective nature of the disease, from the mental health problems which are often associated, as well as their social group.

Provision of palliative care in HIV and CJD requires attention to the course of the disease, need for antiretroviral medication, drug interactions, particular social and psychological issues, and associated mental health problems. A patient-centered approach attends to all of these and allows the patient full choices. The support of the multidisciplinary team leads to a high standard of palliative care for patients with these complex conditions.

INTRODUCTION

Many infectious diseases in neurology have a short and even fulminating course, with death or recovery following intensive medical intervention, rather than a clearly palliative phase. Two notable exceptions to this pattern are both 'new' diseases, unheard of 20 years ago— the acquired immune deficiency syndrome (AIDS) due to human immune deficiency virus (HIV); and variant Creutzfeldt–Jakob disease (vCJD). Both affect young people at the productive period of their lives, are incurable, are associated with stigma due to fear of infection, and may have major psychiatric disorders preceding or concurrent with other neurologic signs.

HIV/AIDS

CASE HISTORY

A 37–year-old male health care worker was admitted in 1997 to an HIV/AIDS hospice for symptom control. He had been diagnosed HIV positive five years previously following which he had troublesome depression treated with venlafaxine. He had esophageal candidiasis three years previously, and was then found to have adrenal insufficiency and began replacement therapy. He had positive sputum cultures for mycobacterium kansasii, for which he continued rifabutin and ethambutol. Two years previously he developed peripheral neuropathy, for which he had fentanyl patches, ketoprofen, and sodium valproate, but which continued to cause significant problems. He also developed cytomegalovirus (CMV) retinitis and colitis, but despite systemic treatment including cidofovir, and intravitreous ganciclovir, he was left with very impaired vision. He also had troublesome intermittent diarrhea for which he was taking dihydrocodeine. He was taking antiretroviral therapy with zidovudine (AZT), zalcitabine (ddC), and indinavir. He lived alone in an apartment and had only occasional visits from family and friends.

His severe visual impairment meant that he could distinguish only large objects with sharply contrasting colours. He expressed strong denial of the degree of his visual impairment, and despite being found in a local station lost and bewildered, he still refused to see an occupational therapist (OT) to work on strategies to improve safety in his activities.

Peripheral neuropathy caused severe pain in his lower limbs. His toes were covered in minor injuries from objects which he could not see. He had hyperesthesia below the knee bilaterally, and reported severe pain from the lightest touch. In the hands, pain was less severe but reduced sensation led to difficulty in distinguishing small objects by touch. He would take some of his medications unaware that he had knocked others on to the floor.

His loose stools were not present every day. After some days with normal stools, he would have watery stools which led to incontinence. Loperamide controlled the diarrhea but at times led to constipation sufficiently severe to require lactulose.

Over some weeks his neuropathic pain was controlled by adjustment of the dose of fentanyl with sodium valproate as adjuvant. His antiretroviral regime included indinavir, which is a protease inhibitor and interacts with cytochrome P450; therefore carbamazepine and phenytoin were avoided because of interactions (for the same reason he had rifabutin rather than rifampicin for his mycobacterial disease).

He insisted he wished to go home to his apartment and could manage alone. He adamantly refused any offer of a carer or an OT assessment. His lack of insight into his need for help and the limitations imposed by his physical disabilities probably represented some degree of cognitive impairment but this could not be more fully assessed because he would not co-operate with cognitive testing. His mental state was not disturbed enough to require compulsory detention in a psychiatric unit under the provisions of the Mental Health Act. We therefore had no powers to restrain him and decided to allow him to return home in a planned

way with all his medication and close liaison with his community clinical nurse specialist. After four weeks, he was readmitted dirty and dishevelled. He had not been eating properly or taking his symptom control medications adequately, and had pain and diarrhea.

He discussed his prognosis and that it was unlikely that his vision would improve with any treatment. He was considering whether to stop active treatment when he started vomiting; and was found to have been refusing all medication apart from analgesics. Restarting steroid replacement therapy controlled the vomiting. He chose to continue on symptomatic treatment only, which now included steroid replacement. He stated that he did not wish to have further active treatment in hospital in any circumstances, but would come into the palliative care unit when necessary. He wished to return home.

His pain, diarrhea, and constipation were controlled and he agreed to have the help necessary to allow discharge home to succeed. The multidisciplinary team assessed him and planned assistance with activities of daily living. He went home with a full-time carer who was acceptable to him and the support of community-based nurses. He remained at home for six months, with short admissions for planned respite, and died peacefully at home as he had wished.

Case Discussion

For the patient with a neurological complication of HIV, problems in management are not confined to those of the neurological problem alone, but to a variety of other issues, some of which interact to produce a greater effect on the patient (see Table 7–1):

1. *Onset of mental health problems after HIV diagnosis.* In this patient depression was severe enough to require specialist psychiatric advice, and continued to be a problem five years later. He was at the peak of his career in a job requiring skill and training, and suffered considerable loss because he could not work again.

2. *Multiple infections.* He had esophageal candidiasis, CMV retinitis and colitis, and mycobacterium kansasii representing opportunistic infections with fungi, viruses, and bacteria.

3. *Multiple body sites affected.* Esophagus, lungs, adrenals, retinas, colon, peripheral nerves.

4. *Fluctuant course.* His first AIDS-defining illness was five years previously, after which

Table 7–1. Issues in HIV Palliative Care from Case History

- High incidence of mental health problems
- Multiple infections and complications in the same patient
- Fluctuant course
- Pain a common symptom—usually neuropathic
- Diarrhea may be severe
- Antiretroviral therapy still taken in advanced illness
- Cognitive impairment often a problem
- Many drug interactions with antiretrovirals
- Patients usually actively involved in decision to stop active treatment
- Multidisciplinary team plan care
- Many patients wish to die at home

he improved before developing other complications.

5. *Neuropathic pain may be severe.* His pain was not fully controlled on strong opioid (fentanyl patches), non-steroidal anti-inflammatory (NSAID, ketoprofen) and anticonvulsant (sodium valproate). He required additional oral morphine. Newer anticonvulsants such as gabapentin and lamotrigine may also be used.

6. *Diarrhea may be severe.* Few patients now become severely debilitated by profuse uncontrollable pouring diarrhea—a common pattern in HIV prior to the use of highly active antiretroviral therapy (HAART). But intermittent symptoms may be severe enough to cause fecal incontinence. One loose stool in the morning may not meet the physician's definition of diarrhea; but the patient, devastated by the social implications of fecal incontinence, rates diarrhea as the most troublesome symptom.

7. *Antiretrovirals (ARVs) are still used at late stage of disease.* ARVs may control symptoms particularly due to opportunistic infections (e.g. CMV) as well as those directly due to the HIV virus. Other specific treatments may be the best palliation, in this case steroid replacement to relieve vomiting due to hypoadrenalism.

8. *Cognitive impairment is often a problem.* Detailed cognitive testing can be completed only if the patient co-operates. HIV-related dementia frequently affects the frontal lobes,

and patients may have behavioral problems and lack of insight while verbal and motor skills are preserved.

9. *Medications interact.* Indinavir and other protease inhibitor ARVs interact with cytochrome P450, contraindicating use of carbamazepine and phenytoin for neuropathic pain and use of rifampicin for mycobacterial disease. An alternative ARV combination would include a non-nucleoside reverse transcriptase inhibitor (NNRTI). NNRTIs such as nevirapine and efavirenz affect hepatic metabolism and may significantly alter levels of opioids.

10. *The patient is actively involved in the decision to stop treatment.* Patients often wish to evaluate each of their medications, to understand the benefit to be expected from it, the possible side effects, and the advantages and disadvantages of stopping it. The patient who knows they will not live long may choose to omit all medications where the benefit is only in the medium or long term.

11. *Multidisciplinary team plan care.* A team including medical, nursing, occupational therapy, physiotherapy, massage therapy, counseling, social care, and chaplaincy meets to plan patients' care, and is available for individual sessions as necessary.

12. *Many patients wish to die at home.* This can be achieved by careful planning with assessment of needs by the multidisciplinary team and close liaison with family and carers as well as nurses and social workers based in the community, who will have continuing responsibility for the patient at home.

Presentation and Course of HIV and AIDS

The HIV virus is an ribonucleic acid (RNA) virus. The virus binds to CD4 receptors on the surface of cells, and therefore selectively to cells which have these receptors, particularly CD4 lymphocytes. Once a host cell is infected, the viral enzyme reverse transcriptase produces viral DNA (deoxy-ribonucleic acid) which becomes incorporated into the host DNA in the cell nucleus to become part of the cell genome. The cell then produces millions of copies of viral RNA and viral proteins, which are assembled into virus particles by the viral enzyme protease.

Most effects of HIV virus are not due to direct virus damage. HIV virus in CD4 cells damages the cells, and the number of CD4 cells is reduced. From a normal of 500 to 1000×10^6/litre, the CD4 count may fall below 200×10^6/litre, which allows infections such as pneumocystis carinii pneumonia or esophageal candida, which would not occur with normal immune responses; these are opportunistic infections (OIs). When the CD4 falls as low as 50 or less, particular OIs are more likely to develop, such as mycobacterium avium-intracellulare complex (MAI, MAC) and retinitis due to cytomegalovirus (CMV). The virus may also directly affect the nervous system centrally causing HIV dementia, or peripherally leading to neuropathy.

HIV is associated with disorders of brain, meninges, spinal cord, and peripheral nerves; some related directly to the HIV virus, others to opportunistic infection or tumors such as lymphoma.[1] HIV affects all organs or systems of the body, and in any combination. A patient with neurological complications of HIV will usually have other body systems involved and a variety of symptoms due to different pathologies (see Table 7–2).

Antiretroviral Therapy

Most ARVs block the action of one of the viral enzymes reverse transcriptase or protease; a newer generation of fusion inhibitors have their effect on the initial fusion of the virus to the CD4 receptor (see Table 7–3). ARV combinations may reduce the replication of new virus particles to the level where none is detectable in blood by polymerase chain reaction (PCR) and other tests for viral DNA; this is known as 'undetectable viral load'. Long-term maintenance of an undetectable viral load has become the objective of treatment since it is associated with persistence of the immune response and improved survival. But the ARVs are not effective against viral DNA incorporated in the genome of a quiescent cell in other organs, and since this cannot be eradicated with current medication, HIV cannot be cured.

The use of highly active ARV therapy (HAART) has been widespread since 1996. HAART delays immune damage, so that the patient does not progress to develop AIDS. The number of new AIDS diagnoses in the United Kingdom fell from 1187 in 1994 to 507 in 1999.[2] The mortality from AIDS also fell, despite increasing numbers of people living with HIV. HAART may improve HIV-related symptoms including fevers, night sweats, and weight loss, and AIDS-defining illnesses including Kaposi's sarcoma, cryptosporidiosis, and PML.[3–5] However, the immunereconstitution occurring with HAART may produce a more exuberant cellular response to infection, which has an adverse effect such as worsening hepatitis.[3] HAART drugs have many interactions with symptom-control

Table 7–2. **Neurological Infectious Disorders in HIV/AIDS**

	Infecting/Associated Agent	Diagnosis
Encephalitis	HIV virus	HIV encephalopathy, HIV dementia
	Cytomegalovirus	CMV encephalitis
White matter of brain	JC virus	Progressive multifocal leukoencephalopathy (PML)
Cerebral abscess	Toxoplasma gondii	Toxoplasmosis
	Mycobacterium tuberculosis	Tuberculoma
Meninges	Mycobacterium tuberculosis	TB meningitis
	Cryptococcus neoformans	Cryptococcal meningitis
	Listeria monocytogenes streptococcus pneumoniae	Bacterial meningitis
Spinal cord	HIV virus	Vacuolar myelopathy
Peripheral nerves	HIV virus	HIV neuropathy

Table 7–3. **Antiretroviral Drugs**

Nucleoside analogues (NAs) (Nucleoside reverse transcriptase inhibitors, NRTIs)	Zidovudine (AZT, ZDV) Stavudine (d4T) Didanosine (ddI) Zalcitabine (ddC) Lamivudine (3TC) Abacavir (ABC)
Nucleotide analogue	Tenofovir
Non-nucleoside reverse transcriptase inhibitors (NNRTIs)	Nevirapine (NVP) Delavirdine (DVD) Efavirenz (EFV)
Protease inhibitors (PIs)	Indinavir (IDV) Ritonavir (RTV) Saquinavir (SQV) Nelfinavir (NFV) Amprenavir (AMP, APV) Lopinavir (LPV)
Fusion inhibitor	Enfuvirtide T20
Immunesuppressive	Hydroxycarbamide (Hydroxyurea)

medications as well as direct side effects (see Table 7–4).[6]

The dramatic improvement of people when they start HAART has been labelled the 'Lazarus effect'. The improvement may be against all expectations. We found that of 15 patients admitted for terminal care to a hospice unit for HIV-related brain impairment, the three who could take HAART recovered and were rehabilitated to live independently in the community.[5] The prognosis for HIV dementia had previously been accepted as almost invariably poor, with a survival of three to six months.[7]

Adherence to HAART is a major factor in determining its effectiveness. Adherence to 95% or more of doses is necessary for optimal response. Paterson found that patients with 90%–95% adherence had a failure rate of 32% at three months, and this rose to 50% failure rate for 80%–90% adherence.[8] In most chronic diseases adherence is at best 60%, and this may be the level of adherence for many patients with HIV.[3] The principal reason for poor adherence is side effects of the HAART drugs; appropriate symptom control may greatly improve adherence.

Some protease inhibitors (PIs) are poorly absorbed, and when used alone must be given eight-hourly in large doses. The addition of a small dose of another PI, ritonavir, serves to boost the level of the PI used in treatment such that twice daily dosage at a lower overall dose is effective. Lopinavir is produced in capsules where it is combined with ritonavir, the dosage regimen allowing for the boosting effect. Other patients may have a regime with four ARVs—two nucleoside agonists (NAs) and a PI such as indinavir, with levels boosted by ritonavir. Ritonavir is unpleasant to take, with frequent nausea and other gastrointestinal side effects. If ritonavir alone is stopped, levels of the other PI will be inadequate, resulting in reduced effectiveness. Replication of virus would increase, bringing increased risk of mutation and of development of resistance to NAs and PIs in the regime. Thus, stopping one drug in a four-drug regime readily leads to treatment failure and persistence of resistant virus, which greatly reduces future treatment options.

Since HAART reduces symptoms due to HIV and other pathologies, there is a case for continuing HAART even in some patients with advanced disease where there is little prospect of recovery. Psychological factors play a large part in the final decision to stop HAART; the patient may see the decision as

Table 7–4. **Symptoms in HIV/AIDS**

Symptoms	Cause	Treatment
Mouth discomfort/ dysphagia	Candida mouth/esophagus	Fluconazole, itraconazole, IV amphotericin
	Kaposi's sarcoma of mouth/pharynx	Radiotherapy, chemotherapy
	Herpes simplex of mouth/pharynx	Aciclovir, famciclovir, IV foscarnet
	Aphthous ulceration	Thalidomide if intractible Difflam, tetracycline mouthwash
	Gingivitis	(Metronidazole) amoxycillin Chlorhexidine mouthwash
Nausea, vomiting	Raised intracranial pressure	Dexamethasone and treat cause
	Opportunistic infections e.g. CMV	Treat cause and metoclopramide, cyclizine, haloperidol, levomepromazine
	Medication load	Discontinue any medications no longer essential
	Antiretroviral drugs—didanosine (ddI)	Change to enteric-coated formulation Antiemetic before morning dose
	Antiretroviral drugs—ritonavir (RTV)	Check being given with food Haloperidol first line Levomepromazine often effective
Weight loss	Cognitive impairment (e.g. HIV dementia)	HAART, specific treatment for infections plus dietary measures
	Opportunistic infections (e.g. MAI, TB)	Specific treatment plus dietary measures
	HIV wasting syndrome	Check for infections such as MAI; dietary measures—provide food patient will accept even if not balanced diet, add supplements most acceptable to patient, consider nasogastric or gastrostomy tube feeding to supplement oral intake. Possibly megestrol up to 80 mg daily; dronabinol poorly tolerated; stanozolol and anabolic steroids; thalidomide may be effective
Diarrhea	Cryptosporidia/microsporidia	HAART may give remission; antibiotic (e.g. paramomycin) may improve; antidiarrheals
	Viruses (e.g. CMV)	HAART, cidofovir, antidiarrheals
	Shigella, salmonella	Antibiotics always indicated (e.g. ciprofloxacin)
	Antiretrovirals (e.g. nelfinavir)	Insoluble calcium salts orally (e.g. calcium carbonate 500 mg bd) Antidiarrheals
	Pathogen negative (no cause detected)	Loperamide up to 8 mg qds, codeine phosphate 10–60 mg qds, oral morphine, subcutaneous diamorphine, subcutaneous octreotide

Continued on following page

Table 7–4—*continued*

Symptoms	Cause	Treatment
Pain	Neuropathy following antiretroviral therapy	Consider change of regime Analgesia
	Neuropathy HIV-related	HAART may bring remission Regular analgesia—WHO ladder adjuvant at steps 2 and 3 e.g. gabapentin, valproate (compatible with HAART), amitriptyline 10–75 mg daily; methadone may be more effective than morphine
	Cholangitis, pancreatitis, malignancies	Regular analgesia—WHO ladder
Malaise/withdrawal	Pain, pyrexia, nausea, discomfort, diarrhea	Treat cause and specific symptoms
	Depression and anxiety	Paroxetine
	Depression alone	Citalopram, venlafaxine
		Tricyclic antidepressants second line
	HIV-related brain impairment (HRBI)	Diagnose only when above causes excluded or treated; may respond to HAART
Mania/hallucinations	Relapse of pre-existing mental illness	Antipsychotics—haloperidol, chlorpromazine; ask psychiatrist's advice
	New diagnosis of psychosis	Often onset of HRBI/HIV dementia Acute treatment; haloperidol or other regime as advised by psychiatrist. Once stable, olanzapine, risperidone best in HRBI

meaning that they have 'given up' and have nothing to live for, or that they are not worth treating. Such patients may wish to continue HAART even when they are very frail and using a syringe driver for symptom control medication, stopping only when they become unable to swallow the capsules. Other patients, conscious of the side effects of HAART, are keen to stop taking it as soon as long-term benefit becomes unlikely. There is no one recommended strategy for ARVs in terminal care; for each patient their own cost–benefit analysis must be worked out, taking into account virological, pharmacological, and psychological factors.

Mental Health Issues

Many people with HIV have coexisting or pre-existing mental health problems. In 80 patients admitted to an HIV palliative care unit in 1988–9, we found 20 (25%) had clinical depression.[9] In HIV brain impairment patients admitted in 1997–8, 10 of 15 (66%) had a pre-existing mental health problem.[5] In the same palliative care unit in 2001, 80% of patients admitted had a history of a mental health problem.[10]

A psychotic episode may be the first manifestation of HIV, and may lead on to a more typical dementia pattern. Everall states that a new episode of hypomania may be an initial presentation of HIV dementia.[11] HIV dementia occurs when immune deficiency has already occurred and the CD4 count is usually below 200 and frequently below 100. There is the difficult management problem of the patient who is acutely psychotic but also has the likelihood of developing severe physical illness. Infection control may be a real or perceived risk, as a disturbed patient may bite others, cut themselves, or struggle when given injections, putting staff at risk of a needlestick injury.

If a patient with cognitive impairment remains well physically on HAART, while remaining unable to be responsible for financial and other affairs, it may be necessary to follow legal requirements to allow a designated person or persons to administer their affairs. In the United Kingdom this is through the Court of Protection. The procedures are slow and inflexible, and informal arrangements are to be preferred wherever the patient's condition permits.

Antipsychotic medication such as phenothiazines interact with protease inhibitors, particularly ritonavir. Where dosage is titrated to a patient's needs whilst on HAART this creates no problem; but where a patient, stable on phenothiazines, starts a HAART combination including a PI, then phenothiazine levels may rise to become severely toxic.

Symptoms in HIV/AIDS

In the pre-HAART era, the most common symptoms found in an HIV hospice were debility/weight loss in 61% and anorexia in 41% of admissions.[9] With HAART these are much less common problems,[5] although still an issue for some patients, particularly those unable to take HAART. Many patients who would previously have been assumed to have HIV wasting syndrome are now found to have MAI, as diagnostic techniques and awareness of the diagnosis have improved. This can be treated with antimycobacterial agents, although rifampicin must avoided if the patient is on a regime including protease inhibitors. Rifabutin, in a 50% reduced dose, is used instead. Better supplementary feeding regimes and increased use of nasogastric tube and percutaneous endoscopic gastrostomy (PEG) feeding have greatly improved patients' nutritional status. The dietician is an essential team member when caring for HIV patients.

Diarrhea is a common symptom in HIV. With HAART very few patients now suffer from the debilitating pouring diarrhea which was common in 1988; Moss found 18% of patients had diarrhea on admission.[9] Most diarrhea is controlled by loperamide, up to 32 mg daily, or codeine. Octreotide and/or diamorphine subcutaneously usually control the resistant diarrhea, and can be continued at home once a patient is stabilized.

Pain in HIV is often underestimated. Pre-HAART, Moss found neuropathic pain in 22% of patients, pressure sore pain in 12%, and visceral pain in 10% of patients, and six other types of pain.[9] These figures would be lower now; but pain in people with HIV remains underrated and undermedicated, particularly in women, less-educated patients, and intravenous drug users. Neuropathic pain remains the predominant pain in HIV. Where it is present at diagnosis, then treatment with HAART may bring about an improvement. More commonly, the pain occurs while the patient is taking HAART, particularly regimes including stavudine (d4t). Assessment of pain in HIV should include careful examination, appropriate investigations, and a stepwise approach to treatment, titrating only one drug at a time (see Table 7–4 for a more detailed list of symptoms and treatment).[12]

Psychological Factors

The diagnosis of HIV has considerable implications for a person's psychological well-being. Most adults are diagnosed at an age where they are independent, with their identity and self-image established around work, relationships, and leisure activities. HIV may necessitate leaving work because of malaise and lack of energy, an unsightly change in appearance, or mental health problems and impaired cognition. This results in loss of status, role, income, and contact with colleagues, as well as dependence on family, partner, or professionals. Relationships may be affected by blame around who introduced the infection, fear of transmission to a negative partner, and worries for the future of dependents. Those not in long-term relationships may find themselves unable to initiate contact with others because of reduced opportunity and fear of rejection. Loss of income and reduced stamina may have a profound effect on leisure activities. A person with a relaxed and spontaneous lifestyle finds that the promise of future health is tied to frequent hospital attendances and regular medication—a routine which itself becomes oppressive, leading to low mood and feelings of hopelessness. Those who have had HIV since the late 1980s have survivor guilt as they remain alive while many friends and acquaintances have died. There may be considerable fear—of ill-health, disfigurement, and death; of loss of relationships and rejection; of infecting others—which may lead to a feeling of uncleanness and unworthiness.

Many patients with HIV have already been traumatized by their experiences before they discover they are HIV positive—gay men still are victimized, harassed, and physically assaulted; drug users (IVDUs) are treated with suspicion and disdain; refugees may have escaped war zones, witnessed woundings and killings, suffered injuries, or been infected with HIV during a rape; African people experience racism. The diagnosis of HIV may lead to the person becoming very depressed and even suicidal. Moss describes 'a heightened potential for self destruction, whether it be in the form of an active response such as suicide, or a more passive response, such as self destructive hate or self-pity'.[13] The essence of palliative care is to provide acceptance and to reduce fear and anxiety.

Stigma, Isolation, Fear, and Infection Control

When HIV is diagnosed, there may then be added stigma and discrimination due to unnecessary fear of infection. Many people are now better informed, but still there are families and others who bleach the bath, who will not use the same toilet, who insist on separate crockery and cutlery, who will not have any physical contact such as shaking hands.

People who have discovered that they have HIV are already deeply shocked, anxious, and vulnerable. They most need reassurance, support, and comfort. Omitting unnecessary precautions is as important as observing those which are necessary. Patients need not be isolated and it is inappropriate for staff to wear masks or gloves for everyday contact. Normal hygiene measures are sufficient for bathrooms and toilets as well as cups and crockery. There is no risk of infection from examining a patient, sitting on their bed, holding their hand, or hugging them.

Sharps injuries can transmit the HIV virus. Staff have become infected by a needlestick injury where the needle has previously been used for a patient with HIV, particularly when the needle has been in a vein and is still attached to a syringe with blood in it. To reduce the risk of transmission of HIV, sharps and intravenous injections should be reduced to those which are essential, and practical measures taken to minimize the risk of injury. Disposal boxes for needles should be nearby; injections and blood sampling should be done by experienced staff. For procedures involving sharps, gloves should be worn. This does not prevent the injury, but the rubber has the effect of wiping the needle which reduces the inoculum of blood to the injured staff member. If there is a sharps injury from a known HIV-positive patient, then post-exposure prophylaxis (PEP) is recommended. United Kingdom national guidelines[14] specify that prophylaxis is given within one hour of the needlestick, starting with zidovudine, lamivudine, and either nelfinavir or indinavir (see Table 7–5). Prophylaxis should be continued for one month, but it is preferable for the staff member to be reviewed by an HIV specialist within one or two days with details of virology on the 'donor' patient. If the donor, for instance, had virus resistant to AZT and 3TC then this is likely to be the resistance profile of any virus infecting the staff member. Prophylactic medication should be changed to a regime likely to be effective against that virus.

Table 7–5. **Post-exposure Prophylaxis After Sharps Injury from HIV-positive Source**

- Start within one hour, or as soon as possible
- Zidovudine 250 mg or 300 mg BD plus
- Lamivudine 150 mg BD plus
- EITHER nelfinavir 1250 mg BD OR indinavir 800 mg fasting 8-hourly
- Subsequent regime adjusted on reviewing donor's virology
- One-month course
- Blood for HIV test on day one (but can be after first dose of PEP)
- Subsequent blood for HIV test at three and six months

CREUTZFELDT–JAKOB DISEASE

Creutzfeldt–Jakob disease (CJD, subacute spongiform encephalopathy) is one of the group of diseases known as transmissible spongiform encephalopathies (TSE). CJD exists in two main forms: sporadic CJD, which includes familial CJD; and variant CJD (vCJD). Both are associated with a self-replicating agent which is a prion, or protease-resistant protein. This prion is an abnormal configuration of the cellular protein sialoglycoprotein, encoded by a gene on chromosome 20. Newly synthesized abnormal protein forms deposits in the central nervous system leading to spongy degeneration and neuronal damage. The basal ganglia, caudate nuclei, and cerebellum are most often affected. Brain biopsy reveals abnormal amyloid.

Sporadic CJD

Sporadic CJD is present in many countries. In most cases the route of infection is unknown, but some cases are related to contaminated neurosurgical instruments, and use of cadaveric corneal transplants, dura mater, or pituitary hormones account for 5% of cases. Familial cases constitute 10%–15% of sporadic CJD; they have an autosomal dominant pattern with changes in the gene for the specific protein involved. Familial CJD has an onset around 40 years of age, but 80% of other cases of sporadic CJD have an onset between 50 and 70 years of age.

The onset of CJD often involves memory loss or confusion, but there may also be depression, anxiety, or abnormal behaviour.[15] Focal neurologic signs occur at an early stage in one third of patients, with ataxia, aphasia, visual loss, or hemiparesis. Myoclonic jerking is often a feature, particularly in response to any stimulus. Late in the disease, the patient is mute and akinetic, and myoclonic jerks subside. Deterioration may occur rapidly, changes being detectable from one day to the next. Progress from first symptoms to death occurs with a median duration of 4.5 months.[16]

Variant CJD

Epidemiological surveillance of CJD in the United Kingdom was set up in 1990 following an epidemic of bovine spongiform encephalopathy in cattle. By 1996, 10 cases of vCJD were detected in the United Kingdom, although none had appeared in other European countries.[17] By the end of December 2001 a total of 113 cases had been reported in the United Kingdom (60 male and 53 female), with 104 deaths at a median age of 28 years.[18] The duration of vCJD was a median of 12 months (7.5 to 22.5 months), three times that of sporadic CJD.

Biopsy or necropsy in vCJD shows changes distinct from sporadic CJD, with spongiform changes throughout the brain, neuronal loss, and astrocytosis, particularly in the basal ganglia and thalamus. In all cases of vCJD prion protein plaques were distributed extensively through the cerebrum and cerebellum.

A striking feature of the vCJD patients was the presentation of their disease; in nine of the 10, behavioral change was an early clinical feature and the patient was referred to a psychiatrist. All patients developed progressive dementia but memory impairment was a presenting feature in only two. Nine developed ataxia early in the course of the disease. Other prominent symptoms were pain, dysesthesia, myoclonus, and choreoathetosis. Early presentation of psychiatric symptoms and ataxia, and marked sensory symptoms are all features of vCJD.

Douglas carried out in-depth interviews with families of 19 patients with vCJD, and found that many families were angry that their relatives had been given an initial psychiatric diagnosis, and often stated that early physical signs were underestimated.[19] Patients who were very dependant physically and also had marked psychiatric symptoms were not managed well on medical or psychiatric wards, and families felt the patients' rapid deterioration was not adequately assessed or treated unless specialist palliative care services were involved.

Infection Control in CJD

Sporadic CJD has been transmitted medically and experimentally by brain, spinal cord, and eye tissue. Prions are resistant to destruction by conventional methods of autoclaving or chemical sterilization. There is no evidence of direct transmission to staff or family members involved in caring for a patient, and universal precautions are sufficient, with no additional requirement for gowns, gloves, or other specific infection control measures. However, once the brain has been disturbed at autopsy, it is a usual precaution to suggest that family members and staff have no further direct contact with the body.

Palliative Care Issues in CJD

Management of depression, personality change, hallucinations, and delusions is needed, alongside management of pain, immobility, mutism, involuntary movements, and cognitive impairment. Nurses find care of these patients challenging and may require counselling.[18] Where care is provided at home, frequent reassessments of needs are required because of rapid deterioration. Families require support and encouragement, particularly where a late diagnosis leaves the prognosis uncertain until a late stage of the illness.

REFERENCES

1. Simpson D, Tagliati M. Neurologic manifestations of HIV infection. Ann Intern Med 1994;121:769–785.
2. Communicable Diseases Surveillance Centre. AIDS infection in the United Kingdom; monthly report. The effect of highly active antiretroviral therapy (HAART) on progression to AIDS. Commun Dis Rep CDR Weekly 2000;10:123–4.
3. Easterbrook P, Meadway J. The changing epidemiology of HIV infection: new challenges for palliative care. J Roy Soc Med 2001;94:442–448.
4. Rackstraw S, Conley A, Meadway J. Recovery from progressive multifocal leukoencephalopathy following directly-observed highly active antiretroviral therapy in a specialised brain impairment unit. AIDS 2000;14(suppl. 4):S 129.
5. Stephenson J, Woods S, Scott B, Meadway J. HIV-related brain impairment: from palliative care to rehabilitation. Int J Pall Nursing 2000; 6:6–11.
6. Brogan G, George R. HIV/AIDS: symptoms and the impact of new treatments. CME Bulletin Palliative Medicine 1999;1:104–110.
7. McArthur J, Harrison MJG. HIV associated dementia. Curr Neurol 1994;14:275–320.
8. Paterson DL, Swindells S, Mohr J, et al. Adherence to protease inhibitor therapy and outcomes in patients with HIV infection. Ann Intern Med 2000;133:21–30.
9. Moss V. Patient characteristics, presentation and problems encountered in advanced AIDS in a hospice setting—a review. Pall Med 1991;5:112–116.
10. Rackstraw S, Dodhia M, Meadway J. Psychiatric comorbidity and substance use prevalence amongst patients in an HIV palliative care unit: impact on service provision. XIV International AIDS Conference MoPeB3178, 2002.
11. Everall I. Neuropsychiatric aspects of HIV infection. J Neurol Neurosurg Psychiatry 1995;58:399–402.
12. Pickhaver K. Palliative care. In Gazzard B, ed. Chelsea and Westminster AIDS Care Handbook. Mediscript Ltd, London, 1999:229–245.
13. Moss V, Sims R. Palliative Care for People with AIDS, 2nd Ed. Edward Arnold division of Hodder Headline PLC, London, 1995.
14. HIV Post-Exposure Prophylaxis: Guidance from the UK Chief Medical Officers' Expert Advisory Group on AIDS. UK Health Departments, July 2000.
15. Will RG, Ironside JW, Zeidler M, et al. A new variant of Creutzfeldt-Jakob disease in the UK. Lancet 1996;347:921–925.
16. CJD Insight: Sporadic CJD. http://www.cjdinsight.org/Deana/sporadiccjd.html, 22 July 2002.
17. World Health Organization: Variant Creutzfeldt–Jakob Disease (vCJD). Fact Sheet No.180, http://www.who.int, revised June 2001.
18. Andrews NJ. Incidence of Variant Creutzfeldt–Jakob Disease Onsets and Deaths, January 1994–December 2001. Public Health Laboratory Service, Statistics Unit. http://www.cjd.ed.ac.uk/cjdq31.html, 11 January 2002.
19. Douglas MJ, Campbell H, Will RG. Patients with New Variant Creutzfeldt–Jakob Disease and Their families: Care and Information Needs. Report of UK Creutzfeldt–Jakob Research Unit, University of Edinburgh. http://www.cjd.ed.ac.uk/carerep.html, February 1999.
20. Bailey B, Aranda S, Quinn K, Kean H. Creutzfeldt–Jakob disease: extending palliative care knowledge. Int J Pall Nursing 2000;6(3):131–139.

Chapter 8

Diseases of Motor Nerves

David Oliver
Gian Domenico Borasio

INTRODUCTION
PALLIATIVE CARE
DIAGNOSIS-RELATED ISSUES
DISEASE PROGRESSION
Physical Aspects

Psychological Aspects
Social Aspects
Spirituality
TERMINAL STAGES
SUMMARY

Motor neuron disease (MND)/amyotrophic lateral sclerosis (ALS) is a progressive disease with no curative treatment and a prognosis of three or four years for most people. Thus, the care of patients with MND/ALS requires a palliative care approach from the time of diagnosis, with the involvement of the wider multidisciplinary team. It is essential to consider all the aspects of the patient and family's care, including the physical, psychological, social, and spiritual. As the disease progresses, the management of the various symptoms, including dysphagia, dyspnea, dysarthria, pain, and drooling, becomes increasingly important, to maintain the person's quality of life. The support of the person with MND/ALS and their family and carers is essential, as fears and concerns may develop as the disease progresses. There are often fears of a distressing death but, with this approach to care, actively managing and anticipating the potential problems, the majority of patients are able to die peacefully, with their symptoms controlled.

CASE HISTORY

Mr AA was a 72-year-old man who had been widowed five years ago and lived with his daughter and her family, comprising her husband and two children aged 12 and 15 years. He was a very active churchgoer and an elder in his local church community. He had developed weakness of his legs two years previously and had fallen on several occasions. Initially he had been investigated at a rheumatology clinic, but he had then developed slurring of his speech. A referral had been made for speech therapy and the speech and language therapist had asked for a neurological opinion. Further investigations had confirmed the diagnosis of MND (ALS).

In August 2000 he had become less mobile and was seen by the physiotherapist; by October he required a frame; and by December was regularly using a wheelchair. The house in which he lived had two large rooms downstairs and one was converted into a bedroom for Mr AA. The children found the loss of their television room, where they met their friends, very difficult.

His speech deteriorated and was barely understandable, and he started to cough and splutter with meals. He was able to take puréed food, although this took his daughter longer time to prepare, and the family started to refuse to eat with him. After discussion he was admitted for the insertion of a percutaneous endoscopic gastrostomy and he was fed enterally at night. The grandchildren found it increasingly hard to spend time with Mr AA as they could not understand his speech and found the drooling of saliva offensive.

He continued to weaken but the friends from the local church visited regularly and allowed his daughter days away from the home. The drooling was eased by anticholinergic medication. He became more breathless but did not want to consider respiratory support, and the symptom was eased by regular oral morphine.

As he deteriorated further the friends from the church continued to visit and took him to services regularly. The minister visited and was a great support to him and his family, as was the local palliative care team who visited regularly. The social worker met with the grandchildren and allowed them to talk about their fears and then to spend some time with their grandfather. One evening he became more breathless and a community nurse gave him an injection and arranged for further injections over night. He died peacefully at home, with his daughter with him, during that night.

INTRODUCTION

ALS (MND in the United Kingdom and Lou Gehrig's disease or ALS in the United States) is the most common degenerative disorder of the motoneuronal system occurring in adult life. The estimated incidence of ALS is 1.5–2 per 100,000 per year; the prevalence is around 6–8 per 100,000.[1] While rare cases may begin before the age of 20 years, most cases begin after age 40, the mean age at onset being around 58. For the majority of people the etiology is unknown, although in about 5% there is a family history and about 20% of these people have been shown to have a recognizable gene mutation—the superoxide dismutase (SOD 1) gene on chromosome 21.[2]

The clinical picture is characterized by fasciculations and slowly progressing paresis of voluntary muscles, coupled with hyperreflexia and spasticity due to concomitant involvement of upper and lower motor neurons. Bulbar onset with slurred speech (dysarthria) and/or difficulty in swallowing (dysphagia) occurs in 20%–30% of all cases, particularly in older females.[3] Extraocular movements and sphincter continence are usually spared, and sensation is normal. Although subtle neuropsychological deficits can be detected upon careful examination, frank dementia is a rare occurrence (about 5%–10%). The main symptoms of ALS are shown in Table 8–1. The rate of disease progression in ALS is remarkably variable. Average disease duration

Table 8–1. **Symptoms Associated with MND/ALS**

Directly:	*Indirectly:*
Weakness and atrophy	Sleep disturbances
Fasciculations and muscle cramps	Constipation
Spasticity	Drooling
Dysarthria	Thick mucous secretions
Dysphagia	Symptoms of chronic hypoventilation
Dyspnea	Pain
Pathological laughing/crying	

is around 3–4 years, 10% of patients survive >10 years, and single cases may run over several decades.[4]

The available disease-specific treatment options for ALS are still unsatisfactory. Riluzole, a drug with antiglutamatergic properties, is the only treatment that has been shown to be effective in MND/ALS. It prolongs life by about three months.[5] However, therapeutic nihilism is not justified as a large array of palliative measures is available to enhance the quality of life of patients and their families.[6]

PALLIATIVE CARE

As there is no curative treatment for MND/ALS, the care provided for patients and their families is palliative from the time of diagnosis. The aim of palliative care is to consider the 'whole patient' in the context of their social support system, which is often their family. This holistic approach is crucial in the care of someone with MND/ALS and is relevant from the time of investigation, before the diagnosis has been confirmed, and throughout the progression of the disease.[7]

A multidisciplinary team approach is essential as there are so many aspects of care that need to be addressed. The team approach can enable these concerns to be considered and the management can then be as effective as possible. The team will include:

- Physician
- Nurse
- Occupational therapist

- Physiotherapist
- Speech and language therapist
- Chaplain
- Social worker/counselor
- Dietitian

This team approach for the person with MND/ALS and their family will need to be co-ordinated and supported so that the care can be optimized and aspects of care are neither missed or duplicated.

Within the progression of MND/ALS there are times of increasing need and concern:

- At the time of diagnosis
- At the time when there is a particular loss associated with the disease progression and a new intervention is necessary—such as the use of a wheelchair or the insertion of a gastrostomy
- In the terminal stages

At all these times there will be the need to look at every aspect of the person's care and concerns—physical, psychological, social, and spiritual.

However, the changes may not be so clearly defined, as all people with MND/ALS progress at different rates and in different ways. They all face losses as the disease progresses and have to cope with these challenges, together with their family and carers.

DIAGNOSIS-RELATED ISSUES

There are particular issues to be faced at the time of diagnosis.

PHYSICAL ISSUES

These will vary greatly according to the presentation and the possible delays in diagnosis. Some people will have few physical problems at this time, having presented with mild weakness or fasciculation; but some may have experienced delays in diagnosis and may therefore be disabled and have severe progression of the disease.

The various symptoms experienced will be discussed below.

PSYCHOLOGICAL ISSUES

The diagnosis of MND/ALS is usually a shock to the person and family. The way the news is broken can greatly influence the way they cope with the disease as it progresses. If there has been little information imparted or even if the information has been inaccurate, the person may lose faith in the professional carers involved, whereas the empathetic approach will allow the person and family to feel more confident and able to ask for further advice and help later. Suggestions for how the news should be imparted[8,9] include the evidence-based Practice Parameter which has recommended that:

- The physician should give the diagnosis and discuss its implications, respecting the cultural and social background of the patient
- The diagnosis should always be given in person
- Printed materials should be available to support
- The withholding of the diagnosis, insufficient information, callous telling, and the taking away of hope should be avoided

SOCIAL ISSUES

The reactions of the person and family may vary greatly. For many, the diagnosis of MND/ALS is an unknown, and, unfortunately, coverage of the disease in books and the media is alarming and stresses the risk of a distressing death—although the available evidence does not support this. Many families may try to shield the person with MND/ALS from the diagnosis, but experience has shown that this may be harmful and, in the longer run, reduces communication within the family and may actually reduce the care offered.[10]

DISEASE PROGRESSION

Physical Aspects

As the disease progresses, and often from the time of diagnosis, the person with MND/ALS faces increasing losses and problems due to muscle weakness. Some of these changes are directly due to the disease itself and others are related to disability and alterations in lifestyle as a result of the disease, but primarily part of the process itself. These symptoms and problems require careful multidisciplinary team assessment and a carefully co-ordinated team approach.[11,12]

Table 8–1 shows the various symptoms and problems faced by a person with MND/ALS. There are particular symptom changes that will lead to alteration in the person's life and may require an intervention—such as the provision of a walking aid or an intervention such as a gastrostomy. There may be particular needs for the person in coping with these changes.

WEAKNESS

Increasing muscle weakness is a major symptom of MND/ALS and most people with the disease will find the progressive weakness difficult. A physiotherapist will be helpful in allowing the person to retain as much activity as possible, with active exercise. Passive physiotherapy is important as the weakness increases to prevent contractures and stiffness.[13]

In conjunction with the occupational therapist, the physiotherapist is able to advise and provide additional devices to aid mobility and comfort. These may initially include a walking stick but, as the disease progresses, a frame or wheelchair may be necessary to maintain independence and mobility.[14] The provision of this equipment should take into account the psychological readiness of the person, and family, to cope with these changes as the use of an aid, and especially a wheelchair, will emphasize the increasing progression of the disease and its use may initially be resisted.

DYSPHAGIA

Over the progression of the disease up to 87% of people will have swallowing problems[12] of variable severity, due to disturbed motility of the tongue, pharynx, and esophagus. Swallowing, especially of fluids and crumbling foods, becomes increasingly difficult, and initially changes in the consistency of foods, to a custard consistency, may be helpful. The involvement of the speech and language therapist and dietitian is very important in providing advice and ensuring that the dietary intake is adequate and the risk of aspiration is minimized.[15]

As swallowing deteriorates, and weight is lost or mealtimes become increasingly fraught, a percutaneous endoscopic gastrostomy (PEG) may be inserted.[15,16] This should be considered before there is appreciable respiratory deterioration or distress, as there is evidence that the morbidity and mortality is increased if the forced vital capacity (FVC) is less than 50% expected.[9] The early discussion of a PEG is useful and it should be stressed that the presence of a PEG does not stop oral intake continuing, which may be possible for many weeks or months.[15] A PEG does seem to improve quality of life but there is no clear evidence as to whether life is extended.[17]

DYSPNEA

Dyspnea becomes a problem for up to 85% of people with MND/ALS and it is often feared by patients and families. Many publications on MND/ALS discuss respiratory distress as the terminal event.[12] There is usually associated anxiety and a calm approach is essential to prevent a vicious circle of anxiety increasing the dyspnea. Benzodiazepines, such as sublingual lorazepam, can be given for an acute dyspneic episode.[18] Regular opioids, such as oral morphine (as oral direct-release solution or modified-release tablets or capsules), are very helpful in relieving the distress of dyspnea.[19] Benzodiazepines such as diazepam may be added to relieve anxiety.

Chronic hypoventilation may develop as the respiratory muscles weaken. The symptoms are shown in Table 8–2. Non-invasive ventilation (NIV), using a face mask, can relieve these symptoms and improve the quality of life.[20] However, there is a need to discuss the issues of ventilation fully with the person. As the respiratory weakness increases the person may find that NIV is required for longer each day, until it may be in use 24 hours a day, requiring a decision on whether to progress to invasive ventilation.

If patients are not fully informed about their disease, invasive ventilation with tracheostomy is often started without the opportunity for full discussion, as the changes occur rapidly and there is insufficient time to make a fully informed decision.[21] People with invasive ventilation can be maintained for long periods of time—there are reports of over 10 years—but there are increasing care needs

Table 8–2. Symptoms of Chronic Respiratory Insufciency

- Daytime fatigue and sleepiness, concentration problems
- Difficulty falling asleep, disturbed sleep, nightmares
- Morning headache
- Nervousness, tremor, increased sweating, tachycardia
- Depression, anxiety
- Tachypnea, dyspnea, phonation difficulties
- Visible efforts of auxiliary respiratory muscles
- Reduced appetite, weight loss, recurrent gastritis
- Recurrent or chronic upper respiratory tract infections
- Cyanosis, edema
- Vision disturbances, dizziness, syncope
- Diffuse pain in head, neck, and extremities

for the person whose physical needs increase as the muscle weakness progresses. This can impose excessive care loads on family carers, and their quality of life can be greatly affected. There is also the risk of the weakness progressing to such an extent that there can be no communication from the person— the 'locked-in' syndrome. This may occur in up to 10% of people undergoing long-term invasive ventilation, and there are obvious ethical and legal problems as discontinuation of ventilation may be considered. Before the start of ventilation (NIV or invasive) these risks and the possibility of increasing disability should be discussed and consideration given to the completion of advance directives.[22] In this way everyone—person, family, and professional carers—are clear as to the plan of care, including agreement on the conditions when ventilatory support should be withdrawn.

DYSARTHRIA

Speech problems are very common (up to 71% of people) and cause much distress for the person with MND/ALS and their carers.[12] The involvement of a speech and language therapist is important early in the disease progression, and before speech is too greatly affected.[23] They will be able to help the person continue to communicate, using simple aids like an alphabet board to more complex communication aids, including computer systems. The person with MND/ALS may find the adjustment to these aids very hard to come to terms with and much support and practice may be necessary. Support is also important for the carers, both family and professionals, so that they can be aware as to the best way to help the person communicate effectively using the communication aid.

MUSCLE FASCICULATIONS

One of the early symptoms of MND/ALS is muscle fasciculation, due to degeneration of the intramuscular motor axons. These may, on occasions, be distressing and may be helped by the use of medication, such as quinine sulphate, carbamazepine or phenytoin.

PSEUDOBULBAR AFFECT

Pseudobulbar affect (pathologic laughing/ crying; emotional lability) may affect up to 50% of people with MND/ALS.[24] It may be related to frontal lobe damage, which can be seen in up to 35% of people when appropriate testing is performed.[25] It is often very disturbing for people with MND/ALS, as they feel out of control and fear that they are 'going mad'. Friends, family, and some carers may also treat them as if they are of reduced intelligence. The explanation of the symptom is crucial, and knowing that it may be part of the disease process is often very helpful. Amitriptyline can help, as can fluvoxamine and lithium.[26]

PAIN

Pain may be experienced in up to 73% of people with MND/ALS, although there is no evidence of sensory nerve involvement.[12] Pain may occur because of:

- *Muscle spasticity and cramps*, which can be treated with baclofen and quinine sulphate, respectively (see Table 8–3). However care must be taken in the use of antispasticity drugs, as increased muscle tone may allow the person with MND/ALS to remain mobile, and so careful monitoring is essential. Dantrolene, in particular, may increase

Table 8–3. **Symptomatic Medication in ALS**

	Dosage°
Fasciculations and muscle cramps	
If mild:	
Magnesium	5 mmol qd-tid
Vitamin E	400 IE bid
If severe:	
Quinine sulphate	200 mg bid
Carbamazepine	200 mg bid
Phenytoin	100 mg qd-tid
Spasticity	
Baclofen	10–80 mg
Tizanidine	6–24 mg
Memantine	10–60 mg
Tetrazepam	100–200 mg
Drooling	
Glycopyrrolate	0.1–0.2 mg sc/im tid
Transdermal hyoscine patches	1–2 patches
Amitriptyline	10–150 mg
Atropine/benztropine	0.25–0.75 mg/1–2 mg
Clonidine	0.15–0.3 mg
Pathologic laughing/crying	
Amitriptyline	10–150 mg
Fluvoxamine	100–200 mg
Lithium carbonate	400–800 mg
L-Dopa	500–600 mg

°Usual range of adult daily dosage; some patients may require higher dosages (e.g. of antispastic medication).

weakness, although in the terminal stages, extreme spasticity may be relieved by intravenous dantrolene.

- *Joint pain* due to loss of the protective muscle sheath or abnormal muscle tone or spasm around a joint. This may respond to physiotherapy and non-steroidal anti-inflammatory medication.
- *Skin pressure pain* from immobility and continuous pressure on areas of skin. The person with MND/ALS may deny that they are experiencing pain and talk only of 'discomfort', but with regular analgesia they realize that there was the need for pain relief. Regular simple analgesics, such as paracetamol, may be sufficient but, if necessary, analgesia should be increased according to the WHO analgesic ladder—to regular weak opioids, such as tramadol or codydramol, and for many people, strong opioids, such as morphine.[12,19] Fears of respiratory depression should not prevent appropriate analgesia, and studies have shown that, with careful titration, morphine can be used safely and effectively—the median dose was 60 mg morphine per 24 hours and the mean duration of use was 95 days.[19]

DROOLING

As swallowing deteriorates the drooling of saliva may occur, as it is no longer possible to swallow the volume of saliva produced. Anticholinergic medication, such as hyoscine hydrobromide (scopolamine) or glycopyrronium bromide and amitriptylline, starting at a low dose and slowly increasing, can be useful (see Table 8–3). Botulinum B toxin injections into the salivary glands has been shown in initial studies to be effective, although larger trials are awaited.[27]

THICK MUCOUS SECRETIONS

Some people with MND/ALS produce thick tenacious secretions, which are difficult to cough up, particularly with reduced respiratory effort. These secretions can cause great distress and they may become retained in the pharynx. Moistening the mucosa by humidifying the atmosphere (by steam or a nebulizer of saline)—may be of help, and fruit juices, especially those with mucolytic enzymes like grape or pineapple, may help.[23] Anticholinergic medication may reduce the amount of the secretions but increase the tenacity. Propranolol has been suggested.[27] Physiotherapy may help in aiding the clearing of the secretions.[28] A mechanical cough-assisting device has shown some effectiveness ('In-Exsufflator', J.H. Emerson Co., Cambridge, Mass., www.jhemerson.com).

CONSTIPATION

Reduced dietary intake, especially of fibre, and reduced physical activity, can lead to constipation. Dietary measures of increasing fibre and ensuring an adequate fluid intake

Table 8–4. Causes of Sleep Disturbance

- Psychological disturbances, anxiety, depression, nightmares
- Inability to change position during sleep due to weakness
- Fasciculations and muscle cramps
- Dysphagia with aspiration of saliva
- Respiratory insufficiency with hypoxia and dyspnea
- Insecurity

may be helpful and the advice of the dietitian should be sought. Aperients, such as lactulose with sennoside, may be necessary and if there is severe weakness, local rectal measures, of suppositories and enemata, may be required.

INSOMNIA

There may be many differing causes of poor sleep (see Table 8–4). These need to be assessed and treated appropriately. Simple measures, such as the provision of a sensitive call system so the person can summon help, may be very effective in reducing anxiety at night. If there is evidence of respiratory insufficiency and hypoventilation, non-invasive ventilation should be considered. Sedatives, such as benzodiazepines, may be helpful for many people.

Psychological Aspects

As the person with MND/ALS faces the progression of the disease they may experience many different emotions. The fears about the disease itself may become greater, as they are less able to speak or swallow. They also face increasing disability and dependence, and the acceptance of extra help, either from family and carers or as additional aids are used, may lead to frustration and non-acceptance of this help initially. This extra care may need to be introduced gradually and with sensitivity, so the person, and their family, can become adjusted to these changes. MND/ALS is a disease characterized by continual loss and the person may need time to grieve the loss of their abilities as they are lost.[10]

Many people with MND/ALS fear dying, especially as there is often misinformation about the distress of the dying process, with discussion of 'choking to death' and 'suffocation'. This is not the case in MND/ALS, as a recent study has demonstrated.[29] These issues need to be discussed openly and, if possible, while the person can still communicate easily. To discuss these issues using a communication aid can be very hard, as the nuances of oral communication are lost. Discussion of these issues emphasizes the importance of preparing the person for the deterioration and death from MND/ALS from soon after the diagnosis; palliative care should start at this time, not when the person is disabled and less articulate.[7]

Social Aspects

Most people with MND/ALS are members of families or other small social groups. These other people are very significant in the care of the person with MND/ALS and their fears and needs should be considered—with the consent of the person with MND/ALS. They may have particular concerns.[10]

DIAGNOSIS

The family may also fear the diagnosis and the progression of the disease, and know very little about it, apart from the information in books and the media. They may become fearful of the future and benefit from the provision of information and the opportunity to discuss their own concerns. This may allow more open discussion and sharing with the person with MND/ALS.

ISOLATION

As the person with MND/ALS becomes more disabled, and perhaps communication is reduced, the person and their family may become more isolated. The care needs increase and the family members may take on more of these activities, and feel that only they can provide this care. In this way they become more isolated and may need help and encouragement to take time for themselves, for if they do not they may become increasingly tired and eventually be less able to provide the care. The involvement of a social worker or counsellor may facilitate these discussions and allow the family to look at their involvement in the care of the person.

FINANCES

As the disease progresses there may be increasing financial problems, as the person with MND/ALS may be unable to work and the carers may also be forced to leave paid employment. These issues can cause great distress and frustration and the involvement of a social worker and financial advisor may allow the problem to be controlled and anticipated.

CHILDREN

Many younger families will include children or grandchildren, and they will be affected by the disease. Often there is a reluctance to include children in the discussion about the disease progression, although in most cases their lifestyles will have been dramatically altered and they will have concerns and fears about what is happening. There is a need to involve children in the care of the person with MND/ALS and to listen to their concerns and fears, as they will sense the anxiety within the family, overhear conversations or gossip, and will notice the practical alterations within the household. Children need extra support and the opportunities to express their concerns, in particular:

- Respect and acknowledgement of their concerns
- Information about what is happening in simple terms they can understand
- Reassurance e.g. that they have not caused the disease or could catch the disease
- Appropriate involvement in the care
- Opportunities to express themselves—this may be in drawing or games
- Opportunities to reflect and remember the person[10]

SEXUALITY

This area of care is rarely considered, although people with MND/ALS may wish to discuss these issues. The sexual function will usually remain unaltered but there may be a need to look at a couple changing their usual sexual activity to accommodate the increasing disability. Couples may benefit from the opportunity to discuss these changes—of different sexual positions or consideration of mutual masturbation—and all professionals involved in the care of people with MND/ALS should be aware of these issues and open to discuss them. Counselors or other therapists may be of help and the involvement of the physiotherapist or occupational therapist to advise on mobility or aids for comfort may be helpful.[30]

DEATH AND DYING

Families may have their own fears about the future and often these are not shared with the person with MND/ALS, for fear of upsetting them. However, open discussion can help in the reduction of these fears and enable clearer planning and anticipation of the future.[18]

Spirituality

Often, issues about the deeper meaning of life come to the fore when a person is faced with a progressive disease and death. Palliative care should provide opportunities to address these deeper issues and help the person, and their family, consider 'the need to find within present existence a sense of meaning'. This may not necessarily be religious and may relate for some people in terms of a more 'natural religion' and belief system.[10,18] The concerns about meaning and fears for the future, before and after death, should be heard and the opportunity to discuss these in greater depth offered. This may be with a religious leader or with a counsellor or social worker.[10]

It is always important to ensure that cultural aspects of care are considered. These may not necessarily be related to the religion or ethnic background of the person and family. Many families will have their own cultural norms and professional carers should be aware of the need to listen and respond to everyone as individuals—not assuming that all people from a certain ethnic or religious background share the same cultural mores (see Chapter 40).

TERMINAL STAGES

Although many people with MND/ALS, and their families, fear the final stages of the

Table 8–5. **Causes of Death**

Respiratory failure	143 (86%)
Heart failure	10 (6%)
Pneumonia	8 (5%)
Suicide	1 (0.5%)
Other	5 (2.5%)

disease, there is evidence that the majority, over 90%, die peacefully and choking to death is very rare.[29] The terminal phase varies greatly—for most people there is a gradual deterioration, then a sudden change over hours to a few days, usually following a respiratory tract infection or a silent aspiration. Between 48%–72% of patients deteriorate rapidly and die within 24 hours. The causes of death are shown in Table 8–5. Without the intervention of ventilatory support most people with MND/ALS have increasing hypercapnia and slip from drowsiness to sleep and then coma.

PHYSICAL ASPECTS

It is increasingly important that symptoms are controlled as effectively as possible, in particular:
- Pain—by regular analgesia, and often morphine
- Dyspnea—by regular morphine and benzodiazepines
- Drooling and chest secretions—by anticholinergic medication such as hyoscine hydrobromide (scopolamine) or glycopyrronium bromide
- Anxiety—with benzodiazepines, such as lorazepam sl, midazolam sc, or diazepam pr

The medication may need to be given parenterally, as swallowing deteriorates due to bulbar symptoms and/or increasing weakness and coma. The use of intramuscular or subcutaneous injections may be necessary, and a continuous subcutaneous infusion by syringe driver can allow medication to be continued easily and with minimal discomfort to the patient. The following medications can be given subcutaneously:
- Morphine for analgesia, and help with cough and dyspnea
- Midazolam for sedation and muscle relaxation

- Glycopyrronium or hyoscine hydrobromide (scopolamine) to reduce chest secretions[12,18]

Studies have shown that opioids can be given safely and, in this terminal phase, symptoms can be managed and reduced to the minimum.[19] However, some patients may become distressed and care should be given to minimize this—the most common forms of distress being dyspnea and restlessness.[18,29]

It is important to ensure that medication is readily available at home so that if there is a crisis or sudden deterioration then it can be given quickly, without delay. In the United Kingdom the Motor Neurone Disease Association has developed the Breathing Space Programme, which aims to help in the anticipation of problems at home.[12] There are leaflets about death and dying for the person with MND/ALS, his family, and professional carers to discuss, and a box is provided in which medication can be stored at home, in particular:
- Morphine
- Midazolam
- Hyoscine hydrobromide (scopolamine) or glycopyrronium bromide
- Buccal midazolam, for family members to give while awaiting help
- Injections and needles

The pack ensures that medication is readily available and its use has been discussed and is understood by all involved, so that an emergency situation can be managed effectively.[12,18]

PSYCHOLOGICAL ASPECTS

Some people with MND/ALS may become more distressed as their condition deteriorates. There may be particular fears or concerns that need to be addressed, and on some occasions increased sedation may be necessary (see Chapter 33).

SOCIAL ASPECTS

Families may find the period of deterioration particularly difficult and they may need increased support (both practical and emotional) at this time. Regular contact and visits are supportive, and time is necessary for the family to talk about their concerns and fears.[10] The provision of the Breathing Space Programme box (see above) can be very reassuring for families, as they may be more comfortable that they can cope if there is an emergency situation.[12]

The majority of people with MND/ALS wish to remain at home and, with the involvement of the primary health-care team and specialist palliative care/hospice team, this is often possible. The involvement of hospice teams should be as early as possible, so that relationships can be developed and preparations can be made to support the person at home. Admission to a hospice may be possible in the terminal stages.

The support of the family may continue after the death, as they may benefit from bereavement support. As families have faced so many losses throughout the disease progression they may be more prepared for the death. However, although they may feel relieved that the person is no longer facing the disease, they may also feel guilt that they feel this way. Bereavement support and counseling may help many families.[31]

SUMMARY

Patients with MND/ALS witness their progressing debilitation with a fully clear mind. This situation is regarded as a nightmare by most neurologists. However, the intact mentation offers patients with MND/ALS the possibility to develop coping mechanisms which can lead to a surprisingly serene acceptance of the disease. As physicians, it is a privilege to work with these patients and to witness the formidable amount of inner strength that often develops in the wake of seemingly unbearable adversity. Patients and their families usually wish to be actively involved in the decision processes regarding symptomatic treatment. It is the physician's responsibility to establish a working relationship with patient and family that may enable their full participation in all aspects of palliative care.

REFERENCES

1. Borasio GD, Miller RG. Clinical characteristics and management of ALS. Sem Neurol 2001; 21:155–166.
2. Rosen DR, Siddique T, Patterson D, et al. Mutations in Cu/Zn superoxide dismutase gene are associated with familial amyotrophic lateral sclerosis. Nature 1993;362:59–62.
3. Li TM, Alberman E, Swash M. Clinical associations of 560 cases of motor neuron disease. J Neurol Neurosurg Psychiat 1990;51:778–784.
4. Mulder DW, Howard RM. Patient resistance and prognosis in amyotrophic lateral sclerosis. Mayo Clin Proc 1976;51:537–541.
5. Lacomblez L, Bensimon G, Leigh PN, Guillet P, Meininger V (for the Amyotrophic Lateral Sclerosis/Riluzole Study Group II). Dose ranging study of riluzole in amyotrophic lateral sclerosis. Lancet 1996;347:1425–1431.
6. Oliver D, Borasio GD, Walsh D, eds. Palliative Care in Amyotrophic Lateral Sclerosis (Motor Neurone Disease). Oxford University Press, Oxford, 2000.
7. Oliver D. Palliative care. In: Oliver D, Borasio GD, Walsh D, eds. Palliative Care in Amyotrophic Lateral Sclerosis. Oxford University Press, Oxford, 2000:23–28.
8. Borasio GD, Sloan R, Pongratz DE. Breaking the news in amyotrophic lateral sclerosis. J Neurol Sci 1998;160(Suppl. 1):S127–S133.
9. Miller RG, Rosenberg JA, Gelinas DF, et al. (and the ALS Practice Parameters Task Force: Practice Parameter). The care of the patient with amyotrophic lateral sclerosis (an evidence-based review): report of the Quality Standards Subcommittee of the American Academy of Neurology: ALS Practice Parameters Task Force. Neurology 1999;52:1311–1323.
10. Gallagher D, Monroe B. Psychosocial care. In: Oliver D, Borasio GD, Walsh D, eds. Palliative Care in Amyotrophic Lateral Sclerosis. Oxford University Press, Oxford, 2000:92–103.
11. O'Brien T, Kelly M, Saunders C. Motor neuron disease: a hospice perspective. Brit Med J 1992;304:471–473.
12. Oliver D. The quality of care and symptom control—the effects on the terminal phase of ALS/MND. J Neurol Sci 1996;139(Suppl):134–136.
13. O'Gorman B. Physiotherapy. In: Oliver D, Borasio GD, Walsh D, eds. Palliative Care in Amyotrophic Lateral Sclerosis. Oxford University Press, Oxford, 2000:105–111.
14. Kingsnorth C. Occupational therapy. In: Oliver D, Borasio GD, Walsh D, eds. Palliative Care in Amyotrophic Lateral Sclerosis. Oxford University Press, Oxford, 2000:111–117.
15. Wagner-Sonntag E, Allison S, Oliver D, Proseigel M, Rawlings J, Scott A. Dysphagia. In: Oliver D, Borasio GD, Walsh D, eds. Palliative Care in Amyotrophic Lateral Sclerosis. Oxford University Press, Oxford, 2000:62–72.
16. Smith RA, Gillie E, Licht J. Palliative treatment of motor neuron disease. In: de Jong JMBV, ed. Handbook of Clinical Neurology, Vol. 15: Diseases of the Motor System. Elsevier, New York, 1991:459–473.
17. Mazzini L, Corra T, Zaccala M, et al. Percutaneous endoscopic gastrostomy and enteral nutrition in amyotrophic lateral sclerosis. J Neurol 1995;242:695–698.
18. Sykes N. End-of-life care in ALS. In: Oliver D, Borasio GD, Walsh D, eds. Palliative Care in Amyotrophic Lateral Sclerosis. Oxford University Press, Oxford, 2000:159–168.

19. Oliver D. Opioid medication in the palliative care of motor neurone disease. Palliat Med 1998;12:113–115.

20. Lyall R, Moxham J, Leigh N. Dyspnoea. In: Oliver D, Borasio GD, Walsh D, eds. Palliative Care in Amyotrophic Lateral Sclerosis. Oxford University Press, Oxford, 2000:43–56.

21. Gelinas D. Amyotrophic lateral sclerosis and invasive ventilation. In: Oliver D, Borasio GD, Walsh D, eds. Palliative Care in Amyotrophic Lateral Sclerosis. Oxford University Press, Oxford, 2000:56–62.

22. Borasio GD, Voltz R. Advance directives. In: Oliver D, Borasio GD, Walsh D, eds. Palliative Care in Amyotrophic Lateral Sclerosis. Oxford University Press, Oxford, 2000: 36–41.

23. Scott A. Foulsom M. Speech and language therapy. In: Oliver D, Borasio GD, Walsh D, eds. Palliative Care in Amyotrophic Lateral Sclerosis. Oxford University Press, Oxford, 2000: 117–125.

24. Gallagher JP. Pathologic laughter and crying in ALS: a search for their origin. Acta Neurol Scand 1989;80:114–117.

25. Abrahams S, Goldstein LH, Kew JJM, et al. Frontal lobe dysfunction in amytrophic lateral sclerosis. A PET study. Brain 1996;119: 2105–2120.

26. Iannaccone S, Ferini–Strambi L. Pharmacologic treatment of emotional lability. Clin Neuropharmacol 1996;19:532–535.

27. Newall AR, Orser R, Hunt M. The control of oral secretions in ALS/MND J Neurol Sci 1996;139(Suppl):43–44.

28. Giess R, Naumann M, Werner E, et al. Injections of botulinum toxin A into the salivary glands improve sialorrhoea in amyotrophic lateral sclerosis. J Neurol Neurosurg Psychiatry 2000;69:121–123.

29. Neudert C, Wasner M, Borasio GD. Patients' assessment of quality of life instruments: a randomised study of SIP, SF-36 and SEIQoL-DW in patients with amyotrophic lateral sclerosis. J Neurol Sci 2001;191:103–109.

30. Wasner M, Enody U, Borasio GD. Sexuality in patients with amyotrophic lateral sclerosis (ALS) and their partners. ALS 2001;2(Suppl 2):108.

31. McMurray A. Bereavement. In: Oliver D, Borasio GD, Walsh D, eds. Palliative Care in Amyotrophic Lateral Sclerosis. Oxford University Press, Oxford, 2000:169–181.

Chapter 9

Muscular Dystrophy and Related Myopathies

Ian Maddocks
Leon Stern

INTRODUCTION
**ISSUES ARISING IN THE TERMINAL
   CARE OF MUSCULAR DYSTROPHY**
The Site of Care
The Burden of Care
The Burden for Siblings
The Transition from Child to Adult Services
The Transition to a Palliative Care
   Approach

Multiplicity and Fragmentation of Care
The Management of Respiratory Failure
PRACTICAL ASPECTS OF HOME CARE
Introducing Palliative Care Services
What Palliative Care Services and Skills
   are Appropriate?
Assisting the Final Stages
Bereavement Support
SUMMARY

The management of muscular dystrophy and the various related myopathies presents particular challenges in the maintenance of effective professional oversight during the transition from adolescent to adult (which often entails a change in institutional and professional relationships) and in assisting caring family members face the inevitability of deterioration and death after long years of intense loving effort in the promotion of positive attitudes and optimal function. Some of the skills learnt in the more usual settings of palliative care can be appropriate to this situation, but sensitivity will be necessary if, in introducing them, they are regarded as appropriate only to the terminal phase. A broad coalition of professional skills will best meet the complex physical and emotional needs of patient and family as the terminal period draws on.

CASE HISTORY

B.S. and K.S. were siblings who both developed Duchenne muscular dystrophy. No family history

had been known, and the elder child, B.S., was not recognized as having the disease until he was three years old, when an apparent reluctance to walk and an increasing difficulty in running, getting up from the floor, and climbing stairs was noted. By that time his younger brother, K.S., had already been born, and the condition was diagnosed in him before he began to walk.

Progress of the disease differed in the two boys; in B.S. cardiac involvement was more apparent from the age of 14 years, evidenced by ECG changes and clinical signs of left ventricular failure. B.S. was regarded also as having a mild degree of intellectual disability. By the age of 16 years B.S. was confined to a wheelchair and had developed flexor contractures of hips and forearms and a marked scoliosis. Recurrent chest infections had precipitated many admissions to hospital. He had experienced progressive weight loss and had suffered frequent morning headache associated with sleep apnea and carbon dioxide retention at night. Nasal positive pressure ventilation was tried, but he tolerated the nasal mask poorly. Dyspnea was regarded as predominantly due to cardiac failure by this time, and exacerbated by pulmonary infection. During an episode of major respiratory difficulty he was admitted again to hospital, where active ventilatory support was initiated; tracheostomy was considered but declined by the family. Antibiotics were prescribed, but no improvement was apparent and after three days active ventilatory support was ceased at the request of the parents, and he died the following day.

K.S. remained able to walk for much longer than his brother, having had more active interventions during childhood, with muscle-strengthening exercises, passive stretching of muscles to counteract contractures, and several tendon-lengthening operations. At the age of 21 he was employed in a clerical position and had married a muscular dystrophy care attendant who maintained regular stretching and massage support at home. When his ventilation effort began to fail two years later, he was able to establish a regular regimen of nocturnal ventilatory support with bilevel positive airway pressure (BiPAP) at home, and access to a coughing ventilator which facilitated clearance of bronchial secretions, helping him to avoid recurrent pulmonary infection. He was later able to tolerate BiPAP throughout much of the day and night. K.S. and his wife were determined to avoid hospitalization. Increasingly they recognized that while he did not have the strength to manage without the BiPAP, and though it had allowed him to continue a considerable degree of normal functioning at first, it was now seeming to prolong his discomforts. One evening, therefore, the couple agreed to discontinue the ventilation, and with the use of small doses of oral and subcutaneous morphine he died at home in no obvious distress.

INTRODUCTION

The story of these siblings illustrates several features of the muscular dystrophies. The MOST common, Duchenne muscular dystrophy (DMD), is transmitted as an X-linked recessive trait, and so occurs predominantly in males; it occurs also as a spontaneous mutation, and 30% of cases will have no family history. The condition affects first the pelvic girdle muscles, later the pectoral girdle and upper limbs. Ocular, facial, and bulbar muscles are usually spared, and smooth muscle is not affected. The heart is commonly involved to some degree. Some degree of intellectual disability is observed in many cases. Death is usually the result of pulmonary infections and

respiratory failure, and occurs during late adolescence, fewer than 25% of those affected surviving beyond 25 years.

Other, less common, muscular dystrophies differ in numerous ways from Duchenne, as (for example): having a later onset, milder course, and longer life expectancy (Becker type); adult onset and affecting small muscles of the hand and face (dystrophia myotonica); affecting muscles of the face and shoulders (facio-scapular-humeral muscular dystrophy); or affecting both sexes (Erb type dystrophies). Some forms are found predominantly in one population group (e.g. severe childhood autosomal recessive muscular dystrophy in Tunisia, others in the Amish of the United States, or in particular family groups in Holland or North America).[1]

ISSUES ARISING IN THE TERMINAL CARE OF MUSCULAR DYSTROPHY

The two cases also exemplify some of those issues arising in the management of the condition during the final stages of its progressive course. Family concern usually has focused primarily on the maintenance of physical function, with a determination to extend length of life. A positive and encouraging attitude is encouraged in the face of progressive deterioration. Looking ahead to further disability and deterioration can be seen as negative thinking and will commonly be avoided. It will not be easy for either patient or caregivers to recognize openly the inevitability of death or speak about it or prepare for it. Such discussions are within the province of palliative care, and it is not surprising that relatively little liaison with palliative care is usually effected.[2,3]

Nevertheless, issues learnt by palliative care services in the care of terminal cancer have some relevance in the final stages of muscular dystrophy.[3]

The Site of Care

It is commonly felt that it is best for a child to die at home. One study found better adaptation and return to previous social involvement plus fewer pathological grief reactions in families who had managed their child's death at home, compared with families who had used hospital care.[4] Studies of child death in hospital have reported major grief reactions, clinical depression, work-related problems, marital discord, and school difficulty for siblings among family members. If families have come to rely upon emergency hospital care for the management of exacerbations of respiratory infection, they may have acquired a dependency on hospital care and have little confidence in their ability to undertake terminal care at home. Nevertheless, with appropriate equipment, practical education, and adequate support, the option of home death may be achieved with no greater stress than attends a hospital death, and be a source of real satisfaction and comfort for the caring family.

The Burden of Care

The physical burden of daily care at home is considerable and commonly falls disproportionately upon the mother. The emotional burden can be even more difficult. One component of that difficulty is the need to continuously redefine the illness and the changes which arise from the progressive nature of the child's condition. These can be new and frightening as terminal stages are reached, and carers may feel inadequate, unsure if they are able to do all that is necessary at this time. A mother may have to cope with the intrusion of additional equipment and new carers into the home and feel unable to give sufficient attention to her other children or herself. Knowledge of the genetic basis of the condition can lead to a persistent feeling of guilt and an anger which is hard to displace on others.

The patient may exhibit behavioral difficulties, and parents often feel ill-prepared or unsupported in offering appropriate developmental guidance. Marital conflict is common; divorce has been described in up to 24% of parents of children with DMD. Whether to tell the reality of the diagnosis to the affected child can be a source of great stress. Where more than one child is affected the repetition of events is particularly upsetting, and parents may feel blamed for having not availed themselves of genetic counseling or prenatal screening.[5,6]

The social effects of the diagnostic label, the prolonged time between diagnosis and death,

and the rehearsal and anticipation phenomena which must accompany a diagnosis in more than one child, also add to the burden for family caregivers. There is some advantage in bringing affected children together in special facilities to provide realistic encouragement, to facilitate education, and promote mutual support among family members. Close and helpful relationships will form, but the death of one child then affects all.

The Burden for Siblings

Siblings of individuals who have required consistent or increasing supportive care over long periods have their own long-term issues, feeling sometimes that their needs have been ignored, with the focus on the one child whose care takes such an effort by the family. Emotional stress has been reported in up to 60% of siblings, and the consequences of feeling passed over in the allocation of interest and attention in the family can continue for many years on into adult life.

The Transition from Child to Adult Services

As with all chronic pediatric conditions which continue on into adult life, a child with DMD who moves into the adolescent or adult age range may experience a break between pediatric and adult services and a change in supervision at the very time that physical deterioration begins to become more apparent. This can lead to the loss of a relationship with the physician and care team who best understand the individual and the family needs, and whose support might prove very welcome during the terminal phases of care, compounding the burden of care with a sense of isolation, of losing the supports which were previously so important. Adult services may be poorly versed in the necessary information about the disease, and less confident in meeting patient and family needs. At any stage of care, communication between the various professional services involved is of great importance, and the transition from the child service to the adult service, in particular, needs careful coordination, which has often been lacking.

The Transition to a Palliative Care Approach

For most of the course of DMD, extending over more than a decade, efforts are made to encourage, to the greatest degree, a full range of life experiences and a positive, active engagement with the disability. The discipline of controlling contractures with regular passive stretching exercises and prescribed periods of standing, and the judicious use of tendo achilles or tensor fascia lata tenotomy operations and night plasters are examples of the positive effects of skilled interventions which maintain a sense of holding back the inexorable progress of decline.[7] Family activity and identity can be largely defined by the condition and by the success of such interventions, and mothers will usually endeavor to make positive reports on progress.

Denial of reality is itself a form of coping. To then be asked to accept a previously denied reality—the inevitability of approaching death—can be a difficult and testing transition. Many health professionals whose work has been that of active encouragement will not be comfortable with the different role of assisting a family to cope with that inevitability and that grave prognosis. Yet it is a time when steady and skilled support and compassionate attention is much needed. Staff trained in palliative care are well-prepared to offer such skill and attention, but may be seen as a threat, a representation of death itself. If early referral can be made, before the threat of death seems imminent, the implementation of palliation may be better accepted if presented as 'supportive care'.

Multiplicity and Fragmentation of Care

Recurrent episodes of acute distress (as with respiratory infection) call for emergency and intensive measures undertaken in acute care settings. There is a separation from the long-term care which has been based principally in the home.[8] Who does the family call in times of uncertainty? Whom do they trust? If a palliative care team becomes involved, it may add to the confusion. The availability of a single key worker, possibly an experienced nurse, who is able to remain in contact with the family and the patient through successive crisis admissions and transfers to various sites of care, and who can coordinate, liaise, and advise, is a great advantage. In which service such an individual belongs may be irrelevant; the important thing is that he or she can maintain a comprehensive and coordinating role for the family, ready at all times to suggest and/or arrange further interventions, reviews, and strategies, as new features evolve.

The Management of Respiratory Failure

The decision to undertake assisted ventilation is one which calls for intensive preparatory counseling for both affected individual and family. Too often, however, the decision is taken in an emergency situation, and often by a physician who has not had prior opportunity to engage with either patient or family, or be aware of expressed preferences. If no advance preparation has been made and no advance direction is available, most physicians will feel obliged to initiate assisted ventilation. Once established, the suspension of ventilation will usually require a direct request by the patient, and often this is seen as very difficult, even impossible—a deliberate action to end life.

In approaching the decision about ventilatory support in the terminal stages, it is important that all the options are presented, if possible with sufficient time and consideration to prevent the decision having to be made in a crisis of dyspnea and hypoxia. Symptoms of headaches and tiredness will encourage intervention. A sleep study demonstrating a fall in oxygen levels and a rise in carbon dioxide during the night will be useful.[9] Preventive ventilation has not been shown to improve discomfort or prolong survival.[10] Where a special clinic has been established for the management of incipient respiratory failure, it has been possible to form guidelines for raising the issue of ventilation in advance and encouraging open discussion of the options of life-sustaining treatment or a natural death.[11,12] Because palliative care tends to focus on acceptance of a natural death and to avoid heroic interventions, staff from that background may need additional instruction so that they are ready to offer full and open advance consideration of supported ventilation. Not all individuals will choose mechanical ventilation, but for those who do, quality of life is often reported as improved. But situations change, and decisions also change:

> It ended up being a bit of a curse, I think, because it prolonged the suffering that he went through in the end. So many times he said...he wanted to take it off and you'd take it off and he'd be struggling to breathe. He'd get so angry with himself that he couldn't cope without it and then he'd have to have it straight back on again, because it was hard for him to breathe without it...I think he was wanting to move things along instead of having it drawn out, but he didn't have the strength to be without the Bi-PAP, and the Bi-PAP really did end up making the suffering longer. So it was wonderful at first, but then at the end it was really hard to stop, and made him suffer more. (Wife of a DMD patient)[3]

There is a transition from nocturnal ventilation to day periods being also necessary, and finally there may come a time when BiPAP is not sufficient to maintain adequate ventilation. Then tracheostomy with positive pressure respiration may be regarded as the only additional option. This is a difficult choice; it requires additional equipment and carer support, it further compromises quality of life (for example, through the need for tracheal suctioning), and it has been stated that 'patients almost invariably prefer non-invasive aids over tracheostomy for safety, convenience, appearance, comfort, facilitating effect on speech, sleep, swallowing and general acceptability'.[13] Although a respirator can be mounted on a wheelchair, the effort and cost involved in maintaining this level of care puts a considerable strain on patient, family, and carers.

PRACTICAL ASPECTS OF HOME CARE

The physical needs of young individuals with progressive muscle diseases call for readily available basic nursing skills, and do not require the regular involvement of trained professional staff. Caregivers with minimal formal training can be invaluable in assisting and relieving the family in the persistent demand for bathing, toileting, feeding, positioning, and mobilizing,

24 hours a day. They can quickly learn management of lifters and other equipment. But the balance of responsibility allocated between untrained carers and skilled professionals may need to shift as function deteriorates and assessment and management demands greater knowledge, skill, and confidence.[3] Less experienced caregivers can lose confidence and feel inadequate, fearful that they cause further distress to the patient, poorly prepared to cope with the death of one whom they have come to know intimately.

Introducing Palliative Care Services

Palliative care services usually support an individual and family members for a relatively short time, often an average of three to four months. Judging the appropriate time for referral to palliative care of a person with a long-standing chronic condition will always be difficult, and may only be accepted at the very last stages, when death is imminent, allowing little opportunity for palliative care staff to provide the support they would hope to give. On the other hand, if presented with an earlier referral, the palliative care inpatient unit may feel that it is being exploited in ways for which it was not intended.

One way of initiating a discussion about the terminal phases of a chronic condition is to invite consideration of advance directives concerning the type and level of care which will be sought, given progress of the condition and deterioration in function. In South Australia, the concept of 'good palliative care' orders as an alternative to 'do not resuscitate' orders has found wide support, and has the advantage of focusing on positive aspects of care—what will be done, rather than what will not be done.[14] When such a discussion is introduced, by whom and in what way demands great sensitivity and no small measure of experience.

What Palliative Care Services and Skills are Appropriate?

Palliative care services are familiar with death and dying, and should be able to convey a quiet sense of calm and acceptance in situations of great distress and anticipatory grief for those intimate with the dying patient. An ability to demonstrate compassion through presence, steadiness, listening, and waiting may be the major contribution of a palliative care professional. There is also useful experience in symptom control and family counseling for advanced cancer which can appropriately be brought to the final stages of care for a younger person with muscular dystrophy.

Palliative care staff need to recognize that their appearance in the care situation may be interpreted as a threat, as a symbol of an inevitable finale against which all effort has been mobilized over many years. One wife of a patient commented: 'When you're in a hospice, you know what a hospice is, don't you. They're reminding you that your're on your way out, and you don't need that.'[3]

If palliative care services are to be useful, therefore, it is important that their staff are sensitive to the long-standing emphasis on fighting back the decline of function. They should be well-informed about how the needs of patient and family are different from those of cancer patients, and should have opportunity to develop skills which can be recognized and accepted by client families. Those skills may be in the management and coordination of new services as symptom needs change in the terminal phase, in facilitating and supporting respite placements, in offering support to family members who find the reality of deterioration difficult to accept, in listening to siblings, and in arranging and participating in bereavement care.[2]

If a children's hospice is available, it may have been used for respite in the past, and can prove a desirable site for terminal care. If no such facility is available, if hospital care is not desired, and if home care has become too demanding, a decision must be made as to whether an adult hospice will be appropriate for the terminal care of children or adolescents.

Assisting the Final Stages

Hypoxia and carbon dioxide retention may be associated with an obtunding of awareness and consciousness, but there may also be times of choking, of panic, and of frantic ineffectual effort. The use of small doses of opioids, administered via an indwelling subcutaneous cannula or by a continuous subcutaneous infusion, will relieve respiratory distress without influencing prognosis noticeably. Doses as small as 1–2 mg and up to 5 mg every 2–4 hours, or 10–15 mg over 24 hours are suggested.[2] Alternatively, or in addition, small doses of an injectable benzodiazepine such as midazolam 2–5 mg every 2–4 hours, or 10–15 mg over 24 hours, will assist calm and relaxation.

Families may need reassurance that the aim and effect of such measures is to ease the course of what is now a final phase of care. The stigma sometimes felt by nurses of having administered 'the last injection', which was followed soon after by the death of the patient, may need to be addressed.

End-of-life decision making in muscular dystrophy and related myopathies has been little studied. Sensitive communication about the realities which will be faced, and the best opportunity to explore necessary decisions before they become urgent is clearly desirable. This is a skill learnt in palliative care, but the circumstances are different from those familiar to palliative care teams, and their approach requires careful modification if it is to meet the end-of-life issues in muscular dystrophy.

Bereavement Support

Bereavement care is well established in many palliative care programs but is often lacking in the support service for progressive disorders such as muscular dystrophy, and not provided for or funded as a responsibility of that service. When the 24-hour responsibility undertaken by family caregivers is removed by death, it is at the one time a relief, but also a trigger for a grief which can be powerful and persistent.

Support groups which gather together family members who have shared a common experience of prolonged care of a child and final loss of an adolescent or young adult may be one of the most effective ways of assisting the grieving process. In work with cancer, it has been found best to see such group work as a defined program, offering a 'course', with sessions which work through aspects of grief to a final 'graduation', perhaps to a less formal social environment which does not focus so intently on loss and grief, but still offers companionship and shared activity.

SUMMARY

There has often been a distance between neurology and palliative care which has prevented families caring for individuals with muscular dystrophy and other myopathies from availing themselves of the best available mix of supportive services. A flexible team approach is recommended, with the skills and resources of neurology, respiratory medicine, psychology, and palliative care working in harmony. This offers a comprehensive oversight with timely and appropriate interventions geared to patient and family need.

REFERENCES

1. Adams RD, Victor M, Ropper AH. The Muscular Dystrophies. Principles of Neurology. Chapter 50, p. 1414. McGraw Hill, New York, 1997.
2. Maddocks I. Palliative Care: A Guide for General Practitioners. International Institute of Hospice Studies, Adelaide, 2001.
3. Maddocks I, Stern L, Parker D. The Palliative Care of Advanced Muscular Dystrophy and Spinal Muscular Atrophy. Palliative Care Unit, Flinders University of South Australia, 1998.
4. Lauer M, Mulhern R, Wallskog J, Camitta B. A comparison study of parental adaptation following a child's death at home or in hospital. Paediatrics 1983;71:107–112.
5. Buchanan D, LaBarbera C, Roelofs R, Olson W. Reactions of families to children with Duchenne muscular dystrophy. Gen. Hosp Psych 1979;1: 262–268.
6. Botvin Madorsky J, Radford L, Neumann E. Psychosocial aspects of death and dying in Duchenne muscular dystrophy. Arch Phys Med Rehab 1984;65: 79–82.
7. Vignos PJ, Wagner MB, Karlinchak B, Katirji B. Evaluation of a program for long-term treatment of Duchenne muscular dystrophy. J Bone Joint Surg 1996; 78:1844–52.
8. Hilton T, Orr R, Perkin R, Ashwal S. End of life care in Duchenne muscular dystrophy. Pediatric Neurol 1993;9:165–177.
9. Khan Y, Heckmatt JZ, Dubowitz V. Sleep studies and ventilatory treatment in patients with congenital muscle disorders. Arch Dis Child 1996;74:195–200.
10. Raphael J–C, Chevret S, Chastang C, Bouvet F. Randomised trial of preventive nasal ventilation in Duchenne muscular dystrophy. Lancet 1994;343: 1600–1604.
11. Gilgoff I, Prentice W, Baydur A. Patient and family participation in the management of respiratory failure in Duchenne's muscular dystrophy. Chest 1989;95: 19–524.
12. Miller JR, Colbert AP, Osberg JS. Ventilator dependency: decision-making, daily functioning and quality of life for patients with Duchenne muscular dystrophy. Dev Med and Child Neurol 1990;32:1078–1086.
13. Bach JR, Ishikawa Y, Kim H. Prevention of pulmonary morbidity for patients with Duchenne muscular dystrophy. Chest 1997;112:1024–1028.
14. Maddocks I. Good palliative care orders. Palliative Medicine 1993;7:35–37.

Chapter 10

Epilepsy

Sabine Weil
Soheyl Noachtar

INTRODUCTION
EPIDEMIOLOGY
SUDDEN UNEXPLAINED DEATH IN
   PERSONS WITH EPILEPSY
EPILEPSY SYNDROMES
SOCIAL INTEGRATION

FAMILY PLANNING
Inheritance Risk
Complications and Adverse Outcomes of
   Pregnancy
Contraception
SUMMARY

Epilepsy is a chronic disorder which affects about 1% of the population and their relatives. Mortality in patients with epilepsy is nearly three times higher than in the standard population and includes causes such as trauma suicide and SUDEP (sudden unexpected death in epilepsy patients). Counseling about special risk situations is required. Social integration, education, employment, family planning, and family life are affected and may recurrently be impaired by epileptic seizures. Beside optimization of antiepileptic therapy, integrational work preventing social stigmatization of patients with epilepsy is a great challenge to physicians and lay groups.

Discussion

Special instructions were given to the parents of this patient in order to prevent seizure-related injuries or suffocation, including not to use big soft pillows, to avoid swimming, and to wear a crash helmet during clusters of seizures or when riding a bicycle. For many years no serious trauma-related injuries occurred. Further security measures (e.g. sleeping next to the patient, 24-hour observation) may have an enormous impact on both the patient's and the relatives' quality of life.

CASE HISTORY

A 30-year-old man had been suffering from epilepsy since his early infancy because of a chromosomal aberration. He was mentally handicapped and was attended lovingly by his parents. Every fourth to sixth month he had a cluster of generalized tonic clonic seizures, despite antiepileptic drug therapy. In October 2000 he was found dead in bed, lying in a supine position with a swollen tongue. Autopsy revealed asphyxia. Precise circumstances of this death have not been clarified retrospectively.

INTRODUCTION

Epilepsy is a chronic disorder comprising a large group of syndromes with the common symptom of epileptic seizures. Epileptic seizures are transient events due to epileptiform activity in the brain with hyperexcitabilitiy of neurons as underlying mechanism. Epileptic seizures are characterized by a variety of signs and symptoms, which depend on the area of brain involved in the generation and spread of the epileptic activity. For the list of different types see Chapter 18, Table 1. Most epileptic syndromes are characterized by different epileptic seizure types.

Table 10–1. **Etiology of Seizures**[8]

Idiopathic	Probably genetic
Symptomatic	
Neoplastic	Brain tumors, metastasis
Infectious	Encephalitis, meningitis, abscess
Vascular	Cerebral infarction, hemorrhage, sinus thrombosis
Toxic	Neuroleptics, penicillin, theophyllin, immunsuppressives, etc.; withdrawal of alcohol, benzodiazepines, or barbiturates
Metabolic	Disturbances of electrolytes, uremia, liver dysfunction, thyroid disturbances, hypoglycemia,etc.
Traumatic	Contusion, hemorrhages
Degenerative	Alzheimer's disease, leucodystrophies, etc.
Unknown	

Epileptic seizures can be caused by a variety of etiologies affecting the cerebral cortex directly or indirectly (Table 10–1), some of which are age dependent. Epilepsy is defined as spontaneously recurring epileptic seizu——res. Thus, single epileptic seizures occurring exclusively in the setting of another brain or systemic disorder is not considered epilepsy. Most genetic and metabolic etiologies of epilepsy usually manifest in early life, whereas degenerative brain disorders, and vascular and neoplasms are more common in the older age group.

EPIDEMIOLOGY

About 5 % of the population sustain an epileptic seizure at least once in their life. However, only 0.5%–1% of the population have recurrent seizures and thus chronic epilepsy.[1] The prevalence is age dependent, with peaks in early childhood and old age.[2] Following neurovascular diseases, epilepsy is the second common group of neurological diseases. About 60% of epilepsies are focal and 40% are generalized (see below).[3] Although most patients with epilepsy respond well to medical treatment and become seizure free (60%–70%), about 20%–30% of patients with epilepsies continue to have seizures despite maximum tolerable doses of antiepileptic drugs (AED).[4]

Mortality in patients with epilepsy is nearly three times higher than in the standard population.[5] This is due to trauma during seizures or status epilepticus (serious drops, drowning, asphyxia, etc.), hypoxia during status epilepticus, or an unknown cause named SUDEP (see below). A few epilepsy syndromes, such as West syndrome and Lennox–Gastaut syndrome, are associated with poor prognosis and high mortality rate. The prognosis of focal epilepsies depends on the underlying etiology. Major malformations of the brain like hemimegencephaly and lissencephaly, and epilepsies due to severe congenital metabolic disorders, usually occur in early life and respond poorly to medical treatment. Epileptic status in these patients occurs frequently and constitutes a major life-threatening condition.

Counseling about special risk situations (swimming, hiking in exposed locations, etc.) should be done carefully.

SUDDEN UNEXPLAINED DEATH IN PERSONS WITH EPILEPSY (SUDEP)

SUDEP is a recognized though not well understood phenomenon. In the typical case, a person with a history of seizures is found dead in bed or elsewhere at home and autopsy does not disclose physical evidence for the cause of death. Commonly the death is attributed to epilepsy, asphyxia, or heart failure, even though no evidence exists to determine the cause.[6]

In a large cohort with 4578 patients, Walcazak et al.[7] found a incidence of 1.21

per 1000 patient years with a female preponderance. Generalized tonic clonic seizures, polytherapy with more than two antiepileptic drugs, and full-scale IQ less than 70 were independent risk factors of SUDEP. This constitutes another reason to avoid polytherapy and systematically try to reduce seizure frequency. As no specific prevention of SUDEP is known, patients and relatives should only be confronted with the SUDEP risk on special demand in our opinion.

EPILEPSY SYNDROMES

Epileptic syndromes are divided into focal and generalized epilepsies.[8] Identification of the epilepsy syndrome and its underlying etiology determines the therapy and prognosis. Therapeutic conceptions in general, and in palliative care, are discussed in Chapter 18 on epileptic seizures. Table 10–2 lists the commonly accepted epileptic syndromes. Epileptic syndromes usually have different etiologies. For the assessment of prognosis and therapeutic options the etiology is crucial.

Table 10–2. **Epilepsy Syndrome Classication[8]**

Focal epilepsy
Temporal lobe epilepsy (TLE)
   Mesial TLE
   Neocortical TLE
Frontal lobe epilepsy
   Supplementary sensorimotor epilepsy
Perirolandic epilepsy
Parieto-occipital lobe epilepsy
Rassmusen syndrome
Benign focal epilepsy of childhood

Generalized epilepsy
Absence epilepsy
Juvenile myoclonic epilepsy
Grand mal epilepsy
West syndrome
Lennox–Gastaut syndrome
Progressive myoclonic epilepsy

SOCIAL INTEGRATION

Patients with epilepsy frequently encounter social stigmatization, which may lead to depression, impaired self confidence, and social isolation. Seizure occurrence is usually unpredictable, which therefore usually impairs patients' independence. On the other hand, overprotection by the patient's family is a common phenomenon. Social integration is a great challenge to physicians, social workers, and lay groups. The main tasks are optimization of antiepileptic therapy (best seizure control with avoidance of side effects), optimization of education, vocational guidance, and knowledge about legal assistance.

Disabling seizure with loss of consciousness and motor manifestations precludes patients with epilepsy from a number of jobs. A common error is to assume that computer screens generally precipitate seizures. In fact this is a rare phenomenon restricted to patients with photo- or pattern-sensitive epilepsy syndromes. Counseling the patients and employers is very important in these cases.

FAMILY PLANNING

In general epilepsy is no impediment to family planning. There are however a few points which should be discussed with the patients.

Inheritance Risk

Considerable evidence supports a genetic contribution to the etiology of epilepsy. This is particularly true for idiopathic generalized epilepsies and the benign focal epilepsy of childhood. Furthermore, a genetically transmitted susceptibility seems to exist in symptomatic epilepsies.[9] A number of studies have determined the prevalence of epilepsy in relatives of affected patients. If one of the parents suffers from epilepsy, the overall risk for a direct offspring to develop epilepsy is 3%–12% and is higher in parents with idiopathic generalized epilepsies than in parents with focal epilepsies. If both parents have epilepsy, the inheritance risk increases to about 25%.[11,12]

Complications and Adverse Outcomes of Pregnancy

The children of mothers with epilepsy are at greater risk for a variety of adverse outcomes of pregnancy. Fetal death and perinatal mortality rates were slightly elevated for infants of mothers with epilepsy versus controls (10% versus 9% and 21% versus 15%, respectively).[13] Infants of mothers with epilepsy exposed to AEDs in utero have a greater risk of developing congenital malformations than do non-exposed infants of mothers with or without epilepsy.[10] The overall risk of birth defects in exposed infants is between 4% and 6% and is twice as high in exposed than in unexposed infants.[13]

All commonly used AEDs cross the placenta and are present in the fetal circulation. They are associated with more or less congenital malformation. Specific major malformations have been described for valproic acid, which is associated with a 3% risk for spina bifida—a risk which seems to be lowered by folic acid supplementation during early pregnancy. Generalized convulsions pose a risk of maternal injury and miscarriage.

Although women with epilepsy have an increased risk for complication during pregnancy, more than 90% of women with epilepsy will have a normal delivery of a healthy child.[13,14] However, maternity care and delivery is best performed in hospitals with close co-operation of obstetricians, neurologists, and pediatricians.

Contraception

If women with epilepsy choose to take oral contraceptives, liver enzyme induction due to antiepileptic drugs such as carbamazepine or phenytoin has to be considered, which may lower the estradiol levels and thus the contraceptive effect.

SUMMARY

Although epilepsy is a chronic, potentially disabling disease, most epilepsy patients, with adequate medical and social care, can live a normal life. In severely handicapped epilepsy patients, relatives need special counseling and support.

REFERENCES

1. Keränen T, Riekkinen P. Severe epilepsy: diagnostic and epidemiological aspects. Acta Neurol Scand 1988;57:7–14.
2. Hauser AW, Annegers JF, Anderson EV, Kurland LT. The incidence of epilepsy and unprovoked seizures in Rochester, Minnesota. Epilepsia 1993;34:453–463.
3. Gastaut H, Gastaut JL, Concalves e Silva GE, Fernandez Sanches GR. Relative frequency of different types of epilepsy: a study employing the classification of International League against Epilepsy 1975;16:457–461.
4. Juuel Jensen P. Epidemiology of intractable epilepsy. In: Schmid D and Morselli PL, eds. Intractable Epilepsy. Raven Press, New York, 1986:5–11.
5. Henriksen P, Juul–Jensen P, Lund M. The Mortality of Epileptics. Epilepsy and Insurance. Social Studies in Epilepsy, Vol. 5. International Bureau for Epilepsy, London, 1967.
6. Tennis P, Cole TB, Annegers JF, Leestma JE, McNutt M, Rajput A. Cohort study of incidence of sudden unexplained death in persons with seizure disorder treated with antiepileptic drugs in Saskatchewan, Canada. Epilepsia 1995;36:29–36.
7. Walczak TS, Leppik IE, D'Amelio MD, et al. Incidence and risk factors in sudden unexpected death in epilepsy. A prospective cohort study. Neurology 2001;56:519–525.
8. Lüders HO, Noachtar S, eds. Atlas of epileptic seizures and syndromes. W.B. Saunders, Philadelphia, London, New York, 2001.
9. Treiman LJ, Treiman DM. Genetic aspects of epilepsy. In: Wyllie E, ed. The Treatment of Epilepsy: Principles and Practice, 2nd Ed. Williams & Willkins, Baltimore, 1996:152–153.
10. Holmes LB, Harvey EA, Coull BA, et al. The teratogenicity of anticonvulsant drugs. N Engl J Med 2001;344:1132–1138.
11. Annegers JF, Shirts SB, Hauser WA, Kurland LT. The risks of seizure disorders among relatives of patients with childhood onset epilepsy. Neurology 1982;32:174–179.
12. Doose H, Baier W. Genetic factors in epilepsies with primarily generalized minor seizures. Neuropediatrics 1987;18:2–64.
13. Yerby MS. Treatment of epilepsy during pregnancy. In: Wyllie E, ed. The Treatment of Epilepsy: Principles and Practice, 2nd Ed. Williams & Willkins, Baltimore, 1996:785–798.
14. Practice parameter: management issues for women with epilepsy (summary statement). Report of the Quality Standards Subcommittee of the American Academy of Neurology. Neurology 1998;51:944–948.

Chapter 11

Pediatric Neurology

Eric Bouffet
Phyllis McGee
Deryk Beal

In pediatrc neurology, the time taken for the transition into palliative care differs according to the underlying disease (e.g. brain tumor, CNS degenerative disease, neuromuscular disorders). Symptom management, to alleviate, for example, nausea, constipation, convulsions, or pain, is paramount. Whereas the management of pain does not differ much from adults, it is expressed very differently by children, and may just present as a 'too quiet a child'. Communication with a neurologically impaired child may be an everlasting struggle for relatives and caregivers. For this, setting up new communication systems may be very helpful. Other issues in neurologic palliative care for children are intellectual deterioration, swallowing impairment, and withdrawal of life-sustaining medical treatment.

CASE HISTORY AND DISCUSSION

A seven-year-old boy presented to the Pediatric Brain Tumor Clinic with evidence of tumor progression eight months after diagnosis with a diffuse intrinsic pontine glioma. At diagnosis, he had been treated with six weeks of radiation therapy. During the course of radiation, his symptoms had resolved, and he spent an uneventful six-month period going to school, playing hockey, camping and traveling during the summer with his family. At follow-up, two weeks prior to the aforementioned clinic, he had been symptom free with a normal neurologic examination. Since one week prior, he was having symptoms similar to those he had had pre-diagnosis; he was emotionally labile, tired, sad, withdrawn, with short episodes of sudden laughing in his sleep, loss of confidence in his ability to play hockey, and complaining of occasional double vision, headache, and dizziness. His neurologic exam was normal except for nystagmus in the lateral gaze and a brisker left-sided Achilles reflex. MRI confirmed tumor progression.

The parents were presented with the fact that most children with diffuse pontine glioma succumb within three months from the time of clinical progression, and that surgery and re-irradiation were not an option because of the location of the tumor and the previous radiation treatment. His parents wanted to know what else could be done, stating 'We can't give up, what else can we try?' Low-dose dexamethasone was started with the aim of achieving some attenuation of symptoms. Palliative chemotherapy with temozolomide was offered, to which parents agreed with some reluctance, fearing side effects at a time every minute was precious. The parents also wished to explore alternative therapies, which was not discouraged. The dexamethasone was weaned quickly once chemotherapy was started because of the unwanted side effects of weight gain and emotional irritability. Referrals were made to community health services for palliative care and to a local hospice for family support. A weekly conference call was made between the parents, social worker, staff physician, and clinic nurse to review symptoms, alter interventions, support parents in their grieving, and reaffirm the care they were giving their son.

The first course of chemotherapy did not alter the progression of the neurologic symptoms. As the tumor progressed, behavioral and neurologic symptoms increased. Initially, he had anxiety and temper tantrums that were attenuated somewhat by hydroxyzine. He voluntarily wore an eye patch for double vision. Codeine was prescribed for headaches. A bowel regime of lactulose and bisacodyl was established. He had a steady loss of mobility from clumsiness, to unsteadiness, to crawling, to left-sided paralysis, to complete paralysis. His parents learned how to turn and position him, and transfer him from the bed to a wheelchair. Communication became increasingly frustrating as he lost the ability to speak. A referral was made to the speech language pathologist to assist the family in implementing alternative communication strategies, such as the use of a picture board and eye blinking. With the loss of speech also came difficulty in handling fluids and secretions. Transdermal scopolamine was used to minimize secretions and transdermal fentanyl was used with good effect for pain control. Near the end, fluids offered on a sponge were a source of comfort.

The child was extremely limited physically, though still intellectually sharp. He expressed the wish to see a fashionable play with his family. His wish was supported by a local charity. He went to the play in an ambulance, saw the play lying on a couch, and could achieve his dream a few days before his death despite his extreme neurologic handicap. Just before his ninth birthday he died at home, surrounded by his family, three months after the tumour progressed, eleven and a half months following diagnosis.

The concept of a dying child has become part of the unthinkable in our western industrial society.

Death is associated with a label of failure, and modern medicine often challenges its own limits in refusing patients the right to die peacefully. The right to die with dignity is, regardless of the age, the primary objective of the care to the palliative patient. The death of a child is associated with an emotional component and a feeling of discomfort and deception which make attempts at heroic resuscitation a tempting solution. Acknowledging the palliative status of a child is to some extent a success. Providing appropriate palliative care is another challenge for caregivers, as information and training is limited and the number of professionals with expertise in this area is small.

Amongst the variety of palliative care situations, the care of children with primary neurologic illnesses is unique and deserves special consideration.

PALLIATIVE CARE IN NEUROLOGIC DISEASES: ETIOLOGY

Classifying pediatric health states into subcategories has many advantages and some limitations. In our context—the palliative care of the child affected by a neurologic illness—the extent of the neurologic disorders involved may vary according to whether this definition includes only primary neurologic diseases and neurodegenerative disorders or, more broadly, any illness which alters the function of the brain. As an example, a child with a brain tumor will qualify according to these criteria, whereas a child with a primary bone tumor and secondary brain metastases may not. In this chapter, we will focus on the main issues associated with the care of a dying child with progressive neurologic deterioration, regardless of the etiology.

Brain tumors account for a significant subgroup, making up 25% to 30% of all childhood cancers. The survival rate in childhood brain tumor still lags far behind survival rates observed in many other malignant conditions such as lymphoma and leukemia. Brain tumors continue to be the leading cause of death by cancer in children less than 15 years old. Some brain tumors, such as diffuse pontine gliomas, are still incurable and their management will be palliative from the time of diagnosis.

The grouping of other CNS degenerative processes is complex, as they represent an enormous range of neurologic diagnoses, individually rare, but accounting for a significant number of children in total.[1,2] Batten's disease, adrenoleukodystrophy, and metachromatic leucodystrophy are the most common diagnoses of progressive degenerative neurologic disease. Some neuromuscular disorders such as Duchenne's muscular dystrophy are reported under the neuromuscular label and may be included in this list, as some features of their palliative care are not dissimilar from other children affected with primary neurologic degenerative diseases.

Care at the end of life in children with neurologic diseases may differ according to their etiology. In oncology, in most situations, a transition between therapeutic and palliative care can be established, which determines the main focus of the intervention. For an oncology patient, the decision to offer another trial of chemotherapy may be a temptation for the physician and/or the family, even when cure is not the endpoint. The morbidity of this intervention may affect the quality of the palliative care, and there is a fine line between a positive (even unsuccessful) phase I or phase II experience and unacceptable toxicity. In chronic neurodegenerative diseases, no clear transition between therapeutic care and palliative care can be demonstrated, and the care provided at the end of life is a mixture of preventive, therapeutic, and palliative care. Unlike the chemotherapeutic option, therapeutic interventions available for children with neurodegenerative disorders have relatively low morbidity. Parents will favor the continuing use of anticonvulsants to better control seizure activity if their child has severe epilepsy. The use of antibiotics may be potentially effective for chest or urinary tract infections. The discontinuation of standard treatment for common complications of the underlying illness is not a care paradigm or prerequisite for appropriate palliative care.

SYMPTOM MANAGEMENT

No symptom is specific to palliative children with neurologic illness. Convulsions may be observed in all palliative circumstances, whether or not the child has a primary neurologic illness. Pain may or may not be an issue, with some children experiencing complex and sometimes uncontrolled thalamic or neuropathic pain, especially oncology children. When the child's condition is acknowledged to be, or becomes palliative, the original diagnosis often becomes secondary, with a new need to concentrate on the child's symptoms. As an example, the use of a CT or MRI scan will become exceptional during the palliative care of a child with a brain tumor. Symptom management becomes more a priority than the documentation of the underlying cause. Symptoms may be related to the primary disease itself, or to adverse effects of the treatment, or to incurrent illness. The understanding of the symptoms and the assessment of the discomfort caused by these symptoms may be limited by communication difficulties (see the section 'Communicating with neurologically impaired children') or the age of the child.

Pain (see table overleaf)

Pain is expressed differently in children, and a child who does not complain is not necessarily pain-free (see Chapter 19). Chronic pain can cause developmental regression and immobility. Physicians and nurses should always question pain control in a 'too quiet child'. Specific pain assessment tools have been developed in recent years but no, or limited comparison, is available between these tools, and the choice depends on the child's age, the clinical situation, and the physician's experience.[3,4]

As far as pain management is concerned, there is no difference between children and adults with relation to the drugs used for pain management and their indications, especially with regard to the opioids. One of the limiting factors may be that some opioids are not licensed for pediatric use in some countries, especially with infants. Many physicians nowadays bypass these outdated regulations as there is an extensive literature providing evidence of benefit at any age when simple to strong analgesia is required. The route for strong opioids is oral (by mouth or via nasogastric tube), intravenous (IV), subcutaneous, transdermal, or by suppository. The starting dose is prescribed according to the child's age and weight, but there is no upper dose limit

Table 11–1. Dosage of Common Analgesics, Co-analgesics, and Anti-sickness Medications Used in Pediatric Palliative Care, According to the Route of Administration

	Dose Orally	Dose IV	Dose sc
Pain			
Paracetamol	Maximum 60 mg/kg/day		
Dihydrocodeine	0.5–1 mg/kg/4 hours		
Morphine	Starting dose: 0.1–0.25 mg/kg/4 hours	Starting dose: 0.02–0.05 mg/kg/day	Starting dose: 0.02–0.05 mg/kg/day
Co-analgesics			
Amitriptylline	0.5–1.0 mg/kg/day		
Carbamazepine	5–10 mg/kg/12 hours (start at 2.5 mg/kg/12hours)		
Gabapentin	10 mg/kg/8 hours (start at 10 mg/kg/day)		
Dexamethasone	0.2 mg/kg/day	0.2 mg/kg/day	
Nausea, vomiting			
Methotrimepazine		0.25–05 mg/kg/day	0.25–05 mg/kg/day
Haloperidol	25–50 micrograms/kg/day	50 micrograms/kg/day	50 micrograms/kg/day
Metoclopramide	300 micrograms/kg/day	300 micrograms/kg/day	
Cyclizine	3 mg/kg/8 hours		3 mg/kg/day
Dexamethasone	0.2 mg/kg/day	0.2 mg/kg/day	
Ondansetron	0.2 mg/kg/8 hours		

and dose adjustments are made according to the child's needs (Table 11–1). Overall, there is no such thing as a standard dose of morphine and no rigid guideline for pain management in the dying child.

The route of administration may change as the clinical condition evolves. Swallowing disorders or persistent vomiting, for example, may affect the intake of oral analgesics. The physician should be aware of dose conversions from oral morphine to IV (usually the dose is divided by three) and conversion from oral morphine to transdermal fentanyl patch. Active morphine metabolites are excreted renally and accumulate in the case of renal impairment. Neuropathic pain may require specific medications for symptoms such as burning, stabbing, or shooting, which tend to show little or incomplete response to opioids. Drugs active on neuropathic pain (Table 11–1) include antiepileptics such as carbamazepin or gabapentin, or antidepressants such as amitriptyline. There is evidence of synergism between opioids and drugs used for neuropathic pain, and pain control often requires a combination of both agents. In refractory neuropathic pain,

IV infusion of ketamin has been proposed with apparent success.[5]

Muscle spasms are common in children with neurologic illnesses and can be extremely painful. Muscle relaxants such as diazepam are offered as a first option, and can eventually be combined with dantrolene and/or baclofen.

When communication is impossible with a comatose child, symptoms such as agitation, sweating, or grimacing should be considered as a possible manifestation of pain. Routine continuous subcutaneous administration of opioids is never excessive in that context. The recommended starting dose of morphine when pain assessment is limited or impossible is 0.5–1 mg/kg/day.

The use of steroids in palliative patients with brain tumors may be useful for pain control.[6] Steroids may also produce temporary neurologic improvement when new symptoms develop. Various schedules and doses can be considered, such as daily low dose, pulsed high doses, or daily high doses. The side effects of the prolonged administration of steroids, especially when used at high doses, are the main limits of their use during palliative care.

The cosmetic effects of massive weight gain, 'moon face', and stretch marks can be devastating to the child's self-esteem and eventually the parents' recollections during their bereavement process. Steroid-induced behavior changes, especially aggressiveness, are also common in children, and may ultimately affect the child's and family's quality of life, despite some evidence of neurologic benefit.

Constipation

As a common complication of immobility in a child with a primary neurologic illness, constipation may become a serious adverse problem (see Chapter 24). Other factors, such as the use of opioids, low-fiber diet, and low fluid intake may contribute to severe constipation. The recording of bowel motions and regular use of laxatives and stool softeners are recommended in order to avoid acute discomfort when action has not been taken preventively. The help of a dietician is helpful in providing advice on diet and fluid intake.

Nausea and Vomiting

Nausea and vomiting are commonly experienced problems in the dying child. Their cause may be multifactorial—raised intracranial pressure, brainstem dysfunction, chronic constipation, pain, medications (chemotherapy, opioids)—and this should be taken into account in the plan for management. Medications should be chosen according to the presumed cause of vomiting. Metoclopramide is often prescribed as a first-line medication, but the incidence of extrapyramidal side effect during chronic administration in children is a limiting factor. Haloperidol and methotrimarazine are used for drug-induced and metabolic causes. Oral cyclizine is the drug of choice for raised intracranial pressure related vomiting. For children with severe uncontrolled vomiting, the use of regular ondansetron may be beneficial. Drug combinations may be necessary, especially in children with brain tumors with chronic increased cranial pressure. When oral administration is not possible, cyclizine and/or haloperidol are

the drug of choice and can be administered intravenously or subcutaneously.

Sialorrhea

Sialorrhea and drooling are secondary to swallowing disorders and can be responsible for considerable discomfort, skin irritation, loss of self-esteem, and social embarrassment. Transdermal scopolamine can be used to reduce the amount of secretion. However, the side effects of this anticholinergic medication may lessen the benefit of the reduction in sialorrhea. Finally, regular mouthwashes may aid the prevention of infections, especially in children receiving steroids.

Convulsion

Epilepsy may be pre-existing in relation to the underlying neurologic illness or seizures may develop as the child's condition deteriorates (see Chapter 18). In any case, a seizure is a distressing event, especially when the family has opted for home palliative care. Children with known epilepsy are generally on anticonvulsants, but their use in children who may develop a seizure is not routine. If the risk of seizure is considered to be significant, an emergency package and specific training in administering diazepam rectally is always a useful prevention. For children with severe and prolonged seizures, midazolam or phenobarbitone can be administered subcutaneously through a syringe driver or a pump and the dose adjusted to achieve optimal control.

Alimentation

Most children with neurologic impairment experience swallowing difficulties (see Chapter 16). The inability to feed their dying child may become an additional source of guilt for parents. In the case of severe swallowing impairment, withdrawal of hydration and nutrition may become an issue (see Chapter 32). The implementation of such a decision requires intensive attention to the child's comfort. There is no published information on the effect of dehydration on the comfort of the dying child, but the decision to withdraw alimentation, especially fluids, may be traumatic for parents and affect them in their grieving process.[7]

COMMUNICATING WITH NEUROLOGICALLY IMPAIRED CHILDREN

As the child shows more neurologic impairment, his capacity to communicate with his loved ones may become affected (see Chapter 17). Determining whether the child is in pain, thirsty, or uncomfortable, or generally trying to ascertain what he wants, is an everlasting struggle for relatives and caregivers when communication is altered. This difficulty may be related to either a limitation in speech, limitation in the ability to understand or use language, or degradation in intellectual capability. The difference between the former and the latter sometimes may be difficult to accurately appraise and the situation may change as palliative care evolves.

Communication difficulties deserve specific consideration as management of the child's symptoms requires a good understanding of his personal feelings. Communication skills may be impaired with or without concomitant intellectual or cognitive impairment. In either situation, the guidance of a speech–language pathologist is key in setting up new communication systems. There are many options, according to the physical capability of the child. The use of a computer is often suggested, but other confounding handicaps may limit the possibility of using the keyboard. Simply asking the child to write his ideas on paper is also used, but may be confounded by his ability to use language, his intellectual capacity, or his motor skills. If a child is unable to speak, write, or point, auditory scanning of the alphabet may be used. This technique involves the parent or caregiver reciting the alphabet and the child indicating with a signal (e.g. blink, hand squeeze) when the desired letter is reached. The parent or caregiver records the letters on paper, spelling a word or short sentence. Lip reading may be used when a child is intubated and unable to produce voice but retains the motor ability to posture the speech pattern for words on his lips. Eye gaze towards letters of the alphabet, words, or pictures may be used to communicate if the child is unable to talk or point. One may remember the book 'The Diving Bell and the Butterfly',[8] which highlights the sometimes phenomenal discrepancy between physical limitations and intellectual sharpness.

This time-consuming exercise is an essential part in the palliative care of neurologically affected patients. The skills of the speech–language pathologist are essential to supporting the child's communication with the family during the dying process.

This limitation in communication may affect the family work on the approaching death. To tell the truth regarding the coming death is always more difficult to achieve in practice than in theory, and the presence of speech or language difficulties may impinge on the family desire and ability to deal with this issue. Physicians must remind parents that feelings can be well understood through non-verbal communication and that they will not be judged for what they have said or not said. There is always a fine line between what the parents can say and will not accept to say, based on their culture, their recognition of the situation, their persisting expectations, the family set up, and many other factors. Physicians can often provide only limited support and accurate advice, and the help of social workers and/or psychologists is often critical.

REHABILITATION

Advanced disability results in bed rest and subsequent aggravated physical weakness. Children may require specific equipment such as a wheelchair, a hospital bed, and/or a stair lift to fulfil their physical requirements. The role of rehabilitation in palliative care has been established, and its benefit demonstrated.[9,10] The goal of rehabilitation in patients with neurologic impairment has to be tailored to each individual situation. Regular needs assessment by the rehabilitation team and appropriate modifications may help to adjust the environment to the patient's requirements. Range of motion exercise and regular frictions can help prevent pressure sores, muscle spasms, and joint stiffness. Massages contribute to better pain control and can be taught to the parents at the bedside.

HOME OR HOSPITAL?

Although the spectrum of underlying neurologic illnesses is diverse, the principle and the spirit of care is the same for all terminally ill children. Most children wish to spend the time remaining at home.[11] Admission to hospital may be dictated by medical requirements, social constraints, inadequate home health-care support, or cultural issues. The difference between health-care systems with regard to the site of care is striking, but the reasons for these differences remain unclear. More than 70% of children admitted to a palliative care program in England or the United States die at home, compared to 30% in Canada.[12]

When home is the site chosen for palliative care, the development of a care plan is essential, acknowledging that most of the care at home is provided by family members. The choice of the medications, the route of administration, the frequency of diagnostic tests, if necessary, and the organization of follow-up visits are prerequisites for a successful care plan. Planning ahead in anticipation of potential problems such as pain, seizures, swallowing problems, is important, especially in the context of home palliative care. It may be helpful to prepare the family for the process of dying, with practical explanations on the changes in breathing patterns, heart rhythm, or skin coloration, in order to reduce their anxiety. When home care is offered, the family and the community services should ideally have 24-hour access to expertise in pediatric palliative care and immediate access to hospital if needed.

OTHER ISSUES

Assistance to a palliative child may involve many different activities including music therapy,[13] art, and school.[14] These activities will give the child a short-term objective and reduce his fears and anxiety. The intellectual deterioration may be a limiting factor to these activities.

Many families wish to consider complementary therapies during the palliative care of their child. The hope is often that complementary medicine will achieve what conventional medicine has failed to achieve. There is also some expectation that alternative therapies will improve the child's well-being and reduce his suffering. The role of the palliative care specialist should be to share the information and as much as possible to guide and advise families. Some families may be approached by questionable therapists who make unrealistic claims, charge high prices, and subject children to unpleasant treatments, and thus the primary physician should not consider complementary and alternative medicine as an exclusive and independent choice made by families.

WITHDRAWAL OF LIFE-SUSTAINING MEDICAL TREATMENT FOR CRITICALLY ILL CHILDREN

Advances in intensive care have resulted in successful management of many pediatric disorders including acute complications of chronic conditions. It is not exceptional to consider life-sustaining medical treatment for a patient who inevitably dies if such treatment is withdrawn. The decision to maintain or withdraw life-sustaining medical treatment should be made in the child's best interest, following an assessment of benefit and burdens. Such a decision requires a careful team approach with the opportunity for open discussion. Full parental comprehension is crucial, and the decision may involve additional family members, close friends, and/or spiritual advisors. The decision should take into account the medical situation, the treatment options, their risks and benefits; decision making issues on the one side, ethnic and cultural traditions, customs, beliefs, and values on the other side.

The decision to withdraw life-sustaining medical treatment is hardly ever an emergency. Parents should be supported in the decision-making process with advice and opportunity to discuss thoroughly the various options. In the process of decision making, assurance should be given that the fundamentals of care will be maintained despite the withdrawal of life-sustaining medical treatment.

SUMMARY

Providing care to a dying child is always a technical and emotional challenge. Children with neurologic illness have specific needs, which may affect their care and symptom management. The use of a palliative care consultation provides a way to address the needs of the child and his family. Even if a palliative care service is not available, a focus on reassessing the child's environment, advance directive planning, providing comfort, planning alternative communication with the patient, limiting futile and painful medical interventions, as well as providing psychological support to the family, could facilitate an improved end-of-life care experience for the child and the family.

REFERENCES

1. Feudtner C, Hays RM, Haynes G, Geyer JR, Neff JM, Koepsell TD. Deaths attributed to pediatric complex chronic conditions: national trends and implications for supportive care services. Pediatrics 2001;107(6):E99.
2. Feudtner C, Christakis DA, Connell FA. Pediatric deaths attributable to complex chronic conditions: a population-based study of Washington State, 1980–1997. Pediatrics 2001;106:205–209.
3. Collins JJ, Devine TD, Dick GS, et al. The measurement of symptoms in young children with cancer: the validation of the Memorial Symptom Assessment Scale in children aged 7–12. J Pain Symptom Manage 2002;23:10–16.
4. Collins JJ, Byrnes ME, Dunkel IJ, et al. The measurement of symptoms in children with cancer. J Pain Symptom Manage 2000;19:363–377.
5. Klepstad P, Borchgrevink P, Hval B, Flaat S, Kaasa S. Long-term treatment with ketamine in a 12-year-old girl with severe neuropathic pain caused by a cervical spinal tumor. J Pediatr Hematol Oncol 2001; 23:616–619.
6. Glaser AW, Buxton N, Walker D. Corticosteroids in the management of central nervous system tumours. Kids Neuro-Oncology Workshop. Arch Dis Child 1997;76:76–78.
7. Liben S. Pediatric palliative medicine: obstacles to overcome. J Palliat Care 1996;155:24–28.
8. Jean–Dominique Bauby. The Diving Bell and the Butterfly. Knopf Publishing Group: New York, 1998.
9. Santiago–Palma J, Payne R. Palliative care and rehabilitation. Cancer 2001;92:1049–1052.
10. Hopkins KF, Tookman AJ. Rehabilitation and specialist palliative care. Int J Palliat Nurs 2000; 6:123–130.
11. Liben S, Goldman A. Home care for children with life-threatening illness. J Palliat Care 1998;33–38.
12. Feudtner C, Silveira MJ, Christakis DA. Where do children with complex chronic conditions die? Patterns in Washington State 1980–1998. Pediatrics 2002;656–660.
13. Daveson BA, Kennelly J. Music therapy in palliative care for hospitalized children and adolescents. J Palliat Care 2000;16:35–38.
14. Bouffet E, Zucchinelli V, Costanzo P, Blanchard P. Schooling as a part of palliative care in paediatric oncology. Palliat Med 1997;11:133–139.

PART **2**

NEUROLOGIC OUTCOME AND PALLIATIVE CARE

Chapter 12

Persistent Vegetative State

Rudolf Töpper
Wilhelm Nacimiento

The term 'persistent vegetative state' was coined in 1972 and has since been used to describe patients who respond to stimulation only in a reflex way but show no signs of awareness. Diagnosis is made by repeated clinical examination. The two most common causes of the vegetative state (VS) are trauma and cerebral hypoxia following cardio-pulmonary arrest. The prognosis for patients in the VS depends on the time a patient has remained unresponsive. Overall, only 15 % of patients regain consciousness. Although neuro-physiological and neuroimaging studies have some prognostic value, there are no reliable prognostic markers which are able to predict the clinical outcome of patients in the VS. At present there is no medical treatment of proven efficacy in promoting clinical recovery in these patients. Good palliative care is the mainstay of therapy in VS patients. Additionally, the therapeutic concept of sensory stimulation has gained some popularity in the treatment of VS patients and is widely used in neurorehabilitation units.

The management of patients must always include the patient's family who should be provided with sufficient medical knowledge to understand the patient's condition. Because of the particularly poor prognostic outlook in patients who have remained in the VS for months and years, the issue of withdrawing life support therapy in these patients has been hotly debated in recent years. The question of whether or not to terminate treatment in VS patients is strongly influenced by the cultural background and cannot be answered on medical grounds alone. Guidelines and clinical practice, therefore, differ considerably from country to country.

CASE HISTORY

A 47-year-old man with no remarkable prior medical history collapses while playing tennis. After failing to palpate a pulse his tennis partner calls for help and immediately initiates cardiopulmonary resuscitation. An ambulance team arrives seven minutes later. ECG monitoring reveals ventricular fibrillation. Electrical defibrillation is applied, and the apneic and unconscious patient is intubated. An adequate cardial rhythm is finally achieved and the patient is rushed to a nearby hospital. On arrival the patient is severely acidotic and the ECG reveals signs of an extensive myocardial infarction. The patient is transferred to a coronary care unit, where immediate revascularization procedures are carried out successfully. The cardiopulmonary situation stabilizes over the following 24 hours, but the patient remains comatose. A CT scan of the head shows signs of cerebral hypoxia. A severe aspiration pneumonia develops which requires artificial ventilation. Antibiotic therapy is started. After seven days a tracheostomy is performed, and over the next three days the patient is weaned from the ventilator. However, the patient remains unresponsive. An EEG shows diffuse slowing bilaterally while median nerve somatosensory evoked potentials are present with decreased amplitude. A repeat CT scan three weeks later shows progressive cerebral atrophy. A consultant neurologist makes the diagnosis of a persistent VS and the patient is transferred to a specialized neurorehabilitation unit. Intensive physiotherapy is performed but the clinical condition remains unchanged. Four months later the patient is transferred to a long-term care facility. Sixteen months later he develops a severe pulmonary infection which is not treated pharmacologically. He dies from pneumonia without having regained consciousness. An autopsy is not performed.

Comment

This case illustrates the typical clinical course of a patient who develops a VS following cardiopulmonary resuscitation. The initial stages are characterized by intensive diagnostic and therapeutic procedures. As it becomes apparent that the neurologic situation remains unchanged, therapeutic interventions are increasingly restricted. This case also illustrates the lack of reliable prognostic indicators to determine the clinical outcome of patients in a VS.

INTRODUCTION

Trauma and cerebral hypoxia following cardiopulmonary arrest are by far the most common causes of the persistent VS. With the sophisticated rescue systems available in most developed countries, many patients survive accidents and cardiopulmonary arrests which would have been fatal 30 years ago. As the brain's hypoxia tolerance is limited many patients surviving the initial incident remain incapacitated by the cerebral consequences of hypoxia. The brain stem in general is more resistant to hypoxia than supratentorial structures such as the cortex. Following cerebral hypoxia structures essential for bodily homoestasis are likely to survive, whereas the structures responsible for cognitive functions are often permanently lost. The ensuing clinical syndrome, characterized by preserved brain stem function and loss of consciousness has been named the 'persistent vegetative syndrome'.[1]

As suggested in the case history, the prognosis regarding recovery of consciousness is rather poor in these patients, despite active rehabilitative efforts. Up to now there has been no therapy which effectively improves the course of disease. No reliable prognostic indicators are available which would enable the treating physicians to identify patients likely to show a more favorable outcome. The longer a patient remains in the persistent VS, the more unlikely it becomes that he will regain consciousness.[2,3] Because of the poor prognostic outlook for patients remaining in the persistent VS for months and years, concepts of withholding or withdrawing therapy in these patients have been discussed in recent years.

PROBLEMS OF TERMINOLOGY

The term best suited to describe the syndrome of the VS has been much debated. The term 'persistent vegetative state' was first used by Jennett and Plum in 1972 in an article which was entitled 'Persistent vegetative state after brain damage: a syndrome in search of a name'.[1] It was an attempt to describe the behavioral features of patients with severe brain lesions. The term 'vegetative state' was meant to describe a syndrome rather than a single clinical entity. The adjective 'persistent' has been the reason for some confusion among relatives and physicians caring for these patients because 'persistent' is often thought to be equal to 'permanent' or 'irreversible'. In Jennett and Plum's original article, however, the term 'persistent' was not meant to carry any prognostic meaning. Rather, they wished to characterize a clinical condition which has persisted for some time. Nevertheless, to avoid any prognostic implications it would be more prudent to speak simply of the 'vegetative state' (VS), a recommendation which we follow in this article. The term 'vegetative' has also been critizised as being derogatory and not appropriate for a human being.

Before 1972, when the condition under review was named the 'persistent vegetative state', a number of other terms such as 'neocortical death' had been used in the medical literature. In German-speaking countries the term 'apallic syndrome', which goes back to an article published by Kretschmer in 1940, is still widely used.[4] This term is derived from the Latin word 'pallium' meaning 'cortex' and suggests that a complete cortical loss is the pathological substrate of this condition. As we will review later in this article, both neuropathological and functional imaging studies have found evidence that this is not always the case.

Because of the negative connotations which many associate with the term 'vegetative state', a number of alternatives, such as 'prolonged postcomatose unawareness', have been proposed. None of these newer terms, however, have received wider acceptance. As the term 'vegetative state' is firmly established in clinical medicine, it is in our opinion always advisable for physicians to stress the descriptive rather than prognostic aspect of this term when communicating with people.

CONSCIOUSNESS AND AROUSAL IN NEUROLOGY

Before discussing the clinical presentation of the VS it is appropriate to devote a short paragraph to the concepts of consciousness, awareness, and arousal as they are utilized in clinical medicine. In neurology, the terms 'consciousness' and 'awareness' are often used synonymously. They describe the subject's ability to perceive, interact, and communicate with the environment. To be conscious presupposes that the subject is awake and can be aroused.

The brain stem and the thalamus play the key roles in the anatomy and physiology of arousal. The so-called 'ascending reticular activating system', including the formatio reticularis of the brain stem and its thalamic targets, has been regarded as the most important activating system in the brain. In recent years, however, there has been overwhelming evidence that the cerebral systems mediating arousal comprise of a variety of pathways using a whole range of neurotransmitters. Systems which play a role in the maintenance of wakefulness include cholinergic pathways from the brain stem to the basal forebrain, noradrenergic pathways from the locus coeruleus, and dopaminergic and serotonergic pathways from the brain stem.[5]

Conscious perception is supplied primarily by the co-ordinated activity of several cortical areas. This has been studied mainly in the visual system. Studies in patients with brain lesions have made a tremendous impact on our understanding of the neuroanatomy of visual awareness. Destruction of parts of the visual cortex may lead to visual perception without awareness, a phenomenon which has been termed 'blindsight'.

CLINICAL PRESENTATION

The essential clinical features of the VS are the loss of any meaningful cognitive responsiveness, the lack of awareness and, therefore, of consciousness, while spontaneous breathing and a range of reflex responses are preserved.

Patients in a VS are not able to interact with others in a meaningful way. That they are unaware of themselves or the environment can be assessed by the absence of meaningful voluntary behavioral responses to visual, auditory, tactile, or noxious stimuli. There is no evidence of language comprehension or language expression in these patients. Contrary to comatose patients, patients in a VS show evidence of periodic but irregular sleep–wake cycles. They show arousal responses to painful stimuli which include opening of the eyes, changes in the breathing pattern, and occasional grimacing. Autonomic functions including cardiovascular reflexes, temperature regulation, and gastrointestinal function are largely intact, but they are incontinent for stools and urine. Reflexive swallowing is usually possible, but in the absence of the voluntarily regulated initiation of swallowing, patients depend on a nasogastric tube or a percutaneous gastrostomy for adequate nutrition. Cranial nerve reflexes and spinal reflexes are also usually preserved.[2,3,6]

Table 12–1. **Summary of Behavioral Responses Compatible and Incompatible with the Diagnosis of a Vegetative State**

Behavior compatible with the vegetative state	Behavior incompatible with the vegetative state
• Random eye movements	• Patient fixates and follows objects in his visual fields
• Orienting responses to visual and acoustic stimuli	• Avoidance reactions to frightening gestures
• Random limb movements; flexor synergies to painful stimuli	• Co-ordinated motor responses (e.g. active grasping)
• Grimacing; yawning	• Appropriate facial emotional responses
• Occasional vocalization without evidence of language comprehension and expression	• Patient consistently follows simple commands (e.g. 'open your eyes', 'move your head')

Patients with persistent VS (PVS) show intact auditory and visual orienting responses. They do not, however, fixate a person or follow movements with their eyes. They also fail to react to frightening gestures.

Patients in the VS usually move their limbs in a non-purposeful way unless the limbs are paralysed due to other neurological conditions. Patterned movements, such as flexion synergies of the arms or legs, are sometimes observed in response to external painful stimuli.

Any evidence of voluntary movements or behavior must be taken as a sign of cognition and is therefore incompatible with the diagnosis of a VS. Any evidence of communication, in whatever form, between the examiner and the patient, including a consistent response to commands, also rules out the diagnosis. To make the diagnosis of a VS, careful prolonged observation is mandatory and should take into account the observations of nurses and family members (Table 12–1).

The diagnosis of cognitive ability in the presence of profound physical disability can be very difficult. Studies performed in neuro-rehabilitation units have found a considerable degree of misdiagnosis in patients admitted with the diagnosis of a VS. Physicians making the diagnosis of a VS should therefore be experienced in the appropriate assessment of brain-damaged patients. In addition, the diagnosis should only be made after a period of observation over several days.[7,8]

DIFFERENTIAL DIAGNOSIS

To make the diagnosis of the VS other disorders of consciousness must be differentiated.

Coma describes a brain state which is characterized by unconsciousness *and* a lack of arousal. Even the most vigorous stimulation cannot evoke awakening in these patients. Patients have their eyes closed and no cyclical sleep–wake changes are observed. To distinguish coma from brief transient states of unconsciousness such as syncope or concussion, the state of unconsciousness must persist for at least one hour. Coma results from structural injury to the brain's arousal mechanisms (described above) or from pharmacological anesthesia.

Akinetic mutism is a rare clinical syndrome which is due to extensive bilateral lesions of the frontal lobes or to lesions of the paramedian thalamic nuclei, the basal ganglia, or the basal forebrain. Patients are characterized by an absence of movement and a loss of speech. Wakefulness and consciousness are preserved in these patients, but in the absence of movements and speech, this can be difficult to detect. The ability to fixate the examiner is sometimes the only clinical sign of preserved consciousness.

Consciousness is also preserved in the locked-in syndrome (see Chapter 14). This rare neurologic condition results from lesions in cortico-spinal and cortico-bulbar tracts at the level of the pons. The bilateral pontine lesion leads to complete quadriplegia and pseudobulbar palsy. Due to the lack of voluntary movements it can be sometimes quite difficult to differentiate a locked-in syndrome from the VS. Patients with the locked-in syndrome have preserved vertical eye movements and sometimes preserved voluntary movements of the eyelid, which make communication via eye movements and blinks possible. A similar clinical picture can be seen in patients with severe inflammatory polyneuropathy with cranial nerve involvement, such as the Guillain–Barré syndrome.

Brain death is defined by the irreversible loss of all brain functions. In contrast to the VS, the brain stem is also affected, leaving the patient comatose and without brain stem reflexes. In most countries it is accepted that a person is dead when his or her brain is dead. The diagnosis of brain death should be made according to standard clinical criteria. After brain death has been diagnosed, organ removal for transplantation may be performed if consent is obtained from the next of kin.

These neurologic conditions of disturbed consciousness and/or arousal can usually be clinically differentiated from the VS. In selected cases, however, the use of brain imaging (CT, MRI) and neurophysiological methods (EEG, evoked potentials) may be helpful in the differential diagnosis.

DIAGNOSIS OF THE VEGETATIVE STATE

While protocols have been devised for diagnosing brain death, there has been no such protocol, either nationally or internationally, for the diagnosis of the VS. It is common practice that the diagnosis is made by a single physician who has no requirement either to justify the reasons for his diagnosis or to document the diagnosis. Since the diagnosis of the VS may determine the patient's future management, it is essential that the physician making the diagnosis is experienced in treating patients with altered states of consciousness.

The clinical assessment should only be performed when medical or pharmacological causes of sedation are excluded. The physician has, therefore, to take into account current medication with sedative effects, such as benzodiazepine, anticonvulsant drugs, and analgesics. The patient should not be septic, or in a state of cardiopulmonary shock, since these conditions are also known to severely reduce the level of consciousness. As it is known that patients in the VS undergo cyclic sleep–wake cycles, the examiner must be sure that the patient is not sleeping during the examination.

Wade and Johnston have published careful descriptions of the clinical approach to patients suspected to be in the VS.[9] To test for visual awareness, the examiner first must make sure that spontaneous eye movements are present and, by checking the pupil reflex, that the primary sensory pathways are intact. The examiner should then look carefully for signs of visual fixation or visual tracking of objects moving in visual field. To test language comprehension, the examiner has to establish whether loud noises cause general startle responses, as these are usually intact in patients in the VS. If this is the case, the examiner should give simple instructions to perform movements such as closing the eyes or moving the arm. Responses to other noises such as familiar voices or music must also be taken into account. Spontaneous motor activity such as grasping an object, co-operative motor responses during routine nursing, or appropriate facial emotional responses should be looked for. The examiner should not restrict himself to direct examination of the patient but should try to collect relevant information from both nursing staff and the family members. The examiner must be aware, however, that the interpretation of behavior by family members is often biased. Orienting responses to visual cues or noises may be mistaken for signs that the patient recognizes the visiting family members. It is therefore essential for the examiner to separate observation from interpretation.

The diagnosis of the VS may be difficult in patients who show equivocal signs of responsiveness. It has been established that there are no sharp boundaries between the VS and states of awareness. For conditions in which clinical examination has found signs of minimal awareness in one modality or the other, the terms 'low awareness state' and 'minimally conscious state' have been established. A definition and diagnostic criteria of the minimally conscious state has been published recently.[10]

NEUROPATHOLOGY OF THE VEGETATIVE STATE

The causes of the VS are manifold. In the majority of patients, the VS is the result of a traumatic or non-traumatic acute brain insult. Acute non-traumatic causes include hypoxic or ischemic brain injury resulting from cardiopulmonary arrest, prolonged hypotension, near drowning, carbon monoxide poisoning, or hypoglycemia. In addition to these acute forms of brain injury, the VS may characterize the end stage of progressive dementing conditions such as Alzheimer's disease, Creutzfeldt–Jakob disease, and some metabolic disorders in children such as ganglioside storage disease and adrenoleukodystrophy. Some severe congenital brain malformations such as anencephaly, lissencephaly, and severe microencephaly may also prevent the development of awareness and may therefore lead to the VS.

In cases with acute brain injury the structural changes responsible for the VS may be rather subtle. Although clinically the VS is characterized by a loss of cortical brain function, the underlying neuropathology in the majority of cases affects mainly the white matter and/or the thalamus.

Following blunt head trauma, autopsy cases with the VS are characterized by severe bilateral white matter damage secondary to diffuse axonal injury (DAI). DAI is difficult to diagnose with brain imaging techniques. In severe cases petechial hemorrhages in the white matter can be seen on CT scan, but DAI often goes undetected by imaging techniques. Histologically, the early stages of DAI are characterized by axonal retraction bulbs, with microglial scars and Wallerian degeneration appearing after longer survival times. Axonal damage is thought to be due to shearing strains secondary to angular accelerations of the head. In addition, focal lesions in the corpus callosum and in the rostral brain stem are common in these patients. Since the occurrence of thalamic damage is dependent on the length of survival, a transneuronal origin has been suggested as the cause of thalamic injury.

In patients with a VS due to circulatory arrest, laminar necrosis in the cortex and diffuse neural necrosis in hippocampal and thalamic structures is often seen. In selected cases the thalamus is disproportionally involved, with cortical lesions being limited and focal. In traumatic as well as non-traumatic acute brain injury cases the damage to the brain stem is rather small. Extensive brain stem damage typically results in coma and is usually fatal in a relatively short time.

The features common to acute cases of the VS are therefore extensive destruction of the white matter of the cerebral hemisphere as well as thalamic damage. Cortical dysfunction in the VS is mainly due to a disruption of connections between different cortical areas, as well as damage to afferent and efferent cerebral connections[11,12]

NEUROPHYSIOLOGICAL PROGNOSTIC EVALUATION

Considerable interest has been centered around the prognostic evaluation of patients in a VS. Recovery in VS patients must be differentiated into two categories: recovery of function and recovery of consciousness. Three factors seem to be relevant in the prognosis: underlying etiology; the results of neurophysiological studies; and structural brain imaging. Despite all efforts the prognostic value of these methods is still rather limited. The prognostic evaluation of patients in a VS has been carefully reviewed by the Multi Society Task Force on PVS.[2,3] Overall, only 15% of patients regain consciousness at some point after the insult, and recovery of function is mostly poor. Recovery of consciousness is unlikely in patients with traumatic brain injury who have remained in the VS for more than 12 months, although there have been occasional case reports of traumatic patients regaining consciousness after 12 months. All these patients, however, had a poor functional outcome. In patients with non-traumatic causes recovery is unlikely when patients have remained unresponsive for more than three months.

It is therefore reasonable to consider the VS as permanent after three months in patients with non-traumatic brain injury, and after 12 months in traumatic brain-injured patients. The experience in children is rather limited, but there do not seem to be important differences in the prognosis.

Neurophysiological studies have been used to aid in the prognostic evaluation in patients at early stages following brain injury. Somatosensory evoked potentials (SEP) are the most widely used neurophysiological test in patients in a VS.[13] The most reliable indicator is the bilateral absence of the cortically generated responses. If cortical SEP are absent within one week after the insult, then the recovery of consciousness is highly unlikely. However, many patients with preserved cortical SEP remain in the VS. It may therefore be concluded that the loss of cortical SEP is an indicator of a poor outcome, but preserved SEP may not be taken as an indicator of a favorable outcome. If the SEP are used for prognostic evaluation it is necessary to record the cervical N13 with electrodes over C2 to demonstrate intact somatosensory transmission up to the level of the brain stem. It has also been stated that SEP recording should not be obtained in the acute stage of the disease, in order to exclude transient dysfunctions. So far, however, this has not been studied in detail.

Motor evoked potentials obtained with transcranial magnetic stimulation may also serve as a prognostic indicator. Although larger studies have yet to be performed, the loss of cortically evoked motor potentials may indicate a poor prognostic outcome.

The EEG is of limited usefulness in the VS: EEG findings are unspecific. In most patients diffuse activity in the delta or theta band predominates, which is usually not attenuated by sensory stimulation. In some patients in the VS a continuous alpha rhythm is recorded which, unlike normal alpha activity, is not responsive to eye opening or stimulation. The various EEG types found in the VS have, however, no prognostic significance.

In conclusion, the combined use of some neurophysiological parameters (SEP, MEP) allows VS patients with a particularly poor prognosis to be identified at a relatively early stage of the disease.

IMAGING STUDIES

In recent years the results of imaging studies have contributed most to our increasing understanding of the VS. CT and MRI are valuable tools to visualize the extent of brain injury. A typical sequence of characteristic changes has been described following global cerebral hypoxemia. Loss of the normal grey-white matter differentiation is usually the first sign which can be detected with CT following cerebral hypoxia.[14] This is followed by signs of global brain swelling, which include compression of the lateral and third ventricle and the perimesencephalic cistern, as well as abnormal appearance of deep grey matter nuclei (Fig. 12–1). In some patients with anoxic encephalopathy, non-enhanced CT shows increased density of the falx, the

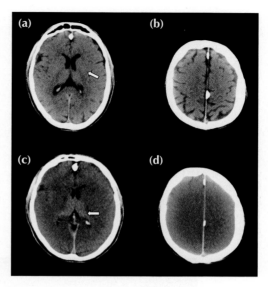

Figure 12–1. CT scans of a 40-year-old patient following cardiopulmonary arrest. Sixteen hours after the incident (a, b) there is discrete effacement of the basal ganglia (arrow in a). The brain parenchyma appears otherwise normal. Eight days later (c, d) there is massive swelling of the brain. With the exception of the thalamus (arrow in c) and the infratentorial structures (not shown), the parenchyma is hypodense with loss of the normal grey-white matter differentiation. After initial coma the patient has remained in the vegetative state for three years.

tentorium, and in the basal cistern, which can mimic the CT appearance of subarachnoid hemorrhage. These changes diminish over several days and atrophic changes, with widening of the ventricle and cortical sulci, appear over time. There are no established correlations between the results of imaging studies and the development of the VS. However, most patients who have not recovered consciousness have abnormal CT scans.

The use of newer MRI techniques, such as diffusion weighted imaging, may provide an earlier and more reliable indicator for the extent of neuronal damage following global cerebral hypoxemia.

Metabolic changes in patients in a VS have been studied using positron emission tomography (PET) and single photon emission computed tomography (SPECT). A global reduction of cerebral glucose consumption has been found in PET studies investigating patients in the VS.[15] This technique is not, however, able to make a reliable differentiation between functional inactivation and irreversible structural brain damage. To overcome this limitation a more recent study has used radioactively labelled benzodiazepine receptor ligands (flumazenil), the reduction of which has been found to be correlated with irreversible structural damage in stroke patients.[16] In VS patients who had a poor clinical outcome the flumazenil binding at cortical sites was severely reduced compared to normal subjects (Fig. 12-2).

New imaging techniques such as diffusion weighted MRI and PET scanning may, therefore, be used in the future as prognostic markers, in patients in a VS, at an earlier stage.[17] Before the use of these techniques for prognostic purposes can be recommended, however, rigorous prospective studies must be performed in well-defined patient populations.

A whole new field in the study of patients in a VS has been opened up with development of so-called 'activation studies'. Functional MRI and PET allow the imaging of specific task-related cortical and subcortical activations. These techniques may allow the objective assessment of residual cognitive function, which can be extremely difficult to perform clinically in VS patients with minimal motor responses. These methods have the power to demonstrate distinct and specific physiological responses to controlled external stimuli and may shed some light on the question of remaining awareness in VS patients.

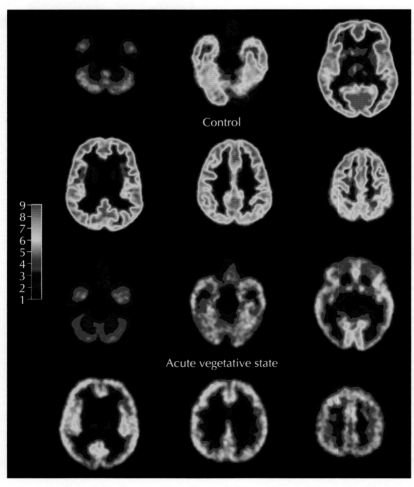

Figure 12-2. Cortical flumazenil binding in a healthy control and a patient in an acute vegetative state. Note that flumazenil binding is severely diminished in all cortical areas compared to the control subject. (Reprinted with permission from Rudolf et al. Lancet 2000;354:115–116).

In recent years some reports have found evidence for preserved residual cortical processing in VS patients. Laureys and co-workers studied a group of five VS patients who had a markedly reduced resting glucose metabolism.[18] During auditory stimulation (click stimuli) the primary auditory cortices were activated bilaterally, as revealed by PET. Compared to normal subjects, however, there was no evidence for activation in the auditory association areas located in the temporoparietal junction area. Another report described an activation in the right fusiform gyrus and extrastriate visual association areas in response to the presentation of familiar faces in a VS patient who recovered consciousness over the next months[19] These observed metabolic changes are therefore compatible with the presence of isolated modules of cognitive processing. In contrast to normal subjects these activations remain disconnected from higher order multimodal association areas, which makes it unlikely that the observed activations represent conscious perception. This preliminary evidence for isolated perceptual processes without awareness in patients in the VS may be comparable to the concept of blindsight in patients with visual cortex lesions.

What then constitutes awareness? Are specific and anatomically defined circuits necessary for consciousness, or is awareness dependent on the preservation of an adequate number of such functional modules? Is it possible that residual cognitive processing can be integrated enough to provide some level of consciousness, but still has no access to output? These are important questions for future research and will have both implications for the question of the biological basis of consciousness as well as ethical implications for the treatment of patients in a VS.[20]

INTERACTION WITH FAMILY MEMBERS

Active communication with famliy members and relatives is an essential part of the palliative care of patients in the VS. The burden which a VS patient imposes on a family cannot be overestimated. The relatives must be provided with a basic medical knowledge of the concepts of the VS in order to understand the patient's condition. Differences in the relatives' intellectual background must be taken into account when the medical facts are explained. It is important that relatives understand the distinction between a patient in the VS and a patient with brain death—two concepts which are often confused in public discussions. The relatives should be instructed that the patient's centers for the control of bodily functions such as breathing are intact but that his capabilities to interact, as well as all features which have characterized the personality of their loved one, have been compromised by the disease or the accident. It should be stressed that the patient is not aware of his condition and, despite possible signs of distress, is not suffering.

The inevitable question of prognosis is the most difficult to answer to relatives of patients in the initial stages of the VS. Since statistics are only rarely understood by relatives, information regarding the prognostic outlook should be balanced in a way that relatives are aware of the seriousness of the condition without leaving them with no hope. It is important to inform them that there are no diagnostic procedures available at present to make accurate prognostic statements and that there are, as yet, no effective treatment options to promote recovery.

Interaction with relatives requires a high degree of empathy in order to detect the hidden hopes and anxieties and to react accordingly. Professional psychological and/or spiritual counseling should be offered to all close family members.

If the patient does not regain consciousness within the first few weeks, issues of further treatment must be discussed with the relatives. The question of guardianship regarding medical as well as financial matters must be solved together with the family members. Ideally, a family member should take the responsibility as legal guardian of the patient. The question of transfer to specific rehabilitation units or to nursing homes must be discussed. Some families might wish to care for the patient at home. These families should be informed that care for a VS patient requires specific equipment such as hospital beds and a basic nursing expertise. Families also have to consider that patients in the VS, unlike terminally ill cancer patients, might live in this state for years. A family which plans to provide care for a VS patient at home must therefore be made aware of the enormous psychological as well as temporal burden which the patient's care places on them.

Information to relatives may be given by physicians or nursing staff. It is of paramount importance, however, that those giving information agree in their statements. Ideally, conversations with relatives should include members of the medical team and the nursing staff. In large families it may be advisable that the family chooses a 'speaker' who conveys the information given to him to the rest of the family.

MANAGEMENT

The issue of management in the VS has a number of different features. It includes aspects of pharmacological and behavioral methods to reverse the state of unconsciousness and medical treatment of the patient confined to the VS, as well as issues of terminating the treatment in patients in a permanent VS.

Treatment to Reverse the VS

At present there is no therapy available which has the proven effect of reversal of the VS. Studies have been performed to investigate the efficacy of L-dopa, bromocriptine, or amphetamines, but placebo-controlled or double-blind studies are up to now lacking. Since the published evidence for a pharmacological treatment is weak, specific pharmacological therapy in patients in a VS cannot be recommended at present.

There have been occasional case reports in the medical literature which have described successful deep brain electrical stimulation of different areas such as the mesencephalic reticular formation or the dorsal column of the spinal cord leading to patients in a VS subsequently regaining consciousness. These reports, which were published in the late 1980s and early 90s have not been substantiated by further case-controlled studies.

In contrast to medical therapy or electrical stimulation methods, the concept of sensory stimulation has gained a lot more popularity. Specific techniques are intended to 'stimulate' vegetative patients. The methods are aimed at achieving arousal, raising levels of consciousness, and promoting recovery. These techniques range from constant background stimulation, such as a radio or television, and the placement of items with a personal significance for the patient, to detailed multimodal stimulation programs. Published protocols describe one-hour sessions where vision, hearing, touch, smell, and taste are stimulated in sequence, separated by time for nursing care (polymodal stimulation). In other forms of treatment just one sense is selected, on a random basis, and is treated in any one session (unimodal stimulation). Each of the senses is stimulated up to the level at which responses can still be obtained. Visual stimulation, for example, includes shining a light into the patient's eye to induce pupillary constriction, inducing a withdrawal response by threatening movements, testing tracking responses by moving objects in the patient's visual fields, and, finally, letting the patient perform simple visual discrimination tasks. The level of responses to each sensory modality is recorded.[21]

The concept of sensory stimulation is based on the idea that such an 'enriched environment' promotes recovery of function. There is indeed evidence from human and animal research on the adverse effects of environmental deprivation, both for normal psychological development and for recovery from experimentally induced brain lesions in animals. The proponents of sensory stimulation have argued that a stimulating environment promotes synaptic re-innervation. A critique of sensory stimulation, however, has been that it leads to an increase of habituation, which as a result would generally diminish response capabilities.

Some form of sensory stimulation is practised in most rehabilitation units treating patients in the VS. It is conceivable that practising sensory stimulation increases the contentment of those caring for the patient. It has been argued that it is insufficient to care only for the maintenance of bodily functions, leaving other aspects of the human being unattended, which makes the practice of sensory stimulation also important for the patient's family. There is, however, no published evidence at present that sensory stimulation actually improves the clinical outcome in patients in the VS. Most studies which measured effectiveness of sensory stimulation are of limited value because of the lack of appropriate control groups and small sample size. Meaningful studies are urgently needed.[22]

Palliative Care

Palliative care consists of medical, nursing, social, psychological, and spiritual care, which all VS patients are entitled to receive. Good standards of nursing care should be applied to all chronically ill patients confined to bed. Prevention of pressure sores which may lead to infection is important. To control bladder function, the placement of a suprapubic catheter is usually indicated. Chronic constipation resulting in electrolyte disturbances should be prevented. In the initial phase of the VS, the patients are often in a hypercatabolic state with high nutritional demands. Adequate nutrition at this point is therefore important. The complications associated with long-term feeding via a nasogastric tube (e.g. gastric pressure ulcers) are usually prevented when a percutaneous gastrostomy is applied.

The majority of patients who develop a VS are initially comatose and require artificial ventilation. To secure long-term ventilation most patients undergo tracheotomy, which facilitates weaning from the ventilator, as well as nursing care of the airways. Tracheostomy care should be performed by experienced personnel. If bronchial secretions are not very distinct, the removal of the tracheostomy may be considered when the patient has sufficient spontaneous breathing.

Contractures should be prevented by physiotherapy performed over the passive range of movements.

The use of analgesics is a matter of controversy in VS patients. Clinical experience and neuropathological examination suggest that VS patients are unaware of pain. Since the nociceptive pathways in the spinal cord and the brain stem are usually intact, patients react to pain stimuli with a variety of behavioral motor reponses. These nociceptive responses do not, however, necessarily reflect the perception of pain. The conscious experience of pain is mediated by the integrated activity of different cortical areas. This makes it unlikely that patients in the VS are capable of experiencing pain. There are, up to now, no functional imaging data on pain processing in VS patients which could further substantiate this claim. Recommendations on using or withholding analgesics in VS patients are therefore usually based on the individual physician's judgment. If significant vegetative responses such as tachycardia or sweating in response to pain stimuli are observed, the use of analgesics may be appropriate to prevent vegetative hyperactivity.

Whether, and to what extent, concurring medical problems should be treated in VS patients depends on the prognostic evaluation of the patient. The decision to withhold active medical therapy such as antibiotics (in pneumonia) or anticoagulants (in deep venous thombosis) should only be discussed when all relevant information concerning the patient is available. The reliability of the prognostic assessment increases with increasing time of observation. It is recommended, therefore, to continue intensive therapy until prognostically relevant data such as CT scans and results of evoked potentials studies are available. In patients in a long-standing, potentially irreversible VS, on the other hand, it is common practice not to treat medical complications such as concurrent infections. Rare reports of patients surviving in a reasonably good condition are no argument for the continuation of aggressive medical therapy if the patient remains in the VS for a considerable amount of time. If the diagnosis of an irreversible VS can be made with a high degree of diagnostic certainty it is recommended that preventive therapy such as the subcutaneous application of heparin to prevent thrombotic disease should be terminated.

About 50% of the patients in a VS die within the first year. Most of these patients die within the first weeks. If, however, they survive the first three months, they may survive for years, with a life expectancy ranging from two to five years. Survival for more than 10 years is unusual. The causes of death include infection, the most common being pulmonary and urinary tract infection, generalized systemic failure, and respiratory failure.

Published data indicate that the life expectancy for children in the VS is much better. A large survey from the United States reported that 63% of children in the VS (3–15 years of age) had survived for more than eight years.[23]

Terminating Life Support Therapies

While it is commonly accepted that certain therapies, such as cardiopulmonary resuscitation, should be withheld in patients in a long-standing VS, the concept of withdrawing life support therapies such as nutrition is strongly debated. It has been argued that, in principle, there is no ethical difference between withholding and withdrawing therapy. As in other end-of-life decisions, cultural background and/or religious belief have strong influences on the decisions regarding therapy in VS patients. The attitudes of physicians regarding treatment of the VS vary from country to country. In some countries such as the United Kingdom, the United States, and the Netherlands, medical treatment, including nutrition and fluid substitution, may be stopped if diagnosis of a permanent VS is made. In other countries such as Japan, physicians are very reluctant to abandon therapy for patients in the VS. These differences are reflected in the physicians' therapy preferences if they themselves were in the VS. Whereas in the United States, only a small minority of approximately 10% of physicians would want artificial nutrition, in Japan, only 40% of physicians responding to a questionnaire would opt for the termination of their nutrition.[24] The question of terminating treatment in VS patients is therefore strongly influenced by the cultural background and cannot be answered on a medical basis only. It is ultimately a moral question, which must be discussed openly, from different professional perspectives. Such a discussion may ultimately lead to a redefinition of death, as some have advanced the opinion that the permanent loss of cognitive life should be considered equivalent to brain death.

There are also economic aspects which are often discussed when the issue of terminating treatment in VS patients is debated. Resources in medicine are increasingly limited in almost all countries. It has been argued that the allocation of resources to patients with an exceptionally poor prognosis is against the principles of medical ethics if other patients are denied effective beneficial therapy.

Discussions concerning therapy in VS must always include family members. One of the essential ethical principles in medicine is the patient's autonomy. In most patients in the VS, however, no written documents are available which would enable the physician to determine the patient's wish concerning continuation of therapy. It is therefore imperative to obtain information about the patient's presumed preferences in such situations. Oral evidence, as well as written advance directives, should be considered when the patient's presumed preferences are inquired about through the

relatives. It is appropriate to remind the relatives that it should be the patient's wishes, not their own preferences, which must guide the decisions regarding therapy.

The termination of medical treatment has been very openly debated in the United Kingdom where clear guidelines have been published which specify the procedure which leads to the termination of medical treatment in VS patients.[25] If a patient in whom a clear cause of the VS can be delineated remains in the VS for more than 12 months, the diagnosis of a permanent VS is made. In patients with global cerebral ischemia, the diagnosis of a permanent VS may be made as early as six months. After diagnosis of a permanent VS is made, active medical treatment may be stopped. Following a decision of the House of Lords in 1993, active medical treatment in the United Kingdom includes artificial nutrition and hydration. In order to stop medical treatment, a specific legal process must be followed. After discussing the significance of the diagnosis of the permanent VS with the family, the treating physician usually informs health authorities. The health authority's solicitor then contacts the official solicitor's office acting on behalf of the patient. The official solicitor will examine the applicant's evidence and conduct inquiries of the patient's family. In the court hearing which follows, the identity of the patient, the hospital, and the physicians directly involved are usually protected. Up until the year 2000, active medical treatment has been terminated in approximately 20 patients in the United Kingdom. After court approval has been given, further management remains with the treating physician. It is recommended that the patient should be transferred to a different location, where feeding tubes should be removed. It is not necessary to start intravenous fluids in these patients. This is based on the assumption that dehydration causes analgesia via the release of ketons and endogenous opiates. The patient usually dies within 14 days after withdrawal of artificial nutrition. During this time, staff caring for the patient, as well as family members, should be given emotional support by experienced personnel.

In the United States, termination of feeding is also possible if court approval and consent of family members is obtained. In the Netherlands, a law passed in 2001 decriminalized voluntary euthanasia, ending a paradoxical legal situation in which euthanasia performed by physicians was still subject to criminal laws but was not prosecuted when certain requirements were met. The requirements included the patient's formal voluntary request. Nevertheless, euthanasia has been practiced in incompetent patients including, although rarely, patients in the VS.

In Germany, the discussion is influenced by the crimes committed by physicians during the Nazi regime. Under a so-called 'euthanasia' program of racial purification, thousands of mentally handicapped and chronically ill patients were murdered. This devastating historical experience precludes the acceptance of guidelines which include active withdrawal of nutrition.[26] According to guidelines of the Federal Medical Council only the withdrawal of technical supports may be taken into consideration. Easing hunger and thirst is included in the basic support every human is entitled to. The patient's autonomy must, however, be respected. In cases in which it is the declared or presumed will of the patient not to remain in a state of unconsciousness for a indefinite period of time, the termination of artificial nutrition is possible after evidence has been evaluated in a court hearing.

SUMMARY

Since its introduction in clinical medicine more than 30 years ago, the concept of the VS has remained a valuable tool to describe a clinical entity consisting of severely brain-damaged patients who have an intact arousal system but seem unaware of their environment. Scientifically, the study of these patients has had considerable relevance for discussions concerning the neuroanatomical basis of consciousness. Both neuropathological and, more recently, neuroimaging studies in VS patients have been of help in our understanding of the function of the conscious brain.

In contrast to these advances in our understanding of the neuroanatomy of consciousness, the poor prognostic outlook for these patients has not improved over the years. At present there are no therapies of proven efficacy in promoting the recovery of consciousness. Since the majority of patients never regain consciousness, VS patients are at the center of an ongoing discussion over whether it is justified to terminate nutrition and hydration in a patient unable to communicate

his wishes regarding the continuation or termination of life support therapy. Cultural, religious, legal, as well as economic issues, play an important role in these discussions.

Patients in the VS are objects in a number of discussions. It should never be forgotten, however, that these patients are human subjects who deserve the full range of good palliative care.

REFERENCES

1. Jennett B, Plum F. Persistent vegetative state after brain damage. A syndrome in search of a name. Lancet 1972;1:734–737.
2. Multi-Society Task Force on PVS. Medical aspects of the persistent vegetative state. First of two parts. N Engl J Med 1994;330:1499–1508.
3. Multi-Society Tast Force on PVS. Medical aspects of the persistent vegetative state. Second of two parts. N Engl J Med 1994;330:1572–1579.
4. Kretschmer E. Das apallische Syndrom. Z. ges. Neurol Psychiatr 1940;169:576–579.
5. Schiff ND, Plum F. The role of arousal and 'gating' systems in the neurology of impaired consciousness. J Clin Neurophysiol 2000;17:438–452.
6. Zeman A. Persistent vegetative state. Lancet 1997;350:795–99.
7. Andrews K, Murphy L, Munday R, Littlewood C. Misdiagnosis of the vegetative state: retrospective study in a rehabilitation unit. Br Med J 1996;313:13–16.
8. Freeman E. Personal opinion: protocols for the vegetative state. Brain Injury 1997;11:837–849.
9. Wade DT, Johnston C. The permanent vegetative state: practical guidance on diagnosis and management. Br Med J 1999;319:841–844.
10. Giacino JT, Ashwal S, Childs N, et al. The minimally conscious state: definition and diagnostic criteria. Neurology 2002;58:349–353.
11. Adams JH, Graham DI, Jennet B. The neuropathology of the vegetative state after an acute brain insult. Brain 2000;123:1327–1338.
12. Kinney HC, Samuels MA. Neuropathology of the persistent vegetative state. A review. J Neuropathol Exp Neurol 1994;53:548–558.
13. Rothstein T. The role of evoked potentials in anoxic-ischemic coma and severe brain trauma. J Clin Neurophysiol 2000;17:486–497.
14. Kjos BO, Brant–Zawadzki M, Young RG. Early CT findings of global central nervous system hypoperfusion. Am J Radiol 1983;141:1227–1232.
15. Rudolf J, Ghaemi M, Ghaemi M, Haupt WF, Szelies B, Heiss WD. Cerebral glucose metabolism in acute and persistent vegetative state. J Neurosurg Anesthesiol 1999;11:17–34.
16. Rudolf J, Sobesky J, Grond M, Heiss WD. Identification by positron emission tomography of neuronal loss in acute vegetative state. Lancet 2000;354:115–116.
17. Arbelaez A, Castillo M, Mukherji SK. Diffusion-weighted MR imaging of global cerebral anoxia. Am J Neuroradiol 1999;20:999–1007.

18. Laureys S, Faymonville ME, Degueldre C, et al. Auditory processing in the vegetative state. Brain 2000;123:1589–1601.
19. Schiff N, Ribary U, Plum F, Llinas R. Words without mind. J Cogn Neurosci 1999;11:650–656.
20. Schiff ND, Plum F. Cortical function in the persistent vegetative state. Trends Cogn Sci 1999;3:43–44.
21. Wilson SL, McMillan TM. A review of the evidence for the effectiveness of sensory stimulation treatment for coma and vegetative states. Neuropsychol Rehab 1993;3:149–160.
22. Wood RL. Critical analysis of the concept of sensory stimulation for patients in vegetative states. Brain Injury 1991;5:401–409.
23. Strauss DJ, Ashwal S, Day SM, Shavelle RM. Life expectancy of children in vegetative and minimally conscious states. Pediatr Neurol 2000;23:312–319.
24. Asai A, Maekawa M, Akiguchi I, et al. Survey of Japanese physicians' attitudes towards the care of adult patients in persistent vegetative state. J Med Ethics 1999;25:302–308.
25. Wade DT. Ethical issues in diagnosis and management of patients in the permanent vegetative state. Br Med J 2001;322:352–354.
26. Schmidt P, Dettmeyer R, Madea B. Withdrawal of artificial nutrition in the persistent vegetative state: a continuous controversy. Forensic Science International 2000;113:505–509.

Chapter 13

Quadriplegia and Paraplegia

Walter A. Ceranski

THE SCOPE OF QUADRIPLEGIA AND PARAPLEGIA
Causes of Paralysis
Importance of Acute Management
Acute Stage Complications which can Affect Quality of Life
Functional Level of Injury
Clinical Syndromes

PALLIATIVE CARE
Pain Management
Management of Psychosocial Distress
Decisions Regarding Treatment of Complications
Areas for Research
SUMMARY

Since palliative care in the individual with quadriplegia or paraplegia involves a person with a stable deficit and a nearly normal life expectancy, it requires an understanding of the relationship between a variety of factors (such as level and mechanism of injury) and preserved function. To this end, this chapter begins with a review of those relationships. This is followed by an overview of complications of quadriplegia and paraplegia (along with comments regarding their potential impact on quality of life and productivity). This knowledge can assist in making informed decisions on how (and how aggressively) to treat these complications. Finally, some suggestions are made for areas of research which could contribute to the effectiveness of treatment. The hope remains that advances in research will lead to such restoration of function that the need for palliative care in the person with quadriplegia or paraplegia will no longer exist.

CASE HISTORY

Mr. J.P. is a 67-year-old male injured in a motor vehicle accident when he was 23. His injuries included a cervical spine injury, which resulted in paralysis of all myotomes below the C5 level, except for barely visible contraction of right wrist extensors. Sensory exam was intact to the C5 dermatome, with patchy areas of sensory preservation below (including the perianal area). He satisfies the American Spinal Injury Association (ASIA) criteria, endorsed by the International Medical Society of Paraplegia (IMSOP), of C5 quadriplegia with an impairment scale class B (incomplete).[9]

Neurogenic bladder was initially treated with a Foley catheter, but for the last 10 years he has had a suprapubic catheter. Urinary tract infections have been rare. Neurogenic bowel requires bowel care with glycerin suppositories and a specially formulated 10 mg bisacodyl suppository known as a 'magic bullet'. He takes ephedrine to mitigate postural hypotension and diazepam for muscle spasms. Following his initial hospitalization and recovery from spinal shock, he developed heterotopic ossification, ultimately leading to ankylosis of both hips. Mobility has been maintained with a motorized wheelchair, which he controls with a joystick. He is one of the unfortunate 5%–44% of the spinal cord injury (SCI) population with significant post-injury pain.

Over the ensuing years he has had multiple episodes of autonomic dysreflexia (AD), usually related to a plugged or kinked catheter. He finds these episodes terrifying. Following a dramatic increase in frequency of episodes of AD with no conventional source of noxious stimulus apparent, workup disclosed metastatic lesions in the lumbar vertebrae. The primary lesion was found to be prostatic cancer. Palliative radiation of the metastases has been successful in reducing tumor size and consequently the frequency of episodes of AD. He is now considered end stage and has been admitted to hospice care. His wife—his lifelong caregiver—has expressed a desire to keep him at home until his demise, but wants AD controlled at all costs.

Comment

Palliative care in the individual with quadriplegia or paraplegia presents a significant challenge. A considerable portion of the population with quadriplegia or paraplegia are paralyzed as a result of spinal cord injury. Those with demyelinating disease are the topic of Chapter 3 in this book. According to the American Paralysis Association about 90% of those with SCI who survive the acute injury have near normal life expectancy. For the person with quadriplegia or paraplegia, a large part of the lifelong treatment is palliative in nature, and palliative care in this population does not necessarily equate to end-of-life care. Even when presented with terminal illness (end-of-life care), the cause of approaching death is usually either a complication of the paralysis, the disorder causing paralysis (such as metastatic malignancy leading to spinal cord compression), or an illness completely unrelated to the injury. The challenge, then, is to maintain functional independence and even productivity over the course of a nearly normal life expectancy, while minimizing the impact of any incurable problems on quality of life.

THE SCOPE OF QUADRIPLEGIA AND PARAPLEGIA

Since knowledge of how injury level relates to function and quality of life is important in making decisions regarding palliative care, a discussion of some fundamentals of quadriplegia and paraplegia is appropriate.

Causes of Paralysis

The potential causes of damage to the spinal cord, which can result in quadriplegia or paraplegia include (but are not limited to):

- Direct trauma to the cord (motor vehicle accidents, acts of violence)
- Vascular events (ischemia, hemorrhage)
- External compression (neoplasm, spinal stenosis)
- Demyelinating disease (multiple sclerosis)
- Infection (poliomyelitis)
- Immune complex disorders (Guillain–Barré syndrome).

Of these, only neoplasm and demyelinating disease (both of which are subjects of previous chapters) are truly progressive disorders once the acute phase is concluded. The others can demonstrate deterioration of function with time, but this is usually related to such things as complications, intercurrent illness, and aging.

Importance of Acute Management

Since those with quadriplegia or paraplegia can, for the most part, look forward to a nearly normal life span during which they can remain productive, it is vital that preservation of function (which is a major factor in quality of life) be a high priority during management of the acute stage of injury. Some causes of quadriplegia and paraplegia have specific treatment aimed directly at the disorder (such as oncological management of neoplasms and intravenous immunoglobulins or plasmapheresis for Guillain–Barré). Decompression, along with stabilization of the spine, when appropriate, should be accomplished as quickly as possible. Since the publication of the National Acute Spinal Cord Injury Study (No. 2),[3] initiation of methylprednisolone (30 mg/kg intravenous loading dose given over 15 minutes within eight hours of injury, followed by 5.4 mg/kg/hr intravenously over the next 23 hours) within the first eight hours after acute traumatic spinal cord injury has been considered to be instrumental in preserving function. Methylprednisolone is thought to work by reducing swelling within the injured portion of the spinal canal, and possibly also by providing antioxidant neuroprotection. It should be noted, however, that the methodology and conclusions of this study are currently being questioned.

Acute Stage Complications which can Affect Quality of Life

DEEP VENOUS THROMBOSIS (DVT) AND PULMONARY EMBOLUS (PE)

Vigilance for DVT must be maintained. Physical findings are often unreliable. In an individual with quadriplegia, respiratory effort may already be impaired. A PE is not only life-threatening in the acute phase, but can also contribute to additional long-term impairment of pulmonary function. This can result in a significant diminution of quality of life. The risk of DVT diminishes (but does not disappear) after the first three months. While anticoagulation is appropriate in the acute setting, the reduced risk beyond the first three months generally tilts the risk:benefit ratio against chronic anticoagulation.

HETEROTOPIC OSSIFICATION (HO)

HO usually develops about a joint below the level of injury (usually the hips, knees, shoulders, or elbows) during the first few weeks to months after SCI and can progress for 1–2 years. It is clinically significant in 10%–15% of individuals with SCI (about 20%–30% are actually affected). Long-term functional impairment can result from skin breakdown (poor positioning, bony protuberances), decreased range of motion, or complete ankylosis of the affected joint. Etidronate has proven to be effective in preventing or retarding the development of HO, but apparently has no role in management of HO once it is established. Surgical intervention is sometimes indicated.

Functional Level of Injury

DETERMINATION OF LEVEL

Quadriplegia (although ASIA and IMSOP prefer the term tetraplegia, quadriplegia is probably in wider use throughout the world) is a result of damage to the cervical spinal cord leading to impairment of motor and/or sensory function in the arms, trunk, legs, and pelvis. Paraplegia is a result of damage to the thoracic, lumbar, or sacral spinal cord leading to impairment of motor and/or sensory function in the trunk, and/or legs, and/or pelvis (depending on level of injury), but not the arms.

NEUROLOGIC LEVEL

Sensory (dermatome) level is determined by testing pinprick and light touch. Position sense and awareness, and deep pressure and deep pain testing can also be helpful (as in Brown–Sequard syndrome), but are not used to determine sensory level. Motor (myotome) level is determined by testing muscle strength. Skeletal level is determined radiologically. Zone of partial preservation refers to those dermatomes and myotomes below a *complete* injury that demonstrate *some* preservation of function.

COMPLETE VS. INCOMPLETE INJURY

Any perceived sensation on digital rectal examination constitutes a sensory incomplete injury. Voluntary contraction of the anal sphincter constitutes a motor incomplete injury. ASIA has adopted an impairment scale based on the Frankel scale. ASIA A complete would have *no* sensory or motor function preserved in the S4–S5 levels. ASIA B incomplete has sensory preservation below injury level (*including* S4–S5). ASIA C and D incomplete have less or more motor function respectively preserved below injury level (*including* S4–S5). ASIA E denotes normal motor and sensory function.

HOW LEVEL AFFECTS FUNCTION

See Table 13–1.
- An injury *above C-4* usually results in ventilator dependency. A mouth stick can be used to control an environment control unit. This person is generally dependent on others for all other activities, but can direct care (can speak with cuffless tracheostomy).
- An injury at C5 will usually permit sitting (including shifting of weight and sitting up from a supine position) and rolling with minimum to moderate assistance. Moderate to maximum assistance is required for slide board transfers. Most other activities of daily living (ADLs) can be accomplished with the

Table 13–1. Relationship Between Injury Level and Retained Function

Injury Level	Breathing	Transfers/Turning	ADLs	Wheelchair (WC)/Driving	Ambulation
C-1 to C-3	Dependent on ventilator, phrenic pacer, negative pressure device, may 'frog breathe'	Dependent	Dependent: mouth stick for writing, page turning, environmental control unit	Power WC controlled with mouth, chin, tongue, 'sip & puff'; unable to drive a motor vehicle	None
C-4	Unassisted	Dependent	Dependent	Same as C–1 to C–3	Dependent on use of hydraulic standing frame
C-5	Unassisted	Assisted slide board transfers; dependent bed positioning	Assisted (with set up and equipment)	Manual WC (level surfaces) at home; power WC (joy stick control) elsewhere	Same as C-4
C-6	Unassisted	Independent transfers (except tub); assisted positioning	Independent	Manual WC (no wheelies, curbs); may drive motor vehicle (help getting WC in & out)	Moderate assistance with use of standing frame
C-7	Unassisted	Independent	Independent	Manual WC (some wheelies, no curbs); independent driving	Minimum assistance with use of standing frame
C-8 to T-1	Unassisted	Independent floor to WC	Independent	Manual WC (may do wheelies & curbs)	Independent use of braces, standing table
T-1 to T-4	Unassisted	Independent	Independent	Manual WC or ambulation with devices	May brace ambulate in parallel bars
T-4 to L-2	Unassisted	Independent	Independent	Manual WC or ambulation with devices	Long braces; crutches on level/ assisted on curbs, stairs, ramps
L-3 to L-4	Unassisted	Independent	Independent	Manual WC or ambulation with devices	Short leg braces/ crutches +/− at home, + away
L-5 to S-1	Unassisted	Independent	Independent	Ambulation	Braces +/−; may need cane

proper assistive devices and setup, except for lower extremity dressing, for which the individual is dependent.

- Self-catheterization is possible for most males at *C6*, and females at *C7*. Bowel care may require minimum assistance with adaptive equipment, or may be independent.
- *Below T1*, ambulation becomes more independent as the injury level gets lower.
- Those injuries *below T6* carry little to no risk of autonomic dysreflexia.

Clinical Syndromes

Central cord syndrome: Also known as the 'upside-down quad', is characterized by sacral sensory sparing with motor weakness greater in the upper extremities than in the lower extremities.

Brown–Sequard syndrome: Usually a result of hemisection of the cord. Proprioceptive and motor loss is more pronounced on the side ipsilateral to the injury than on the contralateral side, while pain and temperature loss is more pronounced on the contralateral side than on the ipsilateral side.

Anterior cord syndrome: Variable motor function loss is seen, accompanied by variable pain and temperature loss. Proprioception is not affected.

Conus medullaris syndrome: Injury is to the sacral cord usually causing loss of reflexes in the bladder, bowel, and lower extremities.

Cauda equina syndrome: Injury is below the level of the conus medullaris with losses similar to those seen in conus medullaris syndrome.

PALLIATIVE CARE

Pain Management

As previously stated, the management of pain in the person with quadriplegia or paraplegia is a challenge. Not only will the goals be somewhat different if the individual is not terminally ill, but management strategies are complicated by the complexity of causation of the various pain types seen in this population. Further, even in the absence of consciously perceived pain, the noxious stimulus emanating from such problems as bladder distension or bowel obstruction can serve as a trigger for an episode of AD. Chapter 19 deals with pain management in depth, but some discussion relevant specifically to quadriplegia and paraplegia is warranted.

In 1997, P.J. Siddall proposed a taxonomy, which should be helpful not only in management but in providing a common language for research into how to approach these pain types.[12,16] While he retains the familiar system-oriented categories (musculoskeletal, visceral, and neuropathic), he breaks neuropathic pain down into two categories based on site: 'at level' (the lowest segment with normal spinal cord function) and 'below level'. At level neuropathic pain is further broken down based on source: radicular and central. Finally, there is an 'other' category.

MUSCULOSKELETAL PAIN

Also known as somatic pain, this form of nociceptive pain is characteristically described as aching, dull, gnawing, or throbbing. It tends to be worse with movement and less when at rest. For mild pain or bone pain in the individual capable of tolerating them, non-steroidal anti-inflamatory agents (NSAIDs) remain the first choice. Corticosteroids also play a role. For those unable to take NSAIDs, other non-opioid analgesics, either alone or in combination with weak opioids such as propoxyphene, hydrocodone, oxycodone, or codeine, can be used. Care must be taken when using opioids to minimize the likelihood of resultant constipation.

VISCERAL PAIN

This is also a form of nociceptive pain, usually characterized as pressure, or as deep, dull, aching, cramping, or squeezing in nature. It is usually poorly localized. Prompt evaluation for a cause of visceral pain should be undertaken. If remedial action is appropriate, it should be accomplished quickly. In the absence of a reasonable remedy, non-opioid analgesics alone (although NSAIDs are usually not desirable) or in combination with weak opioids form a starting point. For pain unrelieved by the aforementioned, strong opioids (morphine, hydromorphone, levorphanol, methadone, meperidine, or fentanyl) are required. For special cases, such as pain from a stretched liver capsule, corticosteroids may be useful.

NEUROPATHIC PAIN

Also known as deafferentation pain, neuropathic pain in the quadriplegic or paraplegic is difficult to treat. Words frequently used to describe this type of pain include constant, sharp, burning, or squeezing. Often there are episodes of shooting, stabbing (lancinating), or 'electrical shock' type pain superimposed.[11]

In the case of 'neuropathic at level pain', that of radicular origin (emanating from the peripheral nervous system as opposed to the brain and spinal cord) can frequently be differentiated from that of central origin by an increase in pain on movement of the spine. In this form of pain, the treatment centers on relieving the cause of nerve root compression. What is not determined to be 'neuropathic at level radicular pain' is considered by Siddall to be 'neuropathic at level central pain'. 'Neuropathic below level pain' is central in origin.

First line management of central neuropathic pain in the absence of second degree heart block or a QRS duration >450 msec remains a tricyclic antidepressant (nortriptyline, desipramine, or amitriptyline). In the elderly, amitriptyline is the least desirable because of its relatively greater anticholinergic effect. If, after four weeks on any of the tricyclic antidepressants, satisfactory analgesia has not been achieved, addition of a second line agent (anticonvulsants: carbamazepine, or divalproate) is appropriate. Should the combination of first and second line agents fail, a trial of gabapentin is indicated (see Table 13–2).

At the Third IASP Research Symposium (held April 16–18 2001 in Phoenix, Arizona)[16] a broad range of therapeutic options were reported as being under investigation, but as yet they are not a part of mainstream management. Medications being evaluated include lamotrigine (Finnerup), topiramate (Harden), and gabapentin in combination with dextromethophan or ketamine (Sang). A model for cognitive-behavioral interventions was proposed (Wegener). Intrathecal administration of local anesthetics, opioids, clonidine, and baclofen, as well as clonidine and morphine in combination were discussed (Siddall). A surgical approach involving dorsal root entry zone coagulation (DREZ) was proposed by both Gorecki and Falci.

Table 13–2. **Treatment of Neuropathic Pain**

Drug	Initial Dose	Increase	Maximum Dose	Comments
First Line (Choose One)				
Nortriptyline	10 mg q HS × 5–7 days	10–25 mg q 5–7 days	50–100 mg daily	Less anticholinergic
Desipramine	10 mg q HS × 5–7 days	10–25 mg q 5–7 days	75–125 mg daily	Less anticholinergic
Amitryptyline	10 mg q HS × 5–7 days	10–25 mg q 5–7 days	75–125 mg daily	Most anticholinergic
Second Line (Add One)				
Carbamazepine	100 mg BID × 5–7 days	To 200 mg BID	200 mg TID	To TID only if serum concentration <8 mcg/ml
Divalproate	250 mg BID × 7 days	250 mg each week	500 mg TID	
Third Line				
Gabapentin	100 mg TID × 7 days	300 mg each week	600 mg TID	

OTHER PAIN

This category contains such identifiable types of pain as that associated with syringomyelia, the headache of autonomic dysreflexia, compressive mononeuropathies, and reflex sympathetic dystrophy. Each is treated when appropriate by addressing the underlying cause.

For the terminally ill patient it is acceptable to use strong opioid analgesics in adequate (i.e. high or rapidly increasing) doses. There is no ceiling dose for opioids. Morphine helps pain and breathing, and decreases anxiety. It should be titrated upwards to a level necessary to control pain. Sustained-release morphine sulfate in regularly scheduled doses (po, pr) can be augmented with elixir or tablets for breakthrough pain (q 1–2 hours). For subcutaneous infusion, divide the daily oral ms dose by two to get the daily subcutaneous (or IV) dose, then divide by 24 to get the hourly rate. Usually a 1:1 solution is administered unless very high doses are required.

Management of Psychosocial Distress

Early in the treatment of a person with quadriplegia or paraplegia, a great deal of emphasis is placed on optimizing those abilities still present as opposed to dwelling on those that have been lost. This creates a sense of ability instead of disability. As a result, those who internalize this concept are prepared to approach adversity by attempting to control their destiny rather than acting as victims. This can be an asset in care, but when control issues at the end of life lead to conflict with those caring for the individual, it becomes an impediment. Quality of life in the paralyzed individual is closely linked to mobility[2] (as an expression of independence) and control over the environment. Loss of this mobility and control frequently results in depression. Screening for depression should be undertaken and, when found, should be managed with therapies ranging from compassionate communication (involving nonprofessionals such as family, friends, clergy, and others), to professional counseling and antidepressants. When neuropathic pain is present, tricyclic antidepressants would be a logical choice, but attention must be paid to consequences of their anticholinergic side effects (for example, urinary retention or fecal impaction could trigger an episode of AD). Utilizing a team approach, including such as the clergy (bereavement and spiritual issues), a social worker (financial issues), a psychologist, and others, can serve to identify and address the variety of psychosocial stressors likely to be present.

Decisions Regarding Treatment of Complications

In order to properly inform a person with quadriplegia or paraplegia (or a surrogate decision maker) of the advantages and disadvantages involved in treating complications of paralysis, knowledge is required of the complications seen in these people and how they may be interrelated. Once properly informed, decisions can be made with regard to which complications are to be treated. The decisions made will also be heavily influenced by whether or not the individual is terminally ill and/or actively dying.

PRESSURE ULCERS

For preservation of quality of life, awareness of the risk factors associated with aggressive institution of measures to prevent skin breakdown are essential. The fundamental reason for skin breakdown from pressure ulcers is *ischemia*. The ischemia can be caused by pressure (resulting from immobility caused by the paralysis and loss of sensory input telling the brain of the need for pressure relief), as well as friction and shearing related to repositioning of the paralyzed individual. Malnutrition, when seen in quadriplegics and paraplegics, must be corrected in order to prevent (or heal) pressure ulcers. When present, pressure ulcers can contribute to malnutrition because valuable nutrients can be lost in the exudate coming from the ulcers. Incontinence and perspiration can provide a moist environment leading to skin maceration and increased risk for skin breakdown.

INFECTIONS

For the person with an injury at T6 or higher, one of the possible causes of AD is an infection below the level of injury. The most common infections seen in the paralyzed individual are urinary tract infections and pneumonia, as well as the cellulitis and osteomyelitis one might expect to see as a result of pressure ulcers.

SPASTICITY

Occurs in approximately 35% of paralyzed individuals, and spasms frequently are an indicator of an acute process such as infection, or a noxious stimulus capable of triggering AD. Treatment with such medications as baclofen, clonidine, diazepam, or dantrolene can often significantly contribute to an improved quality of life (see Chapter 15).

HETEROTOPIC OSSIFICATION

This subject is discussed in the previous section 'Acute Stage Complications which can Affect Quality of Life'. Non-steroidal anti-inflammatory agents are sometimes helpful for the palliative care of this complication.

OSTEOPOROSIS; FRACTURES

Bone loss below the level of injury begins within a few weeks after injury. This predisposes to fractures, especially of the long bones. Those with complete injuries are 10 times more likely to sustain fractures than those with incomplete injuries. Relatively minor stress on a bone (for example, normal range of motion) can result in a fracture. In the person with sensory loss, such a noxious stimulus can trigger an episode of AD. The risk of DVT also increases in the presence of a fracture. Treatment includes immobilization and elevation of the extremity. Institution of stringent pressure ulcer prevention and treatment techniques is essential. Prompt and aggressive treatment of spasms may be needed to relieve distressing symptoms. Healing may be markedly prolonged.

UPPER EXTREMITY PAIN

Frequently this is musculoskeletal pain related to wheelchair use; occasionally it is related to syringomyelia, radiculopathy, or rheumatologic disorders. Treatment depends on the cause of the pain, thus an accurate diagnosis is needed. Palliative care of these problems is focused not just on relieving discomfort but also on maintaining independence.

MALNUTRITION

Nutritional status is intimately interrelated with other complications such as pressure ulcers, osteoporosis (as a risk factor for fractures), infection (by its effect on the immune system), and bowel problems. In the absence of advanced cancer, correction of malnutrition may be both possible and desirable. Even in the terminally ill, consideration must be given to the adverse effect on quality of life generated by some of these complications when discussing whether or not to intervene. As suggested above, protein malnutrition can prevent synthesis of components necessary to heal pressure ulcers, and the exudate they produce can serve as a vehicle for loss of nutrients. Increased fluid intake can reduce risk of stone formation by supporting adequate urine volume. In fact, most quadriplegic and paraplegic individuals intentionally have an increased fluid intake throughout their lives to serve just that purpose. It must be noted that serum sodium levels are usually low in this population, and only rarely is the low sodium level indicative of syndrome of inappropriate antidiuretic hormone secretion (SIADH), true water intoxication, or sodium loss.

BOWEL PROBLEMS

Neurogenic bowel can result in delayed gastric emptying, constipation, and/or ileus, any of which can create a noxious stimulus capable of triggering an episode of AD. The life-long management of bowel care is usually decided during the acute management phase following injury. This management can include stimulation of reflex defecation either manually or with a suppository or enema. This is usually done on a regular schedule. Some individuals choose to have a colostomy in order to minimize their dependence on their caregiver. Preventive measures include increased physical activity (if possible), and a diet with sufficient fiber and fluid intake to properly regulate stool consistency.

SEXUAL DYSFUNCTION

Sexual activity, even for the terminally ill person with paralysis, may be possible. It may be one of the few remaining sources of quality of life. Methods for overcoming erectile dysfunction in quadriplegic and paraplegic men include sildenafil, intracavernous injections of papaverine (sometimes combined with phentolamine), devices using a vacuum to draw blood into the penis (sometimes utilizing a penile ring to hold the blood in), and internal penile prostheses. In women, lubrication is sometimes a problem (although in many, stimulation of the genitalia can cause a reflex lubrication and in others, fantasy can cause lubrication). If the woman is unable to lubricate naturally, a water-soluble lubricant is advisable. Without adequate lubrication, sexual activity can produce a noxious stimulus capable of triggering AD.

DEEP VENOUS THROMBOSIS

As stated above, long-term anticoagulation after the acute phase of treatment is rarely seen. During periods of prolonged immobilization, especially at the end of life, frank discussion with the individual and/or surrogate decision maker should be held regarding benefits and risks of anticoagulation.

AUTONOMIC DYSREFLEXIA[5]

This disorder, most likely to be seen in a quadriplegic, or a paraplegic with an injury level of T6 or higher, is triggered by a noxious stimulus (usually with no conscious appreciation of pain sensation) emanating from below the level of injury. It usually presents with pounding headache, a metallic taste in the mouth, a feeling of impending doom (often the most terrifying symptom), and an urge to void. Findings usually include a rapidly rising blood pressure and can include bradycardia (but absence of bradycardia does not rule out the diagnosis). Systolic blood pressures greater than 140 require immediate control with potent agents, while a search for the source of the noxious stimulus may have to wait until lower blood pressures are obtained or another person becomes available to conduct the search. From 85%–90% of all episodes of AD are caused by a noxious stimulus in the genitourinary tract (distended bladder, urinary track infection (UTI), ureteral calculus, urethritis, prostatitis, salpingitis, endometritis, tubal pregnancy, labor). The next most likely source is the bowel (fecal impaction, bowel obstruction, impacted gall stones, appendicitis, diverticulitis, penetrating ulcer, perforated viscus). The next place to look is the skin (sun-burn, cellulitis, hyperthermia, pinched or punctured skin); then the long bones (osteoporosis makes fractures likely).

GENITOURINARY PROBLEMS

As with bowel problems, neurogenic bladder management is usually decided during the acute stage of treatment. Most often, those who are unable to manage their neurogenic bladder with assisted voiding techniques utilize intermittent catheterization, condom catheters, suprapubic catheters, or indwelling catheters. Problems associated with catheters, such as kinked or plugged catheters, urinary tract infections, and stone formation can produce noxious stimuli capable of triggering AD.

Areas for Research

AUTONOMIC DYSREFLEXIA

Much has been done in the realm of treatment of AD and in minimizing the frequency of occurrence of many of the sources of the noxious stimuli that trigger AD. What would be more effective, however, would be a method for blunting or minimizing the autonomic *response* (vasoconstriction) that results from stimulation of the below level autonomic ganglia by the ascending pain fibers from the location of the noxious stimulus. While other complications may be more frequent, none are more terrifying.

NEUROGENIC BOWEL AND BLADDER

This constellation of problems presents a major source of impairment of quality of life. A large part of the person's day is devoted to bowel and bladder care, and it is often a major cause of dependency on others. New techniques for stimulation of bowel evacuation and for management of neurogenic bladder are the subjects of intense research, but solutions remain elusive.

PAIN

This is another area that has a profound impact on quality of life. The meeting previously mentioned, which brought together some of the best researchers involved in pain control with their counterparts in spinal cord injury, promises to begin a dialogue leading to improved methods of SCI pain management (especially the vexing area of central neuropathic pain).

HETEROTOPIC OSSIFICATION

A method for dissolving the calcifications once they have developed would be most welcome.

SUMMARY

Palliative care in the patient with quadriplegia or paraplegia presents an unusual challenge. Since they present with a stable deficit and a nearly normal life expectancy, the focus of management cannot be on alleviation of discomfort to the exclusion of such factors as function and productivity. Quality of life must be balanced with the ability to earn a living. As a consequence of these considerations, most of the research suggested above must overcome specific limitations:

- Pain management must be effective, but must not cloud the senses.
- Bowel and bladder management must not detract from the ability to remain productive in the workplace.
- Methods of blunting the response to a noxious stimulus would be far more desirable than having to treat AD once it develops.
- Vocational rehabilitation, not traditionally viewed as a tool used in palliative care, has obvious value in this setting.

REFERENCES

1. Blissitt PA. Nutrition in acute spinal cord injury. Critical Care Nursing Clinics of America 1990;2:3.
2. Bozzacco V. Long-term psychosocial effects of spinal cord injury. Rehabilitation Nursing 1993;18(2):82–87.
3. Bracken MB, Shepard MJ, Collins WF, et al. A randomized controlled trial of methylprednisolone or naloxone in the treatment of acute spinal cord injury. New England Journal of Medicine 1990;322:1405–1411.
4. Delisa JA, et al. Rehabilitation Medicine: Principles and Practice, 3rd Ed. Lippincott–Raven: Philadelphia, 1998.
5. Karlsson AK. Autonomic dysreflexia. Spinal Cord 1999;37:383–391.
6. Katz RT. Management of spasticity. American Journal of Physical Medicine and Rehabilitation 1988; 67:108–116.
7. Kottke FJ, Lehmann JF. Krusen's Handbook of Physical Medicine and Rehabilitation, 4th Ed. W.B. Saunders, Philadelphia, 1990.
8. Lee B, et al. The Spinal Cord Injured Patient—Comprehensive Management. W.B. Saunders, Philadelphia, 1991.
9. Marino RJ. International Standards for Neurological Classification of Spinal Cord Injury, 5th Ed., revised. American Spinal Injury Association: Chicago, 2000.
10. Merritt's Textbook of Neurology, 10th Ed. Lippincott Williams & Wilkins, Philadelphia, 2000:416–423.
11. Rousseau P. Hospice and palliative care. Disease-a-Month 1995;XLI(12):769–844.
12. Siddall PJ, Taylor DA, Cousins MJ. Classification of pain following spinal cord injury. Spinal Cord 1997;35:69–75.
13. Stover SL, Delisa JA, Whiteneck GG. Spinal Cord Injury: Clinical Outcomes from the Model Systems. Aspen, Gaithersburg, Maryland, 1995:Chapters 9, 13.
14. Subbaro JV, Garrison SJ. Heterotopic ossification: diagnosis and management, current concepts and controversies. Journal of Spinal Cord Medicine 1999; 22(4):273–283.
15. Tator CH. Experimental and clinical studies of the pathophysiology and management of acute spinal cord injury. Journal of Spinal Cord Medicine 1996;19(4):206–214.
16. Yezierski RP, Burchiel KJ. Spinal Cord Injury Pain: Assessment, Mechanisms, Management Progress in Pain Research and Management, Vol. 23. IASP Press. Seattle, 2002.
17. Zejdlik C. Management of Spinal Cord Injury, 2nd Ed. Jones & Bartlett, Boston, 1992.

Chapter 14

Locked-in Syndrome

Heinz Lahrmann
Wolfgang Grisold

INTRODUCTION
CLINICAL PICTURE AND
   NEUROANATOMY
DIAGNOSIS AND DIFFERENTIAL
   DIAGNOSIS
PROGNOSIS AND OUTCOME
CARE

COMMUNICATION
Non-electronic Communication Aids
Electronic Communication Aids
CARE OF RELATIVES
ETHICAL ASPECTS
SUMMARY

In this chapter the neurologic symptoms, the neuroanatomical and pathophysiological background, and the palliative management of patients with locked-in syndrome (LIS) is presented. Most often LIS is caused by basilar artery thrombosis. The patient becomes completely paralysed with only vertical eye and upper lid movements spared. Consciousness, sensation, and hearing are most often intact. Emphasis is put on the explanation of the diagnosis and its implications to the patient, the relatives, and the caring team. Of major importance is to establish a sufficient mode of communication with the LIS patient. Different methods and technical solutions are presented. The ethical point of this condition, which belongs to the nightmares of human beings, is discussed.

CASE HISTORY

A 60-year-old male army officer without any neurologic history experienced dizziness and vertigo for some days, which he had never experienced before. He was hospitalized. Two days later he fell into a coma-like state. When a neurologist was consulted he saw a tetraplegic patient with bilateral incomplete facial palsy. However, the patient was able to open his eyes on command. Pupillary reaction was normal. A lesion of pontine structures was suspected. Computerized tomography showed bilat-

eral ischemic lesion of pontine structures which extended to the medulla oblongata on one side. LIS was diagnosed. Because respiration deteriorated the patient was transferred to an intensive care unit (ICU), where he was intubated and put on mechanical ventilation.

The neurologist took much effort to establish a 'basic' communication by eye opening at least—one opening signaling 'yes' and two blinks for 'no'. With this reduced form of communication it was hardly possible to investigate the patient's needs concerning pain, distress, and ventilation. He was not informed about his diagnosis and any discussion of his will regarding prolongation of life-sustaining therapies was not undertaken. He died a few weeks later because of uncontrollable pneumonia, despite maximal antibiotic therapy.

At the ICU the major problem was to explain the conscious state and the intact awareness of the patient to the staff and the relatives. They believed he was in coma, unaware of his environment, because he was unable to speak or show any facial expressions. In the beginning they were not cautious to avoid frank discussion of the patient's bad state and prognosis in his presence. As he was unable to react, ostentatively he was assumed to be unaware. The nurses were not aware that he perceived pain, which can be assumed as his lemniscal tracts were intact (also proven by somatosensory evoked potentials (SEP)). However, he was unable to signal his perceptions, in particular pain, to the caring team.

135

Sudden address, touch, and pain caused vegetative reactions with an increase in heart rate. A crucial point was to explain to the caring team and the relatives that the same simple code of communication had to be used by all of them in order to avoid confusion and frustration of the patient.

Comment

From this case history we may learn how much caution and effort has to be taken to improve the horrible situation of a patient with LIS and all persons involved. Early establishment of the best possible way of communication is necessary. As LIS is very rare, full and repetitive explanation to the caring team and the relatives has to be achieved. It is the experience of many neurologists that it may take several days until the medical staff believes in the patient's awareness of almost everything in his environment.

INTRODUCTION

With good reason LIS may be called the nightmare of all possible outcomes of modern medicine. Being initially often in a comatose state, the patient awakens into a life without any voluntary motor control, while hearing, vision, and often sensation are unimpaired. The only voluntary movements possible in classical LIS are vertical gaze and upper eyelid movements.[1] Cognition is retained in most patients with LIS. The underlying neuropathological condition is usually an extensive bilateral lesion of the ventral pons as a result of basilar artery thrombosis.

After the patient has survived the acute phase and the diagnosis of LIS has been established, palliative intensive care is challenged. The neurologist has to transfer the information to the medical staff and relatives and remind them regularly that, despite the 'locked-in'state, the patient is fully aware of his environment and feels, sees, and hears in an almost normal way.

One major problem in caring for these patients is to differentiate between loss of consciousness and loss of responsiveness. Symptom control is very difficult and requires much intuition and active attendance of the caring team. In order to infer the patient's needs, wishes, and will, adequate communication has to be established quickly using any device available and suitable. The patient should be informed about his situation at the earliest possible time. Most patients die in the acute phase. However, as long-term survivors can live for up to 27 years, and improvements in motor function have been reported in the literature, rehabilitation therapy should be initiated as early as possible and in a vigorous manner.[2-4]

In 1966, Plum and Posner introduced the term LIS for the first time.[1] However, LIS was vividly and accurately described 120 years earlier in the novel 'The Count of Monte Cristo' by Alexandre Dumas. One character, Monsieur Noitier de Villefort, was depicted as 'a corpse with living eyes'. Mr Noitier had been in this state for more than six years, and he could only communicate by blinking his eyes.[5]

Despite the fact that LIS is mentioned in many textbooks and scientific articles on neurology and intensive care medicine, most often only 'classical' medical aspects are reported, as neuroanatomy, neurological symptoms, electrophysiology, neuroimaging, and intensive care management. Palliative care concerning the patient's and his relatives' needs for sympathetic understanding and communication has rarely been considered. The only patient's report we are aware of was written by J.D. Bauby who communicated without the assistance of any technical device by just lifting his left eyelid.[6] In this very impressive and sensitive book, which is highly recommended to everyone interested in the problem, the author writes about the needs, fears, pains, and daydreams (oneroids) of a man living in a locked-in state. Being a formerly socially very active man he had to learn infinite patience to cope with this state of being locked in himself. He describes the lack of communication with his relatives and the caring team as one of his major problems. Future palliative care investigation will have to address the problem of communication with LIS patients and possible forms of its realization.

CLINICAL PICTURE AND NEUROANATOMY

Most patients experience a prodromal period days to weeks prior to the acute event. In a review of 139 cases, Patterson and Grabois found dizziness, vertigo, headache, and hemiparesis to be the most frequent.[4,6] Initially, the patient may lose consciousness and become comatose.[7] After days to weeks the patient will regain consciousness. Yet, the total motor de-efferentiation results in paralysis of limbs, neck, jaw, and facial muscles. Initially, spasticity and pyramidal signs are often absent. As other central structures may be involved, disorientation and/or vegetative dysfunction such as respiratory failure and/or arrhythmia may be present. On the other hand, the lesion may be incomplete and some voluntary movements may be retained.[8]

Sensation in LIS may vary from normal to absent.[4] This variation, described in literature, may be explained partly by the difficulty to perform an adequate sensory examination in these patients and partly by the variation in size and location of the lesion. However, as it has to be assumed that sensation of pain should be normal in most LIS patients, this fact has to be communicated early and repeatedly to the caring team and relatives to avoid any painful passive movements of the patient's limbs and body. The sensation of visceral pain caused by the bladder and/or bowel has to be taken into account, as the patient himself cannot signal his needs. Of equal importance for care is the functional integrity of vision and often hearing in most patients.[6] Sleep is often disturbed with abnormalities in REM and non-REM sleep.[4]

Another issue in the care of LIS patients are involuntary motor phenomena, as they may be misinterpreted for voluntary movements of the patient. Ocular bobbing, crying, and trismus are the most frequent.[4] Bauer and co-workers described stimulus-evoked oral automatisms and involuntary cries.[9] Furthermore, groaning, facial grimace, yawning, palatal myoclonus, sighing, coughing, bruxism, and laughing have been observed.

Respiration is often impaired. Death in chronic LIS patients is most often caused by respiratory complications, such as pneumonia, respiratory arrest, and pulmonary emboli. Particularly in chronic LIS, with impaired swallowing and cough reflexes, secretion management and pulmonary hygiene are of major importance. In their review on 139 cases Patterson and Grabois reported abnormal breathing patterns in many patients, including

Cheyne–Stokes, ataxic, involuntary/diaphragmatic respiration, hyperpnea, and apnea.[4]

Bauer and co-workers have suggested a tripartite classification for LIS:
1. Classical, according to the criteria of Plum and Posner: quadriplegia, lower cranial nerve paralysis, and mutism with preservation of only vertical gaze and upper eyelid movements[1]
2. Incomplete LIS, with retained movements other than vertical movements of the eye and the upper lid
3. Total LIS, without any voluntary movements.[8]

A fourth condition has been described by Zwarts and coworkers.[10] It is regarded as a state of brain stem death with absent cortical function but preserved EEG activity and visually evoked potentials (VEP). In this very rare condition the ethical issue of life-sustaining therapies is even more difficult.

Classically, an extensive bilateral lesion of the ventral pons, which interrupts cortiospinal and cortico-bulbar tracts, is the neuroanatomical substrate of LIS.[1,11] In Figure 14–1 we schematically present the anatomical features of LIS. More than 80% are caused by thrombosis of the basilar artery. As a consequence of the anatomy of the basilar artery and its branches, thrombosis often causes ischemic lesions in the cerebellum, thalami, and territory of the posterior

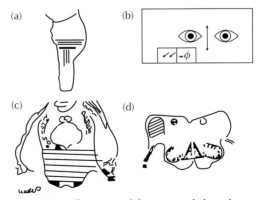

Figure 14–1. Illustration of the neuropathological lesions and eye movements of our patient, drawn from clinical records and the neuropathological findings: (a, c, d) sagittal extension of the lesion shows large transverse lesion of the lower pons (c) with a column-like extension in the lateral medulla oblongata (d); (b) vertical eye movements only were possible, at the onset also spontaneous nystagmus (see arrows indicating direction) occurred.

cerebral artery. The resulting loss of function may confuse the clinical picture. A review of the neuroanatomic literature shows that 15%–28% of all cerebrovascular lesions involve the brain stem.

DIAGNOSIS AND DIFFERENTIAL DIAGNOSIS

The first and most important step in the diagnosis of LIS is the clinical investigation. Often much neurologic experience is needed to detect the subtle signs of the patient signaling cognition and retained efferent functions. A close observation of the eye and lid movements after calling the patient's name or speaking to him may give the first diagnostic hint. Pain may cause dilatation of the ipsilateral pupil (cilio-spinal reflex), but this is of no diagnostic value. Sometimes slight voluntary movements of the facial muscles or minimal voluntary innervations of extremities (fingers, toes) upon verbal instruction may be detected by close inspection. Automatisms, synergistic extensor and flexor movements, and isolated facial contractions after painful stimuli do not signal voluntary control as they are seen in patients with vegetative state too. Stimulus-evoked oral automatisms have been described.[9]

MRI has contributed much to the early and exact diagnosis of brain stem lesions, which may not be achieved with cranial CT. In some cases angiography of intracerebral arteries has to be performed to achieve the exact diagnosis. The value of electrophysiological investigations is discussed controversially. With intact median lemniscal tract one should assume SEP and magnetically evoked potentials (MEP) to be normal. However, Gütling and co-workers reported on electrophysiological findings in five patients with LIS of different origin. They concluded that there is no specific pattern of SEP abnormalities characteristic for LIS and that positive EEG response to stimuli cannot be taken as the only measure of consciousness.[7] Therefore one has to be cautious with the interpretation of these parameters when assessing the diagnosis and prognosis of LIS patients, particularly with respect to the differential diagnosis of vegetative state.

Other diseases to be considered for differential diagnosis are: pontine hemorrhage, brain stem tumors, and demyelination due to central pontine myelinolysis, encephalitis, and traumatic lesions, which have also been described.[3,11] Severe bilateral hemispheric stroke, heroin abuse, viral brain stem encephalitis, intrathecal cytosine–arabinoside therapy, and fibro-muscular dysplasia with dissection of basilar artery are very rare causes of LIS. Severe forms of polyradiculitis Guillain–Barré, poliomyelitis, and myasthenic syndrome have to be considered for differential diagnosis—particularly as these conditions may have a more favorable prognosis.

PROGNOSIS AND OUTCOME

Most patients with LIS do not survive longer than a few weeks or months.[12] Extension of the lesion is reported as the primary cause of death during the first week after onset.[4] Pulmonary complications represent the most frequent cause of death after the first week. However, some patients have been reported to survive with chronic LIS for up to 27 years.[2,3,12] No systematic studies on the recovery, morbidity, and mortality of patients with LIS exist. Many of the published case reports were post-mortem studies and did not, or only very superficially, report on neurologic function and course of disease.

In a cohort study of 27 patients with LIS, Haig and co-workers found very long survival times. Twenty-four patients were still alive up to 12.8 years after onset, with a mean survival time of 4.9 years (range 1.2 to 12.8 years).[2] In this study only patients with definite LIS (anarthria, quadriplegia, and preserved consciousness) lasting for more than one year were included. None of these patients achieved recovery of motor control sufficient to move a limb against gravity. Some did make minor improvements, which helped them to control electronic devices such as wheelchairs and communication systems, by hand, head, or tongue movements. The long survival times within this patient group is in contrast to most of the published case reports. When reviewing the literature the same authors found that 67% of 117 published cases were post-mortem reports.[13] In this review they state that 75% of 44 reported reasons of death were pulmonary complications. However, in their series of 27 patients with an average follow-up of 4.9 years, only 11% mortality (three patients) occurred, one due to pulmonary problems. Maybe the rather young age of their patients may have biased their results (mean age at onset 32 years, standard deviation (SD) 15 years). According to our experience most patients die shortly after the acute event (unpublished observation).

Following 29 patients with chronic LIS for a further five years, Katz from the same group reported survival times between 2.02 and 18.2 years.[3] The most common etiology of LIS was cerebrovascular disease (52%) followed by trauma (31%). All patients were in stable condition for more than one year before they were included into the study. Life table analysis revealed that 82% of LIS patients who survived the first year would be expected to survive the five- and ten-year follow-up. Their data clearly suggest that once a patient has clinically stabilized in LIS for more than one year, the life span can be prolonged dramatically.

Although minimal late neurologic recovery occurs in chronic LIS, survival may be prolonged with adequate care.[3] It is extremely important to start a rehabilitation program early to help the patient attain the highest level of function possible in the most expeditious manner.[4] As there are reports on late functional recovery, intensive rehabilitation programs should be performed over at least a period of one year after onset of LIS. However, significant improvement of motor function after one year of disease has rarely been reported. Furthermore, we stress again the overall importance of establishing adequate communication with these patients in order to make ethical and long-term care decisions *with* the patient rather than *for* the patient.

CARE

In chronic LIS, care, either at the patient's home, in a nursing home, or in hospital, is very laborious and costly. It has to be planned carefully and in advance (e.g. before the patient is discharged from the ICU). Care is one of the main contributing factors not only to the survival of the patients but, most of all, to their quality of life. The most important point is to speak to the patients, touch them, and give them a warm feeling of human proximity to relieve their isolation. If there is any mode of communication established, take time to listen to the patient before beginning to care for him. Most of the issues discussed shortly in the following paragraph are explained in more detail elsewhere and are only mentioned for completeness.

Bulbar structures are affected in LIS. Therefore chewing and swallowing is impaired and most patients are nourished by percutaneous gastric tubes (PEG). Feeding should provide adequate caloric intake and contain enough bulking agents to ensure normal digestion. Feeding at regular meal times is preferable to continuous infusion via PEG. It gives a more physiologic feeling of satiety. Enough fluid intake is essential, particularly in a hot environment (e.g. if an air mattress is used). Care must be taken to avoid or at least reduce contractures and calcification of joints by regular appropriate passive movements. Carers must be advised to be very careful when moving the patient to avoid rupture of joint capsules. Prevention of skin ulcera often requires special anti-decubital beds and extensive care of the exposed parts of the skin. The same holds true for care of corneal ulcera, which arise quite frequently because eye blinking may be reduced. Particularly during the night, eyes have to be occluded by a watch-glass bandage, and special eye fluids may be applied. Bauby reports on the shocking and painful experience of having his right eyelid sewn up one morning without having been informed properly.[6] This measure should be considered a last resort, because vision is the only communicational aid left to LIS patients. Cramps and spasms develop regularly in these patients and should be treated early and adequately. The medical treatment of pain syndromes is explained in Chapter 19 in detail.

The respiratory system is affected in a significant number of patients and pulmonary complications represent the leading cause of death after the first week after onset of LIS.[4] Some of the patients with acute LIS, and many with chronic LIS, have to be tracheotomized and ventilated mechanically either because of secretion problems or ventilatory failure. Home care of tracheotomized and ventilated patients puts a great burden on the family. However, Haig and colleagues reported that in many of their patients with chronic LIS gastrostomy, tracheotomy tubes and indwelling catheters could be removed.[2] Yet, no statistically significant relationship could be found between medical complications and the presence of the tubes or catheters. The most frequent causes of morbidity in their sample were urinary tract infections (14 of 24 patients), pneumonia, pressure sores, urinary tract stones, gastrointestinal bleeding, and deep venous thrombosis.

The issue of patient's depression has been discussed often. Patients are at great disadvantage if facial muscles are paralysed because their ability to express emotions is lost. Depression may be common in patients with speech disorders.[14] However, as no objective measures exist, no general recommendations on the application of antidepressant drugs in this patient population can be given at the moment.

Mucus, secretion problems, and sialorrhea, which are a great problem in patients with impaired bulbar function, may be alleviated by medical treatment (anticholinergic drugs, amitriptyline, beta-blocking agents) or radiation of the parotid glands. Some authors reported injection of botulinum toxin A into the parotid glands to be effective. Upper airway suction may be effective in tracheotomized patients. However, care has to be taken not to cause bleedings by lesion of mucosal vessels.

COMMUNICATION

Effective symptom control is impossible without effective communication. Thus, communication has to be a major issue in the palliative care of LIS patients. It is the basic concept of palliative care to respect the individuality and freedom of the patient. But in order to fulfil the free will of the patient, communication is the most essential point. As LIS develops as a result of an acute event (e.g. thrombosis of the basilar artery), there will be hardly any statement of the patient concerning his will regarding prolongation of life (advance directive). In LIS, vertical gaze and eyelid movements are possible. Based on these voluntary movements it should be possible to establish a meaningful conversation with a patient whose mental status is undisturbed.

Clark states in the 'Oxford Textbook of Palliative Medicine' that 'inability to communicate is not a loss of life but a loss of access to life'.[14] Further on, the author mentions that the specific role of a speech therapist is to ensure that patients are using all communication modalities available, that communication aids are introduced at the correct time, and to educate carers to change their communication strategies in order to optimize communication with the patient. It should also be remembered that listening is tiring for carers because they invest a lot of energy in return for poor communication from the patient. Listeners should allow patients time to communicate, they should not interrupt or finish sentences for them, and they should not shout, for the patients are not deaf.

Non-electronic Communication Aids

Yes/No answers to questions: This is the simplest form. A common communication code has to be established (e.g. one eye blink signalling 'yes' and two for 'no').[6]

Communication board: This simple communication aid has to be developed by the patient and his carers to meet their individual needs. It may contain commonly used words, phrases, pictures, numbers, and/or the alphabet.

Communication booklet: It is a small book with several 'chapters' separated by thumb-tabs on which the symbol of the particular category is printed (e.g. food, clothing, emotions). The caregiver turns the appropriate page and points to the symbols waiting for the agreement of the patient using his most reliable movement.

E-tran frame: This is a colour-coded alphabet to spell out words, using eye pointing only. A rectangle with the centre cut out is placed between the patient and the listener. Letters of the alphabet are drawn in groups of four to five around the rectangle and they are colour-coded. To indicate a letter the user looks at the corresponding group and then to the corner representing the appropriate colour. It is very easy to use, cheap, and appropriate for LIS patients. The disadvantages are that it has no voice, no written or printed output, and the user is dependent on the communication partner to pick up the messages.

Electronic Communication Aids

A multitude of different electronic devices are available, either based on a PC or stand-alone. The rehabilitation engineer must ensure that the appropriate device for the patient and the caregiver is chosen. A highly sophisticated computer-based device may be useless for people not accustomed to using a computer. Regular maintenance of the device must be provided. Input may be achieved by suck–puff, air pad, touch, squeeze, eye blink, or even EEG. In EEG-controlled communication the patient has to learn to generate special EEG potentials, mostly recorded from the frontal or parietal cortex. Complete alertness and a certain degree of intelligence are prerequisites to learn this method. Because only few reports exist and we have no experiences of our own, no recommendations can be given regarding EEG-based communication in LIS patients at the moment. Memory facilities, word prediction, and a variety of speech synthesizers are available. Even access to telephone and extensive environmental control is theoretically possible. Future palliative care research will have to show which communication devices are useful and for which patient group.

CARE OF RELATIVES

Another important issue is the care of the relatives, as they bear a huge psychological and financial burden. Information about the state and perception of the patient has to be provided early and repeatedly. Extensive discussion of the prognosis and absence of any curative treatment is necessary. The fact that the patient hears, sees, and feels everything has to be reiterated. A frequent misunderstanding is that people who do not speak cannot hear either.

Whether home care is possible depends on the patient's state, the family structure, the social medical system, and the possibility to provide technical aids, as there are special beds, wheelchairs, feeding tubes, suction devices, etc. Additional help by neurologists, physicians or hospice doctors, home care nurses, physiotherapists, psychologists (if necessary), and speech therapists has to be organized. For the mental and physical health of the primary caregivers, it is necessary that he/she has some spare time and vacations for regeneration. This has to be considered in the planning of home care too. Otherwise a 'burn out' syndrome may develop in a short period of time. Most of all it is important to give the caring relatives the feeling that they are not left alone with their fate. There must be someone with whom they can share the responsibility, their sorrows, and grief. The professional health carers must bear in mind what it means to be alone at home with a seriously ill and handicapped person. The caring person must be equipped with 24-hour emergency telephone numbers where they can reach a physician or nurse they know.

ETHICAL ASPECTS

Ethical aspects are explained in more detail elsewhere (see also Part 5 of this book).[15] Here we will focus on the particular situation found in LIS. These patients, who are mostly people without any serious disease in their history, will usually not have any advance directive concerning their will about mechanical ventilation and other life-sustaining therapies. In the acute phase the need for mechanical ventilation may arise. Having survived the acute phase, and once the diagnosis of LIS has been established, questions concerning withdrawal of ventilator, antibiotics, etc. will be inevitable. If the patient is completely awake and any kind of communication has been established, his will and needs may be inferred. Then, the question asked in the Hastings Centre Report, 'Who speaks for the patient with LIS?', will be obsolete. In any other case (e.g. the patient has to be sedated, does not regain consciousness) his presumptive will has to be inquired from the relatives. If this is not possible, or there exists doubt on the attitude of the relatives towards the patient, a responsible person can be named by the court.

SUMMARY

LIS is the nightmare of all possible outcomes in modern neurology, as it means a totally paralysed person with intact cognition and senses. Most often it is caused by bilateral pontine infarction due to basilar artery thrombosis.

Diagnosis and care management are a great challenge for the neurologist, the intensive care physician, and the caring team. The state of the patient with loss of motor control, yet mostly unimpaired sensation, vision, and hearing has to be reiterated to the team and the relatives to avoid physical and mental injury to the patient. Establishment of a meaningful communication is another issue for all people involved in the care of a LIS patient. Every technology available (up to EEG-controlled computer devices) should be used to infer the needs and pains of the patient. As most LIS patients have only short survival times (their prognosis is, in general, fatal) and many of their problems may occur in other terminal neurological diseases (e.g. bulbar and respiratory involvement in ALS), it seems appropriate to include them into the palliative care program for neurologic diseases.

REFERENCES

1. Plum F, Posner JB. The Diagnosis of Stupor and Coma. F.A. Davis Company, Philadelphia, 1966.
2. Haig AJ, Katz RT, Saghal V. Mortality and complications of the locked in-syndrome. Arch Phys Med Rehabil 1987;68:24–27.
3. Katz RT, Haig AJ, Clark BB, DiPaola RJ. Long-term survival, prognosis, and life-care planning for 29 patients with chronic locked-in syndrome. Arch Phys Med Rehabil 1992; 73:403–408.
4. Patterson JR, Grabois M. Locked-in syndrome: a review of 139 cases. Stroke 1986;17:758–64.
5. Dumas A. The Count of Monte Christo. Collier & Son, New York, 1910.
6. Bauby JD. Le scaphandre et le papillon, Editions Robert Laffont, Paris, 1997.
7. Gütling E, Isenmann S, Wichmann W. Electro-physiology in the locked-in-syndrome. Neurology 1996;46:1092–1101.
8. Bauer G, Gerstenbrand F, Rumpl E. Varieties of the locked-in syndrome. J. Neurol 1979;221:77–79.
9. Bauer G, Prugger M, Rumpl E. Stimulus evoked oral automatisms in locked-in syndrome. Arch Neurol 1982;39:435–436.
10. Zwarts MJ, Kornips FHM, Vogels OM. Clinical brainstem death with preserved electroencephalographic activity and visual evoked potentials. Arch Neurol 2001;58:1010.
11. Virgile RS. Locked in syndrome. Clin Neurol Neurosurg 1984;86:275–279.
12. Thadani VM, Rimm DL, Urquhart RN, et al. 'Locked in syndrome' for 27 years following viral illness. Neurology 1991;41:498–500.
13. Haig AH, Katz RT, Sahgal V. Locked-in syndrome: review. Current Concepts in Rehab Medicine 1986;2:12–16.
14. Clark SD. Speech therapy in palliative medicine. In: Doyle D, Hanks GWC, MacDonald N, eds. Oxford Textbook of Palliative Medicine, 2nd Ed. Oxford University Press, Oxford, 1998:847–854.
15. Bernat JL. Ethical Issues in Neurology. Butterworth–Heinemann, Boston 1994:201–220.

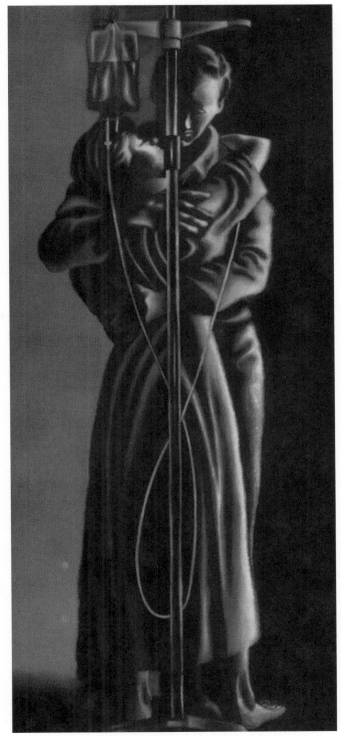

Plate 3 'Hug' by Robert Pope, 1990. (Acrylic on canvas, 182.9 × 78.7 cm)

PART **3**

COMMON SYMPTOMS

Chapter 15

Spasticity

Johannes Noth
Gereon R. Fink

Spasticity—an increased stretch resistance of the passive skeletal muscle with exaggerated tendon jerks—is a common neurologic symptom in palliative care and can result from any lesion (e.g. due to a stroke or a brain tumor) of the long corticospinal tract. The clinical variety of spastic syndromes results from the topology of the CNS lesion and the subsequent differential involvement of the descending pathways. The overall approach to the management of spasticity includes reversing any noxious stimulus, using physical interventions before adding pharmacotherapy, and reserving more invasive techniques (e.g. nerve blocks, orthopedic or neurosurgical procedures) to a few exceptional situations. The aim of the treatment is to prevent joint contractures, decubiti, and orthostatic hypotension. Current pharmacological treatment is based on substances that act as muscle relaxants including baclofen, tizanidine, diazepam, and botolinum toxin.

CASE HISTORY AND DISCUSSION

A 49-year-old, right-handed, bedbound female was admitted to hospital because of an acute deterioration of her general condition, as well as her longstanding spastic tetraparesis resulting from primary progressive multiple sclerosis which first had affected her when she was 19 years old. On physical examination there was an increased temperature which disappeared following antibiotics given because of an urinary tract infection. In addition, a severe spastic tetraparesis with cerebellar signs was observed; spasticity was particularly pronounced in the lower extremeties with painful flexor spasms already elicited by the slightest cutaneous stimulation.

While her general medical condition improved with the antibiotic treatment, the severe spasticity remained. The patient received intensive physiotherapy and was treated additionally with baclofen, which was subsequently increased to a total of 80 mg daily. On follow-up the patient's spastic tetraparesis remained. However, the increased muscle tone was reduced significantly and the pain associated with spasticity was also significantly reduced, thus leading to an important improvement of the patient's quality of life. Spasticity in palliative medicine is not different from spastic syndromes in otherwise healthy subjects, although the mode and the intensity of treatment of the spastic muscle tone may differ. Spasticity is a common neurologic syndrome, observed both in diseases primarily affecting the CNS, such as ischemic stroke, and a number of medical conditions which secondarily affect the CNS (e.g. global brain ischemia following transient heart arrest or septic shock). Any lesion of the long corticospinal (pyramidal) tract can cause spasticity. There are easily recognizable subtypes of spastic syndromes explained by involvement of the adjacent corticobulbar or bulbospinal pathways variously affecting the clinical picture.

Lance describes spasticity as a motor disorder characterized by a velocity-dependent increase in tonic stretch reflexes (muscle tone) with exaggerated tendon jerks stemming from hyperexcitability of the stretch reflex,[1]—a key component of the 'upper motor neurone syndrome'. The term 'upper motor neurone' highlights spasticity as a consequence of any lesion of the corticospinal tract, not only in the primary motor cortex (Brodmann area 4, BA 4) but also in other pericentral areas such as the primary somatosensory cortex (BA 3,1,2) and the premotor areas (BA 6). Discussion continues as to the extent to which other factors such as changes in muscle fiber properties, alterations in spinal neuronal networks not directly related to motoneurone hyperexcitability, and joint contractures contribute to the passive stretch resistance of spastic muscles. No single one of these pathophysiological mechanisms sufficiently explains the variety of clinical features seen in spasticity. The time course and the location of the CNS lesion, the age of the patient at disease onset, and the way the patient is treated all contribute also to the clinical syndrome.

PATHOPHYSIOLOGY

Animal Models of Spasticity

Knowledge about the pathophysiology of spasticity has been based largely on animal experiments. In 1898, Sherrington[2] introduced the intercollicular decerebrate cat with its enhanced muscle tone of anti-gravity muscles and demonstrated that sectioning of the appropriate dorsal roots abolished this enhanced muscle activity. Enhanced γ-motoneurone activity was thought responsible for the exaggerated 'postural tone' of the decerebrate animal. However, in patients with spastic hemiplegia, microneurographic recordings from muscle spindle afferents did

not show enhanced input from Ia fibers (primary muscle spindle afferents) as would be expected.[3] The extensor 'rigidity' of the decerebrate cat therefore seems more like the pathological muscle tone which develops immediately after acute lesions of the brain stem in humans.[4]

The chronic spinal animal is the most frequently used animal model of spasticity and exhibits some of the features seen in human spasticity of spinal origin. Following acute section of the low thoracic spinal cord the animal develops a complete flaccid paresis below the lesion site, which slowly recedes within two weeks.[5] Thereafter, some features of human spasticity may develop. The most characteristic one—the so-called 'clasp-knife phenomenon'—is only observed in spasticity of spinal origin.

The cat motor system displays a lower degree of corticalization compared to the human motor system[6] and may therefore not mimic the full clinical syndrome of spasticity. If so, spasticity caused by lesions of descending motor projections should be more readily obtained in non-human primates than in other vertebrates. However, even in the monkey a complete unilateral or bilateral pyramidotomy results in persistent limb hypotonia and hyporeflexia, but not spasticity.[7,8] Some degree of spasticity with increased tendon jerks and enhanced resistance to passive movements in distal arm and leg muscles can develop after excision of the hand or leg area of the primary motor cortex (BA 4). However, the development of severe spasticity seems to require additional lesions of descending corticobulbar or bulbospinal motor projections.[9]

Sprouting Hypothesis of Spasticity

Following spinal cord lesions, altered excitability and synaptic remodeling of α-motoneurones in the ventral horn below the lesion have been described.[10] To date it remains unclear which systems are involved in such synaptic plasticity. One key candidate is the modulatory serotonergic system known to increase the excitability of α-motoneurones.[11] There is some evidence that serotonergic axons can regenerate from the unlesioned side to the ventral horn of the lesioned side and that they form new synaptic contacts with

Table 15–1. **Changes in Excitability of Spinal Neuronal Networks**

Excitability of Neurons	SPASTIC SYNDROME		
	Cerebral Hemiplegia	Cerebral Diplegia	Spinal
Reciprocal inhibition	⇓	⇓ ⇑	⇓
Ib inhibition	⇓	?	=
Presynaptic inhibition	=	?	⇓ ⇓
Renshaw inhibition	=	?	⇓ ⇑
γ-motoneurones	=	?	?

Changes in excitability of spinal interneurones in different types of human spasticity, based on indirect evidence from monosynaptic reflex testing. Excitability of γ-motoneurones is inferred from microneurographic recordings of primary muscle spindle endings in patients with spastic hemiparesis.

α-motoneurones.[12] However, this does not explain the development of spasticity following spinal shock due to complete spinal lesions, as without experimental therapeutic intervention, sprouting of descending tracts across the lesion site has never been observed in either animals or man.[13,14]

Changes in the Excitability of Spinal Interneurones

The excitability of α-motoneurones, the final common pathway to the muscle fibers, is mainly determined by the state of spinal interneurones, because the bulk of descending fibers synapses on interneurones rather than motoneurones. In addition, even the direct monosynaptic input from segmental afferents is modulated by interneurones (presynaptic inhibition). Alterations of the excitability of these interneuronal circuits have been implicated in the pathophysiology of spasticity.[15] However, the contribution of these networks is difficult to assess, both because direct recordings from interneurones are impossible in man, and because most of the favorable evidence is deduced indirectly from measurements of the conditioned H-reflexes taken mainly under relaxed conditions in which spasticity is not well expressed. Furthermore, conflicting results in the literature may be related to the fact that the various types of spasticity differentially affect these interneurones. An overview of the postulated changes in excitability of interneurones is presented in Table 15–1.

Role of Spinal Stretch Reflexes in Spasticity

For many years it had been generally accepted that the enhanced velocity-dependent stretch resistance of a spastic muscle, which is not voluntarily activated, is due to the enhanced spinal stretch reflex evoked by primary muscle spindle endings, projecting via mono- and oligosynaptic pathways to their α-motoneurones. More recently, this view has been challenged by the observation that during natural movements (i.e. walking of patients with spastic gait disorder), the slowing of muscle shortening could not be explained by enhanced EMG activity of the antagonistic muscles.[16] Neither was the paresis itself responsible for the slowing of movements as the agonistic muscles exhibited a high amount of EMG activity during the (impeded) shortening contraction. An enhanced stretch resistance of the spastic muscle fibers themselves, without any contribution by the spinal stretch reflex, was postulated and prompted a number of further studies, which have changed views about spastic muscle tone.

In relaxed spastic muscles, an individual velocity threshold for eliciting a stretch response exists, which during a ramp stretch ranges from 20°–100°/sec. This 'dynamic stretch reflex' should be distinguished from the 'phasic stretch reflex' that is evoked by a tendon jerk. In initially relaxed spastic muscles, large-amplitude stretches above a certain velocity threshold evoke this dynamic stretch reflex, which at moderate and high velocities lasts for the entire stretching phase. Such behavior cannot be provoked in healthy subjects, even at the highest angular velocities. The presence of an individual velocity threshold explains the failure in detecting increased dynamic stretch reflexes in spastic muscles in those studies in which the applied stretch velocities were (too) low.[17] In spastic arm muscles, the highest stretch-induced EMG activity is developed when the muscle is relaxed prior to the passive stretch being imposed.[18] Accordingly, in spasticity the dynamic stretch reflex gain in antagonists is pathologically enhanced only when the agonist is in a relaxed state, whereas the gain is downregulated with increasing voluntary activation of the agonists. Thus the enhanced dynamic stretch reflex has its major impact in spasticity when patients are examined in the absence of any voluntary muscle activation.

SYMPTOMATOLOGY OF SPASTICITY

The key symptom of spasticity is an increased stretch resistance of the passive skeletal muscle. In contrast to other types of increased muscle tone, the stretch resistance increases with the velocity of the applied stretch. Dynamic stretch evokes a spastic increase in muscle tone and almost no electromyographic activity is present in the resting, non-activated spastic muscle. In most cases the velocity-dependent increase in stretch resistance is accompanied by paresis or plegia of the affected limb and exaggerated tendon jerks. Pathological reflexes such as the Babinski sign, flexor spasms, mass reflexes, and clonus are frequently observed but not obligatory symptoms of spasticity. The 'clasp-knife phenomenon', which is characterized by a sudden decrease in muscle tone during ongoing muscle stretch, is a rather rare observation and only seen in spasticity of spinal origin.

Related to spasticity is the 'detrusor sphincter dyssynergy' of the bladder that develops with a variable delay following complete spinal cord injury. Due to the hyperexcitability of the motoneurones localized in the Onuf's nucleus of the conus medullaris which innervate the external sphincter of the bladder, the initiation of micturition via an increase in the detrusor activity elicits co-contraction of the external sphincter. This results in an inability to empty the bladder. Another complication of such a detrusor sphincter dyssynergy is hypertension with flushing and headache. Similarly, autonomic bowel dysfunction may develop after spinal shock. Fortunately, reconditioning is easier in this case than that for the bladder. In any case, correct treatment of these autonomic disturbances is mandatory.

Beside these autonomic failures, the most striking sequel of spasticity is the patient's motor disability. Depending on the level and the severity of the CNS lesion, the associated spasticity can result in a complete loss of voluntary movements. Even in less severe cases with preserved voluntary movements, the functional motor impairment due to spasticity can be striking, particularly affecting the dexterity of the hands, with an inability to independently use the fingers despite a preserved powerful grip. Other typical symptoms are spastic gait disturbances. In the prone position, patients with mild spastic paraplegia often show absent or only minor spastic muscle tone in their leg muscles. Upon walking they may nevertheless exhibit severe slowing of their gait with impaired dorsiflexion of the foot during the swing phase. The reasons for such a striking discrepancy in the expression of spasticity between the resting state and locomotion remain to be elucidated. At present, the most parsimonious explanation for this phenomenon is that in the upright position preserved fibers of the vestibulospinal tract are activated, which are known to excite preferentially anti-gravity muscles.

Chronic pain is a major complaint of patients suffering from spasticity.[19] In patients with spinal cord injury the prevalence of severe pain is estimated to be as much as 25%. The mechanisms of pain generation in spasticity are far from being fully understood. One likely mechanism is that pyramidal tract lesions will often involve afferent tracts like the lemniscal system or the spinothalamic tract with consecutive structural plastic changes. This may eventually lead to neuropathic pain. This may also provide a plausible explanation for differences in both the prevalence of pain and the time of its onset in spasticity depending on the lesion site.[20] For example, in spinal cord injury ascending and descending long fiber tracts are often damaged together, causing a higher prevalence of pain. The other type of pain in spasticity is of peripheral origin and arises from musculo-tendinous structures and joint receptors. Dystonic muscle tone, frequently seen in longstanding spasticity of any origin, can lead to painful contractures, and phasic flexor spasms and mass reflexes also are normally accompanied by painful sensations.

SPASTIC SYNDROMES CHARACTERIZED BY THE TOPOLOGY OF THE CNS LESION

In palliative neurology only rarely circumscribed lesions are responsible for the spastic syndrome. One way to classify different pathophysiological entities or syndromes of spasticity is to subdivide the spastic syndromes according to the lesion sites along the rostro-caudal extension of the pyramidal tract (Fig. 15–1). The site of the lesion determines directly how many of the pyramidal tract fibers are affected, whether other descending motor systems are involved (such as the corticobulbar and the corticocerebellar fibers), whether bulbospinal pathways are released from cortical control with intact connections to the spinal cord, and whether these centers

are damaged in the lower brain stem region.[21] In many cases a mixture of these pathophysiologically relevant mechanisms will occur following CNS lesions. This is most evident in severe traumatic brain injury where cortical, subcortical, and brain stem lesions occur, or in ischemic brain stem infarction following basilar artery thrombosis. Nevertheless, there are some principal pathophysiological rules in spasticity, based on animal experiments and on patients with well-defined localized lesions, which can be described.

Cortical Lesions

Circumscribed lesions of the primary motor cortex (BA 4) result in weakness of the affected limb, but not in spasticity. This relatively rare condition is called pure motor plegia. Larger lesions that extend into other parts of the sensorimotor cortex typically induce spasticity in addition to the paresis. Severe spasticity can develop following extensive cortical lesions, caused for example by cerebral hypoxia, although in such cases an additional contribution of brain stem nuclei cannot be excluded.

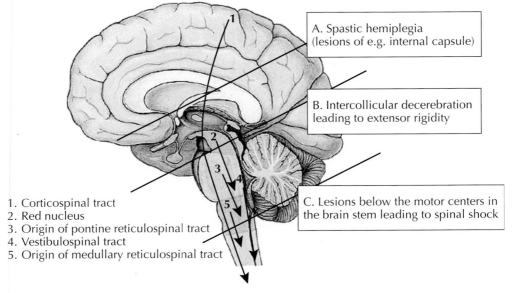

A. Spastic hemiplegia (lesions of e.g. internal capsule)

B. Intercollicular decerebration leading to extensor rigidity

C. Lesions below the motor centers in the brain stem leading to spinal shock

1. Corticospinal tract
2. Red nucleus
3. Origin of pontine reticulospinal tract
4. Vestibulospinal tract
5. Origin of medullary reticulospinal tract

Figure 15–1. Schema of the major descending motor tracts originating in the brain stem. The modulatory descending pathways (serotonergic, noradrenergic, dopaminergic) are not included in this illustration. In humans, the rubrospinal pathway has lost its significance. Brain stem lesions rostral to the origin of the vestibulospinal tract result in extensor spasms, corresponding to the extensor rigidity of the intercollicular decerebrate animal.

In large lesions of the primary sensorimotor cortex that extend into adjacent areas, spasticity develops slowly as an 'adaptation' process to the pyramidal tract injury.[22] It is preceded by a state of 'cerebral shock' with paresis of the affected limb, muscle hypotonia, and an absence of deep tendon jerks. By contrast, spastic muscle hypertonia can develop immediately when the lesion site involves the premotor cortex (BA 6). This is typically observed in patients with ischemic infarction in the territory of the anterior cerebral artery. As spasticity resulting from pyramidal tract lesions is in most cases preceded by a flaccid stage, the muscle hypertonia following damage of the frontal/prefrontal cortex, with its immediate onset, is a distinct pathophysiological phenomenon due to release from inhibition of subcortical motor centers.

Capsular Lesions

The fibers of the corticospinal and corticobulbar tracts are gathered into compact bundles in the posterior and anterior limbs of the internal capsule. Relatively small lesions in these areas can damage multiple voluntary motor pathways, resulting in hemiplegia of the contralateral face and limbs. The hemi-spastic syndrome associated with such lesions develops slowly over days and weeks.

Brain Stem Lesions

On the way from the internal capsule to the spinal cord, the corticobulbar fibers leave the pyramidal tract and cross the midline at different levels in the brain stem to reach their respective motor nuclei. Depending on the level of the brain stem lesion a number of clinical pictures can be encountered. For example, ipsilateral lesions of the facial nucleus and/or other cranial nuclei and contralateral hemiplegia can be observed. These so-called 'crossed brain stem syndromes' are easily recognizable, distinct clinical syndromes of high localizing value. More important with regard to spasticity is the degree of involvement of the descending brain stem pathways in the lesion. These pathways originate at different levels between the midbrain and the lower pons. Hence, the lower the brain stem lesion,

the more pathways are damaged.[6] Since these bulbospinal neurones are under steady control by higher centers, deafferentation of these neurones by more rostral lesions can induce disinhibition and thus hyperexcitability of descending motor pathways.

The animal model of this type of spasticity is the decerebrate cat.[2] From this model it is known that small variations in the height of the cross-section can change the type of muscle hypertonia. The reason for these sometimes dramatic changes is the proximity within the brain stem of the neurones where the main descending motor pathways originate (see Fig. 15–1). Most important in this context is the vestibulospinal tract that originates in the pons. It has predominantly excitatory connections to the motoneurones that support posture. Lesions cranial to the vestibular nuclei evoke muscle hypertonia preferentially in extensor muscles, because the intact vestibulospinal neurones are released from the inhibitory control of higher centers. Higher brain stem lesions destroy the neurones of the more rostrally localized lateral reticulospinal tract, which mainly subserves excitation of flexor muscles. This explains why, in brain stem lesions in man in some cases, extensor spasms prevail, while in others flexor spasms prevail.

Spinal Lesions

Most of the corticospinal fibers cross in the pyramidal decussation at the level of the medulla oblongata and then descend in the spinal cord in the lateral funiculus, an area lateral to the dorsal horn. A smaller portion of the corticospinal tract descends uncrossed in the spinal cord in the ventral funiculus, reaching the target neurones after crossing the midline at the respective segmental level. Damage of these uncrossed fibers has not been reported to cause spasticity. Spasticity of spinal origin can develop following any kind of unilateral or bilateral lesion of the lateral funiculus. Unilateral destruction of the lateral funiculus at high cervical level (e.g. by a mediolateral disc prolapse) causes ipsilateral hemiplegia; lesions at thoracic level above the motor nuclei of the leg muscles lead to ipsilateral monoplegia of the leg. In most cases, however, lesions of the spinal cord affect both sides, resulting in tetraplegia or paraplegia, respectively. Since the corticospinal fibers in the lateral funiculus intermingle with other descending fibers from bulbospinal pathways, complete destruction of the lateral funiculus invariably results in severe denervation of the segmental interneurones and motoneurones.

Even more disastrous is a complete spinal cord lesion with interruption of all descending motor fibers, which causes the 'spinal shock' syndrome. It is characterized by a flaccid tetraplegia (or paraplegia, again depending on the level of the lesion), accompanied by autonomic failure and complete sensory loss. While the loss of descending facilitation is the major pathophysiological mechanism in spinal shock,[23] the reason for the delayed recovery of excitability of motoneurones below the lesion and the development of spasticity remains obscure. Even in complete spinal cord lesions, the final degree of spasticity can vary between patients, and most severe spasticity is seen in conditions in which some supraspinal descending input to the spinal cord is preserved (e.g. in multiple sclerosis).

THERAPY OF SPASTICITY

When planning the therapy for patients with spasticity, it is most important to appreciate the patient's functional disability. Here, the treatment of palliative care patients does not differ from the treatment of other neurologic patients with spasticity. Accordingly, before any treatment of spasticity is initiated, detailed exploration and investigation of the patient's abilities and disabilities is mandatory. Patients with spastic hemiplegia do not necessarily need pharmacotherapy when they are able to walk, using the spastic/dystonic muscle tone as a 'substitute' for the lost physiologic muscle tone during the stance phase of walking. However, antispastic treatment is indicated whenever the high muscle tone results in an impairment of the activities of daily living or personal hygiene.

Typically, treatment is needed for patients with myelopathies who experience painful spasms or involuntary flexor or extensor trunk or leg movements (which, as described in the case history, are often associated with transfer or minor cutaneous stimulation). In spastic paraplegic gait, for example, when

circumduction of the legs is impaired, spastic muscle tone can severely impede walking, so that pharmacological treatment may be beneficial. The need for pharmacotherapy is even more evident when patients are chairbound or bedridden with painful spastic muscle spasms. Any pain resulting from spasticity should be treated. In palliative care, the sedative effect of some antispastic drugs may also prove useful. Even with optimal nursing care and hygiene, spasms resulting from spasticity normally cannot be controlled without muscle relaxants and /or botolinum toxin. The latter is also indicated in palliative care, as the improvement of the patient's quality of life is the main aim of therapy.

Physiotherapy

The basic therapy for any kind of spasticity is physiotherapy. Even in the acute flaccid state following a CNS lesion, physiotherapy has to be employed immediately to prevent contractures of joints, decubitus, and orthostatic hypotension. When spastic muscle tone develops, physiotherapy can prevent pathologic patterns of muscle synergy. Physiotherapy also helps to teach strategies to compensate for lost motor functions and to prevent irreversible shortening of dystonic muscles and the danger of fixed joint contractures. A number of additional therapeutic procedures can be applied, such as local application of ice, the use of biofeedback or functional electric stimulation (FES), and the daily treadmill training of paraplegic patients.

Pharmacotherapy

The evolving view that the functional impairment in spasticity is not primarily caused by the enhanced stretch reflex[15,17,24] has implications for the pharmacological therapy of spasticity. Most antispastic drugs used today have been developed and tested in animal models. Assessment of their therapeutic effectiveness has used their ability to reduce the tonic stretch reflex elicited in animal models of spasticity. The rather disappointing effect of these antispastic drugs on the functional disability of spastic patients supports the notion that the pathophysiologic bases of experimental and human spasticity differ. Moreover, a limiting factor for the use of muscle relaxants is their adverse effect on the residual voluntary force in spasticity.

To stand up and walk requires a considerable power in extensors. In hemiplegics or paraplegics who are deprived of their physiologic muscle tone, the 'pathological' but useful spastic muscle tone substitutes for the lost voluntary power. Pharmacological reduction of spastic muscle tone counteracts this beneficial postural adaptation and thus impedes the patient's functional performance. However, when spastic muscle tone is high in the presence of relatively preserved voluntary power, as can occur in hereditary spastic paraplegia, for example, oral treatment with baclofen, tizanidine, memantine, or benzodiazepines can ameliorate the motor disability. The antispastic action of cannabinoids is the subject of current drug trials. Oral medication with antispastic drugs always starts slowly in order to find the optimal individual dosage that ensures that the benefit of reduced spasticity outweighs the loss of voluntary power. General precautions regarding drug interactions and metabolic effects apply.

The situation is different in patients unable to use their limbs because of severe spasticity, in patients with flexor reflexes and mass reflexes, particularly in those with spinal spasticity, and in unconscious patients. Here the muscle-relaxing action of these drugs and its interaction with voluntary motor action is less problematic, so that doses can be much higher. In these patients the sedative effect of muscle relaxants becomes the dosage-limiting factor. In most severe cases of cerebral spasticity, following head trauma or hypoxic brain lesions in which patients are comatose, parenteral treatment with high dosages of benzodiacepines or barbiturates may be necessary to cope with muscle spasms. Dantrolene, which acts on the muscle fibers themselves by inhibiting the release of calcium into the myoplasm, is also a very effective substance in this situation. When patients survive the initial stage of coma, the spastic syndromes often subside, especially in children, while myoclonic jerks (Lance–Adams syndrome) and epileptic seizures may persist. This necessitates an adjustment of the pharmacotherapy, exchanging barbiturates for drugs such as clonazepam or valproic acid.

Severe spasticity of spinal origin, as frequently observed in advanced multiple sclerosis, can be effectively treated by continuous intrathecal application of baclofen via a subcutaneously implanted pump.[25] This is a safe method to ameliorate dystonic muscle spasms and phasic flexor spasms, in particular when oral treatment with baclofen or other potent antispastic drugs fails to evoke sufficient relief from these symptoms. More recently, the local injection of botulinum toxin into the end-plate region of skeletal muscles was introduced as an alternative antispastic therapy.[26] Botulinum toxin exerts its effect on the neuromuscular junction by reducing the release of acetylcholine from the motor axon terminals, thereby weakening the motor output. The therapeutic effect develops slowly over one or two weeks and lasts for a few months. Injections into the same muscles can be repeated when spasticity reappears. Many clinical trials have shown that botulinum toxin is useful in treating spastic dystonia of cerebral or spinal origin. Because of the need to inject each muscle separately, patients with spastic tetraplegia, generalized flexor spasms, or mass reflexes are not suitable for this type of treatment, as the total amount of toxin needed would exceed the tolerance limit. Treatment with botulinum toxin requires skill and extensive experience and should be limited to specialized centers. Its availability has reduced destructive neurosurgical procedures which nowadays are rarely indicated and confined to those rare cases in which painful muscle spasms are resistant to conservative therapy. Then, microsurgical lesions of the dorsal root entry zone are the treatment of choice. Other possible surgical procedures include tendon lengthening, tenotomy and tendon transfer, and correction of deformities induced by spasticity.

SUMMARY

Spasticity is characterized by an increased muscle tone with velocity-sensitive resistance to passive stretch during the initial phase of excursion; there may then be an abrupt decrease in resistance (the so-called 'clasp-knife' phenomenon). The physiologic basis of spasticity is only in part an increased dynamic stretch reflex. Other factors that contribute to spasticity are the decreased presynaptic inhibition to control the sensory inflow from the periphery, the loss of reciprocal innervation, and a loss of recurrent inhibition mediated by Renshaw cells. Also, an increase in motoneurone excitability from excitatory sources other than muscle spindles and changes in muscle fiber properties may contribute to spasticity.

The clinical syndrome of spasticity varies considerably and is strongly influenced by the topology of the lesion. Despite the disabilitating effects of spasticity, one should keep in mind that sometimes spasticity may be useful to a patient. For example, a patient with hemiplegia may need the increased muscle tone to make use of this spastic leg when walking. In chairbound or bedbound para- or tetraplegics, however, flexor spasms can be very painful and continue to be a major problem in patient management. Treatment strategies combine physiotherapy, to prevent contractures of joints, decubitus, and orthostatic hypotension, and pharmacotherapy, which is based on substances that act as muscle relaxants (e.g. baclofen, tizanidine, diazepam, and botolinum toxin).

REFERENCES

1. Lance JW. Symposium synopsis. In: Feldman RG, Young RR, Koella WP, eds. Spasticity: disordered motor control. Year Book Medical Publishers, Chicago, 1980:485–494.
2. Sherrington CS. Decerebrate rigidity and reflex co-ordination of movement. J Physiol (London) 1898; 22:319–322.
3. Burke D. Critical examination of the case for or against fusimotor involvement in disorders of muscle tone. In: Desmedt JE, ed. Motor Control Mechanisms in Health and Disease. Raven Press, New York, 1983:133–150.
4. Walshe FMR. The decerebrate rigidity of Sherrington in man. Its recognition and differentiation from other forms of tonic muscular contraction. Arch Neurol Psychiatry 1923;2:644–647.
5. Goldberger ME, Murray M. Patterns of sprouting and implications for recovery of function. In: Waxman SG, ed. Functional Recovery in Neurological Disease. Raven Press, New York, 1988:361–385.
6. Kuypers HGJM. Anatomy of the descending pathways. In: Brooks VB, ed. Handbook of Physiology. Williams and Wilkins, Baltimore, 1981:597–666.
7. Freund H–J. Abnormalities of motor behavior after cortical lesions in humans. In: Plum F, ed. Handbook of Physiology I. Williams and Wilkins, Baltimore, 1987:763–810.
8. Tower SS. Pyramidal lesions in the monkey. Brain 1940;63:36–90.
9. Denny–Brown D. The Cerebral Control of Movement. Liverpool University Press, Liverpool, 1966.
10. Nacimiento W, Sappok T, Brook GA, et al. Structural changes of anterior horn neurones and their synaptic input caudal to a low thoracic spinal cord hemisection in the adult rat: a light and electron microscopic study. Acta Neuropathol 1995;30:552–564.
11. Hounsgaard J, Hultborn H, Jespersen B, Kiehn O. Intrinsic membrane properties causing a bistable behaviour of α-motoneurones. Exp Brain Res 1984; 55:391–394.
12. Saruhashi Y, Wise Y, Perkins R. The recovery of 5-HT immunoreactivity in lumbosacral spinal cord and locomotor function after thoracic hemisection. Exp Neurol 1996;139:203–213.
13. Nacimiento W, Brook GA, Noth J. Lesion-induced neuronal reorganization in the spinal cord: morphological aspects. In: Freund H–J, Sabel BA, Witte OW, eds. Brain Plasticity. Lippincott–Raven, Philadelphia, 1997:37–59.
14. Schwab M, Bartholdi D. Degeneration and regeneration of axons in the lesioned spinal cord. Physiological Reviews 1996;76:319–370.
15. Young RR. Spasticity: a review. Neurology 1994; 44(Suppl. 9):S12–S20.
16. Dietz V, Quintern J, Berger W. Electrophysiological studies of gait in spasticity and rigidity: evidence that altered mechanical properties of muscle contribute to hypertonia. Brain 1981;103:431–449.
17. Noth J. Trends in the pathophysiology and pharmacotherapy of spasticity. J Neurol 1991;238:131–139.
18. Fellows SJ, Kaus C, Thilmann AF. Voluntary movement at the elbow in spastic hemiparesis. Ann Neurol 1994;36:397–407.
19. Siddall PJ, Loeser JD. Pain following spinal cord injury. Spinal Cord 2001;39:63–73.
20. Schott GD. Delayed onset and resolution of pain. Brain 2001;124:1067–1076.
21. Fulton JF. Physiology of the Nervous System. Oxford University Press, London, 1943.
22. Burke D. Spasticity as an adaptation to pyramidal tract injury. In: Waxman SG, ed. Functional Recovery in Neurological Disease. Raven Press, New York, 1998:401–423.
23. Nacimiento W, Noth J. What, if anything, is spinal shock? Arch Neurol 1999;56:1033–1035.
24. Dietz V. Role of peripheral afferents and spinal reflexes in normal and impaired human locomotion. Rev Neurol (Paris) 1987;4:241–254.
25. Penn RD. Intrathecal baclofen for spasticity of spinal origin: seven years of experience. J Neurosurg 1992;77:236–240.
26. Davis EC, Barnes MP. Botulinum toxin and spasticity. J Neurol Neurosurg Psychiatr 2000;69:143–149.

Chapter 16

Dysphagia

Mario Prosiegel
Edith Wagner–Sonntag
Gian Domenico Borasio

Dysphagia is a major problem in neurological patients requiring palliative care. An accurate assessment of swallowing problems and of dysphagia-related symptoms based on clinical, videofluoroscopic, and videoendoscopic evaluation is a prerequisite for appropriate treatment. Management of dysphagia in palliative patients comprises many pharmacological and non-pharmacological interventions. It should be performed on a team basis and should include the patient and his/her relatives in all important decisions such as augmented feeding techniques.

CASE HISTORY

Hans, aged 69, was admitted to our day clinic with swallowing problems, hypersalivation, drooling, and slurred speech due to a bulbar form of amyotrophic lateral sclerosis (ALS), the diagnosis of which was made six months previously. He was able to eat and drink quite normally, but the meals took longer than usual and there were recurrent episodes of choking on liquids. There was bilateral atrophy of the tongue with fibrillations and reduced motility in all directions, a delayed swallowing reflex, a weak voice, and slurred speech. Respiratory function was 60% of the predicted value. Hans was able to eat food which was soft but of almost normal consistency. Drinking was more difficult, and episodes of choking occurred whenever Hans was distracted. Endoscopic evaluation showed residues in the valleculae and piriform sinuses, but adequate voluntary and reflexive cough. During the next few weeks, while the physiotherapist and speech–language pathologists tried to optimize respiratory function and speech, there was a decline in swallowing function. The use of very soft food and thickened drinks and the insertion of a percutaneous endoscopic gastrostomy (PEG) were recommended. In order to save time and effort, Hans decided to use the PEG as a supplement on demand, especially for liquids. Hypersalivation and drooling were successfully reduced by the use of transdermal scopolamine without anticholinergic side effects.

INTRODUCTION

Dysphagia is defined as any difficulty in 'clearing the food and drink through the oral cavity, pharynx, and esophagus into the stomach at an appropriate rate and speed'. It is a frequent syndrome in patients with neurological diseases who need palliative care. Diseases causing swallowing disorders are listed in the International Statistical Classification of Diseases and Related Health Problems (ICD-10); more relevant to palliative care are the resulting consequences for the individual patient described in the International Classification of Functioning, Disability, and Health (ICIDH-2, ICF) of the World Health Organization. The ICF lists the following differentiation:

- Impairment (problems in body structures or body functions such as a significant deviation or loss)
- Activity limitation (difficulties an individual may have in executing activities)
- Participation restriction (problems an individual may experience in life situations)

The predominant activity limitation is difficulty in eating and/or drinking safely, as well as dependence on tube feeding and/or a tracheostomy. Participation restriction in dysphagic patients comprises loss of enjoyment of food and drink, an important domain of quality of life. Accordingly, management of dysphagia and of dysphagia-related symptoms is an important part of palliative care. The principles of intervention for neurogenic dysphagia in palliative medicine are similar to those in rehabilitation, since they are 'mainly focused on disability but aimed at handicap'.[1]

The different interventions for neurogenic dysphagia depend on the anatomical lesions as well as on the diseases which cause them.

ANATOMY

Neurogenic dysphagia may be caused by anatomical lesions at the following levels:

- Cerebral cortex

- Descending fibers from the cerebral cortex to the cranial nerve nuclei in the brain stem (corticobulbar fibers)
- Cranial nerve nuclei and swallowing centers (pattern generators for swallowing) of the brain stem
- Motor and sensory fibers of cranial nerves V (N. trigeminus), VII (N. facialis), IX (N. glossopharyngeus), X (N. vagus), and XII (N. hypoglossus)
- Neuromuscular junction
- Swallowing musculature

The swallowing musculature is represented on the cerebral cortex of both hemispheres, mainly within the inferior part of the sensorimotor cortex (fronto-parietal operculum) and the anterior part of the insula. In the majority of individuals there is asymmetric representation for swallowing between the two hemispheres, independent of handedness.[2]

In patients with bilateral lesions of the swallowing cortex or of the corticobulbar tracts, the cranial nerve nuclei of both brain stem halves are isolated from all cortical inputs with the net result of severe dysphagia. Clinical examples are:

- *Bilateral operculum syndrome* (Foix–Chavany–Marie syndrome) due to bilateral infarctions of the fronto-parietal operculum with 'anarthria and bilateral central facio-linguovelo-pharyngeo-masticatory paralysis'
- *Pseudobulbar palsy* due to bilateral affection of the corticobulbar tracts, caused by stroke lesions or fiber degeneration (e.g. in primary lateral sclerosis)

Because of inter-hemispheric asymmetry, unilateral lesions of the cerebral cortex and/or its descending (corticobulbar) fibers cause dysphagia in those patients in whom the hemisphere with the larger ('dominant') swallowing cortex is affected. The most frequent clinical example is unilateral hemispheric stroke.

Neurogenic dysphagia occurs also after unilateral or bilateral damage to structures at the other anatomical levels: medullary and pontine cranial nerve nuclei, medullary central pattern generators (CPG) for swallowing (dorsomedial CPG near the nucleus of the solitary tract, ventrolateral CPG in the vicinity of the nucleus ambiguus), cranial nerves, neuromuscular junction, and swallowing muscles.

DISEASES

Of particular importance with respect to palliative care are brain tumors and neurological complications resulting from cancer, infection with the human immunodeficiency virus type-1 (HIV-1), degenerative motor neurone disease, stroke, and degenerative diseases of the CNS including different kinds of dementia, as well as old age.

Brain Tumors and Neurological Complications Resulting from Cancer

Brain tumors, including brain metastases, occur in 20%–40% of cancer patients and may cause dysphagia, especially when affecting the brain stem and the base of the skull (see Chapter 4). Other complications of cancer which are relevant to swallowing disorders are meningeal metastases, metabolic encephalopathy, cerebrovascular complications (due to direct invasion, coagulation disorders, chemotherapy side effects, and non-bacterial thrombotic endocarditis), and paraneoplastic syndromes. The latter may present as bulbar encephalitis/paraneoplastic encephalomyelitis, Lambert–Eaton myasthenic syndrome, or inflammatory muscle disease (dermatomyositis (DM); polymyositis (PM); inclusion body myositis (IBM)). The association with malignancy is more frequent in DM than in PM, and more common in PM than in IBM. The frequency of dysphagia in PM or DM is reported to vary between 12%–54% and is not yet known in IBM.[3]

Human Immunodeficiency Virus Type-1 (HIV-1)

Infection with HIV-1 may compromise swallowing through one of many possible complications, including:
- HIV encephalitis
- HIV leukoencephalopathy
- HIV-associated dementia or AIDS dementia complex (ADC)
- Opportunistic infections such as cryptococcosis, toxoplasmosis, cytomegalovirus (CMV) infection, progressive multifocal leukencephalopathy (PML) caused by a papova virus called JC (initials of a patient), herpetic encephalitis, tick-borne encephalitis, herpes zoster multifocal encephalitis, and bacterial (lues, metastatic encephalitis connected with heart valve lesions) or fungal (candidiasis) infections

Primary CNS lymphoma is an important differential diagnosis. Neurogenic dysphagia is very common in PML. In CMV infection of the CNS a polyneuritis cranialis with dysphagia may occur. Esophageal candidiasis and bacterial or CMV esophagitis should be considered also as the sole or contributory cause of dysphagia in HIV-infected patients (see Chapter 7).

Stroke

With a reported incidence of about 240 in 100,000 per year and a prevalence of 900 in 100,000, stroke is the most frequent cause of dysphagia. Brain infarction accounts for 80% of stroke causes. In the acute and subacute phase of stroke, dysphagia occurs in about 50% of patients; about two thirds of aspirations are 'silent'. Since about 50% of dysphagic stroke patients die or recover spontaneously within two weeks, about one half will present chronic swallowing problems.[4] Predominant dysphagic symptoms after stroke are delayed pharyngeal swallow, disturbed lingual movements, and reduced tongue base retraction; in patients with left-hemispheric stroke, signs of swallowing apraxia may additionally be found. In patients with unilateral brain stem stroke, unilateral pharyngeal weakness, unilateral vocal cord paresis, and reduced laryngeal elevation with dysfunction of the upper esophageal sphincter (UES) may occur (see Chapter 2).

Degenerative Motor Neurone Disease

In 25% of patients motor neurone disease begins with bulbar signs such as dysarthria and dysphagia; this rapidly 'progressive bulbar palsy' is caused by degeneration of motor neurones of cranial nerve nuclei V, VII, IX, X, and XII. Clinically the disease is characterized by a mixture of upper motor neurone (UMN) signs such as spasticity, central paresis, pyramidal signs, and hyperreflexia, and lower motor neurone (LMN) signs such as weakness, with atrophy and fasciculations of limb muscles and fibrillations of the tongue. Mean duration of the disease is 3–5 years. During the disease progression nearly 100% of ALS patients show oral and/or pharyngeal involvement. In the later stages of ALS, dysphagia is very common and aspiration pneumonia, either on its own or in conjunction with respiratory insufficiency, may lead to death.[5,6] Dysphagic symptoms comprise reduced lingual control, reduced tongue base retraction, delayed pharyngeal swallow, reduced laryngeal closure, and UES dysfuntion.

Dysphagia in ALS almost invariably progresses as respiratory function declines. Patients should be informed at an early stage about the possibility of supplementing the intake of food and fluid using PEG, since the risk of the procedure increases in patients with vital capacity less than 50% of the predicted level.[7] For answers to more detailed questions on the management of dysphagia in ALS patients, the review by Wagner–Sonntag et al. is recommended (see also Chapter 8).[8]

Degenerative Diseases of the CNS, Age, and Dementia

Parkinson's disease (PD) is a frequent neurodegenerative disorder and constitutes the most common extrapyramidal syndrome (see Chapter 5). Its histological characteristics are depletion of pigmented neurons in the substantia nigra of the midbrain with typical intracellular inclusions called Lewy bodies. The clinical features consist of rigor, tremor, akinesia, postural disturbances, cognitive decline, and vegetative signs. Dysphagia occurs in about 50% of patients with PD.[3] Predominant dysphagic symptoms are pumping motions of the tongue, disturbed tongue base retraction, delayed pharyngeal swallow, reduced laryngeal closure, and UES dysfunction. Motility disturbances of the esophagus and the gastrointestinal tract are also frequent associated findings.

Progressive supranuclear palsy (PSP, Steele–Richardson–Olszewski syndrome) is sometimes difficult to distinguish from PD, especially in the early stages. PSP is a progressive neurodegenerative disease with a mean duration of several years. Besides features of Parkinsonism the following symptoms can be found: axial dystonia and nuchal rigidity, vertical gaze paralysis (especially in the downward direction), dementia, and pseudobulbar signs. Dysphagia occurs frequently in PSP.

Multiple system atrophy (MSA) is a progressive neurodegenerative disease which can be divided into three clinicopathologically overlapping syndromes: olivopontocerebellar atrophy (OPCA), striatonigral degeneration (SND), and Shy–Drager syndrome (SDS). The main clinical features are cerebellar signs, Parkinsonism, and autonomic failure. In early disease stages it is, therefore, often difficult to distinguish between MSA and PD. Death occurs after a mean disease duration of 7–9 years and is caused in most patients by aspiration pneumonia or respiratory insufficiency. The frequency of dysphagia in patients with MSA is reported to be as high as 50%. In MSA patients with stridor the survival time is shorter and tracheotomy has to be considered.

In patients with extrapyramidal syndromes, the average time to onset of dysphagia varies greatly (from 42 months for PSP to 130 months for PD), but after the onset of dysphagia the survival time is consistently 15–24 months for all extrapyramidal disorders.[9] These data reinforce the importance of this symptom from both a clinical and a prognostic point of view in neurological palliative care.

The causes of dysphagia in *elderly patients and/or those with dementia* are very different and comprise stroke, Parkinsonian syndromes, white matter lesions, bad dental status, diminished production of saliva, and cognitive decline (see Chapter 6). Additionally, protein-energy malnutrition is of importance in the elderly, leading to weakness of the deglutitive and respiratory musculature and a reduced immune status favoring aspiration pneumonia.

Multiple Sclerosis

Multiple sclerosis (MS) is an inflammatory demyelinating disease of the CNS (see Chapter 3). In the pathogenesis of MS autoimmune mechanisms play an important role, but the etiology is still unknown. Dysphagia occurs in about 40% of MS patients and the symptoms are similar to those found in ALS, with the addition of sensory disturbances. Aspiration pneumonia is a frequent cause of death.

Iatrogenic Causes

A variety of drugs and other iatrogenic measures may cause swallowing disorders or aggravate existing dysphagia. Examples comprise:

- Disturbed elevation of hyoid and larynx after irradiation of oropharyngeal/laryngeal tumors
- Ipsilateral vagal nerve paresis as a result of carotid endarterectomy
- Weakness of pharyngeal muscles due to botulinum toxin injection into neck muscles for torticollis. Pharmacological side effects of many drugs: benzodiazepines (sedation due to GABAergic effect on CNS), neuroleptics and the antiemetic drug metoclopramide (CNS dopamine antagonist), various agents with CNS anticholinergic properties, aminogylosid antibiotics (affection of the neuromuscular junction), steroids, colchicine, cholesterol-lowering agents, and L-tryptophan (myopathy).

ASSESSMENT OF DYSPHAGIA

Specific interventions for dysphagia require a careful assessment of swallowing function comprising history, observation of signs of aspiration, clinical examination, and swallowing examination. The most important clinical signs predicting about two-thirds of patients who aspirate are: wet phonation, reduced laryngeal elevation, abnormal voluntary cough, abnormal phonation quality, harsh phonation, and breathy phonation.[10]

More trials are needed for more conclusive evidence of the value of screening tests and pulse oximetry. Nevertheless, bedside screening using the 50 ml water test (5 ml aliquots of water; positive result if any coughing or wet voice quality occurs) in conjunction with examination of pharyngeal sensation, which is often reported as being disturbed in patients with silent aspirations, seems to be fairly accurate.[11] The diagnostic gold standard is videofluoroscopic study of swallowing (VFSS) which provides helpful hints for swallowing therapy.[12] Because of the frequent finding of

respiratory dysfunction and the high risk of aspirations in patients with dysphagia, a modified barium swallow should be limited to patients with only mild dysphagia. Hyperosmolar contrast media such as gastrografin may provoke life-threatening lung edema if aspiration occurs; the iso-osmolar contrast agent iotrolan, with no significant side effects in cases of aspiration, is therefore recommended. When VFSS cannot be performed (e.g. in bedridden and/or unco-operative patients), fiberoptic endoscopic evaluation of swallowing (FEES) is a good alternative, allowing direct visualization of the pharynx and larynx. Whether the management of dysphagia is guided by the results of VFSS or of FEES, the outcome with regard to pneumonia incidence seems to be very similar.[13]

MANAGEMENT OF DYSPHAGIA

Co-operation in the therapy of dysphagic symptoms is most important and can usually be achieved by giving as much information as possible about the therapeutic measures being considered. Exercises which are frequently viewed by the patients as being annoying and time-consuming may, after careful counseling, be accepted as helpful measures and as a change from the daily routine.

Pharmacological Interventions for Dysphagia and Dysphagia-related Symptoms

In most patients with severe hypersalivation, anticholinergic drugs (e.g. transdermal scopolamine lasting 24–72 hours) or drugs with anticholinergic side effects (e.g. amitriptyline) are effective.[14] In rare cases, botulinum toxin injection or radiation of the parotid gland may be indicated. When thick secretions are a major problem for the patient, N-acetylcysteine is the drug of choice.

Hiccup is often associated with neurogenic dysphagia. The treatment of choice is a combination of baclofen, a prokinetic drug (e.g. domperidone), and a proton pump inhibitor (e.g. omeprazole).[15] If this combination therapy is not effective or if there are contraindications, other drugs can be applied (e.g. anticonvulsant drugs such as valproic acid, carbamazepine, or gabapentin and/or neuroleptics such as chlorpromazine).

Gastroesophageal reflux disease often causes symptoms such as acid regurgitation and heartburn and may cause or aggravate dysphagia.[16] It should be treated with proton pump inhibitors (e.g. pantoprazole or omeprazole), and the additional application of a prokinetic agent such as domperidone is sometimes necessary.

In some patients with predominant UES dysfunction, cricopharyngeal myotomy or botulinum toxin injection of the UES (endoscopically or transcervically) may be a successful intervention. The prerequisites for both procedures are the same:[17]

1. UES dysfunction
2. Normal elevation of hyoid and larynx
3. Swallowing therapy not successful in achieving the opening of the UES
4. Pharyngeal pressure sufficient to propel a bolus through the open sphincter

Therefore, manometry is necessary prior to these procedures. They are rarely indicated in palliative care patients.

Functional Swallowing Therapy

Functional swallowing therapy depends on the availability of swallowing therapists (usually specially trained speech and language therapists). It focuses more on the disturbed body functions and less on the underlying disease.[18] Patient's residual symptoms and abilities as well as wishes and habits have to be considered when planning therapy. For example, in the case of an elderly patient with a reduced strength and motility of the tongue (and subsequent leaking and aspiration of fluids), engaging in exercises and learning swallowing techniques may be less realistic than simply thickening the drinks to prevent aspiration. PEG feeding must sometimes be considered in patients who are still able to eat and drink, but for whom the learning of a swallowing technique is too exhausting.

To assess specific deficits and residual capacities, an accurate bedside examination will include evaluation of neuromuscular functions (i.e. motility, range, strength) of lips, cheeks, tongue, velum, and larynx, body mass index (BMI), respiratory function (vital capacity), cognition, and motivation. BMI reflects the nutritional state; the respiratory function predicts whether certain swallowing maneuvers or techniques may be helpful and assists decisions about when to recommend a PEG or when to stop oral intake. Cognition and motivational factors provide clues as to an individual's ability to follow instructions and to perform exercises or compensatory strategies on a regular basis and during mealtimes.

If there is enough neuromuscular capacity, exercises can help to preserve the range of movements necessary for swallowing in palliative patients. In progressive diseases like ALS, compensatory strategies and safety techniques are more important.[8]

Exercises

Exercises aim to stabilize/maintain a patient's condition and to support safe oral feeding for as long as possible, but should not exhaust the patient. They reinforce the patient's ability to perform the movements necessary for swallowing and to compensate progressive deficits.

Fatigue is a very common symptom (e.g. in ALS patients) and occurs very early during exercises. Short periods of training, several times a day, with long breaks in between, are desirable. The choice of exercise(s) to be performed depends on the patient's specific swallowing problem(s).

LIP CLOSURE

Patients should try to press the lips together, hold, and relax. There are a lot of possible variations like, for example, holding a little piece of paper or holding a straw between the lips.

TONIZATION OF THE CHEEKS

Patients should suck the cheeks against the teeth, then hold in that position, and relax.

MASTICATION

Patients should pretend to be chewing on old bread or chewing gum, etc.

VELAR MOVEMENT

Articulatory movements with plosives and nasals in words like 'mamba', 'Bombay',

'Simba', 'Inka' or pronouncing 'i' are suitable for practising velar movement. To provide a sufficient intra-oral negative pressure, lip closure with good tone in the cheeks and velar movement is needed. Adequate lip closure supports mastication and bolus control.

TONGUE MOVEMENTS

Patients should try to lick around the lips, to 'count' the teeth, to press the middle part of the tongue against the hard palate, to push the tongue out and pull it back again, etc. Articulatory exercises will also practise tongue movements: for example, with 't' or 'n' for elevation of the tip of the tongue and 'k' or 'ng' for elevation of the back of the tongue (e.g. 'tea', 'knee', 'cake', 'wing'). A change in rounded/unrounded vowels ('teeth' vs. 'tooth', 'take' vs. 'took') or in the tip of tongue/back of the tongue ('key' vs. 'tea', 'cool' vs. 'tool') practises diadochokinetic movements.

TRIGGERING OF THE SWALLOWING REFLEX

Thermal stimulation of the anterior faucial pillars is effective in triggering the swallowing reflex,[19] as are chewing or sucking activation. Due to the risk of gagging, thermal stimulation should not be used in patients with hyperreflexia. Cold or spicy foods increase sensory input and help trigger the swallowing reflex. Patients with pseudobulbar symptoms can tilt the head back in order to help saliva flow backwards.

IMPROVING THE SWALLOWING RATE

Symptoms like hypersalivation, thickening of oral secretions, and sudden bouts of coughing are often caused by a reduced swallowing frequency. In those cases, the patient should be encouraged to swallow more often voluntarily. Patients who suffer from drooling should be advised to swallow before trying to open the mouth or to speak.

Compensatory Strategies

Compensatory methods aim at overcoming delayed swallowing reflex, deficient glottic closure, or insufficient opening of the UES, to ensure a full oral intake or at least partial oral nutrition.

POSITIONING

The patient should sit in a comfortable, usually upright, position while eating and drinking.

POSTURAL CHANGES

Postural changes aim at guiding the bolus via gravity, making the bolus transport more efficient and preventing aspiration. In patients with pseudobulbar symptoms, impaired tongue movements (and resulting difficulty initiating a swallow), but still intact pharyngeal phase of swallowing, tilting the *head backwards* helps to guide the bolus into the pharynx. In patients with bulbar symptoms who have difficulty in triggering the swallowing reflex, *tilting the head forward* may avoid leaking and subsequent aspiration. By use of this 'chin tuck' the valleculae are widened and epiglottic tilt is supported.

In patients with unilateral paresis of the tongue, pharynx, and larynx, *tilting the head to the stronger side* may guide the bolus in this direction. In patients with unilateral paresis of the pharynx, *turning the head to the affected side* helps in closing the ipsilateral recessus piriformes and prevents retentions.

DIETARY MODIFICATIONS

Dietary modification may help to prevent extremely long mealtimes, fatigue, and dread of meals. Soft textures or puréed food can compensate for poor oral preparation phase and ease oral and pharyngeal transport. Liquids should be thickened when thin drinks cause choking. In ALS patients, a reduced respiratory function results in an increased energy demand. The patient should, therefore, be in contact with a dietitian for advice on how to enrich the meals with calories and protein. Patients and relatives need instruction in the preparation of high caloric food and textures which are easy to chew and swallow (including thickening of liquids in order to avoid dehydration). In ALS patients abdominal weakness and failure of glottic closure can lead to constipation requiring added fiber. Triggering of the swallowing reflex can be enhanced by emphasizing taste or temperature: cooled drinks are often easier to swallow. Recipe books specific for neurogenic dysphagia are available from ALS associations in many countries.

SWALLOWING TECHNIQUES

Swallowing techniques must be performed on every single swallow during meals. They are, therefore, rather challenging and require patients with fairly good cognitive abilities. In patients without these prerequisites, multiple swallows may be sufficient to clear residues in the mouth or pharynx.

Supraglottic swallowing is a technique which helps to close the vocal cords during swallowing. The patient holds his breath while swallowing and exhales at full force immediately afterwards. Food or secretion can be expelled from the laryngeal vestibulum by this technique in order to avoid aspiration. This technique is recommended when laryngeal closure is weak and/or the triggering of the swallowing reflex is delayed. It is appropriate for patients who have a normal or near-normal respiratory function and are able to cough and clear the throat.

The Mendelsohn maneuver is a technique which helps to open the UES and prolong its opening time. The patient has to hold the upward movement of the larynx during swallowing for some seconds. This technique is appropriate for patients with pharyngeal residues or deficient opening of the UES (e.g. due to reduced laryngeal movement or weak tongue base movement).

Therapists often have to practise basic functions first: training the patient to close the glottis or to hold his breath on command before teaching the supraglottic swallow; strengthening the tongue base before training the Mendelsohn maneuver.

Adaptations

Adaptations are modifications of the environment which may ease nutrition (e.g. specially formed cups which enable the patient to drink with the head tilted forwards). In order to improve the swallowing rate, the patient can use a simple timer, which reminds him/her at an individually determined interval (e.g. every 40 seconds) to swallow following a 'beep' signal. Patients without significant cognitive dysfunction very quickly learn to swallow more frequently using this simple aid.

Safety Strategies

It is helpful to create a silent, relaxed atmosphere during mealtimes and to avoid distractions like conversation, TV, radio, or other noisy and stress-inducing situations. When patients show a significant level of fatigue, as is often seen in ALS, they are advised to eat several small meals a day which are enriched with additional calories (e.g. with maltodextrose).

In patients with sufficient bolus control, piecemeal deglutition (the division of the bolus into several small boli which can be successively swallowed) may be helpful also. Patients who suffer from episodes of choking while eating or drinking may feel more secure when carers and the family know how to apply the Heimlich maneuver.

Augmented Feeding Techniques and Tracheostomy

As dysphagia becomes more severe, augmented feeding techniques such as nasogastric tube feeding and PEG have to be carefully discussed. Nasogastric tube feeding should be only used for a short time because of many disadvantages, and PEG is, therefore, in most cases the treatment of choice.[8, 20] For ethical concerns about augmented feeding techniques see Chapter 32.

For patients who cannot swallow their own secretions safely, the decision has to be made whether or not to perform a tracheostomy. The consequences of tracheostomies should be carefully discussed with the patient at an early stage of the disease (e.g. in ALS): tracheostomies have to be regularly suctioned; the tubes have to be changed; a tracheostomy may exert a negative influence on swallowing; tracheostomy hinders speaking, since the cuff has to be blocked in the case of severe dysphagia; even in patients who can wear speaking tubes, the degree of respiratory muscle strength required often cannot be achieved. For details on invasive ventilatory support through tracheostomy ventilation see Chapter 23.

Counseling

One of the most important aspects of interventions for dysphagia is careful advice on how to prevent malnutrition, dehydration, and pneumonia. The patient and his/her relatives should be informed as early as possible, and at regular intervals, about all kinds of available interventions including nutritional supplements, augmented feeding techniques, and tracheostomy.

SUMMARY

Management of dysphagia in palliative care includes an array of measures and requires a multidisciplinary team approach. Physicians, swallowing therapists, dietitians, and the patients and their relatives should work closely together to provide the best management of dysphagia during palliative care. More studies are required to establish the effectiveness and optimal timing of palliative interventions aimed at this important symptom in neurological palliative care patients.

REFERENCES

1. Wade DT, ed. Measurement in Neurological Rehabilitation. Oxford University Press, Oxford, 1992:3–14.
2. Hamdy S, Rothwell JC, Brooks DJ, Bailey D, Aziz Q, Thompson DG. Identification of the cerebral loci processing human swallowing with H2(15)O PET activation. Journal of Neurophysiology 1999;81:1917–26.
3. Kuhlemeier KV. Epidemiology and dysphagia. Dysphagia 1994;9:209–17.
4. Bath PMW, Bath FJ, Smithard DG. Interventions for dysphagia in acute stroke. The Cochrane Library 3. Update Software Ltd.: Oxford.
5. Borasio GD, Voltz R. Palliative care in amyotrophic lateral sclerosis. Journal of Neurology 1997;244 (Suppl. 4): S11–S7.
6. Borasio GD, Gelinas DF, Yanagisawa N. Mechanical ventilation in amyotrophic lateral sclerosis: a cross-cultural perspective. Journal of Neurology 1998;245 (Suppl. 2):S7–S12.
7. Borasio GD, Sloan R, Pongratz DE. Breaking the news in amyotrophic lateral sclerosis. Journal of the Neurological Sciences 1998;160(Suppl. 1): S127–S33.
8. Wagner–Sonntag E, Allison S, Oliver D, Prosiegel M, Rawlings J, Scott A. Dysphagia. In: Oliver D, Borasio GD, Walsh D, eds. Palliative Care in Amyotrophic Lateral Sclerosis. Oxford University Press, Oxford, 2000:62–72.
9. Müller J, Wenning GK, Verny M, et al. Progression of dysarthria and dysphagia in postmortem-confirmed parkinsonian disorders. Archives of Neurology 2001;58:259–264.
10. Linden P, Kuhlemeier KV, Patterson C. The probability of correctly predicting subglottic penetration from clinical observations. Dysphagia 1993;8: 170–179.
11. Martino R, Pron G, Diamant N. Screening for oropharyngeal dysphagia in stroke: insufficient evidence for guidelines. Dysphagia 2000;15:19–30.
12. Logemann JA, Rademaker AW, Pauloski BR, Ohmae Y, Kahrilas PJ. Normal swallowing physiology as viewed by videofluoroscopy and videoendoscopy. Folia Phoniatrica et Logopedica 1998;50:311–319.
13. Aviv JE. Prospective, randomized outcome study of endoscopy versus modified barium swallow in patients with dysphagia. Laryngoscope 2000;110:563–574.
14. Talmi YP, Finkelstein Y, Zohar Y. Reduction of salivary flow with transdermal scopolamine: a four-year experience. Otolaryngology—Head and Neck Surgery 1990;103:615–618.
15. Petroianu G, Hein G, Petroianu A, Bergler W, Rüfer R. Idiopathic chronic hiccup: combination therapy with cisapride, omeprazole, and baclofen. Clinical Therapeutics 1997;19:1031–1038.
16. Cote DN, Miller RH. The association of gastroesophageal reflux and otolaryngologic disorders. Comprehensive Therapy 1995;21:80–84.
17. Kelly JH. Management of upper esophageal sphincter disorders: indications and complications of myotomy. American Journal of Medicine 2000;108(Suppl. 4a): S43–S46.
18. Logemann JA. Approaches to management of disordered swallowing. Bailliere's Clinical Gastroenterology 1991;5:269–280.
19. Kaatzke–McDonald MN, Post E, Davis PJ. The effects of cold, touch, and chemical stimulation of the anterior faucial pillar on human swallowing. Dysphagia 1996;11:198–206.
20. Boyd KJ, Beeken L. Tube feeding in palliative care: benefits and problems. Palliative Medicine 1994;8:156–158.

Chapter 17

Communication Impairment

Amanda Scott
Margaret Foulsum

This chapter examines the nature of communication impairment frequently encountered in palliative care settings and the role of the speech and language therapist in the assessment and management of these problems. The specific components of communication—cognition, speech, language and pragmatics—are examined. The focus of intervention for this clinical population is one of informational counselling and the provision of compensatory management strategies. This intervention involves the patient and their key communication partners and should take into consideration changes in the patient's functional and emotional states.

CASE HISTORY

SD was a 66-year-old man diagnosed with a glioma in the left parietal region. His initial symptom was word-finding difficulties, which he and his wife interpreted as a memory problem. At first the problems were mild and intermittent. SD and his wife were anxious and fearful that the problem may develop into dementia. After a few weeks of worsening word-finding difficulties, SD went to his doctor who quickly referred him to a neurologist. After a series of assessments a diagnosis of a glioma was made and, as the tumor was aggressive, a course of radiation therapy and steroids was begun. The medical focus of the intervention was on a reduction in the size and rate of growth of the tumor. However, because of the presenting problems, a referral for speech–language therapy was made. At first SD was unsure whether it was worth attending because he realistically considered that his prognosis was poor and that any improvement in function would be related to the effectiveness of the radiotherapy and medication.

The initial speech pathology assessment was conducted informally using a conversational technique involving SD, his wife, and the therapist. The characteristics of an anomic aphasia were clearly

165

present. While his speech was fluent, word-finding difficulties were obvious. His responses to questions were circuitous, with descriptions of target words. However, he was able to use gesture to augment his verbal communication. He demonstrated that he was able to comprehend language but was unable to match his thoughts with the appropriate words. The same problems were present when he attempted to write down a message. Although these problems were the cardinal features of his presentation, an informed discussion regarding the specific nature of the communication problems had not taken place. Consequently, fears that the problems represented a dementing process were causing anxiety and increased grief. Sadly, SD died within five months of diagnosis.

Speech and language therapy addressed the need of both SD and his wife to gain an understanding of the nature of the communication problems and enabled them to develop appropriate conversational repair strategies, such as sound and semantic cuing, stopping for clarification, and the use of gesture to supplement speech. The therapy provided an opportunity for SD and his wife to express their fears and frustrations in an informed and supportive environment. The intervention avoided extensive formal assessment, which would have been confronting, or speech drills, which would have been ineffective.

THE CONCEPT OF COMMUNICATION

The quality of communication is a primary concern of those involved in palliative care. The need for quality interactions regarding decision making and informed consent between patients, their families, and health professionals is a key element in palliative care practice and is a frequent topic in the palliative care literature.[2-5] It is, therefore, surprising that the nature and impact of communication impairment during the end stage of life and appropriate assessment and management strategies have received little attention. The role of the speech–language pathologist in the care of people with communication problems in palliative care settings also needs further exploration.

Clinicians and carers, in their engagement with patients, need to recognize that communication is a complex process comprising a number of different activities (Table 17–1). When the majority of interactions are brief episodes of small talk or a quick exchange related to basic needs and wants, subtle communication problems may not be recognized and there is a danger of patients being wrongly labelled as lacking motivation or being difficult.

Breakdowns in the communication process can occur at the level of the listener (receptive) or at the level of the speaker (expressive). An ability to function at all levels of communication is dependent on the integrity of several components of the communication process (Fig. 17–1). Effective communication requires appropriate adherence to a range of behaviors, such as turn taking and topic maintenance.

Disruption of particular components of the communication process leads to specific types of communication problems. The speech–language pathologist uses an analytical approach to impaired communication to better understand the problem and to select targeted strategies.

Table 17–1. **Communication Activities**[6]

Face-to-face conversation. Rapid, informal exchange of thoughts and feelings. Small talk between two or more partners.

Quick basic needs/wants. Quick communication of needs/wants (e.g. change position, change the channel, wipe mouth).

Detailed needs/wants. Conveying at least a few sentences about a need/want to be sure that the partner understands (e.g. indicate what you want to do on an outing).

Detailed information. Conveying considerable information (e.g. tell someone how you feel about him/her, give your opinion on an issue or topic).

Personal stories/anecdotes. Telling a personal story or anecdote during a communication interaction for purposes of illustrating a point, exchanging experiences, telling a joke, etc.

Telephone. Using a voice output device or an interpreter to communicate over the phone.

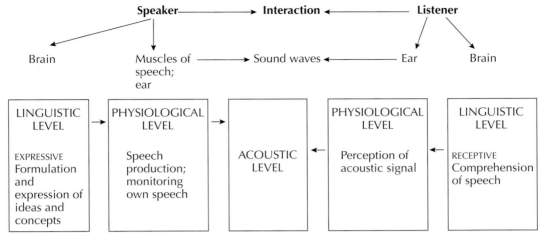

Figure 17–1. Diagram of basic components of the communication process.

Hearing, attention, and comprehension are receptive aspects of communication. Impairment of receptive function impacts on expressive communication because perception and understanding of input are needed to formulate and express ideas. An individual with impaired receptive function may disguise the problem by relying on automatic social interactions or by nodding and smiling and seeming to agree with what is being said. Problems may become apparent only when a response or action, subsequent to discussion, is required.

The expressive aspects of communication impairment are usually recognized. Speech production requires the integrity of several aspects. Table 17–2 provides the basic conceptual framework of the expressive aspects of communication upon which an understanding of impaired communication can be based.

CAUSES OF COMMUNICATION IMPAIRMENT

Communication problems commonly encountered in palliative care settings may result from progressive neurological disease or cerebral tumors, primary or secondary. Primary tumors of the head and neck, breast and lung frequently metastasize to the brain. Investigations into the extent of the spread of the cancer may have ceased by the time a patient reaches palliative care, and secondary

Table 17–2. A Model of Expressive Communication for Adults (Adapted from[7])

Function	Domain	Disorders
Idea	Cognition	Dementia; confusion
Sounds; words; grammar	Language	Aphasia
Motor plan	Motor planning	Apraxia of speech
Speech movements	Speech production	Dysarthria

cerebral tumors causing both behavioral and communication problems escape recognition.

Confusion

Confusion is frequently encountered in palliative care settings, particularly in patients with advanced cancer (see Chapter 22). Confusional states are often transitory and may be related to metabolic problems and medications. Individuals may experience illusions, hallucinations, delusions, excitement, restlessness, and incoherence.[8] The characteristic features of communication during confused states include impaired orientation to the environment, reduced attention span, memory problems, and an inability to think clearly.

Cognitive Impairment and Dementia

There is a wide spectrum of possible deficits from specific cognitive impairment to dementia (see Chapter 6). Dementia represents a global loss of intellectual function that includes learning, memory, motor skills, and social skills. Specific cognitive impairment implies the selective loss of some of these functions and directly impacts on the communication process, often through leading to a paucity of information in the communication process and poor adherence to the rules of interactions, such as turn taking and sticking to the topic.[9]

Cognitive impairments and dementia are very common in patients with advanced cancer. Pereira et al. reported a prevalence of 44% in patients with advanced cancer on admission to a palliative care unit.[8] Dementia is a feature in the latter stages of the progressive neurological conditions, Parkinson's disease, progressive supranuclear palsy,[10] Huntington's disease, and amyotrophic lateral sclerosis.[11] Dementia and cognitive problems may escape recognition in the end stage of these conditions because speech is severely dysarthric.

Aphasia

Aphasia is a specific language disorder that can involve deficits across all linguistic modalities including listening, speaking, reading, and writing. This type of impairment represents the breakdown of the ability to handle symbolic information. Different types of aphasia result from lesions in specific areas of the brain, usually in the left hemisphere, which subserves a range of linguistic functions. Table 17–3 covers the principal aphasic syndromes and demonstrates that specific aphasias have characteristic problems. It is very important to recognize the nature of these deficits because well-meaning attempts to improve the communication of an aphasic person, such as providing a pen and paper or picture board to 'overcome' a 'speech problem', frequently end in failure and frustration on the part of all involved. Similarly, many aphasic individuals may experience frustration and despair when activities such as watching videos or reading are provided.

Agnosia

Agnosia is a brain impairment that, while not specifically linguistic, has a direct impact on communication. The agnosias are a group of disorders of perception in which a person is unable to recognize stimuli, even though the sensory modality is intact. The same stimuli can be recognized through other modalities. For example, a patient with visual agnosia will be unable to recognize objects even though they can see the object. If shown a set of keys, they will be unable to name them; however, if the keys are moved and the typical jingling sound is heard the person is able to name the keys. This disorder was described by the neurologist Oliver Sachs in 'The Man Who Mistook His Wife For a Hat'.[12] Visual agnosias are usually incomplete, intermittent, and inconsistent. The unpredictability of this condition causes great problems for both carers and patients. The problem may only become apparent in new or unfamiliar situations, and the patient may be labelled 'confused'. Visual agnosia is usually caused by bilateral damage to the occipital lobes, posterior parietal lobes, or in the fiber tracts that connect the visual cortex to other parts of the brain.

Other agnosias include auditory agnosia, in which the patient does not appreciate the meaning of sounds. A patient with auditory agnosia is unable to match a sound with the object that is its source (e.g. the sounds of keys jingling or of a match being struck). The inability to recognize objects by touch or palpation, even though the sense of touch is intact, is referred to as tactile agnosia. These conditions can be difficult to recognize and often lead to incidents of confusion.

Speech Apraxia

Apraxia is defined as a disorder of purposeful movement not caused by muscle weakness. Typically an individual with apraxia will be able to perform automatic functions, but as soon as voluntary intent is required, problems with initiation and sequencing of movements become apparent. In the case of apraxia of speech, more automatic functions, such as swallowing and greeting, are preserved; however, the process of transforming thoughts into words is impaired and speech becomes

Table 17–3. **Principal Aphasic Syndromes**

Aphasic Repetition Syndrome	Site of Lesion	Spontaneous Speech	Comprehension	Word Retrieval	Reading	Writing	Repetition
Broca's	Posterior, inferior frontal lobe	Non-fluent, telegraphic	Fair to good	Fair but misarticulated, telegraphic	Fair to good, usually slow	Effortful, usually write in capitals with omissions of words and letters	Effortful with speech sound errors
Wernicke's	Posterior, superior temporal lobe	Fluent but empty of meaning	Poor	Poor, incorrect words and sounds are produced	Poor	Poor, incorrect letters and words are produced	Fluent with sound and word substitutions, very limited retention span
Conduction	Parietal lobe	Fluent with meaning but with frequent sound substitutions	Fair to good	Fair with frequent sound substitutions	Good	Well formed and legible but with spelling errors and transpositions of syllables and words	Fluent with sound and word substitutions, some limitation of retention span
Transcortical motor	Anterior, superior frontal lobe	Non-fluent but sparse with initiation problems and short utterances	Fair to good	Variable with initiation delays	Able to read aloud with fair to good comprehension	Sparse, reduced in amount and complexity	Good

Continued on following page

Table 17–3—*continued*

Aphasic Repetition Syndrome	Site of Lesion	Spontaneous Speech	Comprehension	Word Retrieval	Reading	Writing	Repetition
Transcortical sensory	Posterior parietal, superior lobe	Fluent but empty of meaning, repeat question before responding	Poor	Poor, may give irrelevant responses	Able to read aloud fluently but not comprehend content	Impaired, may have a right-sided visual field deficit	Good
Anomic	Temporal, parietal lobe	Fluent but interrupted by word-finding difficulties	Fair to good	Fair with substitution of generic terms for specific words and circuitous and wordy descriptions for unrecalled words	Fair to good	Fair to good, word-finding problems are evident in written language	Fair to good
Global	Large, perisylvian	Non-fluent, may be mute	Poor	Poor	Poor	Poor	Poor, with severely limited retention span

difficult to initiate and effortful. Difficulties in sequencing the component sounds of words and phrases and a tendency to replace uncommon words with more frequently used words are a feature of apraxia of speech. The problems are characteristically inconsistent and this increases the frustration experienced by the patient and the communication partners.

This disorder is usually caused by damage to the area of the brain that integrates proprioceptive information in the parietal lobe, or the area in the frontal lobe responsible for initiating and sequencing actions. Problems initiating movements are found in other conditions such as Parkinson's disease and multisystem atrophy.

Because the speech errors are inconsistent, there is a tendency for some people to consider that the person with apraxia of speech is not trying hard enough. However, the more an individual attempts to overcome this difficulty, the worse the problem becomes. Often this leads to perseveration where the person becomes stuck on a sound, word, or phrase. Also, when a person, with great effort, accurately produces the correct word, there may be marked difficulty in producing the next word.

Dysarthria

The impairment of the motor component of speech production (dysarthria) can lead to communication problems ranging from a slight slurring of speech to no speech (anarthria). Normal speech production depends on the adequate functioning of the respiratory system, larynx, tongue, pharynx and soft palate, and lips, and breakdown of functioning in any of these areas results in speech problems.

In progressive neurological diseases (e.g. Parkinson's disease, progressive supranuclear palsy, motor neuron disease, and multiple sclerosis), the functioning of the components of the speech system become impaired due to alterations in the rate, range, and strength of muscle movement. Cerebral neoplasms within the areas of the brain subserving speech functions similarly result in a motor speech impairment.

Respiratory Function

Impaired respiratory support for speech causes decreased volume and a reduction in the expressive features of communication such as stress, rhythm, intonation, and rate. Decreased volume of speech leads to difficulties communicating against background noise and impairs ability to socialize in groups and to interrupt others. The reduction in the prosodic features of speech causes a limitation in the expressive elements of communication such as irony or excitement.

Laryngeal Function

The larynx, which contains the vocal cords, is located at the top of the trachea. During respiration, the vocal cords are in an open position. To produce voice or phonate, the vocal cords come together in the midline and vibrate as the airstream passes through them. This is necessary for a strong, clear voice. Changes in pitch depend on the flexibility of the vocal cords, which lengthen as the larynx raises and tilts forwards to produce higher pitch sounds, and shorten when the larynx is in a lowered position to produce lower pitch sounds.

Incomplete vocal cord closure results in a soft, weak voice with a breathy quality. Excessive tension in the muscles of the larynx causes the voice to be harsh and strained. People with phonatory impairment also experience problems communicating against background noise. Vocal fatigue is a common problem, which further restricts conversation. Impaired phonatory function results in a reduction in speech prosody (tempo, rhythm, loudness, and pitch). The functional consequence of this is a loss of expressiveness during communication.

The Articulators

The articulators (lips, tongue, and soft palate) make changes to the airflow to produce the sounds of speech. Weakness and incoordination of these structures can have a dramatic effect on speech intelligibility. Poor articulation results in the speech sounds being distorted and inaccurate.

LIP FUNCTION

Adequate lip function is required to produce a range of speech sounds. Lip closure is required for the production of 'm', while lip rounding is required to produce 'w'. During the production of 'f' and 'v', the lower lip approximates the upper teeth.

Spastic lips have a retracted appearance with the teeth visible, and the person has difficulty achieving lip closure. Flaccid lips result in weak sound production and drooping of the lips at rest. Poor oral closure is associated with drooling, which can cause embarrassment and reluctance to attempt to speak.

The cheek muscles are usually affected when lip impairment is present. When the muscles are spastic, the inside of the cheeks can become pressed against the teeth and problems associated with biting the cheeks can occur. This can become further exacerbated if the person has a bite reflex, when swelling and pain can result.

TONGUE FUNCTION

The tongue can be considered the principal articulator of the speech system. A range of subtle movements are required to produce many speech sounds. During the production of the 'k', 'g', and 'ng', the back of the tongue elevates. The sounds 's', 'z', 't', 'd', 'l', 'r', and 'n' require elevation of the tip of the tongue. The sides of the tongue elevate during the production of 'sh', and to produce 'th', the tip of the tongue projects forward between the teeth.

Generalized tongue weakness is the major cause of reduced speech intelligibility. This is a particular problem in motor neuron disease. Mild tongue impairment is associated with slurring of speech.

SOFT PALATE AND PHARYNGEAL FUNCTION

During the production of most speech sounds, the airflow is directed through the oral cavity. The closure of the naso-pharyngeal opening is achieved through elevation of the soft palate and contraction of the pharynx. During the production of 'n', 'm', and 'ng' (as at the end of song), the soft palate is lowered against the elevated back of the tongue to allow the air to flow through the nose. This results in the nasal quality of these sounds.

Impaired soft palate/pharyngeal closure results in nasalization of all speech sounds and a consequent loss of clarity and reduced intelligibility. Nasal emission reduces the oral airflow, and the resultant inefficient use of air leads to fading at the end of words and phrases, shorter phrases, and a reduction in the number of words per breath. This contributes to fatigue during interactions.

Pathological Laughing and Crying

Pathological laughing and crying, also referred to as emotional lability, often co-occurs with dysarthria. This problem presents as an unconstrained triggering of an emotional response, with the response usually being appropriate in type but excessive in magnitude. However, sometimes the person may vacillate between laughing and crying or may produce the contextually inappropriate emotional response. Once initiated, the response is difficult to stop. Discussing emotive issues is more likely to trigger pathological crying, and in severe cases the person may experience pathological laughter or crying even when discussing mildly emotional topics. Pathological laughing or crying can seriously impede verbal communication and social activity.

Because pathological laughing and crying can be conceptualized as a perseveration of the motor responses for emotion, changing the motor response by focusing on changing the pattern of breathing may enable the person to regain control (e.g. by concentrating on inspiration during uncontrolled laughter and expiration for uncontrolled crying). In mild cases, simple management strategies can include providing a reassuring but not excessive response or a change of topic to help break the pattern. For some people, antidepressant medication can be of assistance.

PRINCIPLES OF SPEECH PATHOLOGY INTERVENTION IN PALLIATIVE CARE

The focus of speech pathology management in palliative care is to enhance quality of life throughout the disease process, maintaining optimal functional communication tailored to individual needs. Speech–language pathologists aim to facilitate optimal communication with staff, family, and friends. This may involve making changes to the environment, training family members and carers, and/or introducing alternative means of communication at the appropriate time. At the same time the speech–language pathologist will provide support to patients and families as they cope with, and manage, the impact of the symptoms of the disease on their lives. Speech–language pathologists in palliative care liaise closely with members of the multidisciplinary team, the family, and community carers to ensure that appropriate adjustments are made as communication needs change.

ASSESSMENT

Formal communication assessment by a speech–language pathologist includes an in-depth evaluation of receptive language skills and expressive language skills. In the palliative care setting, the speech–language pathologist will need to consider the extent to which such formal assessment is undertaken. Evaluating the person's current functional communication status in a less formal way and trying simple communication strategies will provide a less confronting assessment process and more workable management plan.

In palliative care, the clinician is required to shift the focus of intervention towards functional communication rather than rehabilitation, and ensure that the impact of symptoms on daily function and the psychosocial attitudes towards communication are taken into account.

An understanding of the patient's emotional and physical status and an acknowledgement that life experiences and attitudes will influence each person's coping style is very important. The person's state of alertness, levels of fluctuation, rate of disease progression, physical impairments, and cognitive status will influence the timing and length of the assessment, as well as providing valuable insight into the appropriateness of specific assessment and management strategies.

Valuable information is available through the medical history and from medical, nursing and allied health staff, and family members. If there is concern regarding cognitive status and a neuropsychologist's report is not available, a brief cognitive screening may provide valuable information. Discussion with the physiotherapist and occupational therapist will provide information on fatigue levels, sitting balance, as well as dexterity and upper limb function. Using this information, the therapist can begin to shape the assessment protocol to suit the individual and to conceptualize functional communication needs.

An introductory meeting with the patient and family can be a valuable way of gaining preliminary information and also provides an opportunity for the clinician to discuss the assessment process and management goals with the patient and family. Establishing rapport with the patient and their family during this session will open the channels of communication and provide a basis for ongoing interactions. In this session the patient and family should be encouraged to clarify concerns.

The clinician should begin by observing the individual's functional receptive language skills. Expressive language reflects the way patients respond to their environment, how they convey wants and needs, and how they interact socially with those around them. The speech–language pathologist also evaluates an individual's ability to interpret the meaning of both verbal and non-verbal communication. The person's pragmatic behaviors can be observed during a conversation, noting their ability to take turn appropriately, attend to a communication partner, provide appropriate responses, and remain on the topic.

When observing expressive skills, the clinician will note how the person uses speech and language, as well as gesture, facial expression, and other non-verbal means to communicate. The clinician should note whether speech is dysarthric (slurred), dyspraxic (disordered movement), or aphasic (containing jargon, word-finding difficulty, circumlocution) and whether the pragmatic aspects of communication are impaired. These include aspects that overlay speech, such as intonation patterns, facial expression, and communication repair strategies. Noting how the person copes with communication breakdown and individual compensatory strategies will allow incorporation of effective and familiar strategies into the management plan.

In palliative care, the clinician will need to take into account pre-existing conditions and any adverse effects of disease or surgery that may have resulted in damage to hearing and vision. These senses impact directly on a person's receptive language skills.

Hearing

Ask if the person has a hearing aid. Is it working and is it used? If no aid is used, note whether the person appears to hear adequately during conversation. Is there frequent request for clarification? Is there difficulty hearing over the telephone or in background noise such as when the television or radio is turned on? Find out if the person has a history of wax build-up in the ears or has experienced recurrent middle ear infections. If there is still some doubt as to the level of functional hearing, a brief hearing screening should be conducted. The person should be asked to perform simple tasks or respond to simple questions that are uttered at a moderate level while the clinician has the mouth obscured. Results will indicate whether there may be specific language impairment such as aphasia, whether medical examination of the ears is required, or whether use of an amplified listening device may be beneficial. It should be remembered that people have been labelled as cognitively impaired when they simply could not hear the question being asked!

Vision

Establish whether the person uses spectacles. If so, are they with them and are they used often? Has vision been assessed recently? Seeing a person's face during communication provides much of the information required to understand speech. A visual screening can be conducted simply using object selection or alphabet/picture identification with letters and sketches of various sizes. This screening may reveal the presence of agnosia or visual neglect requiring further assessment. The clinician should also be mindful of literacy skills when using alphabet identification and, on occasion, an interpreter may be required. If vision is impaired, strategies such as increasing the size of written material, reducing reading distance, or maximizing other senses such as hearing, touch, and smell can facilitate interaction.

FUNCTIONAL MANAGEMENT STRATEGIES

Speech not only conveys an encoded linguistic message but also expresses elements of personality, such as sense of humor and feelings towards the subject of the conversation. The loss of the ability to converse leads to a loss of control over the environment, change in self-image and self-esteem, and a loss of sense of purpose. These changes impact on relationships within the immediate family, carers, and broader community. It is essential to ensure that these psychosocial changes are not ignored by focusing narrowly on improving speech production rather than addressing the wider ramifications of communication.

Many of the aspects of speech impairment discussed in this chapter respond to traditional speech therapy techniques and this is an appropriate approach in a rehabilitation setting. However, in palliative care, careful consideration should be given to prognosis and anticipated changes in physical and psychological function. The goal of maintaining optimal functional communication for as long as possible must remain at the forefront of planning. The desire to ameliorate speech problems by setting up programs that include repetitive speech and muscle exercises may indeed have a negative effect on the patient and the family by providing a means by which deterioration can be monitored.

People with progressive neurological diseases do not usually lose speech suddenly; rather, there is a gradual decrease in intelligibility. As speech deteriorates, adjustments are made to maintain communication, including reducing phrase length to accommodate a reduction in respiratory support for speech, or slowing speech and using deliberate articulatory movements as the speech muscles become weaker.

Positioning and Comfort

The effectiveness of communication may depend on the physical comfort of the individual. Appropriate positioning is important to decrease abnormal tone, reduce effort required to maintain a sitting position, minimize reflexive responses and clonus, facilitate access to communication devices, and optimize respiratory function. Liaison with physiotherapists and occupational therapists with regard to seating, head, neck and trunk support, and upper limb function is helpful in these situations.

General comfort also relies on basic needs being met. People with complex disabilities may rely on carers to assist them with drinking, toileting, blowing their nose, etc. A quick and efficient method of communicating attention to these tasks should be established for these types of requests and a simple picture communication board at the bedside may be useful.

Environmental Considerations

Impaired speech and language are more difficult to understand when there is background noise and in group settings. Simple listener strategies such as turning off the television and radio, shutting doors, or moving to a quieter location can make speaking and listening easier. When conversing, seating arrangements should facilitate effective communication; this is best done by ensuring that the participants are sitting facing each other. Adequate lighting and the avoidance of back lighting the person with communication impairment (as this makes it difficult for the listener to read facial expression) supplement intelligibility.

Facilitating Techniques

Facilitating techniques such as vibration, brushing, and icing can be used to reduce abnormal muscle tone and improve intelligibility for short periods.[13] The use of these techniques before visitors arrive or before meals has been found to be helpful in some cases.

Augmentative and Alternative Communication (AAC)

When a person has relatively intact language function but has unintelligible speech methods, aids such as pen and paper, an alphabet board, a word and phrase board, or an electronic communication device to augment communication may be useful.

Issues related to the portability, durability, availability, and maintenance of the device should be considered. Simple methods such as voice amplifiers, pen and paper, and erasable whiteboards or magnetic boards can provide a quick, convenient, inexpensive, and portable means of supplementing or replacing speech. If there is advanced physical deterioration or fatigue or cognitive impairment, pre-recorded message boards, alphabet boards, and picture boards may be useful. These methods require little or no training and many people find them entirely suitable.

More technologically advanced systems include dedicated electronic communication devices and personal computers. With appropriate software, these systems have the advantage of providing voice output, giving increased flexibility when communicating with children, using the telephone or the internet, and in group situations. Prediction and memory functions assist people with poor keyboard skills or impaired dexterity, and switch-operated scanner attachments can make these systems more suitable if upper limb function is affected. For people with complex physical impairments, an eye scanning board may be useful. These systems require appropriate training and practice of all potential communication partners.

During normal speech, around 150–250 words are communicated per minute.[14] An efficient electronic communication device user communicates 15–20 words per minute.[15] Communicating with someone with dysarthric speech or who is using a communication device requires concentration and patience by both parties. The amount of time required to communicate should be adjusted to allow for the range of different communication activities. Sometimes family, friends, carers, and health professionals envisage that using an electronic device will be more efficient than dysarthric speech and can become disappointed when the slowness of this type of communication system is realized. If possible, a trial of a range of devices will allow for better evaluation of their potential benefits, and sometimes the relative efficiency of a person's mild to moderate dysarthric speech becomes evident.

Cognitive function needs to be considered when selecting the most appropriate communication device. When cognitive function deteriorates, the communication partner must assume more responsibility during interactions. Inaccurate responses and an inability to write concise messages or key words of a verbal message, resulting from cognitive impairment, is a limiting factor.

The Role of Communication Partners

Effective communication is dependent upon active participation by communication partners. This is not always easy to attain, since many people are unfamiliar and lack confidence when faced with electronic equipment. Introduction of additional equipment can be overwhelming in the daily workload of carers. For these reasons, patients, and their families and carers, should be supported when a communication device is introduced and throughout its use.

Many people find communicating with someone who is difficult to understand or who is using a communication device stressful and there is a tendency to avoid interactions. Training listeners in strategies that assist in the communication process is essential. The clinician should assist the listener to develop skills in asking questions to define a topic, framing 'yes/no' questions in a systematic way, and understanding the differences between communication to meet basic needs versus free conversations and the exposition of issues. It is essential that communication devices, regardless of type, do not become a barrier to communication. If the person has a communication device, training of carers and family should include developing an understanding of the device so that they can provide practical assistance to the patient when required. Family, carers, and friends should be facilitated in adapting to its use and encouraged to involve the person in the full range of normal communicative interactions.

Dependency on others to facilitate communication leads to a loss of control for the person with the impairment and sufficient time needs to be allowed for in-depth discussion and expressions of feelings with supportive carers and staff.

COMMUNICATION IN THE TERMINAL PHASE

During the end stage of life, the patient and their family need reassurance. The fear that they will be unable to convey information is very real. Where possible, efficient methods by which the person can communicate daily needs should be established before they enter the terminal phase. The speech–language pathologist should monitor communication function, including use of an AAC device, and make appropriate adjustments according to need. Details regarding the nature of a person's communication impairment and current methods of communication should be clearly documented in the medical history and at the bedside to inform all communication partners as changes are made. At this time many people will prefer to take a passive role in interactions and will happily allow communication partners to simply sit by, read to them, or provide a narrative of family or social events. This choice should be respected.

In palliative care settings, the provision of staff who are familiar with the patient can become a point of contention. When communication is difficult, either because speech and language impairment make it difficult to understand or the use of AAC requires considerable cooperation from the communication partner, individuals often express a preference for specific staff members, usually those with whom they are best able to communicate. This situation illustrates the importance of the speech–language pathologist's role in education and training to ensure that all staff can communicate effectively with their patients.

The speech–language pathologist's role in the management of communication in palliative care should be guided by the rate of progression and severity of the disease, but more importantly, by the wishes and needs of the person in their care. At present, communication impairment in palliative care has received little attention and there is a pressing need for this aspect to develop and contribute to the important area of palliative care.

SUMMARY

The role of the speech–language therapist in the palliative care setting is often overlooked. This may be because speech pathology is perceived as an active intervention inappropriate for a person who is in the process of losing function. If the goal of intervention was to completely restore communication function, this would be an accurate conclusion.

Speech and language therapy in palliative care involves the facilitation of optimal function within the constraints of a progressive disease process. Furthermore, because communication is such a vital aspect of human existence, skilled intervention in this area is important in cases where communication problems exist.

REFERENCES

1. Bottorff JL, Steele R, Davies B, Garossino C, Porterfield P, Shaw M. Striving for balance: palliative care patient's experience of making everyday choices. Journal of Palliative Care 1998;13(1):7–17.
2. Cooley C. Communication skills in palliative care. Professional Nurse 2000;15(9):603–605.
3. Bottorff JL, Steele R, Davies B, Garossino C, Porterfield P, Shaw M. Facilitating day-to-day decision making in palliative care. Cancer Nursing 2000;23(2):141–150.
4. Scott PA. Autonomy, power and control in palliative care. Cambridge Quarterly of Healthcare Ethics 1999;8(2):149–147.
5. Kruijver IP, Kerkstra A, Bensing JM, van de Weil HB. Nurse–patient communication in cancer care. A review of the literature. Cancer Nursing 2000;23(1):20–31.
6. Mathy P. Outcomes of AAC intervention in ALS. Augmentative Communication News 1998;11:5–9.
7. Yorkston KM, Beukelman DR, Strand EA, Bell KR. Management of Motor Speech Disorders in Children and Adults. Pro-Ed, Austin, Texas, 1999.
8. Pereira J, Hanson J, Bruera E. The frequency and clinical course of cognitive impairment in patients with terminal cancer. Cancer 1997;79(4):835–842.
9. Alpert M, Rosen R, Welkowitz J, Lieberman A. Interpersonal communication in the context of dementia. Journal of Communication Disorders 1990;23:337–342.
10. Aarsland D, Litvan I, Larsen JP. Neuropsychiatric symptoms of patients with progressive supranuclear palsy and Parkinson's disease. Journal of Neuropsychiatry & Clinical Neurosciences 2001;13(1):42–49.
11. Massman PJ, Sims J, Cooke N, Haverkamp LJ, Appel V, Appel SH. Prevalence and correlates of neuropsychological deficits in amyotrophic lateral sclerosis. Journal of Neurology, Neurosurgery, and Psychiatry 1996;61:450–455.
12. Sacks O. The Man Who Mistook His Wife For a Hat and Other Clinical Tales. Simon and Schuster, New York, 1998.
13. Scott AG, Staios G. Oro-facial facilitation. In: H Johnson, A Scott, eds. A Practical Approach to Saliva Control. Communication Skill Builders, Tucson, 32–43, 1993.
14. Goldman–Eisler F. Cycle Linguistics: Experiments in Spontaneous Speech. Academic Press, New York, 1986.
15. Foulds R. Guest editorial. Augmentative and Alternative Communication 1987;3:169.

Chapter 18

Epileptic Seizures and Myoclonus

Sabine Weil
Soheyl Noachtar

Epileptic seizures and myoclonus are bothersome for both patients and relatives. They occur in a variety of syndromes and different diseases. Myoclonus can be of epileptic origin, but there are a lot of other etiologies also involved. Non-epileptic myoclonus and epilepsy have to be distinguished because therapy and prognosis are different.

Acute therapy of epileptic seizures secondary to acute etiologies differs from chronic antiepileptic treatment of chronic epilepsy. Almost any type of seizure may occur in a prolonged or repetitive manner (status) and thereby constitutes a potentially greater threat than a single seizure. Both therapy of single epileptic seizures and status epilepticus, as well as therapy of myoclonus, are discussed, with special regard to palliative care medicine.

CASE HISTORY

A 57-year-old male patient was admitted to our hospital because of acute onset aphasia, nausea, and vomiting. Eleven months previously, a left parieto-occipital glioblastoma had been diagnosed and resected. Repeat MRI showed no tumor progression since that time. He had had radiotherapy and, one month before admission, he underwent a first cycle of chemotherapy (procarbacin/vincristine/lomustine). The patient was on valproic acid

(900 mg) following a previous generalized tonic clonic seizure.

On examination the patient presented with a fluctuating global aphasic syndrome with varying impairment of spontaneous speech and speech comprehension, and semantic and phonemic paraphasias. There was no impairment of motor activity. Deep tendon reflexes were slightly exaggerated on the right side but there was no paresis. Visual fields, perception, and co-ordination could not be tested due to difficulties in communication. Neurological examination was otherwise normal.

MRI revealed no evidence of tumor progression, hemorrhage, or increased intracranial pressure. The EEG showed a left occipital status pattern. Intravenous phenytoin caused a bradycardia and was suspended immediately.

Aphasia improved markedly within two days following increase of valproic acid (1200 mg) and prescription of dexamethasone (4 mg tid). Spontaneous speech and speech comprehension fully recovered, but some semantic and phonemic paraphasias persisted. The patient was discharged from hospital after three days.

Discussion

Epileptic seizures are characterized by a variety of clinical features. In this case a fluctuating aphasia was the predominant symptom of status epilepticus (SE). In cases of fluctuating neurological symptoms, one should consider SE, especially in patients with acute or subacute structural cerebral abnormalities.

The therapeutic strategy for SE depends on the impairment of daily activities and the risk associated with the type of SE the patient is suffering and its etiology. Rapid drug loading may lead to adverse cardiac and respiratory events. Because the risks in aphasic SE are very low, and intravenous phenytoin induced bradycardia, in our case there was time to wait for the effect of increased oral valproate doses. Our patient, with an incurable brain tumor, was able to leave hospital after three days. No intensive care or adjustment to other antiepileptic drugs were necessary. Prolonged focal status may cause neuronal damage with an increase of neuron specific enolase (NSE).[1] However, in the setting of an incurable malignant tumor, this is not a major concern.

EPILEPTIC SEIZURES

Introduction

Epileptic seizures are characterized by a variety of clinical features involving consciousness, sensory, motor, and autonomic functions. The signs and symptoms of epileptic seizures depend on the brain region involved in the epileptic discharge. Some seizures involve only one functional system, others involve two or more functional systems. Auras, for instance, involve the perception exclusively, whereas generalized tonic clonic seizures involve consciousness and vegetative and motor functions. The different seizure types[2] are listed in Table 18–1.

Epileptic seizure activity has a tendency to spread. The evolution from one to another seizure type reflects a spread of epileptic activity, varying with the area of seizure onset and the spread pattern. Each seizure type may occur as SE. Epileptic seizures need to be distinguished from epileptic syndromes. Epileptic seizures may occur in a variety of acute syndromes such as metabolic disorders. An epileptic syndrome is defined as chronic epilepsy. Therapy and prognosis depend on the epilepsy syndrome and its etiology and not on a particular seizure type.

The duration of antiepileptic treatment depends on the underlying pathology,

Table 18–1. Seizure Classification[2]

AURA
Somatosensory
Visual-auditory
Auditory
Olfactoric
Gustatoric
Psychic
Abdominal
Autonomic
AUTONOMIC SEIZURE
DIALEPTIC SEIZURE
MOTOR SEIZURE
Simple motor seizure
   Clonic seizure
   Tonic seizure
   Tonic clonic seizure
   Myoclonic seizure
   Versive seizure
   Epileptic spasm
Complex motor seizure
   Automotor seizure
   Hypermotor seizure
   Gelastic seizure
SPECIAL SEIZURE
Atonic seizure
Astatic seizure
Hypomotor seizure
Akinetic seizure
Negative myoclonic seizure

whether rapid therapeutic intervention is necessary, and the risk of seizure recurrence over time.

Acute Therapy

Seizures are usually self-limiting events. During the seizure, the patient should be protected against injury and aspiration and observed until full recovery. The treatment of a first isolated seizure depends on the etiology. If no cause can be identified, no antiepileptic medication is required. Anticonvulsants in patients presenting with a first tonic clonic seizure reduce the risk of seizure recurrence. However, 50% of patients who are not treated will never experience a second seizure. The chance of long-term remission is not influenced by treatment of the first seizure.[3] Antiepileptic drugs will be administered immediately if an increased risk for seizure recurrence is suspected from diagnostic findings suggesting a definite etiology (e.g. a brain lesion is found in imaging studies or focal epileptiform discharges are demonstrated in the EEG). Regardless of these factors, the recurrence rate is about 35%,[4] which for some patients (e.g. patients with bone metastasis) indicates a need for antiepileptic treatment to avoid complications of major motor seizures, such as fractures.[5]

Almost any type of seizure may become prolonged or repetitive (status) and thereby constitute a potentially greater threat than a single seizure. Benzodiazepines are the drugs of choice, characterized by rapid onset of action and relative safety with respect to cardiotoxicity and liver toxicity.[6] Lorazepam, clonazepam, diazepam, and clobazam are the main drugs used. Diazepam is available in oral, rectal, and intravenous applications. Initial doses are 10 mg oral or 5 mg intravenously. Even small doses intravenously can cause respiratory depression. The duration of antiepileptic action of diazepam is short, and subsequent phenytoin loading is necessary. Lorazepam has the advantage of longer antiepileptic effect than diazepam and can be given both orally or intravenously (2–8 mg). The effect of intravenous lorazepam lasts longer than that of diazepam and has probably less depressive effect on respiration than diazepam and midazolam, but lorazepam is not yet approved for SE,[6] although its efficacy has been demonstrated. Clonazepam can be given intravenously (1–4 mg) or orally in SE. Clobazam, probably less sedative than the other benzodiazepines, is available only for oral administration.

If seizures are not controlled with benzodiazepines, phenytoin is the next drug of choice. It is very efficacious in both focal and generalized SE, and is available in oral and intravenous formulations. The usual phenytoin maintenance dose is 300–325 mg daily. For loading, a first dose three to four times the maintenance dose is necessary. Depending on the acuteness of the situation (SE, increase of seizure frequency, single seizure), loading can be done rapidly i.v. with 25–50 mg/min

(generalized tonic clonic SE) or orally, with about 600 mg for three days followed by maintenance dose. In generalized tonic clonic status, i.v. loading will be preferred, whereas in other less severe status types, one would like to avoid the risk of phenytoin i.v. loading (cardiac arrhythmia, 'purple glove' syndrome)[7] provided that the patients are able to swallow the pills. Phenytoin is a strong inducer of liver enzymes and interferes with a number of other drugs, including chemotherapeutics. Intravenous formulation of phenytoin is adjusted to a pH of approximately 11, which is associated with a high risk of venous toxicity, including phlebitis or the serious 'purple glove' syndrome.[7] 'Purple glove' syndrome is characterized by progressive distal limb edema, discoloration, and pain, and is a potentially serious local complication of i.v. phenytoin administration. Further adverse events comprise skin rashes and dose-dependent side effects (nausea, sedation, uncoordination, ataxia). Usually, nystagmus occurs above a phenytoin serum level of 20–25 µg/ml. Most antiepileptic drugs should be given in smaller doses in the elderly because of reduced metabolism in this age group.

Status Epilepticus (SE)

The treatment for SE depends basically on the risk to the patient of ongoing seizure activity and its underlying etiology.[8] A palliative care approach includes consideration of the prognosis of the underlying cause in deciding therapeutic interventions. For example, generalized tonic clonic status epilepticus (GTCSE) constitutes a life-threatening event that puts any patient at risk of neurological, cardiac, respiratory, and surgical complications, and should be stopped rapidly. However, the management of terminally ill patients with GTCSE should avoid intubation.

Treatment of focal status other than generalized tonic clonic seizures is done with less vigor than treatment of GTCSE. Especially in patients with brain tumors or metastasis, it may be difficult to stop unilateral clonic status of the face or hand area (epilepsia partialis continua), and drug therapy at tolerable doses is often unsatisfactory. Twitching of face, thumbs, or other body parts is not dangerous, but impairs quality of life and frequently disturbs relatives even if the patient may cope with it. For terminally ill patients, in whom side effects of antiepileptic therapy are to be avoided, injection of small doses of botulinum toxin in selected muscle groups may bring symptomatic relief.

Absence SE probably poses no risk for neuron damage and initial attempts at its termination should probably not include agents that are likely to affect respiration and blood pressure. So-called non-convulsive SE (NSE), characterized by confusion (and, more or less, automatisms), may be clinically indistinguishable from generalized absence status. Ictal EEG is needed to make a diagnosis. The therapeutic approach depends on the diagnosis. In generalized absence status, valproate is the drug of choice if benzodiazepines are not effective. For loading, 1200 mg i.v. over 1–2 hours, followed by maintenance doses, can be given. Treatment of non-convulsive focal status should allow for the fact that these patients may have sequelae of the status with neuropsychological impairment, which outlasts the status. Increase of NSE has been described in these patients.[1] Therefore, treatment will be more aggressive than in generalized absence status and include benzodiazepines and phenytoin.

Therapy of SE should follow the steps shown in Table 18–2. Initially, benzodiazepines such as lorazepam are given either i.v. or via rapidly absorbing oral formula. If status continues, phenytoin should be given (see

Table 18–2. **Treatment of Status Epilepticus**

Ongoing Status	Treatment
1	Pulsoximetry, cardiac monitor, secure venous catheter (in GTCSE)
	• Bolus of 50% glucose + 100 mg thiamin i.v. unless normal blood glucose is established
⇓	• i.v. injection of 2–8 mg lorazepam or 2–4 mg clonazepam or 10–20 mg diazepam (followed by phenytoin)
2	• i.v. phenytoin: infusion of up to 50 mg phenytoin/min i.v. until cessation of seizures, cardiac adverse side effects, or up to a maximum of 20 mg/kg body weight/24hours; after cessation of SE continue with maintenance dose (300–325 mg/d)
⇓	• Valproic acid up to 20 mg/kg loading dose with infusion rate of 3–5 mg/kg/min
3	Further therapy may require intubation and intensive care (GTCSE). Consequences of intubation have to be considered individually.
⇓	• Phenobarbital: bolus of 10 mg/kg at a rate of 100 mg/min
	• Disoprivan (e.g. Propofol®): starting dose 50–80 mg/h. Increase in steps of 40 mg under EEG monitoring until cessation of EEG seizure pattern or development of burst suppression pattern.
	Maintain burst suppression for 12 hours; discontinue when sufficient doses of other antiepileptic drugs are reached.
4	Thiopental narcosis: consider risks such as arterial hypotension, sepsis, and renal failure.
	• Thiopental: 200 mg bolus ⇒ 200 mg/h maintenance dose
⇓	Increase in steps of 200 mg/h after new bolus of 200 mg until cessation of EEG seizure pattern or development of burst suppression pattern
	Maintain burst suppression muster for 12 h; then stepwise withdrawal.

Table 18–2). Phenytoin administration should not exceed 50 mg/min because cardiac arrhythmias may result, particularly in elderly patients with heart diseases. Valproic acid is a new option if this regimen fails. There is little data on status therapy with rapid i.v. valproic acid administration. The loading dose lies between 15 and 20 mg/kg and can be given in 10 minutes, which leads to therapeutic serum levels of valproic acid in 10–20 minutes. Maintenance dose lies between 1 and 3 mg/kg/hour. Available studies showed no adverse events except slight hypotension.[9,10] Valproic acid may rarely cause toxic encephalopathy, which is reversible after cessation of the drug. Valproate encephalopathy is associated with increased serum ammonium levels. If SE does not cease with the above mentioned regimen and a more aggressive approach is justified, intensive care measures are needed (see Table 18–2) because the treatment may lead to respiratory failure requiring ventilation.

Continuing Therapy

Some seizures occur only with specific precipitating factors. In an adult population, sleep deprivation and withdrawal of sedatives and alcohol are the most common precipitating factors. Treatment aims to avoid these precipitating factors. In the setting of palliative care, other factors such as metabolic dysfunction or drug toxicity have to be considered (Table 18–3).

Furthermore, increase of seizure frequency or induction of SE can occur in severely ill patients because of an inability to swallow medication, vomiting, diarrhea, or confusion. Indications for aggressive therapies, especially those making intubation necessary, should be weighted carefully, but symptomatic causes of epileptic seizures have to be treated whenever possible.

There are a few antiepileptic drugs which can be given i.v. (phenytoin, valproate, benzodiazepines, barbiturates). Intravenous use of phenytoin requires secure venous catheters because of vein toxicity and can present problems if central lines should be avoided. A stomach tube in a sedated or unconscious patient is probably less intrusive than multiple i.v. catheter attempts or a painful phlebitis. Intravenous application is often not indicated in terminal care at home. However, motor seizures are a burden for both patients and

Table 18–3. **Diseases Associated with Epileptic Seizures**

	Diagnostics	Therapy
Encephalopathy due to:	EEG	
Hepathopathy	Ammonia ⇑, liver enzymes ⇑, coagulation parameters	Lactulose, bowel decontamination
Nephropathy	Urea , creatinine, osmolarity ⇑	Diuretics, hemofiltration, dialysis
Drug intoxication (Immunosuppressive/ chemotherapeutic agents; antidepressive/antipsychotic drugs)	Drug screening—therapeutic levels	Drug monitoring, dose adjustment, attention to drug interactions. Control of urine, excretion, liver, and kidney function
Endocrinological diseases:		
Diabetes	Blood glucose, HbA1s, glucose tolerance	Avoidance of hypoglycemia, optimization of blood glucose levels
Hyperthyreosis, hyper/hypoaldosteronismus	TSH, FT3, FT4, Cortisol, ACTH test	Hormone adjustment, possible surgical therapy
Hypoparathyroidism	Calcium/phosphate levels, parathyroid hormone	

relatives. Valproate, diazepam, and primidon are available in syrup form, and diazepam can be given rectally with suppositories. Midazolam is available in some countries as nasal spray[11] (not in the EU).

Treatment of recurrent epileptic seizures with antiepileptic drugs depends on the risk of recurrence and seizure-related injury, and the psychosocial consequences of recurrent seizures. Medication choice includes carbamazepine, valproate, phenytoin, phenobarbital, and a number of new antiepileptic drugs (AEDs)—lamotrigine, gabapentin, oxcarbazepine, topiramate, tiagabin, and levetiracetam[6]—and should be guided by the mechanism of action, the pharmacokinetics, and side effect profile of each drug. Therapeutic strategies in focal epilepsies[12] are illustrated in Figure 18–1; side effects and dosages in Table 18–4. In generalized epilepsy, drugs of first choice are valproate, followed by lamotrigine, primidon, and phenobarbital (see Figure 18–1). Ethosuccimide is only efficacious in absence epilepsy. Phenytoin,

carbamazepine, and phenobarbital induce liver enzyme activity. If seizures appear under AED therapy, doses should be increased until seizures subside or side effects occur. If seizures persist in spite of maximum tolerable doses of one drug, a change in drug therapy is indicated. In patients on multiple drugs, especially chemotherapeutics, choice of an antiepileptic drug will focus on compounds with minimal or no liver metabolization and drug interactions (e.g. levetiracetam, gabapentin, topiramate, lamotrigine). AEDs, with dosage and side effects, are listed in Table 18–4.

MYOCLONUS

Introduction

Myoclonus is defined as involuntary single or irregularly repetitive brief movements of one part of the body associated with either muscle contraction (positive myoclonus) or brief loss of muscle tone (negative myoclonus).[13]

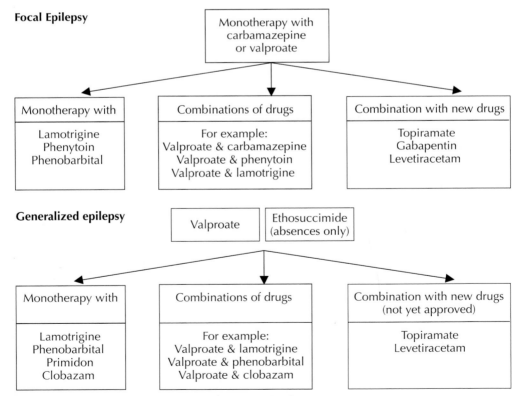

Figure 18–1. Therapeutic strategies in focal and generalized epilepsy.

Table 18–4. Drug Loading and Side Effects

Antiepileptic Drug	Starting Dose	Titration (~Maximum Dose)	Side Effects	Formulation
Carbamazepine	200 mg	200 mg/3d (~1800 mg, in the elderly ~800 mg/d)	Hyponatremia, leukopenia, skin rash, nausea, double vision, ataxia	Oral: tbl, cp
Oxcarbazepine	200–300 mg	200–300 mg/3d (~2500 mg, in the elderly ~1200 mg/d)	Idem carbamazepine	Oral: cp
Valproate (VPA)	300 mg	300 mg/3d (~2000 mg)	Fatigue, hair loss, encephalopathy, nausea, leukothrombopenia, weight gain	Oral: cp, tbl, syrup, sherbet powder i.v.
Phenytoin	300 mg maintenance dose; 1.2 g loading dose (see text)	Rapid: 1.5 g/24 h Medium: 600 mg for 3 days Slow: 300 mg/d	Vertigo, rash, leukothrombopenia, fatigue, purple glove' syndrome	Oral: tbl i.v.
Phenobarbital	100 mg	50 mg/3d (~200 mg/d, in the elderly ~100–150 mg/d)	Fatigue, headaches, ataxia, depression, osteopathy	Oral: tbl i.v.
Lamotrigine	Mono: 25 mg With VPA: 12.5 mg	25 mg/2 weeks With VPA: 12.5/2 weeks (200–400 mg)	Rashes (dosage dependent), nausea, vomiting	Oral: tbl
Gabapentin	300 mg	300 mg/3d (3–4 g, ~2 g in the elderly)	Dizziness, nausea, fatigue	Oral: cp
Topiramate	25 mg	25 mg/1 week (200–1000 mg)	Fatigue, psychosis, depression, nausea	Oral: tbl
Levetiracetam	500 mg	500 mg/3d (3–4 g)	Fatigue, nausea	Oral: cp

Tbl = tablet; cp = capsule

Myoclonic jerks can be elicited by action or stimuli (action myoclonus, reflex myoclonus) or are clinically apparent only when a muscle tone is exerted (negative myoclonus).[14]

Non-epileptic myoclonus has to be differentiated from other involuntary movements such as tics, dystonia, or tremor generated in the CNS and myoclonic movements due to lesions of a peripheral nerve root or plexus.[15,16]

Myoclonus can be classified by etiology, neurophysiological mechanism, or clinical observation. The etiologic classification provides information on prognosis and helps guide specific therapies.[17]

Etiology

Myoclonus can be generated at several levels of the CNS (cortical, subcortical, brain stem, spinal). For differentiation of cortical myoclonus from myoclonus generated from deeper structures, an EEG with simultaneous recording of EMG of the affected muscles is required. Backward averaging of the EEG triggered by myoclonus reveals cortical spikes preceding the myoclonus in cases in which the conventional EEG is non-revealing. The differentiation is helpful for therapeutic concepts and prognosis. Myoclonus is associated with a variety of physiological conditions (sleep myoclonus, singultus, startle reaction) and pathological conditions (various encephalopathies, paraneoplastic syndromes, e.g. opsoclonus myoclonus syndrome, epilepsy, startle disease, storage disease, degenerative diseases, genetic diseases, intoxication).

Prognosis

The prognosis of myoclonus depends on the underlying etiology. In general the prognosis of cortical myoclonus is better than that of subcortically-generated myoclonus. Spontaneous remission is frequently observed in posthypoxic myoclonus.

Treatment

Physiological myoclonus such as singultus or sleep myoclonus is self-limiting and usually does not require medical treatment.

The treatment is usually symptomatic unless the underlying etiology can be treated effectively. Because myoclonus is often a burden for both patients and relatives, it should be treated.

Drugs used in cortical and subcortical myoclonus exert either an increase of inhibition (valproic acid, clonazepam, barbiturates, vigabatrin, baclofen, etc.) or reduce excitation (carbamazepine, phenytoin, lamotrigine, etc.). In some drugs the mechanisms of action are poorly understood (piracetam, oxitriptan, trihexyphenidyl, levetiracetam, dopa agonists). Alcohol may typically improve several forms of myoclonus such as posthypoxic myoclonus, essential myoclonus, and action myoclonus in progressive myoclonus epilepsy.

CORTICAL MYOCLONUS

Valproate and clonazepam are drugs of first choice in cortical myoclonus. Both drugs can be given orally and intravenously.

Valproate can be started with 300 mg/daily and can be increased 300 mg every third day, depending on action and on adverse side effects, up to 600–3000 mg. Starting dose of clonazepam is 0.5 mg tid. Depending on side effects, dose can be increased every third day about 1–2 mg/daily.

Drugs of second choice are piracetam and oxitriptan. An excellent response to piracetam is frequently seen in chronic posthypoxic myoclonus (Lance–Adams syndrome). Starting dose of piracetam is 2.4 g/daily, which can be increased every third day, about 4.8 g, up to 16.8 g a day.[18]

OTHER FORMS OF MYOCLONUS

Myoclonus of brain stem origin is very resistant to drug therapy. The same drugs as in cortical myoclonus can be used but must often be given in combination to exert some effect. In *hyperekplexia* and *spinal myoclonus* carbamazepine and phenytoin can be given. In the *opsoclonus myoclonus syndrome*, steroids or immunosuppressive therapy is helpful when the underlying neoplasm cannot be treated curatively.

SUMMARY

Therapy of epileptic seizures and myoclonus depends substantially on their etiology. Careful diagnosis with EEG and neuroimaging is necessary for optimized therapy. In palliative care, effective reduction of seizure frequency for improvement of quality of life has to be balanced against serious adverse effects of aggressive antiepileptic treatment requiring intubation and intensive care medicine.

REFERENCES

1. De Giorgio CM, Heck CN, Rabinowicz AL, Gott PS, Smith T, Correale J. Serum neuron specific enolase in major subtypes of status epilepticus. Neurology 2001;52:746–749.
2. Lueders HO, Noachtar S, eds. Epileptic Seizures. Pathophysiology and Clinical Seizures. Churchill Livingstone, 2000.
3. Musicco M, Beghi E, Solari A, Viani F. Treatment of first tonic clonic seizure does not improve prognosis of epilepsy. First seizure trial group. Neurology 1997;49:991–998.
4. Annegers JF, Shirts SB, Hauser Wa, Kurland LT. Risk of recurrence after an initial unprovoked seizure. Epilepsia 1986;27:43–50.
5. Noachtar S. Bilateral fractures of the proximal humerus: a rare non-traumatic complication of generalized tonic-clonic seizures following withdrawal of antiepileptic medication. J Neurol 1998;245:123–124.
6. Sillanpää M. Specific antiepileptic medication. In: Wyllie E, ed. The Treatment of Epilepsy: Principles and Practice, 2nd Ed. Williams & Willkins, Baltimore, 1996:808–912.
7. Coplin WM, Rhoney DH, Lyons EA, Murry KR. Incidence and clinical consequence of the purple glove syndrome in patients receiving intravenous phenytoin. Neurology 1999;53:1611–1612.
8. Bleck TP. Management approaches to prolonged seizures and status epilepticus. Epilepsia 1999;40(S1):59–63.
9. Venkataraman V, Wheless JW. Safety of rapid intravenous infusion of valproate loading doses in epilepsy patients. Epilepsy Research 1999;35:147–153.
10. Hodges BM, Mazur JE. Intravenous valproate in status epilepticus. Ann Pharmacother 2001;35:1465–1470.
11. Fisgin T, Gurer Y, Senbil N, et al. Nasal midazolam effects on childhood acute seizures. J Child Neurol 2000;15:833–835.
12. Hufnagel A, Noachtar S. Epilepsy und ihre medikamentöse behandlung. In: Brand T, Dichgans J, Diener HC, eds. Therapie und Verlauf Neurologischer Erkrankungen. Kohlhammer: Stuttgardt, Berlin, Köln, 1998:179–203.
13. Friedreich N. Neuropathologische Beobachtung beim paramyoclonus multiplex. Virchows Arch Pathol Anat Physiol Klin Med 1881;86:421–434.
14. Noachtar S, Holthausen H, Lüders HO. Epileptic negative myoclonus: subdural EEG-video recordings indicate a postcentral generator. Neurology 1997;49:1534–1537.
15. Sotaniemi KA. Paraspinal myoclonus due to spinal root lesion. J Neurol Neurosurg Psychiatry 1985;48:723–724.
16. Banks G, Nielsen VK, Short MP, Kowal CD. Brachial plexus myoclonus. J. Neurol Neurosurg Psychiatry 1985;48:582–584.
17. Hallet M, Topka H. In: Brandt T, Caplan LR, Dichgans J, Diener HC, Kennard C, eds. Neurological Disorders. Course and Treatment. Academic Press: London, New York, San Diego, 2003:1221–1231.
18. Werhahn KJ. Myoklonien. In: Brandt T, Dichgans J, Diener HC, eds. Therapie und Verlauf Neurologischer Erkrankungen. Kohlhammer: Stuttgardt, Berlin, Köln, 1998: 979–992.

Chapter 19

Pain

Eugenia Daniela Hord
Russell K. Portenoy

Pain is a common problem among populations with life-threatening neurologic disorders. Pain usually can be relieved through the systematic application of guidelines adapted from extensive experience in the population with cancer pain. These guidelines are predicated on a comprehensive assessment, which clarifies the nature of the pain, determines whether there is a primarily treatable cause, clarifies the most effective pain management strategies, and provides insight into the degree to which pain is accompanied by other problems that together undermine quality of life. Opioid pharmacotherapy is the mainstay analgesic approach and the most important principle of prescribing is individualization of the dose based on repeated dose titration. The high prevalence of pain in patients with neurologic illnesses warrants controlled trials to help better understand the clinical profile of these syndromes and find the best treatment options.

CASE HISTORY

A 34-year-old woman experienced the sudden onset of paraplegia. A diagnosis of multiple sclerosis was eventually confirmed. Her disease slowly but steadily progressed over the subsequent two years despite treatment with beta interferon and mitoxantrone. Soon after diagnosis, she developed severe burning pain in a band-like distribution around the chest and throbbing pain in the legs. She was given amitriptyline 25 mg at bedtime, which helped her pain and sleep but precipitated several episodes of urinary retention. Gabapentin was tried but provided insufficient relief at the maximally tolerated dose. An oxycodone and acetaminophen combination product, up to two tablets every four hours, was added to the gabapentin. For a few months, her pain was adequately controlled with as many as six tablets per day. As she underwent rehabilitation and trials of primary therapy for the multiple sclerosis, and attempted to maintain function at home, additional deficits occurred. The pain began to increase, and the oxycodone combination product was changed to extended-release oxycodone 20 mg every 12 hours. She continued taking gabapentin and a laxative regimen was added. The oxycodone dose was steadily increased. Each increment improved analgesia for a period of a few weeks to a month or more. She initially experienced no side effects. At a dose of 240 mg three times daily, she became sleepy.

A variety of strategies were discussed with her, including trials of other adjuvant analgesics, opioid rotation, and a trial of a dorsal column stimulator. She requested opioid rotation and the oxycodone was replaced by methadone, at 10% of the calculated equianalgesic dose. The methadone dose was titrated during the next week and pain relief improved substantially. Over the next year, as the disease progressed, the dose of the methadone was increased several times. A psychostimulant, methylphenidate, was added for mild sedation and fatigue. When a lancinating pain began in the ear, oxcarbazepine was added but did not help. However, an increase in her baseline dose of baclofen controlled it. The pain continued to be controlled as her function declined. She was comfortable when she developed urosepsis and died.

INTRODUCTION

There have been very few studies of pain or its management among populations with life-threatening neurologic disorders. As a consequence, the treatment of pain has been largely extrapolated from experience in the cancer population. Cancer pain continues to be poorly managed,[1] despite widespread acknowledgement that its prevalence and adverse impact are great.[2-4] This undertreatment, which is relatively more likely in women, minorities, the elderly, the chemically dependent, and those with impaired cognition or the requirement for multiple other medications, has been attributed to deficiencies in clinician practice, patient underreporting and non-adherence, and system-wide impediments to optimal analgesic therapy.[1,2] Given the likelihood that undertreatment of pain also afflicts populations with neurologic illnesses, it is essential to incorporate a focus on pain management into

a broader approach to palliative care for neurologic diseases.

EPIDEMIOLOGY OF PAIN IN NEUROLOGIC DISORDERS

The epidemiology of pain associated with serious neurologic illnesses is largely unknown. A few surveys have been performed, but relevant data are compromised by small samples and limited information about those with severe or progressive disorders.

Demyelinating Disease

Pain is a problem for more than 50% of patients with multiple sclerosis.[5-7] Although pain may occur at any time, it is associated with evidence of advanced disease. About 1% develop trigeminal neuralgia,[8] which may be identical to the idiopathic syndrome or distinguishable by bilaterality, an association with neurologic deficits, or a response to specific drugs (such as misoprostol or combinations of anticonvulsants).[9,10] Lancinating neuralgias may occur at other sites and continuous dysesthesias, particularly in the lower body, are common. Other syndromes include painful leg spasms, chronic headaches,[11] and musculoskeletal pains.

Extrapyramidal Diseases

Pain is estimated to occur in approximately 40% of patients with Parkinson's disease. In a minority, pain becomes severe enough to overshadow the motor symptoms;[12,13] it is one of the six most frequent causes of emergency department visits.[14] Musculoskeletal pains resulting from dystonia, muscular cramps, and spasms may occur, and some patients experience poorly characterized regional pains, which may represent some kind of central pain syndrome.[15,16] For example, a burning mouth syndrome has been reported to occur in 24% of patients with Parkinson's disease.[17]

Peripheral Neuropathies

Back and leg pain is very common in Guillain–Barre syndrome, affecting 80% to 100% of patients during the acute disorder.[18-20] Few patients develop long-term, clinically relevant deficits following an acute episode, but among those who do, pain continues in 5%–10%.[18] The prevalence and characteristics of pain in progressive demyelinating neuropathies is unknown. Pain appears to be very common, however, among those with progressive sensory or sensorimotor axonal polyneuropathy. The quality of the pain may be dysesthetic or aching, and can become the major reason for functional impairment.

Muscular Dystrophies

There have been no surveys of the symptoms experienced by patients with progressive muscular dystrophies. Nonetheless, anecdotal reports suggest that muscle pains and cramps are common and may occur before muscle strength is affected.[21] Several reports have noted the potential for epigastric pain secondary to acute gastric dilatation or abdominal pseudo-obstruction in patients with Duchenne dystrophy.[22-24] Pain also occurs with bone fractures following falls.[25]

Stroke and Spinal Cord Injury

Following stroke or spinal cord injury, some patients develop stepwise progression of deficits, or comorbid complications, that are best managed from a framework of palliative care. This is certainly true of patients with dementia associated with a multi-infarct state. Central post-stroke pain (CPSP) affects 2%–8% of all stroke patients,[26,27] 25% of patients with Wallenberg infarction,[28] and 17% of those with ventroposterolateral thalamic infarction.[29] Following spinal cord injury, pain affects about 65% of patients,[30] one-third of whom rate the pain as severe. These central pain syndromes are correlated with deficits in pinprick and temperature sensation, but not the size of the neural injury.[28] The pathophysiology is not understood.[28,31]

PAIN ASSESSMENT

The initial steps in a comprehensive pain assessment involve a detailed description of pain characteristics, impact, and comorbidities; an examination; and a review of laboratory and imaging studies.

Definition of Pain

Pain has been defined by the International Association for the Study of Pain (IASP) as 'an unpleasant sensory and emotional experience which we primarily associate with tissue damage or describe in terms of such damage, or both.' This definition underscores the inherent subjectivity of pain and the observation that the experience always incorporates sensory, emotional, and cognitive phenomena. It also highlights the important observation that pain and tissue damage are only loosely associated. The neural processes involved in the transmission and modulation of information about noxious stimuli (collectively termed 'nociception') are neither necessary nor sufficient for the experience of pain. Pain is the perception of nociception, and like other perceptions, can be influenced by many physical and psychosocial factors.

Chronic pain often is defined solely by a temporal criterion, usually 3–6 months. This approach is simple, but may be criticized as too limited. Chronic pain also may be defined as pain that persists for a month beyond the usual course of an acute illness or a reasonable duration for an injury to heal, pain associated with a chronic pathologic process, or pain that recurs at intervals for months or years.

Pain Characteristics

Because pain is inherently subjective, self-report is the gold standard for assessment. Ideally, the description of the pain should characterize its temporal relations, severity, topography, quality, and factors that exacerbate or relieve it (Table 19–1).

TEMPORAL FEATURES

The clinical distinction between acute pain and chronic pain is fundamental (Table 19–2). Temporal features of the pain other than duration (such as onset, daily variation, and course) also may be clinically relevant. These characteristics provide a context for the pain experience and may help guide therapy. For example, patients who experience intermittent episodes of acute pain superimposed on a continuous background pain—a common phenomenon generally termed 'breakthrough' pain[32]—may benefit from analgesic therapy that combines a long-acting analgesic with 'as needed' access to a short-acting analgesic.

Table 19–1. Assessment of Pain Characteristics

Characteristic	Descriptors
Temporal	Acute, recurrent, or chronic
	Onset and duration
	When present, continuous or intermittent
	Course (stable, improving, worsening) and variation (i.e. degree and pattern of fluctuation in pain)
Intensity	Severity on average, at its worst, at its least, right now, measured on a VAS, NRS, VRS, or other tool°
Topography	Focal or multifocal
	Focal or referred
	Superficial or deep
Quality	Varied descriptors (e.g. aching, throbbing, stabbing, or burning)
	Familiar or unfamiliar
Exacerbating/ relieving factors	Volitional (incident pain) or non-volitional

°VAS = visual analogue scale; NRS = numerical rating scale; VRS = verbal rating scale

INTENSITY

Measurement of pain severity is an essential aspect of the pain assessment. Measurement can be performed using simple unidimensional scales or multidimensional questionnaires. The latter scales are typically used in research settings.

The choice of one or another method of pain measurement is probably less important than its systematic application repeatedly over time. The simplest scale is a verbal rating scale (e.g. 'none', 'mild', 'moderate', 'severe'). Both numeric rating scales (e.g. 'On a scale of zero to ten, where zero is no pain and ten is the worst pain imaginable, how severe is your pain right now?') and visual analogue scales (VAS) (e.g. a 10 cm line anchored at one end by 'no pain' and anchored at the other end by 'worst possible pain') are more complicated, but more sensitive to treatment-induced changes. With chronic pain, it may be useful to inquire about the past 1–2 weeks and to inquire about pain in general, pain at its worst, and pain at its least.

Although patients vary in the extent to which any particular pain rating, or change in rating, is clinically important, an analysis of cancer pain scores suggested that the numeric threshold of 5 on a 0 to 10 scale usually

Table 19–2. Acute vs. Chronic Pain

	Acute Pain	Chronic Pain
Temporal features	Recent onset and expected to end in days or weeks	Often ill defined onset; duration unknown
Intensity	Variable	Variable
Associated affect	Anxiety may be prominent when pain is severe or cause is unknown	Irritability or depression
Associated behaviors	Pain behaviors (moaning, rubbing, or splinting the painful part) may occur when pain is severe or very acute	May or may not give any indication of pain; specific behaviors (e.g. assuming a comfortable position) may occur
Associated features	May have signs of sympathetic hyperactivity when severe (e.g. tachycardia, hypertension, sweating)	May or may not have vegetative signs such as lassitude, anorexia, weight loss, insomnia, loss of libido
Biological function	Essential warning; encourages rest and efforts to heal	None

indicates significant functional impairment from pain.[33] In two other analyses, one involving cancer patients, a reduction of 2 points on a 0 to 10 scale, or 30 mm on a 0–100 mm VAS, proved to be a meaningful change.[34,35]

Measurement of pain in the population with dementia can be particularly challenging. Every effort should be made to capture self-report, if possible. For patients who are too impaired to respond to a verbal rating scale or a numeric scale, the use of an illustrated scale, such as the so-called 'Faces' scale, commonly used in pediatric pain assessment, may be successful. For non-verbal patients, behavioral measures that score facial expression or body posture, should be considered. The use of a so-called 'physiologic' measure, such as heart rate and blood pressure, should be pursued only if meaningful communication is not possible.

LOCATION

Pain may be focal, multifocal, or generalized. The term 'focal' also applies to pain that is experienced superficial to the underlying etiology. In the latter sense, focal pain can be distinguished from referred pain, which is experienced at a site remote from a lesion in somatic structures, viscera, or nerves.

Referred pain from neurologic lesions may be complex. An injured peripheral nerve can cause focal pain superficial to the injury or anywhere in the dermatome innervated by the nerve. Pain also may be referred outside a single dermatome. For example, injury to the median nerve can refer pain to the upper arm.[36] Similarly, plexopathy can produce pain that may be segmental, involve multiple dermatomes, or be referred. Again, pain may occur throughout the dermatomes innervated by the injured structures or appear focally anywhere in this distribution. Likewise, injury to a nerve root may cause focal midline back pain or pain referred anywhere into the corresponding dermatome. Polyneuropathy of the axonal type typically produces pain that begins in the feet and may gradually ascend to involve the distal legs, and later the hands. The location of neuropathic pain accompanying lesions of the CNS is particularly varied. Pain related to a lesion of the spinal cord may be experienced as dysesthesias in one or more extremities or the torso, with varying patterns. Pain may mimic radiculopathy or polyneuropathy. A lesion in the brain stem can be complicated by 'crossed' dysesthesias affecting the ipsilateral face and contralateral body. A more rostral lesion can cause chronic pain in the entire contralateral hemibody or a localized site.

QUALITY

The descriptors used by patients to describe the quality of pain may be clues to its underlying mechanisms. Although the pathophysiology that sustains pain in the clinical setting cannot be known with certainty, inferences can be drawn based on these verbal reports and other aspects of the assessment (see below).

FACTORS THAT INCREASE OR DECREASE PAIN

Factors that change the intensity of the pain should be elicited as part of the assessment. This information may be directly applied in treatment, or suggest an etiology or pathophysiology.

Etiology, Inferred Pathophysiology, and Syndromes

The pain history, information from the physical examination, and review of laboratory and imaging studies usually provide sufficient foundation for a more sophisticated understanding of the pain. This understanding, in turn, guides clinical decisions about additional evaluation, prognostication, and therapy.

ETIOLOGICAL CONSIDERATIONS

If the specific disease or structural pathology can be identified, it may clarify the need for additional evaluation, improve classification or staging, suggest prognosis, or highlight the potential use of specific therapies. For example, increasing back pain in the elderly patient with advanced Parkinson's disease may be related to the disease itself, to concurrent degenerative spine disease or osteoporosis, or to some other unsuspected problem. An evaluation that elucidates the cause will guide the use of primary therapy.

The extent to which a patient should be subjected to studies in an effort to identify an underlying etiology for the pain depends on the goals of care. An understanding of the evolving goals of care is a fundamental element in the provision of good palliative care and requires ongoing communication with the patient and family, clear understanding of the nature and severity of the illness, and the extant therapeutic options.

INFERRED PATHOPHYSIOLOGY

Pain can be classified by the set of mechanisms presumed to be involved in sustaining the pain. The broad categories are usually termed 'nociceptive', 'neuropathic', and 'psychogenic'. Although this approach clearly oversimplifies very complex pathophysiological processes, it has clinical utility and has become widely accepted.[37] For example, the observation that some neuropathic pains are relatively poorly responsive to opioids[38] has led to increasing use of the adjuvant analgesics in the clinical setting (see below).

Pain that is believed to be generated by ongoing tissue injury is known as nociceptive pain. The nervous system is believed to be fundamentally intact and the complaints of pain are viewed as an appropriate response to tissue damage. Nociceptive somatic pain is sustained by ongoing activation of pain-sensitive primary afferent nerves that invest tissues such as bone, muscle, and joints. This type of pain is familiar to patients and is usually described as aching, sharp, or throbbing. Nociceptive visceral pain is related to injured viscera and is usually cramping or gnawing if hollow viscus is obstructed, or sharp, aching, or throbbing if other visceral tissues, such as mesentery, are injured.

Pain that is believed to be sustained by aberrant somatosensory processing in the peripheral or CNS is known generically as neuropathic pain. There are diverse subtypes, including a group of disorders presumably related to a set of central mechanisms (sometimes called deafferentation pains), a group related to peripheral mechanisms (painful polyneuropathies and mononeuropathies), and a group sustained by efferent activity in the sympathetic nervous system (sympathetically-maintained pain).[39] The descriptors that characterize these neuropathic disorders are similarly diverse. Some neuropathic pains are familiar, aching, or sharp; others are dysesthetic, often described as burning or electric-like.

The findings on a careful examination are most important in suggesting a diagnosis of neuropathic pain. Abnormal findings on a neurologic examination may support the diagnosis, but are neither necessary nor sufficient. If present, sensory abnormalities are particularly helpful. The term 'dysesthesia' refers to an unfamiliar, abnormal pain response, which may be spontaneous or evoked by a noxious or non-noxious stimulus. Allodynia, which may be considered a subtype of dysesthesia, is pain that is induced by a non-painful stimulus. Another subtype, hyperpathia, is an exaggerated pain response to either a noxious or non-noxious stimulus, which may include temporal or spatial summation, aftersensation, or emotional over-reaction. Other findings may include hyperesthesia (increased sensitivity to a non-noxious stimulus), hypesthesia (decreased sensitivity to a non-noxious stimulus), hyperalgesia (relatively increased pain response from a noxious stimulus), or hypalgesia (relatively decreased pain response to a noxious stimulus). These findings may coexist.

When a careful assessment of the patient yields positive indications that the pain is predominantly sustained by psychological factors, the syndrome is generically labeled psychogenic. These pains can also be described more formally using the psychiatric nomenclature subsumed under the category of the somatoform disorders. In the absence of a clearly diagnosable psychiatric disorder, pain that cannot be explained clinically in terms of nociceptive or neuropathic mechanisms is most appropriately termed 'idiopathic'.

PAIN SYNDROMES

Although the clinical utility of syndrome identification has been well demonstrated in the cancer population,[40,41] little attention has yet been focused on the pain syndromes associated with advanced neurologic illness. Some syndromes have been characterized in the few surveys of pain epidemiology described previously (see above).

Evaluation of Associated Phenomena

The pain assessment should include evaluation of other relevant phenomena. Among the most important are the effects of the pain on the physical and psychosocial functioning of the patient and the patient's family. Most patients with chronic pain also experience comorbidities that may contribute to suffering and become important targets of therapy. Symptoms other than pain should be elicited. Physical impairments, psychiatric disorders and distress, practical needs at home, and spiritual or existential concerns are commonly neglected, yet critical, aspects of the assessment.

PAIN MANAGEMENT

Like the assessment of the pain, the selection of pain management strategies must be guided by the overall goals of care. For patients whose hope for pain control is linked to a desire for better physical or psychosocial functioning, the effectiveness of therapies must be judged by both criteria. For those whose overriding goal is comfort, analgesic therapy may be successful even if it further compromises function. In some cases, aggressive disease-modifying therapies may be pursued, with the intent either to prolong life or to palliate the adverse consequences of the disease.

Primary Therapies

Intuitively, interventions that ameliorate the identified etiology of the pain may have analgesic consequences. Primary treatment for the comorbidities that may cause pain, such as decubitus ulcers, joint contractures, and osteoporosis, can be essential aspects of palliative care. The value of primary treatment for the underlying disease is well established in cancer, and is illustrated by the analgesic effectiveness of both radiotherapy and chemotherapy. In populations with progressive neurologic illness, the availability of primary therapies is more limited and the value of these interventions is supported only by anecdotal observations.

Pharmacotherapy

Analgesic pharmacotherapy encompasses the use of three broad categories of drugs. The first, conventionally known as the non-opioid analgesics, includes acetaminophen (paracetamol), dipyrone, and the nonsteroidal anti-inflammatory drugs (NSAIDs). The second, the so-called 'adjuvant' analgesics, includes a very diverse group of drug classes and refers to those drugs that have been commercialized for indications other than pain, but are analgesic in selected populations. These classes include the antidepressants, anticonvulsants, and many others. The third category comprises the opioid analgesics.

OVERALL APPROACH TO DRUG THERAPY

Advances in the management of cancer pain during the past two decades have had a strong influence on the clinical approach to pain associated with other life-threatening disorders. The established effectiveness of opioid-based pharmacotherapy[42–45] supports the consensus that pharmacotherapy is the mainstay analgesic approach, and that opioid therapy is the first-line if pain is moderate or severe.[46,47] The pure mu agonists, the prototype of which is morphine, are generally preferred, and the overall strategy has been strongly influenced by a World Health Organization guideline for cancer pain known as the 'analgesic ladder' approach.[46]

This analgesic ladder approach suggests that patients with mild pain should be treated first with acetaminophen (paracetamol) or a NSAID. This drug may be combined with an adjuvant drug, which in this context refers to either a drug selected to treat a side effect or to an adjuvant analgesic. For moderate pain, the approach conventionally favors a specific group of opioids, the prototype of which is codeine. In the United States, this treatment typically is accomplished using a combination product containing an opioid (codeine, oxycodone, or hydrocodone) and either acetaminophen or aspirin. The dose of the combination may be increased until the maximum safe dose of the aspirin or acetaminophen is reached (for acetaminophen, this is usually considered to be 4 g per day, and 2–3 g per day in those with known hepatopathy or heavy alcohol use). An adjuvant drug may be added.

Alternative strategies for this second rung of the analgesic ladder include tramadol[48] and the use of a lower dose of a single-entity opioid formulation (like morphine), which is more typically administered for severe pain. Meperidine is occasionally used, but is not preferred for chronic pain management because of the potential for adverse effects (dysphoria, tremulousness, hyperreflexia, and seizures) related to accumulation of an active metabolite, normeperidine.[49]

Patients with severe pain (including those who fail to achieve adequate relief following appropriate administration of drugs on the second rung of the analgesic ladder) are treated with an opioid conventionally selected for severe pain (see below). Again, this treatment may be combined with acetaminophen or an NSAID, or with an adjuvant drug as indicated.

PRINCIPLES OF OPIOID PHARMACOTHERAPY

Guidelines for opioid pharmacotherapy focus on selection of the drug and route, the approach to dosing, and side effect management. Clinicians must also appreciate issues related to the potential for abuse and addiction.

Drug Selection

In the United States, the opioids conventionally used for severe pain include morphine, hydromorphone, fentanyl, oxycodone (used as a single entity), levorphanol, and methadone (Table 19–3). Oxymorphone is available as a suppository and an injectable formulation, and is used rarely. Although morphine has been considered to be the first-line drug for severe pain, there is substantial individual variation in the response to different opioids and no single drug should be considered preferred. For each patient, the balance between analgesia and side effects, and the pattern of side effects, can vary greatly from opioid to opioid, and sequential trials may be needed to identify the drug with the most favorable balance between analgesia and side effects. This technique is known as opioid rotation.[50]

The role of morphine also has evolved with recognition of its active metabolites.[51] Morphine-6-glucuronide is an active metabolite that may contribute to the analgesia and side effects observed during morphine therapy. Morphine-3-glucuronide also may cause toxicity, possibly including myoclonus and worsening pain. These metabolites may accumulate in the setting of renal insufficiency. Patients who develop morphine toxicity can be offered a trial of an alternative opioid, such as hydromorphone or fentanyl, in the hope that lesser metabolite accumulation may contribute to a better response.

Methadone has a unique pharmacology among the opioids. Its half-life is highly variable, ranging from 12 hours to more than 150 hours.[52] Four to five half-lives are required to approach steady-state plasma concentration, and this period can be as brief as several days or as long as two weeks. If the dose is rapidly increased to an effective level, the plasma concentration can continue to rise toward steady-state levels, and late toxicity can occur. Careful monitoring is required for a prolonged period after methadone dosing is initiated or increased.

Methadone is commercially available as the racemic mixture of the d- and the l-optical isomers. The d-isomer does not bind to the opioid receptor and is an antagonist at the N-methyl-D-aspartate (NMDA) receptor. NMDA receptor antagonists can reverse opioid tolerance and produce analgesia via non-opioid mechanisms.[53] The pharmacology of the d-isomer probably explains the observation that methadone as the racemic mixture can have a much greater potency than anticipated from the dose conversions listed on the equianalgesic dose table (see Table 19–3), particularly when given to a patient who is already receiving relatively high doses of an alternative opioid. Based on a growing clinical experience, a trial of methadone is often considered for patients whose opioid requirements are increasing and side effects, such as sedation, confusion, or myoclonus, are compromising therapy.

Route of Administration

For chronic therapy, the oral or transdermal routes for opioid delivery are usually attempted first. Oral controlled-release formulations of morphine, oxycodone, or hydromorphone allow convenient dosing, either once daily (morphine or hydromorphone) or twice daily (morphine or oxycodone). These drugs are

Table 19–3. Opioid Analgesics

Morphine-like Agonists	Equianalgesic Doses[a]	Half-life (h)	Duration (h)	Toxicity	Comments
Morphine	10 i.m. 20–60 p.o.[b]	2–3 2–3	3–4 3–6	Constipation, nausea, sedation most common; respiratory depression rare with chronic use	Standard for comparison for opioids; multiple routes available
Controlled-release morphine	20–60 p.o.[b]	2–3	8–12		Dosing 2–3 times/day
Sustained-release morphine	20–60 p.o.[b]	2–3	24		Once-a-day dosing
Hydromorphone	1.5 i.m. 7.5 p.o.	2–3 2–3	3–4 3–6	Same as morphine	Used for multiple routes
Oxycodone	20–30 p.o.	2–3	3–6	Same as morphine	Combined with aspirin or acetaminophen, or single entity
Controlled-release oxycodone	20–30 p.o.	2–3	8–12	Same as morphine	
Oxymorphone	1 i.m. 10 p.r.	— —	3–6 3–6	Same as morphine	
Meperidine	75 i.m. 300 p.o.	2–3 2–3	3–4 3–6	Same as morphine plus normeperidine toxicity	Not preferred because of toxic metabolite, normeperidine
Levorphanol	2 i.m. 4 p.o.	12–15 12–15	3–6 3–6	Same as morphine	
Methadone	10 i.m.[c] 20 p.o.[c]	12–>150 12–>150	4–>8 4–>8	Same as morphine	Risk of delayed toxicity from accumulation; potency may be much higher than predicted.
Codeine	130 i.m. 200 p.o.	2–3 2–3	3–4 3–6	Same as morphine	
Propoxyphene HCL	—	12	3–6	Same as morphine	Toxic metabolite accumulates and seizures with overdose, but not significant at doses used clinically
Propoxyphene napthsylate	—	12	3–6	Same as above	
Hydrocodone	—	2–4	3–6	Same as morphine	Only available combined with acetaminophen or aspirin

Continued on following page

Table 19–3—*continued*

Morphine-like Agonists	Equianalgesic Doses[a]	Half-life (h)	Duration (h)	Toxicity	Comments
Dihydrocodeine	—	2–4	3–6	Same as morphine	Only available combined with acetaminophen or aspirin
Fentanyl	—	7–12	—	Same as morphine	Can be administered as a continuous infusion; based on clinical experience, 100 µg/h is equianalgesic to morphine 4 mg/h
Fentanyl transdermal	—	16–24	48–72		Based on clinical experience, 100 µg/h is roughly equianalgesic to morphine 4 mg/h; alternatively, a mg:mg ratio of oral morphine:transdermal fentanyl of 100:1 can be used

[a]Dose that provides analgesia equivalent to 10 mg i.m. morphine. These ratios are useful guides when switching drugs or routes of administration (see text). In clinical practice, the potency of the i.m. route is considered to be identical to the IV and subcutaneous routes.
[b]Extensive survey data suggest that the relative potency of i.m.:p.o. morphine, which has been shown to be 1:6 in an acute dosing study, is 1:2–3 with chronic dosing.
[c]When switching from another opioid to methadone, the potency of methadone is much greater than indicated on this table.

more expensive than the immediate-release formulations, but are generally preferred in developed countries.

The transdermal route for fentanyl is a widely accepted alternative, which offers a 48- to 72-hour dosing interval. The latter formulation is particularly useful for patients who are unable to swallow or absorb an orally administered opioid, are candidates for a trial of fentanyl during opioid rotation, or have problems with adherence to therapy. In open-label studies, transdermal fentanyl produced less constipation than oral morphine,[54] suggesting that severe constipation may be another indication for a trial. The use of the transdermal system is limited by the difficulties involved in delivering high doses and the need for an alternative route to provide supplemental doses for breakthrough pain. Because drug delivery is influenced by temperature, frequent fever spikes could potentially lead to unstable absorption from the transdermal system.

The oral transmucosal formulation of fentanyl (oral transmucosal fentanyl citrate or OTFC) is effective for breakthrough pain.[55] This formulation has an onset of effect faster than oral doses.

The rectal route is used occasionally, particularly at the end of life. In addition to the commercially available formulations, which may require relatively frequent dosing, rectal administration of a controlled-release oral morphine preparation and specially compounded methadone suppositories has been effective.

Patients who are unable to swallow or absorb opioids are candidates for other approaches to long-term parenteral dosing. Continuous infusion techniques are preferred and can be implemented with any opioid available in an injectable formulation. Long-term intravenous administration is possible if the patient has an indwelling venous access device. Continuous subcutaneous infusion can be simply performed using a 25-gauge butterfly needle, which is usually changed weekly.

A variety of techniques for intraspinal drug delivery have been adapted to long-term treatment and properly selected patients can benefit greatly.[56-58] The clearest indication is intolerable somnolence or confusion in a patient who is not experiencing adequate analgesia during systemic opioid treatment of a pain syndrome located below the level of midchest. Continuous intrathecal infusion using an implanted pump should be considered for patients with life expectancies longer than a few months. Drug combinations are commonly used. A study of epidural clonidine confirmed its efficacy in cancer patients and highlighted its utility for those with neuropathic pain.[59]

Dosing Guidelines

Fixed scheduled dosing is preferred for continuous or frequently recurring pain and it is common practice to combine this 'around-the-clock' therapy with an as-needed 'rescue dose' to treat breakthrough pains. As-needed dosing alone should be considered at the start of therapy in relatively opioid-naive patients.

Except during therapy with methadone or transdermal fentanyl, the rescue drug is usually the same drug as that administered on a fixed schedule basis. An alternative short-acting opioid, such as morphine, is typically co-administered with methadone or transdermal fentanyl. With the exception of OTFC, the size of the rescue dose is usually 5% to 15% of the total daily dose, and the dosing interval in the ambulatory population is usually 1–2 hours, as needed. Controlled studies of OTFC yielded guidelines for the use of this new formulation that include a low starting dose in all cases (200 mcg or, perhaps, 400 mcg), followed by dose titration.

The goal of dose titration is to identify a dose associated with a favorable balance between analgesia and side effects. As titration proceeds, the size of each dose increment usually is selected as either the total quantity of 'rescue' drug consumed during the previous day or 30%–50% of the current total daily dose. The increment can be larger (75%–100% of the total daily dose) if pain is severe, or smaller if the patient is already experiencing opioid toxicity, is predisposed to adverse effects because of advanced age or coexisting major organ dysfunction, or is relatively opioid-naive.

An extensive clinical experience in the cancer population suggests that opioid dose titration usually identifies a dose that yields a favorable balance between analgesia and side effects, which in the absence of disease progression, remains stable for a prolonged period. This phenomenon belies the inevitability of tolerance as a problem in the long-term administration of opioid drugs.[60]

Some patients fail to benefit during opioid therapy because side effects supervene. This poor opioid responsiveness may be related to any of a large number of processes, each of which either limit the analgesic response or increase the likelihood of side effects (Table 19–4).[61,62]

Guidelines for the management of poor opioid responsiveness are based on clinical experience, and may be categorized into four strategies (Table 19–5). Opioid rotation is one common approach. Equianalgesic dose tables, which are based on well controlled relative potency trials performed over more than four decades, provide the starting point for dose conversion.[63] When switching from one drug to another, the equianalgesic dose of the new drug is calculated from the table. This calculated dose is typically cut by 25%–50% to account for inter-individual variablity and incomplete cross-tolerance. There are two important exceptions to the latter rule: usually, the dose is usually not reduced when switching to the transdermal fentanyl system (the 'safety margin' was built into the published dose conversion formula); the dose is reduced more, as much as 75%–90%, when the switch is to methadone.

Side Effect Management

The management of side effects is an essential element of treatment and can both improve the likelihood of a favorable response and enhance comfort overall.[64] Opioids are associated with numerous potential side effects. Although many, such as nausea, itch, urinary hesitancy, and sedation, are time-limited in a large majority of patients, each of these problems can persist in some patients. For many, the management of constipation and cognitive impairment are major issues over time. Clinical trials evaluating various treatments for these problems have been very limited. There are numerous options for laxative therapy and the best treatment strategy for the individual patient is based on a careful assessment and clinical judgment (Table 19–6). The use of psychostimulant therapy is an advance in the management of opioid-induced cognitive impairment.[65] The most extensive experience is with methylphenidate, but other drugs,

Table 19–4. **Potential Reasons for Poor Opioid Responsiveness**

Increasing nociception
- Rapid progression of a painful lesion

Development of new, less responsive, mechanisms
- Worsening inflammation
- Development of neuropathic mechanisms

Psychological or psychiatric processes
- Increasing anxiety or depression
- Delirium

Tolerance

Table 19–5. **Therapeutic Strategies for Managing Pains that are Poorly Responsive to an Opioid Regimen**

Approach	Example
More aggressive side effect management (open the 'therapeutic' window)	Use of psychostimulant for opioid-related sedation, cognitive impairment
Identify an opioid with a more favorable balance between analgesia and side effects	Opioid rotation
Use a pharmacologic approach to reduce the systemic opioid requirement	Co-administer a NSAID or an adjuvant analgesic; consider intraspinal opioid therapy
Use a non-pharmacologic approach to reduce the systemic opioid requirement	Anesthetic approaches (e.g. nerve blocks); surgical approaches (e.g. cordotomy); physiatric approaches (e.g. an orthotic); psychological approaches (e.g. biofeedback); alternative medicine approaches (e.g. acupuncture)

Table 19–6. **Management of Constipation**

General approaches	Increase fluid intake
	Increase dietary fiber
	Use a bulk laxative or increase dietary fiber (unless debilitated or bowel obstruction is suspected)
	Ensure that impaction has not occurred
Specific approaches	Intermittent use (every 2 or 3 days) of osmotic laxative such as magnesium hydroxide, magnesium citrate, or sodium phosphate
	Daily softening agent (docusate sodium) alone
	Intermittent use (every 2 or 3 days) of a contact cathartic such as senna, bisacodyl, or phenolphthalein
	Daily contact cathartic (with or without concurrent softening agent)
	Daily lactulose or sorbitol
Alternative approaches in refractory cases	Rectal approaches, including contact cathartic or enemas
	Intermittent or daily use of colonic lavage with polyethylene glycol
	Daily treatment with a prokinetic drug such as cisapride or metoclopramide
	Daily treatment with oral naloxone

including dextroamphetamine and modafinil, are also used.

Non-opioid Analgesics

The term 'non-opioid analgesic' is conventionally applied to acetaminophen (paracetamol), dipyrone, and all the NSAIDs (Table 19–7). The NSAIDs all have anti-inflammatory effects, but can provide analgesia independent of this action. The non-opioid analgesics are used alone when pain is mild to moderate in severity, and are combined with opioids during the management of more severe pain.

Clinical Pharmacology

All of the non-opioid analgesics inhibit the enzyme cyclo-oxygenase (COX) and thereby lower tissue levels of prostaglandins (PG) (compounds that sensitize primary afferent neurons, mediate the inflammatory cascade, and are involved in central nociceptive processing). Cyclo-oxygenase has two isoforms: the constitutive variety known as cyclo-oxygenase-1 (COX-1) and an inducible variety known as cyclo-oxygenase-2 (COX-2).[66]

COX-1 is involved in the normal physiology of the stomach, kidney, platelets, and presumably other organs and tissues. COX-2 is constitutive in some tissues (e.g. brain and kidney), but is largely produced in response to injury and is a key element in the inflammatory cascade. NSAIDs that are relatively COX-2 selective have an improved gastrointestinal toxicity profile without loss of anti-inflammatory or analgesic effects.

Several highly selective COX-2 inhibitors are now available, including celecoxib, rofecoxib, and valdecoxib. These drugs are associated with a relatively reduced risk of NSAID-induced gastrointestinal toxicity. They have no effect on platelet function, but appear to have renal toxicity equivalent to the non-selective COX-1 and COX-2 inhibitors.

This reduced risk of gastrointestinal and platelet toxicity supports the preferential use of the selective COX-2 inhibitors in medically frail populations. The overall cost–benefit of these drugs is not known, however. At this time, the choice of NSAID is a matter of clinical judgment and should be based on an assessment of medical comorbidities, planned duration of therapy, prior experience, and cost.

Table 19–7. Nonsteroidal Anti-inflammatory Drugs

Chemical Class	Generic Name	Approximate Half-life (h)	Dosing Schedule	Recommended Starting Dose (mg/d)[a]	Recommended Maximum Dose (mg/dl)	Comment
P-aminophenol	Acetaminophen[b]	2–4	q 4–6h	2600	6000	Overdosage produces derivative hepatic toxicity. Not anti-inflammatory. Lack of GI and platelet toxicity.
Non-selective COX-1 and COX-2 Inhibitors						
Salicylates	Aspirin[b]	3–12[c]	q 4–6h	2600	6000	Standard for comparison. May not be tolerated as well as some of the newer NSAIDs.[d]
	Diflunisal[b]	8–12	q 12h	1000 × 1	1500	Less GI toxicity than aspirin.[d]
	Choline magnesium trisalicylate[b]	8–12	q 12h	1500 × 1 then 1000 q 12h	4000	Believed to have less GI toxicity than other NSAIDs.. No effect on platelet aggregation, despite anti-inflammatory effects.[d]
	Salsalate	8–12	q 12h	1500 × 1 then 1000 q 12h	4000	
Propionic	Ibuprofen[b]	3–4	q 4–8h	1600	4200	Available over the counter acids in the United States.[d]
	Naproxen[b]	13	q 12h	500	1500	Available over the counter in the United States and available as suspension.[d]
	Naproxen sodium[b]	13	q 12h	550	1375	[d]
	Fenoprofen	2–3	q 6h	800	3200	[d]
Propionic	Ketoprofen	2–3	q 6–8h	100	300	Available over the counter acids in the United States[d]
	Flurbiprofen[b]	5–6	q 8–12h	100	300	Experience too limited to evaluate higher doses, though it is likely that some patients would benefit.[d]
Acetic acids	Oxaprozin	40	q 24h	600	1800	Once-daily dosing may be useful.[d]
	Indomethacin	4–5	q 8–12h	75	200	Available in sustained-release and rectal formulations in the United States. Higher incidence of side effects, particularly GI and CNS, than propionic acids.[d]

					Comments
	Tolmetin	1	q 6–8h	600	2000	[d]
	Sulindac	14	q 12h	300	400	[d]
	Diclofenac	2	q 6h	75	200	[d]
	Ketorolac (IM)	4–7	q 4–6h	30 (loading)	60	Parenteral formulation available in the United States. Long-term use not recommended.[d]
	Ketorolac (PO)	4–7	q 6h	40	40	Long-term use not recommended.[d]
	Etodolac	7	q 8h	600	1200	[d]
Oxicams	Piroxicam	45	q 24h	20	40	Administration of 40 mg for >3 weeks is associated with a high incidence of peptic ulcer, particularly in the elderly.[d]
Naphthyl-alkanones	Nabumetone	24	q 24h	1000	1000–2000	Appears to have a relatively low risk of GI toxicity. Once-daily dosing may be useful.
Fenamates	Mefenamic acid[b]	2	q 6h	500 × 1 then 250 q 6h	1000	Not recommended for use longer than 1 week, and therefore not indicated in cancer pain therapy.[d]
	Meclofenamic acid	2–4	q 6–8h	150	400	[d]
Pyrazoles	Phenylbutazone	50–100	q 6–8h	300	400	More toxic than other NSAIDs. Not preferred for cancer pain therapy.
Selective COX-2 Inhibitors						
	Celecoxib		q 12h	200	400	Significantly less risk of GI toxicity.
	Rofecoxib		q 24h	12.5	25	Lesser risk of renal toxicity not established.
	Valdecoxib		q 24h	10–20	20	

[a] Starting dose should be one-half to two-thirds recommended dose in the elderly, those on multiple drugs, and those with renal insufficiency. Doses must be individualized. Studies of NSAIDs in the cancer population are meager; dosing guidelines are thus empiric.

[b] Pain is approved indication in the United States.

[c] Half-life of aspirin increases with dose.

[d] At high doses, stool guaiac, liver function tests, BUN, creatinine, and urinalysis should be checked periodically.

Adverse Effects

Adverse effects are common during NSAID therapy. Gastrointestinal symptoms occur in about 10% of patients who receive the non-selective COX inhibitors, and ulcers occur in about 2%.[67] Nausea and abdominal pain are poor predictors of serious NSAID-related toxicity and as many as two-thirds of patients being treated with NSAIDS experience no symptoms before serious ulceration occurs. The factors associated with an increased risk of ulceration are advanced age, the use of higher NSAID doses, concomitant administration of a corticosteroid, and a history of either ulcer disease or previous gastrointestinal complications from NSAIDs.[67] Heavy alcohol or cigarette consumption, and infection with Helicobacter pylori, also have been implicated as factors in NSAID-related gastropathy.

The risk of NSAID-induced ulcer disease can be reduced by co-administration of gastro-protective drugs. The evidence of this effect is strong for both misoprostol, a prostaglandin analog,[68] and the proton pump inhibitors.[69] Although studies of H2 blockers have not been uniformly favorable, there is evidence that these drugs also may be beneficial, at least at higher doses.[70] Other agents, such as antacids and sucralfate, have never been shown to reduce NSAID risk.

NSAID Administration

Drug selection is empiric. If there is access to selective COX-2 inhibitors, a case can be made to select one of these drugs first in patients with serious medical illnesses.

All non-opioid analgesics produce dose-dependent analgesic effects, and have dose–response relationships characterized by a minimal effective dose and a ceiling dose for analgesia. There is large individual variation in the dose–response relationship. Recommended doses have been developed from studies performed in relatively healthy populations and, for this reason, guidelines should be implemented cautiously when using these drugs in the medically ill and the elderly. Dose titration from low starting doses may be prudent.

ADJUVANT ANALGESICS

The term 'adjuvant analgesic' refers to any drug that has a primary indication other than pain but is known to be analgesic in specific circumstances. The adjuvant analgesics comprise numerous drugs in diverse drug classes (Table 19–8).[71] In populations with life-threatening illness, these drugs typically are added to an opioid regimen to enhance analgesia, or to allow opioid dose reduction and thereby lessen side effects. In this setting, the most common use is in the management of challenging neuropathic pain syndromes, which may be relatively less opioid responsive than other types of pain.[38,39]

Some classes of adjuvant analgesics have been studied in varied types of pain and are best considered multipurpose analgesics; others are conventionally used for specific types of pain. The multipurpose analgesics include the corticosteroids, the antidepressants, and the alpha-2 adrenergic agonists. Drugs for neuropathic pain include the multipurpose analgesics and numerous other classes, such as the anticonvulsants, local anesthetics, and NMDA antagonists.

Multipurpose Analgesics

In the cancer population, the corticosteroids have been shown to improve multiple types of pain, appetite, nausea, malaise, and overall quality of life.[72,73] This experience has guided use in other populations with serious illness. Current data are inadequate to evaluate drug-selective differences, dose–response relationships, predictors of efficacy, or the durability of favorable effects. Long-term therapy usually involves the administration of relatively low doses to patients with advanced disease. Typically, prednisone, 5–10 mg, or dexamethasone, 1–2 mg, is administered once or twice daily. Dose escalation for worsening symptoms is appropriate if benefits decline with progressive disease, particularly at the end of life. A higher dose regimen, usually administered for a shorter period, may be considered in the setting of rapidly worsening pain related to a nerve injury or bone disease. This regimen may begin with dexamethasone 24–100 mg intravenously, followed by 6–24 mg daily in four divided doses, which is gradually tapered.

Antidepressant drugs are used primarily for neuropathic pain. The tricyclic antidepressants (TCAs) have been most extensively studied and

Table 19–8. **Adjuvant Analgesics**

Class	Examples
Multipurpose Analgesics	
Corticosteroids	Prednisone, dexamethasone
Antidepressants	
TCA's	Amitriptyline, nortriptyline, desipramine, doxepin, imipramine, clomipramine
SSRI and related newer drugs	Paroxetine, citalopram, fluoxetine, venlafaxine
Other	Maprotiline, bupropion, trazodone
Alpha-2 adrenergic agonists	Clonidine, tizanidine
Adjuvant Analgesics Used for Neuropathic Pain	
Anticonvulsants	Gabapentin, carbamazepine, phenytoin, divalproex, topiramate, tiagabine, oxcarbazepine, pregabalin, lamotrigine, levetiracetam, zonisamide
Corticosteroids	See above
Antidepressants	See above
Alpha-2 adrenergic agonists	See above
Oral local anesthetics	Mexiletine, tocainide, flecainide
GABA agonists	Baclofen
NMDA receptor antagonists	Dextromethorphan, ketamine
Miscellaneous	Calcitonin
Topical agents	Capsaicin, lidocaine patch, EMLA

there is strong evidence that both the tertiary amine TCAs (e.g. amitriptyline, doxepin, and imipramine) and the secondary amine TCAs (e.g. desipramine and nortriptyline) can be effective. There are few controlled trials of other subclasses, but the extant data support the analgesic efficacy of several selective serotonin reuptake inhibitors (SSRIs), such as paroxetine, and several drugs with noradrenergic effects or combined serotonin and noradreneric actions, including maprotiline, venlafaxine, and bupropion.

Although amitriptyline is the best studied TCA, it has a relatively high side effect liability and may not be well tolerated by many patients with medical comorbidities. Patients who are unable to tolerate amitriptyline, or are predisposed to its sedative, anticholinergic, or hypotensive effects, should be considered for a trial with a secondary amine TCA, such as desipramine. Given the relatively better side effect profile, trials of the newer antidepressants, such as one of the SSRIs, is appropriate for those who cannot tolerate a secondary amine TCA or are strongly predisposed to side effects from these drugs.

Antidepressants do not exert their therapeutic effects rapidly. Dose titration from a low starting dose is typically necessary. Sequential trials are warranted if pain remains refractory.

The alpha-2-adrenergic agonists, such as clonidine and tizanidine, have established analgesic efficacy in a variety of pain syndromes[74,75] and also may be considered nonspecific analgesics. In the setting of advanced medical illness, however, they are usually considered for patients with pain that has not responded to other drugs. Clonidine is usually considered for refractory neuropathic pain, and tizanidine often is tried for neuropathic pain or pain due to muscle spasm. Given its better side effect profile, tizanidine is usually administered first.

Drugs Used for Neuropathic Pain

The multipurpose analgesics are often used for neuropathic pain. Other drug classes are conventionally considered selectively for this indication.

Numerous anticonvulsants are established analgesics. Gabapentin is prescribed most commonly and has proven efficacy in several neuropathic pain syndromes.[76] It has an acceptable adverse effect profile, is not metabolized in the liver, and has no known drug–drug interactions. Treatment usually starts at 100–300 mg per day, and dose titration usually continues until benefit occurs, side effects supervene, or the total daily dose is at 2700–3600 mg per day. Some patients respond to 600 mg per day in divided doses, whereas others do not reach a maximal response until the dose is increased to 6000 mg per day, or more.

Many anticonvulsant drugs other than gabapentin have been evaluated as treatments for neuropathic pains.[77] The anticonvulsant drugs that have been conventionally used for pain include carbamazepine, phenytoin, divalproex, and clonazepam. More limited data also support the analgesic efficacy of newer anticonvulsants, including lamotrigine, topiramate, tiagabine, zonisamide, and levetiracetam. All anticonvulsants are administered using the dosing schedules typically employed for seizures.

Systemic administration of local anesthetic drugs also is analgesic for neuropathic pain.[78] In the United States, mexiletine (a nonselective sodium channel blocker) has been the preferred drug; in other countries, tocainide or flecainide have been preferred.

Brief intravenous local anesthetic infusions also are analgesic.[79] Treatment usually comprises infusion of lidocaine over 30 minutes in a dose that ranges between 1 mg/kg and 4 mg/kg. In the medically ill, it is reasonable to start with a low dose infusion, which is followed, if unsuccessful, by infusions at incrementally higher doses. There is no evidence that a brief local anesthetic infusion is more effective than oral therapy, but this approach may achieve a rapid analgesic response and be useful if neuropathic pain is severe.

Antagonists of the NMDA receptor are undergoing intensive investigation as potential analgesics.[80–82] Three such drugs—the dissociative anesthetic ketamine, the antitussive dextromethorphan, and the antiviral amantadine—already are commercially available in the United States. Memantine is available in many other countries. Ketamine has a difficult side effect profile, which includes nightmares and delirium, but its efficacy in some challenging patients with neuropathic pain has

encouraged its use, either by continuous infusion or by oral administration, in highly selected patients. Dextromethorphan also has been used at relatively high daily doses. The starting dose can be 120 mg/d, and possibly higher; it is likely that the analgesic dose will be at least 350 mg per day. Experience with amantadine as an analgesic is very limited.

The GABA agonist baclofen has been shown to be effective in the treatment of trigeminal neuralgia[83] and may be a useful drug for neuropathic pain in the medically ill. The therapeutic dose appears to vary widely, ranging from 30 mg to more than 200 mg per day.

Benzodiazepines also may have salutary effects in patients with chronic pain, and it may be impossible to determine the degree to which psychotropic or primary analgesic actions contribute to this outcome. Clonazepam is commonly used to treat neuropathic pain, and a similar role has been suggested for alprazolam in a small survey of cancer pain patients.[84]

Topical Analgesics

Topical analgesics may particularly benefit medically ill patients with chronic pain by providing pain relief that complements a systemic analgesic regimen without the risk of additional side effects. Topical therapies include local anesthetics, NSAIDs, capsaicin, and other drugs.[85]

Topical local anesthetics can be administered by patch or cream. Recently, a lidocaine 5% impregnated patch was approved for use in some countries for patients with postherpetic neuralgia. This formulation is well accepted by patients and should be considered for any patient who is a candidate for topical local anesthetic therapy. A 1:1 mixture of lidocaine and prilocaine known as EMLA (eutectic mixture of local anesthetics), which can produce dense cutaneous anesthesia if applied thickly under an occlusive dressing, and other higher concentration local anesthetic creams or gels (e.g. lidocaine 5%), also can be tried.

There is substantial evidence that topical NSAIDs can be effective for soft tissue pain and perhaps joint pain.[86] A trial of a compounded formulation containing diclofenac, ketoprofen, or another NSAID may be considered, particularly when pain has a superficial element of inflammation.

Patients with neuropathic pain also can be offered a trial of topical capsaicin, a peptide that depletes peptides in small primary afferent neurons, including those that mediate nociceptive transmission. Although anecdotal experience with this compound has been mixed, there is evidence of efficacy from controlled trials.[87,88] An adequate trial requires four applications daily for one month.

Other drugs may also be added to compounded topical formulations. There is limited anecdotal experience with various tricyclic antidepressants and anticonvulsants in chronic pain populations.

Anesthesiologic Approaches

Numerous interventional pain therapies are usually performed by anesthesiologists. The most common are neural blockade, myofascial injections, neurostimulation techniques, and neuraxial drug infusion.

Neural blockade can be temporary (somatic, visceral, or sympathetic nerve block) or neurolytic. Temporary neural blockade can be used for diagnostic, therapeutic, or prognostic purposes before a planned neurolytic procedure. With the advent of the non-destructive alternatives of neurostimulation and neuraxial infusion, neurolytic blocks are now seldom performed.

As described previously, neuraxial infusion can be accomplished through a variety of approaches and offer trials of varied drugs. These infusion systems have the advantage of using very small doses of opioids in patients who cannot tolerate systemic delivery because of side effects.[56–58,89–91] A neuraxial strategy should be considered in selected patients who experience an unfavorable balance between analgesia and side effects during systemic opioid therapy.[56–58,89–91]

Neurostimulatory Approaches

Transcutaneous electrical nerve stimulation (TENS) has been used for many years and there is limited evidence of effectiveness in diverse pain syndromes.[92] The approach reflects a practical application of the theoretical construct known as the 'gate control theory' of pain.[93,94] An adequate trial usually involves several weeks, during which the patient should experiment with different electrode placements and stimulation parameters.

The implantable stimulator systems include percutaneous electrical nerve stimulation, dorsal column stimulation (also called spinal cord stimulation (SCS)), and deep brain stimulation (DBS). The percutaneous electrical nerve stimulation is used in treatment of refractory neuropathic pain in the distribution of a single nerve. SCS has been shown to be effective for patients with refractory chronic low back pain and complex regional pain syndrome, and is sometimes considered for medically ill patients with pain refractory to pharmacotherapy. Deep brain stimulation is rarely used.

Rehabilitative Approaches

Rehabilitative approaches comprise diverse modalities, including medicinal diathermy, cryotherapy, therapeutic exercise, and the use of orthoses and assistive devices. Both superficial and deep diathermy and cryotherapy produce local change in blood flow and other factors, but the relationship between these changes and pain relief is yet obscure. Anecdotally, some patients benefit. Therapeutic exercise may improve function and also prevent the development of secondary sources of pain, such as contractures.

Psychological Approaches

Psychological interventions include a variety of psychotherapeutic approaches and specific cognitive treatments intended to reduce pain. The latter include relaxation therapies like autogenic training, hypnosis, biofeedback progressive muscle relaxation, and guided imagery.[95] Cognitive-behavioral and psychoeducational interventions have been successfully implemented in medically ill populations with chronic pain.[96–98]

Neurosurgical Approaches

Neurosurgeons may perform the invasive neurostimulation and neuraxial infusion techniques. Additionally, a variety of surgical neurolytic approaches have been developed for intractable chronic pain. These include include peripheral neurectomy (e.g. for trigeminal neuralgia), spinal cord ablative procedures (dorsal root ganglia excision, dorsal rhizotomy, cordotomy), and central ablative procedures (mesencephalotomy, medial thalamotomy, cingulotomy, hypophysectomy). With the advent of SCS and neuraxial infusion, all of these approaches are now rarely performed.

Complementary and Alternative Medicine (CAM) Approaches

Numerous complementary and alternative medicine approaches are used for chronic pain. The most common modalities used are acupuncture, massage, chiropractic manipulation, herbal medicine and nutritional supplements, and varied mind–body approaches. Clinicians must be open to those therapies for which there is some scientific support or an extensive experience. Given the widespread acceptance of these therapies, patients will be most supported by a willingness to pursue an 'integrative pain therapy' that embraces selected complementary therapies while aggressively pursuing those supported in the medical literature.

SUMMARY

There are very few studies addressing the epidemiology and treatment of pain in populations with advanced neurologic illnesses. Yet, an extensive experience in other medically ill populations provides an adequate foundation for treatment. Clinicians should be aware of the existing data, and gain the knowledge and skills necessary to provide expert pain assessment and management of pain.

REFERENCES

1. Pargeon KL, Hailey BJ. Barriers to effective cancer pain management: a review of the literature. J Pain Symptom Manage 1999;18:358–368.
2. Cleeland CS, Gonin R, Hatfield AK, et al. Pain and its treatment in outpatients with metastatic cancer. N Engl J Med 1994;330;29:73–83.
3. Portenoy RK, Kornblith AB, Wong G, et al. Pain in ovarian cancer. Prevalence, characteristics, and associated symptoms. Cancer 1994;74:907–915.
4. Larue F, Colleau SM, Brasseur L, Cleeland CS. Multicentre study of cancer pain and its treatment in France. BMJ 1995;310:1034–1037.
5. Moulin DE, Foley KM, Ebers GC. Pain syndromes in multiple sclerosis. Neurology 1988;38(12):1830–1834.
6. Vaney C. Pain in multiple sclerosis. Clinical aspects and therapy. Schweiz Med Wochenschr 1990;120:1959–1964.
7. Warnell P. The pain experience of a multiple sclerosis population: a descriptive study. Axone 1991; 13:26–28.
8. Brett DC, Ferguson GG, Ebers GC, Paty DW. Percutaneous trigeminal rhizotomy. Treatment of trigeminal neuralgia secondary to multiple sclerosis. Arch Neurol 1982;39(4):219–221.
9. Anthony TR, Barry Arnason. Trigeminal neuralgia in multple sclerosis relieved by prostaglandin E analogue. Neurology 1995;45:1097–1100.
10. Solaro C, Messmer Uccelli M, Uccelli A, Leandri M, Mancardi GL. Low-dose gabapentin combined with either lamotrigine or carbamazepine can be useful therapies for trigeminal neuralgia in multiple sclerosis. Eur Neurol 2000;44(1):45–48.
11. Rolak LA, Brown S. Headaches and multiple sclerosis: a clinical study and review of the literature. J Neurol 1990;237(5):300–302.
12. Goetz CG, Tanner CM, Levy M, Wilson RS, Garron DC. Pain in Parkinson's disease. Mov Disord 1986;1(1):45–49
13. Ford B. Pain in Parkinson's disease. Clin neurosci 1998;5:63–72
14. Factor SA, Molho ES. Emergency department presentations of patients with Parkinson's disease. Am J Emerg Med 2000;18(2):209–215.
15. Schott GD. Pain in Parkinson's disease. Pain 1985;22(4):407–411.
16. Chudler EH, Dong WK. The role of basal ganglia in nociception and pain. Pain 1995;60(1):3–38.
17. Clifford TJ, Warsi MJ, Burnett CA, Lamey PJ. Burning mouth in Parkinson's disease sufferers. Gerodontology 1998;15(2):73–78.
18. Moulin DE, Hagen N, Feasby TE, Amireh R, Hahn A. Pain in Guillain–Barre syndrome. Neurology 1997;48(2):328–331.
19. Nguyen DK, Agenarioti-Belanger S, Vanasse M. Pain in the Guillain–Barre syndrome in children under 6 years old. J Pediatr 1999;134(6):773–776.
20. Tripathi M, Kaushik S. Carbamazepine for pain management in Guillain-Barre syndrome patients in the intensive care unit. Crit Care Med 2000;28(3):655–658.
21. Samaha FJ, Quinlan JG. Myalgia and cramps: dystrophinopathy with wide-ranging laboratory findings. J Child Neurol 1996;11(1):21–24.
22. Bensen ES, Jaffe KM, Tarr PI. Acute gastric dilatation in Duchenne muscular dystrophy: a case report and review of the literature. Arch Phys Med Rehabil 1996;77(5):512–514.
23. Camelo AL, Awad RA, Madrazo A, Aguilar F, Award RA. Esophageal motility disorders in Mexican patients with Duchenne's muscular dystrophy. Acta Gastroenterol Latinoam 1997;27(3):119–122.

24. Lunshof L, Schweizer JJ. Acute gastric dilatation in Duchenne's muscular dystrophy. Ned Tijdschr Geneeskd 2000;144(46):2214–2217.

25. Hsu JD. Extremity fractures in children with neuromuscular disease. Hsu JD. Johns Hopkins Med J 1979;145(3): 89–93.

26. Andersen G, Vestergaard K, Ingeman–Nielsen M, Jensen TS. Incidence of central post-stroke pain. Pain 1995;61:187–193.

27. Bowsher D. The management of central post-stroke pain. Postgrad Med J 1995;71:598–604.

28. MacGowen DJ, Janal MN, Clark WC, et al. Central poststroke pain and Wallenberg's lateral medullary infarction: Frequency, character, and determinantes in 63 patients. Neurology 1997;49(1):120–125.

29. Bogousslavsky J, Regli F, Uske A. Thalamic infarcts: clinical syndromes, etiology, prognosis. Neurology 1988;38:837–848.

30. Siddall PJ, Loeser JD. Pain following spinal cord injury. Spinal Cord 2001;39(2):63–73.

31. Vestergaard K, Nielsen J, Anderson G, Ingeman–Nielsen M, Arendt–Nielsen L, Jensen TS. Sensory abnormalities in consecutive, unselected patients with central post-stroke pain. Pain 1995;61:177–186.

32. Portenoy RK, Payne D, Jacobsen P. Breakthrough pain: characteristics and impact in patients with cancer pain. Pain 1999;81:129–134.

33. Serlin RC, Mendoza TR, Nakamura Y, Edwards KR, Cleeland CS. When is cancer pain mild moderate or severe ? Grading pain severity by its interference with function. Pain 1995;61: 277–284.

34. Farrar JT, Portenoy RK, Berlin JA, Kinman JL, Strom BL. Defining the clinically important difference in pain outcome measure. Pain 2000;88:287–294.

35. Farrar JT, Young JP, LaMoreaux L, Werth JL, Pool RM. Clinical importance of changes in chronic pain intensity measured on an 11-point numericall pain rating scale. Pain 2002;94:149–158.

36. Torebjork HE, Ochoa JL, Schary W. Referred pain from intraneural stimulation of muscle fascicles in the median nerve. Pain 1984;118:145–156.

37. Woolf CJ, Decosterd I. Implications of recent advances in the understanding of pain pathophysiology for the assessment of pain patients. Pain 1999;6(Suppl):S141-S147.

38. Portenoy RK, Foley KM, Inturrisi CE. The nature of opioid responsiveness and its implications for neuropathic pain: new hypotheses derived from studies of opioid infusions. Pain 1990;43:2733–2286.

39. Portenoy RK Neuropathic pain. In: Portenoy RK, Kanner RM, eds. Pain Management: Theory and Practice Philadelphia. F.A. Davis, 1996:83–125.

40. Caraceni A, Portenoy R, Working Group of the IASP Task Force on Cancer Pain. An international survey on cancer pain characteristics and syndromes. Pain 1999;82:263–275.

41. Cherny NI. Cancer pain: principles of assessment and syndromes. In: Berger A, Portenoy RK, Weissman DE, eds. Principles and Practice of Palliative Care and Supportive Oncology, 2nd Ed. Lippincott–Raven, Philadelphia, 2002.

42. Takeda F. Results of field testing in Japan of the WHO draft interim guidelines on relief of cancer pain. Pain Clinic 1986;1:83–89.

43. Ventafridda V, Tamburini M, Caraceni A, De Conno F, Naldi F. A validation study of the WHO method method for cancer pain relief. Cancer 1987;59:850–856.

44. Schug SA, Zech D, Dorr U. Cancer pain management according to WHO analgesic guidelines. J Pain Symptom Manage 1990;5:27–32.

45. Grond S, Zech D, Schug SA, Lynch J, Lehmann KA. Validation of World Health Organization guidelines for cancer pain relief during the last days and hours of life. J Pain Symptom Manage 1991;6:411–412.

46. World Health Organization. Cancer Pain Relief, 2nd Ed., with a Guide to Opioid Availability. World Health Organization, Geneva, 1996.

47. Jacox A, Carr DB, Payne R. Management of Cancer Pain. AHCPR Publication No. 94–0592: Clinical Practice Guideline No. 9. U.S. Department of Health and Human Services, Public Health Service, Rockville, MD, March 1994.

48. Grond S, Radburch L, Meuser T, Loick G, Sabatowski R, Lehmann KA. High-dose tramadol in comparison to low dose morphine for cancer pain relief. J Pain Symptom Manage 1999;174–179.

49. Kaiko RF, Foley KM, Grabinski PY, et al. Central nervous system excitatory effects of meperidine in cancer patients. Ann Neurol 1983;13:180–185.

50. Bruera EB, Peireira J, Watanabe S, et al. Opioid rotation in patients with cancer pain: a retrospective comparison of dose ratios between methadone, hydromorphone, and morphine. Cancer. 1996;78: 852–857.

51. Sjogren P. Clinical implications of morphine metabolites. In: Portenoy RK, Bruera EB, eds. Topics in Palliative Care, Vol. 1. Oxford University Press, New York, 1997:163–177.

52. Plummer JL, Gourlay GK, Cherry DA, et al. Estimation of methadone clearance: application in the management of cancer pain. Pain 1988;33:313–322.

53. Woolf CJ, Thompson SWN. The induction and maintenance of central sensitization is dependent on N-methyl-D-aspartic acid receptor activation; implications for the treatment of post-injury pain hypersensitivity states. Pain 1991;44:293–299.

54. Ahmedzai S, Brooks D. Transdermal fentanyl versus sustained-release oral morphine in cancer pain: preference, efficacy, and quality of life. The TTS-Fentanyl Comparative Trial Group. J Pain Symptom Manage 1997;13:254–261.

55. Portenoy RK, Payne R, Coluzzi P, et al. Oral transmucosal fentanyl citrate (OTFC) for the treatment of breakthrough pain in cancer patients: a controlled dose titration study. Pain 1999;79:303–312.

56. Bennett G, Burchiel K, Buchser E, et al. Evidence-based review of the literature on intrathecal delivery of pain medication. J Pain Symptom Manage 2000;20:S12–S36.

57. Du Pen SL, Du Pen AR. Intraspinal analgesic therapy in palliative care: evolving perspective. In Portenoy RK, Bruera EB, eds. Topics in Palliative Care, Vol. 4. Oxford University Press, New York, 2000:217–235.

58. Hassenbusch SJ, Portenoy RK. Current practices in intraspinal therapy: a survey of clinical trends and decision making. J Pain Symptom Manage 2000;20:S4–S11.

59. Eisenach JC, DuPen S, Dubois M, Miguel R, Allin D. Epidural clonidine analgesia for intractable cancer pain. The Epidural Clonidine Study Group. Pain 1995;61:391–400.

60. Portenoy RK. Opioid tolerance and responsiveness: research findings and clinical observations. In: Gebhart GF, Hammond DL, Jensen TS, eds. Progress in Pain Research and Management, Vol 2: Proceedings of the 7th World Congress on Pain. IASP Press, Seattle, 1994:595–619.

61. Mercadante S, Portenoy RK. Opioid poorly-responsive cancer pain. Part 1: clinical considerations. J Pain Symptom Manage 2001a;21:144–150.

62. Mercadante S, Portenoy RK. Opioid poorly responsive cancer pain. Part 3: clinical strategies to improve opioid responsiveness. J Pain Symptom Manage 2001b;21:338–354.

63. Derby S, Chin J, Portenoy RK. Systemic opioid therapy for chronic cancer pain: practical guidelines for converting drugs and routs of administration. CNS Drugs 1998;9:99–109.

64. Portenoy RK. Management of common opioid side effects during long-term therapy of cancer pain. Ann Acad Med Singapore 1994;23:160–170.

65. Bruera E, Brenneis C, Paterson AH, et al. Use of methylphenidate as an adjuvant to narcotic analgesics in patients with advanced cancer. J Pain Symptom Manage 1989;4:3–6.

66. Hawkey CJ. COX-2 inhibitors. Lancet 1999;353:307–314.

67. Simon LS. Nonsteroidal anti-inflammatory drug toxicity. Curr Opin Rheumatol 1993;5:265–275.

68. Numo R. Prevention of NSAID-induced ulcers by the coadministration of misoprostol: implications in clinical practice. Scand J Rheumatol 1992;92(Suppl):25–29.

69. Hawkey CJ. Progress in prophylaxis against non-steroidal anti-inflammatory drug- associated ulcers and erosions. Omeprazole NSAID Steering Committee. Am J Med 1998;104:S67–S74.

70. Taha AS, Hudson N, Hawkey CJ, et al. Famotidine for the prevention of gastric and duodenal ulcers caused by nonsteroidal antiinflammatory drugs. N Engl J Med 1996;334:1435–1439.

71. Portenoy RK. Adjuvant analgesics in pain management. In: Doyle D, Hanks GW, MacDonald N, eds. Oxford Textbook of Palliative Medicine, 2nd Ed. Oxford University Press, Oxford, 1998: 361–390.

72. Bruera E, Roca E, Cedaro L, et al. Action of oral methylprednisolone in terminal cancer patients: a prospective randomized double-blind study. Cancer Treat Rep 1985;69:751–754.

73. Tannock I, Gospodarowicz M, Meakin W, et al. Treatment of metastatic prostatic cancer with low-dose prednisone: evaluation of pain and quality of life as pragmatic indices of response. J Clin Oncol 1989;7:590–597.

74. Fogelholm R, Murros K. Tizanidine in chronic tension-type headache: a placebo controlled double-blind cross-over study. Headache 1992;32:509–513.

75. Byas–Smith MG, Max MB, Muir J, Kingman A. Transdermal clonidine compared to placebo in painful diabetic neuropathy using a two-stage 'enriched enrollment' design. Pain 1995;60:267–274.

76. Rowbotham M, Harden N, Stacey B, et al: Gabapentin for the treatment of postherpetic neuralgia: a randomized controlled trial. J Amer Med Assoc 1998;280:1837–1842.

77. McQuay HJ, Carroll D, Jadad AR, et al. Anti-convulsant drugs for management of pain: a systematic review. Brit Med J 1995;311:1047–1052.

78. Dejgard A, Petersen P, Kastrup J. Mexiletine for treatment of chronic painful diabetic neuropathy. Lancet 1988;1:9–11.

79. Galer BS, Miller KV, Rowbotham MC. Response to intravenous lidocaine infusion differs based on clinical diagnosis and site of nervous system injury. Neurology 1993;43:1233–1235.

80. Nelson KA, Park KM, Robinovitz E, et al. High-dose oral dextromethorphan versus placebo in painful diabetic neuropathy and postherpetic neuralgia. Neurology 1997;48:1212–1218.

81. Nikolajsen L, Hansen PO, Jensen TS. Oral ketamine therapy in the treatment of postamputation stump pain. Acta Anaesthesiol Scand 1997;41:427–429.

82. Pud D, Eisenberg E, Spitzer A, et al. The NMDA receptor antagonist amantadine reduces surgical neuropathic pain in cancer patients: a double blind, randomized, placebo controlled trial. Pain 1998;75:349–354.

83. Fromm GH, Terrence CF, Chattha AS. Baclofen in the treatment of trigeminal neuralgia: double-blind study and long-term follow-up. Ann Neurol 1984;15:240–244.

84. Fernandez F, Adams F, Holmes VF. Analgesic effect of alprazolam in patients with chronic, organic pain of malignant origin. J Clin Psychopharmacol 1987;7:167–169.

85. Rowbotham MC. Topical analgesic agents. In: Fields HL, Liebeskind JC, eds. Pharmacological Approaches to the Treatment of Chronic Pain: New Concepts and Critical Issues. IASP Press, Seattle, 1994:211–229.

86. Vaile JH, Davis P. Topical NSAIDs for musculoskeletal conditions. A review of the literature. Drugs 1998;56:783–799.

87. Tandan R, Lewis GA, Krusinski PB, Badger GB, Fries TJ. Topical capsaicin in painful diabetic neuropathy-controlled study with long term follow-up. Diabetes Care 1992;15:8–14.

88. Ellison N, Loprinzi CL, Kugler J, et al. Phase III placebo-controlled trial of capsaicin cream in the management of surgical neuropathic pain in cancer patients. J Clin Oncol 1997;15:2974–2980.

89. Krames ES. Intraspinal opioid therapy for chronic nonmalignant pain: current practice and clinical guidelines. J Pain Symptom Manage 1996;6(11):333–352.

90. Gestin Y, Vainio A, Pegurier AM. Long term intrathecal infusion of morphine in the home care of patients with advanced cancer. Acta Anaesthesiol Scand 1997;41:12–17.

91. Deer T, Winkelmuller W, Erdine S, Bedder M, Burchiel K. Intrathecal therapy for cancer and non-malignant pain: patient selection and patient management. Neuromodulation 1999;2(2):55–66.

92. Marchand S, Charest J, Li J, Chenard JR, Lavignolle B, Laurencelle L. Is TENS purely a placebo effect? A controlled study on low back pain. Pain 1993;54: 99–106.

93. Melzack R, Wall PD. Pain mechanisms: a new theory. Science 1965;150:971–979.

94. Woolf CJ, Thompson SWN. Segmental afferent fibre induced analgesia: transcutaneous electrical nerve stimulation and vibration. In: PD Wall, R Melzack,

eds. Textbook of Pain, 3rd Ed. Churchill Livingstone, Edinburgh, 1994:884–896.

95. Turner JA, Chapman CR. Psychological interventions for chronic pain: a critical review. I. Relaxation training and biofeedback. Pain 1982;12:1–21.

96. Turner JA, Chapman CR. Psychological interventions for chronic pain: a critical review. II. Operant conditioning, hypnosis and cognitive behavioral therapy. Pain 1982;12:23–46.

97. Spiegel D, Bloom JR. Group therapy and hypnosis reduce metastatic breast carcinoma pain. Psychosom Med 1983;45:333–339.

98. Syrjala KL, Cummings C, Donaldson GW. Hypnosis or cognitive behavioral training for reduction of pain and nausea during cancer treatment: a controlled clinical trial. Pain 1992;48:137–146.

Chapter 20

Nausea and Vomiting

Sebastiano Mercadante

Nausea is an unpleasant sensation of the need to vomit and is associated with autonomic symptoms, including pallor, cold sweats, tachycardia, and diarrhea. It may occur without retching or vomiting and as a result of various stimuli. Although the neural pathways that mediate nausea are not known, evidence suggests that they are the same pathways that mediate vomiting. Different neurologic diseases may produce a disturbance in central control of gut motility, resulting in gastrointestinal syndromes such as vomiting or intestinal pseudo-obstruction with or without gastric stasis. There are no accepted treatment guidelines. The pharmacologic treatment of nausea and vomiting usually involves established drugs chosen and rotated as necessary on a trial basis. Many classes of medications have been employed as antiemetics.

Patients should be re-evaluated at regular intervals to optimize doses or to rotate drugs. The choice of medications depends upon drug receptor selectivity and interactions, as patients are frequently receiving several medications with potential to interact or antagonize antiemetics. The afferent pathway and the neuroreceptors involved and the group of antiemetics that antagonize these are key factors in choosing the first drug. An important principle is to use combinations of antiemetics with different modes of action. On the other hand, antiemetics may have adverse effects in patients with neurologic diseases, and anticholinergic medications antagonize the prokinetic effects of drugs acting via the cholinergic system in the myenteric plexus.

CASE HISTORY

A 72-year-old patient attending a pain clinic for diabetic neuropathy complained for many years of chronic nausea. He also presented with intermittent periods, days or weeks, of vomiting. As a consequence of reduced appetite and nutritive intake he had lost about 10 kilograms. He was receiving gabapentin 1200 mg daily with some benefit. He also had hypertension, and the Type II diabetes, diagnosed 13 years before, was irregularly treated with oral hypoglicemic drugs, and subsequently with insulin. During the attacks, his glycemia was difficult to manage.

Given the history of diabetes, some investigations were required to confirm the suspected visceral neuropathy with consequent gastroparesis. Prolonged retention of barium, mild gastric dilatation with poor peristalsis, and no pyloric obstruction were the main radiologic findings. Gastric manometrics confirmed gastroparesis, which was attributed to diabetic visceral neuropathy.

Cisapride was effective and devoid of adverse effects in the first instance. Then the patient was treated with erythromycin, with some success, as cisapride was removed from the market.

Discussion

Diabetic patients are labelled as having gastroparesis, implying that gastric motor dysfunction with delayed gastric emptying is the cause of chronic nausea and eventually vomiting. The typical diabetic patient with symptomatic gastroparesis is characterized by a long-standing, insulin-dependent diabetes that has been poorly controlled for many years. Peripheral neuropathy is frequently associated with autonomic neuropathy. Diagnosis is on the basis of radiologic and radionuclide scanning. This test appears to be a more sensitive diagnostic test than a gastrointestinal series. Indigestible radiopaque solid markers are helpful for detection of diabetic gastroparesis. There is evidence that vagal autonomic neuropathy may be responsible for gastric motor disturbances. Radiologic, histologic, and gastric manometric similarities between diabetic patients and those who have had vagotomies have been found. Other conditions may produce gastroparesis, including renal failure, connective tissue diseases, and idiopathic conditions.

Cisapride has been shown to improve gastric emptying in several conditions of gastroparesis, probably due to the increased release of acetylcholine from the myenteric plexus. Erythromycin accelerates gastric emptying, probably interacting with motilin receptors, regardless of its antibiotic properties.

INTRODUCTION

Nausea and vomiting are common experiences for patients with neurologic diseases, although the exact incidence has never been reported in epidemiologic studies. These symptoms are demeaning and reduce the patient's quality of life. Central and peripheral nervous system diseases, dysfunction of the neuromuscular junction, and muscle diseases may produce nausea and vomiting through different mechanisms. Table 20–1 summarizes these disorders and the possible mechanisms involved.

DEFINITION

Three components of vomiting are recognized: nausea, retching, and emesis. Nausea is an unpleasant sensation of the need to vomit and is associated with autonomic symptoms, including pallor, cold sweats, tachycardia, and diarrhea. It may occur without retching or vomiting and as a result of various stimuli. It is not clear whether nausea and vomiting represent different points along the spectrum of outputs from the vomiting center, or whether they are related, but independent, phenomena.

Although the neural pathways that mediate nausea are not known, evidence suggests that they are the same pathways that mediate vomiting.[1] It may be that mild activation leads to nausea, whereas more intense activation leads to retching or vomiting. During nausea, gastric tone is reduced and gastric peristalsis is diminished. In contrast, the tone of the duodenum tends to be increased.[2]

While nausea is an expression of autonomic stimulation, retching and vomiting are mediated by somatic nerves. Retching is a spasmodic movement of the diaphragm and abdominal musculature with the glottis closed, and denotes the labored rhythmic respiratory activity that frequently precedes emesis. During retching, the antrum of the stomach contracts, whereas the fundus and cardia relax. It may or may not be associated with nausea, and may occur without vomiting. The vomiting act involves forceful contraction of the abdominal wall musculature, contraction of pylorus and antrum, a raised gastric cardia, diminished lower esophageal sphincter pressure, and esophageal dilatation. Intestinal contents commonly are present in vomited material, implicating a possible reverse peristalsis. Hypersalivation and cardiac rhythm disturbances are frequently associated phenomena.[3]

PATHOPHYSIOLOGY

The complex activities occurring in vomiting suggest central neurologic control—a vomiting center. The stimulation of the dorsal portion of the lateral reticular formation in the vicinity of the fasciculus solitarius produces vomiting. This vomiting center is anatomically adjacent

Table 20–1. **Nervous System Diseases Associated with Nausea and Vomiting**

Disease Groups	Mechanisms
Central nervous system	
Cerebral and brainstem disorders	
Multiple sclerosis	Gastroparesis
Parkinson's disease	Gastrointestinal dysmotility
Cerebral masses	Compression vomiting centre
Spinal cord disorders	
Amyothrophic lateral sclerosis	Gastric atony, ileus
Poliomyelitis	Gastric atony, ileus
Autonomic dysfunction–diabetes	Esophageal dysfunction, gastric atony, pseudo-obstruction
Peripheral nervous system	
Alcohol-related	Neuropathy Oesophageal peristalsis, gastroparesis
Myenteric plexus dysfunction (diabetes–Chagas disease, Hirschsprung' disease, acalasia, ganglioneuromatosis)	Pseudo-obstruction
Neuromuscular junction	
Myasthenia gravis	Oropharyngeal incoordination
Muscle disease	
Myotonic dystrophy	Dysphagia, gastric atony, pseudo-obstruction
Dermatomyositis polymyositis	Dysphagia, gastric atony, pseudo-obstruction
Oculopharyngeal muscular dystrophy	Dysphagia
Duchenne muscular dystrophy	Dysphagia, pseudo-obstruction
Familiar visceral neuropathy	Dysphagia, pseudo-obstruction

to medullary centers that control respiration and salivation, although there is no evidence that any substance that causes vomiting does so by direct stimulation; rather, the center co-ordinates the activities of the medullary structures in a patterned response.

For several decades, the concept of a chemoreceptor trigger zone (CTZ), sensitive to chemical stimuli rather than to electrical stimulation, in the floor of the fourth ventricle in the brain stem and an adjacent vomiting center, has provided a useful model in understanding the central mechanisms involved in the initiation of nausea and vomiting. However, the reality seems to be more complex. The area postrema, corresponding to the CTZ, lies outside the blood–brain barrier and is bathed in the systemic circulation. Thus, this center can be regarded as an emetic chemoreceptor requiring the mediation of the vomiting center.[3] It contains receptors for dopamine (D2), serotonin (5HT3), acetylcholine (ACHr), and opioids (mu2), the stimulation of which is emetogenic via input to the vomiting center sited in the third ventricle. It has no reflex co-ordinating ability of its own. High plasma concentrations of emetogenic substances, such as calcium ions, urea, morphine, and digoxin may stimulate dopamine receptors in this area and there is input also from the vestibular apparatus and the vagus (Table 20–2). Anorexia, dehydration, weight loss, abnormal metabolites, and toxins produced by associated infections may also contribute. In the deeper layers of the area postrema there is the nucleus tractus solitarius, which contains the greatest concentration of 5HT receptors in the brain stem and is considered the main

Table 20–2. Factors Stimulating the CTZ

Glycosides
Opioids
Ergot derivatives
Chemotherapeutic agents, enterotoxins, salicylate
Metabolic abnormalities: uremia, hypercalcemia, hyponatriemia, diabetic ketoacidosis
Hypoxia
Radiation sickness

central connection of the vagus. Therefore, visceral afferent impulses arising from the gastrointestinal tract may reach the medullary vomiting center by way of the vagus, without traversing the CTZ.[3–5]

Finally, the emetic pattern generator is close to the area postrema, but in the third ventricle, lying fully within the blood–brain barrier. It contains D2-receptors, histaminic (H1) receptors, muscarinic cholinergic receptors, serotonin (5HT2 and 5HT3) receptors (which are emetogenic), and opioid mu2 receptors (which are antiemetic at this location). Primary or metastatic brain tumors can directly activate histamine receptors, particularly if they cause increased intra-cranial pressure. Inflammatory responses in meningitis or degenerative diseases cause vomiting. Psychological or emotional factors may also generate nausea at this level.

A group of motor nuclei, including the nucleus ambiguous, ventral and dorsal respiratory groups, and the dorsal motor nucleus of the vagus, acts as a central emetic pattern generator and co-ordinates emetic processes, receiving and integrating input from various sources.

Vomiting is an integrated somato-visceral process. The efferent pathways are mainly somatic, involving the vagus nerve, the phrenic nerves, and the spinal nerves. Changes in tone and motility of the stomach during vomiting are likely to be mediated by visceral efferent neurons.

Once the vomiting center has been suffi-ciently stimulated the vomiting reflex is initi-ated and the following sequence of events occurs:[6]

1. The person takes a deep breath which is held
2. The glottis closes to avoid aspiration of vomitus

3. The soft palate is elevated to close off the nasal passage
4. The diaphragm and abdominal muscles contract—this serves to increase intra-abdominal pressure by squeezing the stomach between the two sets of muscles
5. The gastrointestinal sphincter relaxes, thus permitting the expulsion of gastric contents

RECEPTORS AND NEUROTRANSMITTERS

There is strong evidence that dopamine receptors in the CTZ play a role in mediating vomiting. Thus, dopamine agonists (such as apomorphine, L-dopa, and bromocriptine) can cause vomiting, whereas dopamine antagonists (such as metoclopramide and domperidone) are effective antiemetics. Several drugs used in chronic neurologic diseases may affect the dopaminergic system. In addition to dopamine, other neurotransmitters, including serotonin (via 5HT3 receptors), norepinephrine, GABA, substance P, and enkephalin may produce vomiting either when applied directly to the CTZ or after intravenous administration. This area is also implicated in delaying the reflex of gastric emptying and producing taste aversion, a further contribution to vomiting. In addition to the direct afferent pathways from the gastro-intestinal tract to the vomiting center, the anatomic structure of the area postrema receives emetic impulses from the pharynx, heart, peritoneum, mesenteric vasculature, and bile ducts.

Drugs, particularly aspirin and opioids, directly stimulate the vestibular apparatus, which in turn provides input to the vomiting center. Motion sickness, Meniere's disease, labyrinthitis, acoustic neuroma, bone meta-stases at the base of skull, brain tumors, or metastases affecting the vestibular apparatus are possible other causes of vestibular stimulation of H1 receptors and muscarinic cholinergic receptors.

Receptors in the gastrointestinal tract play an equally important part in the pathogenesis and treatment of nausea and vomiting, parti-cularly 5HT3, 5HT4, and D2 receptors. Acti-vation of D2 receptors produces gastroparesis. Vagus receptors include 5TH3 receptors, which are emetogenic, and 5HT4 receptors, which improve the propulsion resulting in a

Table 20–3. **Receptor Site Afnities of Principal Antiemetics**

	Dopamine D2-antagonist	Histamine H1-antagonist	Acetylcholine Antagonist	5HT2 Antagonist	5HT3 Antagonist	5HT4 Antagonist
Metoclopramide	+ +				+	+ +
Domperidone	+ +					
Cisapride						+ + +
Ondansetron					+ + +	
Cyclizine		+ +	+ +			
Hyoscine			+ + +			
Haloperidol	+ + +					
Prochlorperazine	+ +	+				
Chrorpromazine	+ +	+ +	+			
Levomepromazine	+ +	+ + +	+ +	+ + +		

+ = weak; + + = mild; + + + = strong

prokinetic effect. This effect is mediated by the cholinergic myenteric plexus, so that it could be inhibited by anticholinergics. Various stimuli, notably bowel distension and inflammation, may produce massive release of 5HT from enterochromaffin cells contained in the bowel wall. Slowed gastric emptying and constipation, frequently observed in patients progressively immobilized and anorectic, may activate the same process leading to stimulation of the vomiting center via vagal and sympathetic afferents. There are also corticobulbar afferents to the vomiting center that mediate vomiting in response to some smells, sights, and tastes, and may play a role in psychogenic vomiting. In Table 20–3, the receptor site affinities of principal antiemetics are listed.

Stress, anxiety, and nausea, from any cause, induce delayed gastric emptying via peripheral dopaminergic receptors on the myenteric plexus interneurones.

SPECIFIC CONDITIONS ASSOCIATED WITH VOMITING IN NEUROLOGIC DISEASES

Disorders Affecting the CNS

Different neurologic diseases may produce a disturbance in central control of gut motility, resulting in gastrointestinal syndromes such as vomiting or intestinal pseudo-obstruction with or without gastric stasis (see Table 20–1).

Acute head trauma is associated with a high incidence of upper gastrointestinal tract pathology. Although these lesions fall within the spectrum of stress gastritis, a direct neurogenic reflex with gastric hypersecretion has been postulated. The incidence of these lesions is not correlated with steroid administration.

Traumatic lesions of the spinal cord above T5 may isolate the spinal sympathetic control from the influence of high centers. This results in delay in gastric emptying and duodenal progression. In the early post-injury period, severe gastric stasis and dilatation and ileus are commonly present. Many patients face a different set of problems in the months to years after permanent spinal cord damage. With chronic loss of function, patients who develop quadriplegia are more likely to have gut complications than paraplegics. The incidence of gastroesophageal reflux is increased and gastric emptying impaired. Chronic constipation may worsen the clinical picture inducing nausea and vomiting.[7]

Intra-cranial lesions are an important cause of nausea and vomiting. Increased intra-cranial pressure compresses and stimulates the emetic center on the floor of the fourth ventricle. Circumscribed vascular lesions, neoplasms, or local inflammatory lesions of the brain may affect the emetic centre or its afferent pathways directly. The emetic center may also be stimulated through ventricular dilatation without increased intra-cranial pressure, as occurs in low-pressure hydrocephalus. Symptoms may develop insidiously, and may be the first neuro-logic sign of brain tumors in children, even when other neurologic signs are absent.[8] Infectious diseases in the CNS also produce vomiting.

In labyrinthitis, Meniere's disease, and motion sickness, activation of the vestibular system leads to neural activation of the vomiting center. Vestibular stimulation with resultant activation of the vomiting center can affect gastric motor function secondarily.[2,4] Ictal vomiting is considered a localizing sign indicating non-dominant lateralization in patients with partial seizures of temporal lobe origin.[9]

Metabolic Disorders

Significant gastrointestinal disturbances may be associated with thyroid and parathyroid disorders. Intestinal pseudo-obstruction may develop both in hyperthyroidism and hypo-thyroidism. The role of gastrointestinal hor-mones in disorders of upper intestinal motility remains unclear.[4]

Drug-induced Nausea and Vomiting

Many drugs used in neurologic diseases or concomitant medication given for other chronic diseases or symptoms are common causes of nausea.

Adrenergic agents, such as beta-agonists, generally delay gastric emptying, whereas beta-blockers enhance gastric emptying. Clonidine, an alpha-2 agonist, may induce nausea and vomiting. Anticholinergic agents, such as some tricyclic antidepressants, inhibit contractile activity and delay gastric emptying.

Dopamine agonists, L-dopa, bromocriptine (and related anti-Parkinsonian drugs), opioids, digitalis, and chemotherapeutic agents like cisplatin remain the major offenders. Opioids have central and peripheral actions. Centrally, they may stimulate the emetic center via D2 receptors richly distributed in the area pros-trema. In addition, they induce delayed gastric emptying and a delay in intestinal transit. The narcotic bowel syndrome is characterized by a picture similar to pseudo-obstruction. NSAIDs may induce nausea and vomiting by damaging the gastric mucosa and activating peripheral ascending impulses. A central effect of alcohol on the CTZ has been recognized, in addition to its well-known propensity to damage the gastric mucosa.[1,3]

Disorders Affecting Parietal Structures of the Gastrointestinal Tract

Some neurologic disease may affect parietal structures of the gastrointestinal tract, resulting in motility dysfunction which induces nausea and vomiting. Intrinsic gut motility disorders may be classified into myogenic and neuro-genic, although this distinction is not always applicable. In dystrophia myotonica and pro-gressive muscular dystrophy, there may be involvement of smooth muscle of the entire gut. In some patients the proximal duodenum becomes markedly dilated and flaccid.

Amyloid deposits in the intrinsic and extrinsic nerve supply of the gut may produce a neurogenic-type dysmotility, whereas in late stages, dense infiltration of the gut wall impairs contractility and leads to a picture resembling myogenic pseudo-obstruction. In collagen vascular diseases, commonly asso-ciated with vascular neurologic diseases, there may be impairment of gut tone and propul-sion. Duodenal atony is more common and usually develops earlier than in other distal sites. Autoimmune neurologic diseases, such as the paraneoplastic anti-Hu syndrome, may produce an autonomic neuropathy affecting the gut. Radiation injury is another important cause of gastrointestinal dysmotility. Early vomiting is probably due to direct mucosal injury, whereas late vomiting and gastro-intestinal stasis may be due to radiation-induced inflammation or strictures.[2,6]

Finally, the neurologic population, com-monly aged, may be prone to food poisoning, including acute infectious non-bacterial or bacterial gastroenteritis. Organisms involved include staphylococcus aureas, clostridium perfrigens, and bacillus cereus.[2]

Disorders Affecting Extrinsic Gastrointestinal Innervation

GASTROPARESIS SYNDROMES

Disorders of gastric smooth muscle and of autonomic denervation of the stomach can lead to nausea and vomiting. About 30% of diabetic patients complain of intermittent chronic nausea and vomiting. This has been commonly attributed to gastric motor dysfunction with delayed gastric emptying. Peripheral neuropathy, manifestations of autonomic neuropathy, with bladder dysfunction, a sweat disorder, orthostatic hypotension, impotence, nephropathy, and retinopathy frequently are found, and gastroparesis is commonly reported in patients with long-standing, insulin-dependent, poorly-controlled diabetes.[2] There is evidence that vagal autonomic neuropathy may be responsible for gastric motor disturbances in diabetic patients with gastroparesis. These clinical pictures have similar radiologic and manometric findings. The motility disorder involves not only the stomach, but also the upper small bowel. Symptoms such as functional dyspepsia, paroxysmal nausea and vomiting, or intestinal pesudo-obstruction are common in diabetic patients. Centrally related reflexes triggered by gastric dysrhythmia or other peripheral abnormal signals may contribute to gastroparesis.[2]

Although neurotoxic chemotherapy is most commonly implicated in the cancer population, neuropathy also may be caused by direct or metastatic tumor infiltration of nerves or by paraneoplastic effects of the cancer. Visceral neuropathies are less commonly reported and are difficult to diagnose. However, they can strongly influence the gastrointestinal function and produce motor dysmotility.

INFECTIOUS AND DEGENERATIVE DISORDERS OF THE AUTONOMIC NERVOUS SYSTEM

Several agents, such as clostridium botulinum, herpes zoster, and Ebstein–Barr virus may produce a clinical picture of gastroparesis, pseudo-obstruction, or both. In the poly-radiculoneuritis of Guillan–Barrè, the severity of autonomic involvement and gastrointestinal dysmotility may be independent of the degree of somatosensory and motor disturbances. Pan-dysautonomia is characterized by abormalities of both cholinergic and noradrenergic autonomic systems. The Shy–Drager syndrome and idiopathic orthostatic hypotension are regarded as autonomic system degeneration, with disorganized

contractile activity of smooth muscles, and, in advanced stages, a muscle atony.

Other conditions associated with neuropathy, such as uremia, sclerodermia, polymyositis, and dermatomyositis, may also produce gastroparesis.

Idiopathic intestinal pseudo-obstruction is a heterogeneous condition defined primarily on clinical grounds. Many patients with intestinal pseudo-obstruction exhibit features of gastroparesis. In these circumstances it is difficult to determine whether delayed gastric emptying is caused by direct involvement of the stomach by the same neuropathic or myopathic disorder causing the intestinal dysmotility or whether it is caused by increased gastric outlet resistance offered by the abnormal intestinal motility.[2,4]

ASSESSMENT AND DIAGNOSIS

Like pain, nausea is a subjective experience and presents all the same problems inherent in measuring pain. Nausea is usually followed by visual analogue scales or numerical scales.[10] Vomiting can be objectively recorded employing the methodology used to study chemotherapy emesis.

Many factors should be considered when choosing antiemetic treatment. History, examination, and review of the actual drug regimen generally help find the cause of gastrointestinal symptoms in a neurologic population. A multitude of medications, including opioids, digoxin, antibiotics, imidazoles, and cytotoxics can cause nausea and vomiting, acting on the CTZ. NSAIDs, iron supplements, antibiotics, and tranexamic acid may damage the gastric mucosa. Opioids, tricyclics, phenothiazines, and anticholinergics promote gastric stasis. Finally, selective serotonin re-uptake inhibitors and cytotoxics may induce 5HT3-receptor stimulation. Uncontrolled pain may be, per se, a cause of nausea and vomiting.

Movement-related nausea with vomiting suggests either vestibular dysfunction or mesenteric traction. Vertigo may be helpful in distinguishing the two conditions. Candida infection may produce pharyngeal irritation, activating the afferent arm of the vomiting circuit via the vagus nerve. It should be suspected in patients taking steroids.

Emesis produced with cough occurs at the end or during coughing paroxysm and is associated with chronic pulmonary disease, esophageal fistula, and brain metastases. Morning vomiting, sometime projectile, and associated with cognitive changes or neurologic deficits, alerts clinicians to brain tumors. Papilledema may be present. Neck stiffness and headache are possible signs to address meningitis.

Nausea increasing with head motion, with tinnitus, decreased hearing, or skull tenderness is suggestive of vestibular involvement due to drug toxicity and local lesions. CT or MRI may complete the investigation.

The nausea produced by hyperglycemia or hypercalcemia is associated with polyuria and polydipsia. Vomiting that occurs in relation to meals is frequently of diagnostic importance. Patients with gastric outlet obstruction or gastric atony often will complain of vomiting several hours after eating. In contrast, patients who vomit as a result of viral gastroenteritis or psychogenic causes usually are symptomatic in the immediate postprandial period. A chemistry profile consisting of electrolytes, blood urea nitrogen, creatinine, glucose, albumin, and calcium are appropriate screening tests. Drug levels for patients taking digoxin or anticonvulsants should be considered. A pattern of infrequent large-volume vomitus which relieves nausea suggests a partial bowel obstruction. Abdominal examination and an abdominal X-ray can screen for sub-obstruction situations. Eventually, computerized tomography and ultrasounds may complete the instrumental examination. Emotional experience may trigger psychogenic vomiting. Patients treated for prolonged periods with steroids for their chronic neurologic disease may develop Addison's disease after abrupt suspension of medication.

TREATMENT

Prolonged or repeated episodes of vomiting can lead to dehydration, and it is important to replace fluids lost through vomiting by either the oral or parenteral route (subcutaneously or intravenously). Treating any identifiable cause of nausea and vomiting is the first step. Reversible causes include hypercalcemia, hyperglycemia, hypocortisolism, hyponatremia, uremia, constipation, and increased intracranial pressure. Bisphosphonates for hypercalcemia and dexamethasone for intracranial tumors are the first-line treatments in these specific conditions. Identifiable offending drugs should be stopped. A calm and reassuring environment may be useful, avoiding exposure to foods precipitating nausea. Control of malodour from decubitus ulcers is mandatory.

Generally accepted management guidelines are not available. The pharmacologic treatment of nausea and vomiting in the palliative care setting usually involves established drugs chosen and rotated as necessary on a trial basis. Many classes of medications have been employed as antiemetics. Patients should be re-evaluated at regular intervals to optimize doses or to rotate drugs. The choice of medications depends upon drug receptor selectivity and interactions, as patients are frequently receiving several medications with potential to interact or antagonize antiemetics. The afferent pathway and the neuroreceptors involved and the group of antiemetics that antagonize these are key factors in choosing the first drug. An important principle is to use combinations of antiemetics with different modes of actions. On the other hand antiemetics may have adverse effects in patients with neurologic diseases, and anticholinergic medications antagonize the prokinetic effects of drugs acting via the cholinergic system in the myenteric plexus.[3,11,12]

METOCLOPRAMIDE

Metoclopramide, with D2 antagonist activity, improves gastric emptying and has antiemetic properties. It enhances the transit of gastrointestinal tract contents as far as the jejunum, speeding gastric emptying and decreasing small intestinal transit time, probably by increasing cholinergic activity through activation of 5HT4 receptors. In high doses metoclopramide also has 5HT3 receptor antagonist activity. Domperidone, a D2 antagonist that crosses the blood–brain barrier poorly, acts primarily on gastric D2 receptors and D2 receptors in the CTZ, which are outside the blood–brain barrier, facilitating gastric motor activity and emptying.[1,3] It also stimulates upper bowel activity through activation of the 5HT4 receptors.

Metoclopramide in high doses, 60 mg daily, was quite effective in a cancer population with chronic nausea: 3% of patients required other antiemetics because of extrapyramidal adverse effects.[13] Metoclopramide use confers an increased risk for the initiation of treatment generally reserved for the management of Parkinson's disease in patients with drug-induced Parkinsonian symptoms.[14]

PHENOTHIAZINES AND BUTYROPHENONES

All these drugs belong to the class of D2 antagonists. Haloperidol has a relatively narrow spectrum and is a very potent D2 antagonist with negligible anticholinergic activity, so that it produces less sedation than phenothiazines but greater extrapyramidal reations.[3,10]

Phenothiazines, including prochlorpromazine, promethazine, and chlorpromatine, possess a broader spectrum. They have dopaminergic, cholinergic, and histamine receptor antagonism. Hypotension, sedation, decreased salivary flow are the main adverse effects. Levomepromazine is a phenothiazine closely related chemically to chlorpromazine. Its proven analgesic properties make it unique among the phenothiazines. Doses of 5–12.5 mg day is efficacious and generally non-sedating. It is a potent antagonist at 5HT2, H1, D2, and alpha-1 receptors.[15]

ANTICHOLINERGICS

Hyoscine is a naturally occurring compound which competitively inhibits the action of acethylcholine and other muscarinic agonists. The primary application of hyoscine is for motor sickness and labyrinthic disturbances, as well as reducing intestinal secretions in patients with inoperable bowel obstruction. Unlike the other anti-muscarinic agents, hyoscine produces CNS depression at therapeutic doses, manifesting as drowsiness, euphoria, amnesia, disorientation, restlessness, and hallucinations.[3]

SETRON FAMILY

The effect of setrons on the serotonin-mediated emetic pathways may lend itself to the management of chronic nausea. Drugs active on several subclasses of serotonin receptors may have notable effects on gastrointestinal motility.[16] Ondansetron and other 5HT3 antagonists like granisetron and tropisetron appear to antagonize the depolarizing action of serotonin at 5HT3 receptors in the CTZ, on the terminals of vagal afferent nerves, and in the nucleus

tractus solitarius. They have been shown to be effective against vomiting caused by irradiation and cisplatin chemotherapy, and also some other chemotherapeutic agents not acting via D2 receptors. Ondansetron, a selective 5HT3 antagonist, has been used in palliative care setting for patients not responding to conventional treatments. In nine of 16 patients with advanced human immunodeficiency virus, treatment with ondansetron was effective and well tolerated.[17] Tropisetron-containing combinations or tropisetron as a single agent are much more effective in the control of emesis in patients with advanced cancer than the conventional antiemetic combination of chlorpromazine plus dexamethasone.[18]

Not being anti-dopaminergic, setrons are useful when the risk of extrapyramidal reactions is high, as in children or the aged, particularly those with neurologic diseases with an extrapyramidal component. They appear to have no effect on motion sickness.[3]

Some 5-HT3 active drugs have prokinetic activity stimulating gastric motility and emptying. However, this feature seems to be associated with 5-HT4 agonist activity and may be a mechanism by which prokinetics such as metoclopramide and cisapride enhance gastrointestinal propulsive contraction.

CISAPRIDE

This drug acts on acetylcholine receptors in the myenteric plexus of the gut, improving gastro-duodenal and pyloro-duodenal co-ordination. It also affects colonic transit. As it is not a dopamine antagonist, and has no CNS penetration, it does not cause the central adverse effects of many other antiemetic drugs and can be extremely useful in most neurologic patients with gastrointestinal disorders resulting in nausea and/or vomiting. Its prokinetic effect is not limited to the upper bowel but extends throughout the gastrointestinal tract. The enhancement of gastric motor activity by prokinetics may reduce afferent activity in the vagus nerve and so diminish the stimulus to nausea and vomiting from visceral sensation (for example, distension).[3,6]

ANTIHISTAMINES

Cyclizine is effective in nausea associated with motion sickness, pharyngeal stimulation, bowel obstruction, and increased intracranial pressure. Drowsiness and anti-muscarinic actions are the main adverse effects.[3,4,10]

STEROIDS

Dexamethasone has synergy or additive antiemetic effects in combination with setrons, metoclopramide, or phenothiazines. Dexamethasone's antiemetic actions are not well characterized, unless for use in the treatment of nausea and vomiting due to increased intracranial pressure. Adverse effects include glucose intolerance, myopathy, osteopenia, and infections.[3,4,11]

DRONABINOL

In doses of 5–10 mg this drug is recommended in the United States as an antiemetic, for anorexia/cachexia in the acquired immunodeficiency syndrome and cancer, and for the spasticity associated with multiple sclerosis. The mechanism of the antiemetic effect of cannabinoids is unknown. It has been hypothesized to cause an indirect inhibition of the vomiting center in the medulla as a result of binding to opioid receptors in the forebrain. It has been used for intractable nausea and vomiting unresponsive to conventional antiemetics.[19]

OCTREOTIDE

Octreotide inhibits vasoactive intenstinal peptide, and strongly reduces gastrointestinal secretions. Intestinal migrating complexes increase and bowel motility becomes well co-ordinated with octreotide. It relieves gastrointestinal symptoms in patients with sclerodermia and reduces nausea and vomiting as well as the abdominal cramps associated with malignant bowel obstruction.[20]

SUMMARY

Nausea and vomiting may occur in patients with neurologic diseases. Their exact frequency has not been explored, but common experience suggests that these phenomena often present as complications of many neurologic diseases or other diseases with neurologic complications. Mechanisms are quite different and an appropriate assessment is necessary to find the

mechanism sustaining the clinical condition and, as a consequence, to offer the most specific treatment, also considering that most drugs used symptomatically have also CNS adverse effects. Drugs should be selected on the basis of the presumed mechanism and doses should be titrated to that effect.

REFERENCES

1. Allan SG. Nausea and vomiting. In: Doyle D, Hanksa GW, MacDonald N, eds. Oxford Textbook of Palliative Medicine. Oxford University Press, Oxford, 1993:282–290.
2. Lee M, Feldman M. Nausea and vomiting. In: Slesinger MH, Fordtran JS, eds. Gastrointestinal Disease. W.B. Saunders Co, Philadelphia, 1993: 509–523.
3. Twycross R, Back I. Nausea and vomiting in advanced cancer. Eur J Palliat Care 1998;5:39–45.
4. Fallon B. Nausea and vomiting unrelated to cancer treatment. In: Berger AM, Portenoy RK, Weissman DE. Principle and Practice of Supportive Oncology 1998:179–190.
5. Davis MP, Walsh D. Treatment of nausea and vomiting in advanced cancer. Support Care cancer 2000;8:444–452.
6. Nailor R, Rudd JA. Emesis and anti-emesis. In: Hanks GW, ed. Cancer Surveys, Vol. 21. Palliative Medicine: Problem Areas in Pain and Symptom Management. Cold Spring Harbour Laboratory Press, New York, 1994:117–135.
7. Parkman HP. New advances in the diagnosis and management of nausea and vomiting. Case Manager 2002;13:83–86.
8. Bos RF, Ramaker C, van Ouwerkerk WJ, Linssen WH, Wolf BH. Vomiting as a first neurological sign of brain tumors in children. Ned Tijdschr Geneeskd 2002;146:1393–1398.
9. Achauble B, Britton JW, Mullan BP, Watson J, Sharbrough FW, Marsch WR. Ictal vomiting in association with left temporal lobe seizure in a left hemisphere language-dominant patient. Epilepsia 2002;43:1432–1435.
10. Melzack R. Measurement of nausea. J Pain Symptom Manage 1989;4:157–160.
11. Peroutka SJ, Snyder SH. Antiemetics-neurostransmitter receptor binding predicts therapeutic actions 1982;I:658–659.
12. Lichter I. Which antiemetic? J Palliat Care 1993;9: 42–50.
13. Bruera E, Seifert L, Watanabe S, et al. Chronic nausea in advanced cancer patients: a retrospective assessment of a metoclopramide-based antiemetic regimen. J Pain Symptom Manage 1996;11:147–153.
14. Avorn J, Gurwitz JH, Bohn RL, Mogun H, Monane M, Walker A. Increased incidence of levodopa therapy following metoclopramide use. JAMA 1995;274:1780–1782.
15. Twycross RG, Barkby GD, Hallwood PM. The use of low dose levomepromazine in the management of nausea and vomiting. Progr Palliat Care 1997;5:49–53.

16. Hindle AT. Recent developments in the physiology and pharmacology of 5-hydroxytriptamine. Br J Anaesth 1994;73:395–407.

17. Currow DC, Coughlan M, Fardell B, Cooney NJ. Use of ondansetron in palliative medicine. J Pain Symptom Manage 1997;13:302–307.

18. Mystakidou K, Befon S, Liossi C, Vlachos L. Comparison of tropisetron and chlorpromazine combinations in the control of nausea and vomiting in patients with advanced cancer. 1998;15:176–184.

19. Gonzales–Rosales F, Walsh D. Intractable nausea and vomiting due to gastrointestinal mucosal metastases relieved by tetrahydrocannabinol. J Pain Symptom Manage 1997;14:311–314.

20. Mercadante S. The role of octreotide in palliative care. J Pain Symptom Manage 1994;9:406–411.

Chapter 21

Fatigue

Lynne I. Wagner
David Cella
Nicholas A. Doninger

INTRODUCTION
PATHOPHYSIOLOGY OF FATIGUE
ASSESSMENT OF FATIGUE
CLINICAL MANAGEMENT OF FATIGUE

Alleviating Primary Factors
Pharmacological Approaches
Non-Pharmacological Strategies
SUMMARY

Fatigue is one of the most commonly reported symptoms among medically ill populations and adversely impacts quality of life. In clinical settings, fatigue is often not assessed and, consequently, inadequately treated. Causative factors are likely to be multifactorial in nature, and the underlying pathophysiology of fatigue is poorly understood. Principles for the clinical management of fatigue are similar across medically ill populations for whom fatigue is a prominent feature (e.g. multiple sclerosis, cancer, HIV/AIDS). Comprehensive assessment of fatigue should include an evaluation of fatigue characteristics to understand its functional impact and provide insight into potential etiologies. Treatment of fatigue should address causative factors that are commonly observed in medically ill populations and are easily detected and treated (e.g. anemia). Pharmacological and non-pharmacological interventions have been utilized for the management of fatigue; however, few randomized clinical trials have been conducted.

CASE HISTORY

Mr. L. was a 66-year-old white, married man with metastatic breast cancer, referred to a clinical health psychologist in April 2001 for clinical man-

agement of fatigue. He was self-employed as a product importer/exporter on a full-time basis. He described himself as premorbidly energetic and ambitious and reported that prior to his diagnosis he frequently worked 70 to 80 hours per week and his work required extensive travel. He and his wife of 43 years had three children ages 34–41 years, one of whom was a 34-year-old daughter with breast cancer. Mr. L. was first diagnosed with breast cancer in September 1998. He did not report any other medical conditions.

In January 2001, he presented to the emergency room with multiple symptoms, including profound fatigue, and was determined to have lung, bone, liver, and brain metastases. He began ongoing taxane-based chemotherapy in January 2001. He underwent stereotactic radiosurgery in February and May 2001 for right occipital metastasis. His hemoglobin was monitored on a weekly basis and ranged from 11.5–13.2 g/dL. He was maintained on erythropoetin alfa. Albumin was assessed monthly and ranged from borderline low to normal (3.2–3.8 g/dL). He complained of continuing fatigue in March 2001 and was prescribed prednisone and given an exercise plan, which included daily walks.

Mr. L. was initially referred to a clinical health psychologist for fatigue management in April 2001 by his primary oncologist. His presenting complaints included fatigue and diminished capacity to work. He expressed regret at having spent extensive periods of time away from his family due to work

221

over the last several years. He articulated experiencing a conflict between the desire to continue to be productive professionally and to focus on his relationships with family members. His wife attended his initial session. In August 2001, he returned for a second visit with the primary complaint that he was 'tired of being tired'. He reported anger and frustration with his fatigue, early morning awakening, irritability, and excessive daytime sleepiness. He was prescribed 10 mg methylphenidate b.i.d. in August 2001 and reported that it was not helpful. At a return visit in September 2001, he reported 2–3 hours of sleep per night, continued fatigue, depressed mood, a reduced capacity for physical activity, and a reduced capacity for work (35 hours per week). He reported that his only fear related to dying was leaving his wife. He discontinued methylphenidate and began modafinil, which he described as 'modestly helpful' for his daytime sleepiness. He refused an antidepressant.

Mr. L. attended his fourth visit with the health psychologist in October 2001 and complained of increasing fatigue. He stated that he was no longer concerned with treatment for his cancer and wanted to increase his energy level. He described his mood as variable and it fluctuated with his physical functioning. In November 2001, Mr. L. was referred to a nephrologist for acute renal insufficiency, which exacerbated his weakness and fatigue. He began dialysis in December 2001. He was admitted to a hospice in January 2002 and expired three days post-admission.

Discussion

This case illustrates the multifactorial nature of fatigue, particularly in advanced disease. Mr. L. had several potential causative factors for his fatigue, including disease burden, chemotherapy, multiple brain metastases, nephrotic syndrome, and depression. It is unlikely that anemia was a contributing factor, as his hemoglobin was adequately managed. This case illustrates the importance of interdisciplinary clinical management of illness-related fatigue. Mr. L. obtained some clinical benefit from modafinil, an exercise program, and psychotherapy, while methylphenidate did not improve his fatigue. Psychotherapeutic intervention addressed fatigue management, adjustment to cancer diagnosis and diminishing functional capacity, family relationships, goal setting, and end-of-life planning.

INTRODUCTION

Due to recent medical advances, the life expectancy of people with chronic medical illness has been increasing. Fatigue is a symptom commonly associated with medical illness and has a high prevalence in palliative care settings. Fatigue is multidimensional in clinical expression, manifested in physical, emotional, and cognitive impairments. Fatigue is one of the most prevalent symptoms reported by patients with cancer,[1] AIDS,[2] and multiple sclerosis.[3] The presence of fatigue has been associated with functional limitations and impaired quality of life among chronically ill populations, including AIDS patients[2] and cancer patients,[4] and has been found to interfere with adherence to cancer treatment.[5] The development and implementation of effective strategies for the clinical management of fatigue would reduce the overall symptom burden of many chronic illnesses.

Fatigue is often underrecognized and consequently undertreated in clinical settings despite evidence demonstrating the effectiveness of single-item or brief screening measure techniques for identifying patients who may benefit from clinical attention.[6] Survey data indicate that 80% of oncology providers believe that fatigue is not adequately assessed or treated. Among cancer patients with fatigue, 50% did not discuss treatment options with their oncologist and only 27% had received any treatment recommendations. Seventy-four percent of cancer patients endorsed the belief that fatigue was a symptom they had to endure as a normal consequence of cancer and its treatment.[7]

Research conducted on the pathophysiological mechanisms of fatigue is introduced before reviewing available evidence on the efficacy of various treatment strategies for the management of disease-related fatigue.

PATHOPHYSIOLOGY OF FATIGUE

The pathophysiology of fatigue is poorly understood and causes of fatigue vary based on the presence and severity of medical conditions. Few basic research studies have been conducted to investigate the physiological mechanisms underlying fatigue[8] and most studies conducted to date have been descriptive or correlational in nature. Identifying the etiological factors that contribute to fatigue often proves to be complicated, as multiple causes typically co-exist (see Table 21–1).

Among cancer patients, fatigue can be one of the first indicators of the presence or recurrence of cancer, and it tends to increase with the progression of cancer and cancer treatment.[9] Moderate to severe levels of fatigue are commonly reported by patients receiving interferon therapy.[10] Morrow et al. present four hypotheses for the development of cancer-related fatigue,[11] which include:

Anemia
Abnormalities in adenosine triphosphate

Table 21–1. **Causes of Fatigue**[1]

PHYSIOLOGICAL FACTORS

Direct effects of illness:
Cancer
HIV/AIDS
Multiple sclerosis
Chronic Obstructive Pulmonary
  Disease (COPD)
Congestive heart failure
Treatment effects:
Medication side effects
Chemotherapy
Radiotherapy
Surgery
Comorbid medical conditions:
Anemia
Infection
Pulmonary disorders
Thyroid dysfunction
Malnutrition
Exacerbating factors:
Chronic pain
Sleep disturbances
Deconditioning

PSYCHOSOCIAL FACTORS

Coping with chronic illness
Anxiety
Depression

[1] Adapted from Atkinson et al. (2000),[31] Cella et al. (1998),[4] Portenoy and Itri (1999)[24]

Vagal afferent activation
Interaction of cytokines and serotonin

Cytokine deregulation, specifically erythropoietin, interleukin, tumor necrosis factor, and interferon, has been implicated in cancer-related fatigue and has also been associated with factors that exacerbate fatigue, including anemia, cachexia, fever, infection, and depression.[12] Gustein identifies several disease processes associated with fatigue, including anemia, cachexia, infection, paraneoplastic syndromes, and metabolic disorders.[8] Additional factors that exacerbate fatigue, such as chronic stress, mood alterations, and pain are also discussed. Because the mechanisms of fatigue are poorly understood, it is difficult to determine the extent to which these factors are causative in the development of fatigue. Fatigue has been found to be independent of disease severity indicators among patients with multiple sclerosis[13,14] and Parkinson's disease.[15] Recent evidence suggesting that fatigue among patients with multiple sclerosis is associated with CNS dysfunction[16,17] may further our understanding of its pathophysiology.

ASSESSMENT OF FATIGUE

Given the diverse etiological factors that contribute to fatigue and its multidimensional nature, the comprehensive assessment of patients with fatigue is required for the development of effective treatment interventions. Interdisciplinary evaluation and treatment is recommended to adequately comprehend the complex interaction of the associated medical, psychological, and social factors that impact fatigue characteristics.[18] Comprehensive evaluation should include an assessment of disease status and treatment, as well as an in-depth fatigue assessment. Primary factors associated with fatigue, such as anemia, thyroid dysfunction, pain, and sleep disturbance, should be treated accordingly.

An in-depth assessment of fatigue should evaluate fatigue onset, pattern, duration, change over time, associated or alleviating factors, physical, emotional, and mental symptomatology, and functional interference.[18] Because fatigue is a subjective sensation, there is no gold standard for its

Table 21–2. **Examples of Standardized Measures for Assessing Fatigue**

Brief Fatigue Inventory	Mendoza et al. (1999)[40]
Fatigue Severity Scale	Krupp, LaRocca, Muir–Nash, Steinberg (1989)[41]
Functional Assessment of Chronic Illness Therapy—Fatigue	Cella (1997),[1] Yellen et al. (1997)[42]
Multidimensional Fatigue Inventory	Smets, Garssen, Bonke, deHaes (1995)[43]
Multidimensional Fatigue Symptom Inventory	Stein, Martin, Hann, Jacobsen (1998)[44]
Piper Fatigue Scale	Piper et al. (1998)[45]

measurement.[19] The use of standardized assessment instruments can facilitate the in-depth assessment of fatigue on a routine basis. Several self-report measures for assessing fatigue have been developed for medical populations and are used for clinical research (see Table 21–2). Performance-based measures of motor or cognitive functioning have been used in conjunction with self-report measures to evaluate fatigue among patients with multiple sclerosis.[20]

CLINICAL MANAGEMENT OF FATIGUE

First, causative factors for fatigue which are easily detected and treated (e.g. anemia, hypothyroidism) should be ruled out and, if present, treated accordingly. Patients with continued fatigue after resolution of primary factors and patients without identified causative factors may benefit from pharmacological and non-pharmacological interventions.

Alleviating Primary Factors

Primary factors known to exacerbate illness-related fatigue, including anemia and thyroid dysfunction should receive clinical attention prior to implementing interventions aimed at fatigue management, as summarized in Table 21–3. Anemic cancer patients have reported significantly worse fatigue scores than non-anemic cancer patients.[21] For some patients, treatment of these factors may lead to significant reductions in fatigue. Cancer patients with anemia have demonstrated increased energy and improved quality of life following a course of treatment with erythropoietin.[22,23] Patients completing treatment for etiological

factors who continue to experience fatigue and patients without identified causative factors for their fatigue may benefit from pharmacological and non-pharmacological fatigue management.

Pharmacological Approaches

Treatment strategies for illness-related fatigue include pharmacological and non-pharmacological interventions, which are summarized in Table 21–3. Currently, limited research exists to support pharmacological treatments for the management of illness-related fatigue.[24] Controlled, randomized trials have yielded evidence to support the relative efficacy of psychostimulants in treating fatigue associated with opioid administration among cancer patients,[25] depression in the elderly,[26] and multiple sclerosis.[27] The efficacy of modafinil in treating fatigue was demonstrated in a Phase II trial with patients with multiple sclerosis[28] and in a small pilot study (n = 10) among patients with Parkinson's disease.[29] The efficacy of modafinil in treating cancer-related fatigue is currently under investigation.

Clinical observation and limited data from controlled trials favor the use of low-dose corticosteroids, specifically dexamethasone and prednisone, for symptom management among cancer and AIDS patients.[30] The National Comprehensive Cancer Network (NCCN) Practice Guidelines for cancer-related fatigue recommend consideration of antidepressants for fatigue management when major depression is present.[31] Preliminary data from a randomized, placebo-controlled clinical trial of paroxetine with patients experiencing fatigue secondary to chemotherapy indicate an effect for depressive symptoms, which did not generalize to

Table 21–3. **Treatment Strategies for Managing Fatigue**[1]

CAUSE-SPECIFIC TREATMENTS
Anemia—erythropoetic therapy; blood transfusion
Depression—antidepressant medication; psychotherapy
Thyroid dysfunction—thyroid replacement therapy
Malnutrition—nutritional assessment and appropriate therapy
Dehydration—rehydration
Infection—antibiotic/antiviral therapy

NON-SPECIFIC PHARMACOLOGIC INTERVENTIONS
Psychostimulants:
Methylphenidate
Pemoline
Dextroamphetamine
Low-dose corticosteroid:
Dexamethasone
Prednisone
Selective serotonin-reuptake inhibitors

NON-PHARMACOLOGIC INTERVENTIONS
Education
Exercise
Modify patterns of activity and rest
Stress management
Cognitive-behavioral therapy
Nutritional intervention

[1] Adapted from Atkinson et al. (2000),[31] Cella et al. (1998),[46] Portenoy and Itri (1999)[24]

fatigue.[32] With the possible role of cytokines in the etiology of cancer-related fatigue, drugs that block the elaboration, release, or actions of critical cytokines may hold promise as new treatment approaches.[33]

Non-Pharmacological Strategies

Non-pharmacological interventions include patient education, exercise, modification of activity and rest patterns, stress management, and cognitive therapies. Educating cancer patients and their families regarding the anticipated course of illness and treatment

side effects has been advocated, particularly among nursing interventions.[24] Educational groups adopting a rehabilitation approach to managing cancer-related fatigue have also had success in reducing fatigue distress and increasing quality of life.[34] Non-pharmacological approaches to fatigue management have also been demonstrated to be efficacious among patients with multiple sclerosis.[20]

Graded activity and exercise programs have been demonstrated to improve fatigue among patients with chronic fatigue syndrome,[35] patients receiving high-dose chemotherapy and stem-cell support,[36] and breast cancer patients during the first three cycles of chemotherapy.[9] Patients completing home-based aerobic exercise programs demonstrated reduced intensity of fatigue in comparison to patients who did not exercise.

Psychological interventions, including stress management training and cognitive-behavioral therapy, may offer clinical benefit to patients with fatigue secondary to chronic illness. The effectiveness of psychological interventions for symptom management has been demonstrated with cancer patients[37] and individuals with chronic fatigue syndrome.[35] These studies collectively provide some preliminary evidence on the relative efficacy of various types of interventions. A number of unresolved methodological issues remain in studies addressing the prevalence and treatment of disease-related fatigue.

SUMMARY

In conclusion, fatigue is a symptom commonly associated with medical illness and its underlying mechanisms are poorly understood. Fatigue is multifactorial in its etiology and manifestation. Pharmacological treatments currently in use are based on limited research studies and few randomized, controlled trials with fatigue as a primary endpoint have been conducted. Empirical support for exercise in managing fatigue has been reported, whereas other, non-pharmacological interventions have not been adequately evaluated.

Many challenges to conducting clinical research in the context of palliative care exist, which threaten the reliability, validity, and generalizability of research findings.[38] Obtaining self-report data from individuals with advanced illness in the context of a palliative care setting presents challenges, and the representativeness of participants available for study is compromised by attrition, participation bias, and the heterogeneity of study samples.[39] The use of additional sources of data to corroborate patient report and the use of longitudinal research models, including statistical models for managing missing data and time series analysis, may address some of these challenges.

Future research should lead to more accurate estimations of the prevalence and impact of fatigue, reduce the burden of fatigue, and strive for increased diversity. Randomized, placebo-controlled clinical trials are the gold standard in evaluating treatment interventions. Well-designed clinical trials are urgently needed for the development of empirically supported fatigue management strategies and the reduction of symptom burden among chronically ill populations.

REFERENCES

1. Cella D. The Functional Assessment of Cancer Therapy–Anemia (FACT-An) Scale: a new tool for the assessment of outcomes in cancer anemia and fatigue. Seminars in Hematology 1997;S34:13–19.
2. Vogl D, Rosenfeld B, Breitbart W, et al. Symptom prevalence, characteristics, and distress in AIDS outpatients. Journal of Pain and Symptom Management 1999;18:253–262.
3. Bakshi R, Miletich RS, Henschel K, et al. Fatigue in multiple sclerosis: cross-sectional correlation with brain MRI findings in 71 patients. Neurology 2000;53:1151–1153.
4. Cella D. Quality of life in cancer patients experiencing fatigue and anemia. Anemia in Oncology 1998;March:2–4.
5. Yarbro CH. Interventions for fatigue. European Journal of Cancer Care 1996;5:35–8.
6. Kirsch KL, Passik S, Holtsclaw E, Donaghy K, Theobald D. I get tired for no reason: a single item screening for cancer-related fatigue. Journal of Pain and Symptom Management 2001;22:931–937.
7. Vogelzang NJ, Breitbart W, Cella D, et al. Patient, caregiver, and oncologist perceptions of cancer-related fatigue: results of a tripart assessment survey. The Fatigue Coalition. Seminars in Hematology 1997;S34S:4–12.
8. Gutstein HB. The biologic basis of fatigue. Cancer 2001;92:1678–1683.
9. Schwartz AL, Nail LM, Chen S, et al. Fatigue patterns observed in patients receiving chemotherapy and radiotherapy. Cancer Investigation 2000;18:11–19.
10. Malik UR, Makower DF, Wadler S. Interferon-mediated fatigue. Cancer 2001;92: 1664–1668.
11. Morrow GR, Andrews PL, Hickok JT, et al. Fatigue associated with cancer and its treatment. Supportive Cancer Care 2002;10(5):389–398.
12. Kurzrock R. The role of cytokines in cancer-related fatigue. Cancer 2001;92:1684–1688.
13. Giovannoni G, Thompson AJ, Miller DH, Thompson EJ. Fatigue is not associated with raised inflammatory markers in multiple sclerosis. Neurology 2001;57:676–681.
14. Bakshi R, Shaikh ZA, Miletich RS, et al. Fatigue in multiple sclerosis and its relationship to depression and neurologic disability. Multiple Sclerosis 2000;6:181–185.
15. Friedman JH, Friedman H. Fatigue in Parkinson's disease: a nine-year follow-up. Movement Disorders 2001;16:1120–1122.
16. Leocani L, Colombo B, Magnani G, et al. Fatigue in multiple sclerosis is associated with abnormal cortical activation to voluntary movement–EEG evidence. Neuroimage 2001;13: 1186–1192.
17. Colombo B, Martinelli–Boneschi F, Rossi P, et al. MRI and motor evoked potential findings in non-disabled multiple sclerosis patients with and without symptoms of fatigue. Journal of Neurology 2000;247:506–509.
18. Wagner L, Cella D. Cancer-related fatigue: clinical screening, assessment, and management. In: Marty M, Pecorelli S, eds. ESO Scientific Updates: Fatigue, Asthenia, Exhaustion and Cancer, 5th Ed. Elsevier Science, Oxford, 2001:201–214.
19. Neuenschwander H, Bruera E. Asthenia. In: Doyle D, Hanks GWC, MacDonald N, eds. Oxford Textbook of Palliative Medicine, 2nd Ed. Oxford University Press, New York, 1998.
20. Krupp LB, Christodoulou C. Fatigue in multiple sclerosis. Current Neurology & Neuroscience Reports 2001;1:294–298.
21. Cella D, Zagari MJ, Vandoros C, Gagnon DD, Hurtz H–J, Nortier JW. Epoetin alfa treatment results in clinically significant improvements in quality of life (QOL) in anemic cancer patients when referenced to the general population. Journal of Clinical Oncology 2003;21(2):366–373.
22. Littlewood TJ, Bajetta E, Nortier JW, Vercammen E, Rapoport B, the Epoetin Alfa Study Group. Effects of epoetin alfa on hematologic parameters and quality of life in cancer patients receiving nonplatinum chemotherapy: results of a randomized, double-blind, placebo-controlled trial. Journal of Clinical Oncology 2001;19:2865–2874.
23. Demetri GD, Kris M, Wade J, et al. Quality of life benefit in chemotherapy patients treated with epoetin alfa is independent of disease response or tumor type: results from a prospective community oncology study. Journal of Clinical Oncology 1998;16:3412–3425.
24. Portenoy RK, Itri LM. Cancer-related fatigue: guidelines for evaluation and management. The Oncologist 1999;4:1–10.
25. Wilwerding MB, Loprinzi CL, Mailliard JA, et al. A randomized, crossover evaluation of methylphenidate in cancer patients receiving strong narcotics. Supportive Care in Cancer 1995;3:135–138.

26. Massand PS, Tesear GE. Use of stimulants in the medically ill. Psychiatric Clinics of North America 1996;19:515–547.

27. Weinshenker BG, Penman M, Bass B, et al. A double-blind, randomized, crossover trial of pemoline in fatigue associated with multiple sclerosis. Neurology 1992;42:1468–1471.

28. Rammohan KW, Rosenberg JH, Lynn DJ, Blumenfeld AM, Pollak CP, Nagaraja HN. Efficacy and safety of modafinil (Provigil) for the treatment of fatigue in multiple sclerosis: a two center phase 2 study. Journal of Neurology, Neurosurgery & Psychiatry 2002;72:179–183.

29. Nieves AV, Lang AE. Treatment of excessive daytime sleepiness in patients with Parkinson's disease with modafinil. Clinical Neuropharmacology 2002;25:111–114.

30. Wagner GJ, Rabkin JG, Rabkin R. Dextroamphetamine as a treatment for depression and low energy in AIDS patients receiving a continuous infusion of narcotics for cancer pain. Pain 1997;48:163–166.

31. Atkinson A, Barsevick A, Cella D, et al. NCCN practice guidelines for cancer-related fatigue. Oncology 2000;14:151–161.

32. Morrow GR, Hickok JT, Raubertas RF, et al. Effect of an SSRI antidepressant on fatigue and depression in seven hundred thirty-eight cancer patients treated with chemotherapy: A URCC CCOP study. Proceedings of the American Society of Clinical Oncology. 2001;1531.

33. Burks TF. New agents for the treatment of cancer-related fatigue. Cancer 2001;92: 1714–1718.

34. Holley S, Borger D. Energy for living with cancer: preliminary findings of a cancer rehabilitation group intervention study. Oncology Nursing Forum 2001;28:1393–1396.

35. Jason LA, Taylor RR. Chronic fatigue syndrome. In: Nezu AM, Nezu CM, Geller PA, eds. Handbook of Psychology. Vol. 9: Health Psychology. John Wiley and Sons: Hoboken, NJ, 2003:365–392.

36. Dimeo FC, Stieglitz RD, et al. Effects of physical activity on the fatigue and psychologic status of cancer patients during chemotherapy. Cancer 1999;85:2273–2277.

37. Knight SJ. Oncology and hematology. In: Camic P, Knight S, eds. Clinical Handbook of Health Psychology. Hofgrefe & Huber Publishers, Seattle, 1998.

38. Wilkinson EK. Problems of conducting research in palliative care. In: Bosanquet N, Salisbury C, eds. Providing a Palliative Care Service: Towards an Evidence Base. Oxford University Press, New York, 1999.

39. Wagner LI, Cella D, Peterman AH. Methodological considerations in the treatment of fatigue. In: RK Portenoy, E Bruera, eds. Issues in Palliative Care Research. Oxford University Press: New York, 2003:173–185.

40. Mendoza TR, Wang XS, Cleeland CS, et al. The rapid assessment of fatigue severity in cancer patients: use of the Brief Fatigue Inventory. Cancer 1999;85:1186–1196.

41. Krupp LB, LaRocca NG, Muir–Nash J, Steinberg AD. The Fatigue Severity Scale: application to patients with multiple sclerosis and systemic lupus erythematosis. Archives of Neurology 1989;46:1121–1123.

42. Yellen S, Cella D, Webster K, Blendowski C, Kaplan E. Measuring fatigue and other anemia-related symptoms with the Functional Assessment of Cancer Therapy (FACT) measurement system. Journal of Pain and Symptom Management 1997;13:63–74.

43. Smets EMA, Garssen B, Bonke B, deHaes HC. The Multidimensional Fatigue Inventory (MFI): psychometric qualities of an instrument to assess fatigue. Journal of Psychosomatic Research 1995;39:315–325.

44. Stein KD, Martin SC, Hann DM, Jacobsen PB. A multidimensional measure of fatigue for use with cancer patients. Cancer Practice 1998;6:143–152.

45. Piper BF, Dibble SL, et al. The revised Piper Fatigue Scale: psychometric evaluation in women with breast cancer. Oncology Nursing Forum 1998;25(4):677–684.

46. Cella D, Peterman A, Passik S, Jacobsen P, Breitbart W. Progress toward guidelines for the management of fatigue. Oncology 1998;12:369–377.

Chapter 22

Acute Confusional State

Augusto Caraceni
Marco Bosisio

INTRODUCTION
DIAGNOSIS AND CLINICAL FEATURES
Diagnosis
Differential Diagnosis
Subjective Components
Monitoring and Assessment Tools
Causes; Predisposing and Precipitating
    Factors

A Multifactorial Model
Reversibility and Prognosis
TREATMENT
Environmental Intervention
Communication with Patient and Family
Pharmacological Therapy
SUMMARY

Confusion is one of the most prevalent symptoms in palliative care. Different etiologies such as primary CNS disorders, systemic diseases, and exogenous intoxication or drug withdrawal may converge in a final common pathway probably involving the cholinergic system of the brain stem. Clinically, the differential diagnosis includes dementia and psychosis. The fluctuating nature of delirium may pose a source of controversy for the team. As delirium may present in different shades of altered cognition, attention deficits, changes in affection, and productive symptoms, the routine use of screening instruments in palliative care is recommended. As up to 50% of cases are reported to be at least partially reversible, a concise management is indicated. This includes correcting underlying causes if possible, environmental interventions, close communication with patient and relatives (for whom the situation is especially stressful), and pharmacological therapy. The use of haloperidol as monotherapy will only be sufficient in about 20% of patients; benzodiazepines may be added for their anxiolytic and sedative effects.

The case history reported in this chapter can serve as an example of some emerging problems in the diagnosis of the multifactorial conditions that can lead to delirium in advanced medical illness, and in the difficulties of managing this complex clinical syndrome for relatively prolonged periods of time at the end of life.

CASE HISTORY

The patient, a 69-year-old university professor of chemistry, was active in teaching until recently, when his clinical condition deteriorated. A locally advanced adenocarcinoma of the pancreas was diagnosed, after a few months of unexplained lumbar pain, and treated with radiation therapy in October 1993, followed by IV 5-fluorouracil (5-FU) therapy (April–December 1994). A CT scan then showed local progression of the tumor. 5-FU was discontinued and two courses of gemcitabine were given but stopped due to febrile neutropenia and worsening pain. Until February 1995 scans showed only local progression of pancreatic and retroperitoneal disease, but in May 1995 ultrasound demonstrated liver metastases and peritoneal nodes.

His pain initially responded well to radiotherapy and chemotherapy but, in February 1995, recurred as a mild, non-continuous discomfort in the upper lumbar and lower dorsal spine. Pain worsened in the following months affecting the epigastric region with radiation to the back at about Th12-L1 level, consistent with a retroperitoneal pain syndrome due to pancreatic cancer.

Pain was managed initially with tramadol, and later with morphine slow-release tablets, up to 30 mg t.i.d. by May 1995, when the patient was admitted to the hospital. Relatives reported significant weight loss and anorexia but intact cognitive functions until recently. He had still been giving classes at the university.

After admission, the patient started to be delirious. He was completely disorientated in space and time, and tended to fall asleep while being interviewed. His reasoning was disorganized when awake. The Memorial Delirium Assessment Score (MDAS) was 22/30. Pain was impossible to assess but the patient did not appear to be suffering. Morphine was reduced progressively to 10 mg b.i.d. without improvement of the mental state. His neurological examination showed no focal signs but bilateral palmo-mental reflexes and grasping reflexes. Promazine 50 mg IM injection was given with little effect. After neurological opinion, haloperidol was started, 3 mg/day orally, morphine 10 mg sc p.r.n. for pain, promethazine 50 mg at night for insomnia and night-time agitation.

Over the next four days morphine was increased again, to 30 mg b.i.d. The patient was now awake, orientation to time and space was imperfect, attention and short-term memory impaired, but reasoning was more rational. The patient could sleep at night and his behavior was not agitated (MDAS = 12/30). This situation continued over six more days. The patient requested a few rescue doses of morphine for pain.

On the tenth day from the initial episode the patient again was agitated, confabulating, wandering in the hospital (MDAS = 27/30). An IV injection of 2 mg haloperidol was given followed by continuous subcutaneous 24-hour infusion of morphine 50 mg and haloperidol 4 mg. The patient was calm, awake, and collaborative for five days (MDAS = 18/30).

Further episodes of severe agitation recurred with hallucinations (day 16 from initial episode) (MDAS = 30/30), and the drug regimen was changed to morphine 80 mg and haloperidol 6 mg. Promethazine was stopped, and kept only as a rescue medication for agitation if needed. In the following days the level of consciousness worsened; the patient slept but could be woken by verbal stimulation. On day 22 from the onset of delirium

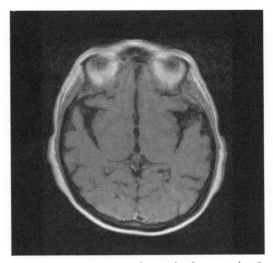

Figure 22-1. Brain MRI during the first episode of delirium experienced by the patient described in the case history (see text). Cortical atrophy is evident especially at the level of the temporal lobe in this section.

the patient could be roused only by intense stimulation and there was multifocal myoclonus. Diazepam was added to treat myoclonus (20 mg/day parenterally). Observation during more alert phases and indications suggesting suffering (e.g. grimacing) led to an increase in the morphine infusion to 120 mg/day. The patient's condition worsened with the onset of tachypnea, fever, and olyguria; he was comatose for three days and died 26 days after admission.

During the last four weeks of life, respiratory, renal, and cardiac functions were within normal limits with the exception of oliguria in the last three days. Hydration and antibiotics were provided as indicated. Fever was remittent and usually of low grade, but in the last days reached 39.5 °C. Laboratory findings showed: low albumin (2.6 g/dl), altered coagulation (PT = 52, PT INR = 1.62, APTT = 53.9, APTT ratio = 1.59), high alkaline phospatase (592), and γ GT (178) with tendency to slightly low levels of potassium, sodium, magnesium, and calcium.

Hemoglobin was 9.5; white cell count 9000 granulocytes with lymphocytes count low to very low (from 17% to 10%). Chest X-rays were normal at the onset of delirium and showed some bilateral basilar findings during the terminal phase. Brain MRI with gadolinium was done at the onset of delirium (Figure 22-1) and showed no metastatic or focal disease but diffuse cortical atrophy with enlarged sulci and ventricles.

Family meetings were frequent throughout the admission and sought to clarify prognosis, potential reversibility of mental function, and symptom control. The family agreed that comfort care was the main goal of therapy given the stage of disease and lack of any correctable causes for higher function impairment.

INTRODUCTION

The experience of neurologists, psychiatrists, geriatricians, and palliative care physicians can all contribute to the understanding of delirium or acute confusional state. Recent views have suggested a global failure of cognitive processes to underlie the etiology of delirium. One hypothetical mechanism explains a 'global failure of cognition' as the consequence of a selective failure of attention;[1] another, noting the compromise in vigilance and level of consciousness, gives more importance to the abnormality in the level of consciousness occurring on the continuum between normal wakefulness and coma.[2]

Acutely altered mental states share an array of different etiologies, and can be characterized by a number of clinical phenomena. In addition, a range of negative and positive phenomena may occur in one individual and fluctuate over time.

Clinical observation commonly uses two terms—'delirium' or 'acute confusional state'. Some authors[3] separate these entities using 'delirium' to describe acute mental status changes characterized by agitation, hyperactivity, and hallucinations (delirium tremens being the prototype) and 'acute mental confusion' to describe those states characterized by confusion without agitation. For many neurologists the term *encephalopathy* conveys the same meaning. In the case described, phases of reduced activity, reduced consciousness, and predominantly negative cognitive findings alternated with phases of agitation, hallucinations, and possibly delusions. Engel and Romano have demonstrated that EEG correlates of most acute confusional states and of deliria are very similar, with the exception of delirium tremens having a prevalence of fast activity EEG pattern.[4]

A unified concept of delirium now underlies the definitions found within the Diagnostic Statistical Manual (DSM) of Mental Disorders and the ICD (International Classification of Diseases) 10.

DSM-IV (see Table 22–1) omitted some of the accessory symptoms listed in the previous manual (DSM-III-R). The new definition underlines the fundamental clinical characteristics of the syndrome as a disorder affecting attention, level of consciousness, and cognitive functions; it may be acute or subacute in evolution, and due to a medical cause.

The tenth revision of ICD (ICD-10) (see Table 22–2) classifies delirium that is not due to alcohol or other psychoactive substances among the 'organic psychic syndromes and disturbances including the symptomatic ones'. If this classification is used, the diagnosis requires that all areas of dysfunction described in Table 22–2 are present, even if in a mild form.

Since the pathophysiology of delirium is unclear, a final common pathway along which multiple different etiologies converge is an attractive hypothesis. One potential candidate for this pathway is the cholinergic system of the brain stem projection to the thalamus and cortex which participates in the regulation of arousal and the sleep–wakefulness cycle.[5] Alternative hypotheses favor a specific role for different neurotransmitter pathways in individual types of deliria.[6]

DIAGNOSIS AND CLINICAL FEATURES

Delirium is one of the most prevalent symptoms encountered in patients with terminal illness, whether in hospices,[7] specialized palliative care units,[8] or home care.[9] In these settings, prevalence ranges between 30 and 40%, incidence increasing with the approach of the end of life.[8]

Diagnosis

The gold standards for clinical diagnosis are the DSM-IV and ICD-10 when applied by trained clinicians such as neurologists and psychiatrists. Clinical examination and laboratory and radiological examination may suggest etiology

Table 22–1. DSM-IV Diagnostic Criteria for Delirium (Modied from DSM-IV and DSM IV-TR, American Psychiatric Press, Washington, 2000. Reproduced with Permission from the American Psychiatric Association.)

A	Disturbance of consciousness (i.e., reduced clarity of awareness of the environment) with reduced ability to focus, sustain, or shift attention.
B	A change in cognition (such as memory deficit, disorientation, language disturbance) or the development of a perceptual disturbance that is not better accounted for by a pre-existing, established, or evolving dementia.
C	The disturbance develops over a short period of time (usually hours to days) and tends to fluctuate during the course of the day.
D	There is evidence from the history, physical examination, or laboratory findings that the disturbance is caused by the direct physiological consequences of a general medical condition.
Diagnostic criteria for delirium due to a general medical condition	
Diagnostic criteria for substance intoxication delirium	There is evidence from the history, physical examination, or laboratory findings that either (1) or (2): 1. The symptoms in criteria A and B developed during substance intoxication 2. Medication use is etiologically related to the disturbance **Note:** This diagnosis should be made instead of a diagnosis of substance intoxication only when the cognitive symptoms are in excess of those usually associated with the intoxication syndrome and when the symptoms are sufficiently severe to warrant independent clinical attention.
Diagnostic criteria for substance withdrawal delirium	There is evidence from the history, physical examination, or laboratory findings that the symptoms in criteria A and B developed during, or shortly after, a withdrawal syndrome. **Note:** This diagnosis should be made instead of a diagnosis of substance withdrawal only when the cognitive symptoms are in excess of those usually associated with the withdrawal syndrome and when the symptoms are sufficiently severe to warrant independent clinical attention.
Diagnostic criteria for delirium due to multiple etiologies	There is evidence from the history, physical examination, or laboratory findings that the delirium has more than one etiology (e.g., more than one etiological general medical condition, a general medical condition plus substance intoxication or medication side effect).

Table 22–2. ICD-10 Diagnostic Guidelines (Reproduced from The ICD-10 Classication of Mental and Behavioral Disorders: Clinical Descriptions and Diagnostic Guidelines, WHO Publications, Geneva, 1992. Reproduced with Permission from the World Health Organization.)

For a definite diagnosis, symptoms, mild or severe, should be present in the following areas:

(a) Impairment of consciousness and attention (on a continuum from clouding to coma; reduced ability to direct, focus, sustain, and shift attention);

(b) Global disturbance of cognition (perceptual distortions, illusions and hallucinations—most often visual; impairment of abstract thinking and comprehension, with or without transient delusions, but typically with some degree of incoherence; impairment of immediate recall and of recent memory but with relatively intact remote memory; disorientation for time as well as, in more severe cases, for place and person);

(c) Psychomotor disturbances (hypo- or hyperactivity and unpredictable shifts from one to the other; increased reaction time; increased or decreased flow of speech; enhanced startle reaction);

(d) Disturbance of the sleep–wake cycle (insomnia or, in severe cases, total sleep loss or reversal of the sleep–wake cycle; daytime drowsiness; nocturnal worsening of symptoms; disturbing dreams or nightmares, which may continue as hallucinations after awakening);

(e) Emotional disturbances, e.g. depression, anxiety or fear, irritability, euphoria, apathy, or wondering perplexity.

The onset is usually rapid, the course diurnally fluctuating, and the total duration of the condition less than 6 months. The above clinical picture is so characteristic that a fairly confident diagnosis of delirium can be made even if the underlying cause is not clearly established. In addition to a history of an underlying physical or brain disease, evidence of cerebral dysfunction (e.g. an abnormal electroencephalogram, usually but not invariably showing a slowing of the background activity) may be required if the diagnosis is in doubt.

Includes:

✓ Acute brain syndrome

✓ Acute confusional state (non-alcoholic)

✓ Acute infective psychosis

✓ Acute organic reaction

✓ Acute psycho-organic syndrome

Differential diagnosis. Delirium should be distinguished from other organic syndromes, especially dementia (F00–F03), from acute and transient psychotic disorders, and from acute states in schizophrenia or mood [affective] disorders (F30–F39) in which confusional features may be present. Delirium, induced by alcohol and other psychoactive substances, should be coded in the appropriate section.

(Table 22–3). Clinical diagnosis can be helped by standardized methods of applying diagnostic criteria, such as the Confusion Assessment Method[10] or the Delirium Symptom Interview,[11] though both are based on earlier versions of the DSM. The EEG, if more often applied to the evaluation of altered states of consciousness, would be a very sensitive diagnostic tool supplementing clinical findings.[12,13]

Among the clinical characteristics of delirium, fluctuating course and reversibility are certainly crucial. Fluctuation is a source of controversy among staff members and, at times, within families, and strongly justifies the use of a formal method of documenting

the mental state. Delirium, in contrast to dementia, is a potentially reversible process, even in the patient with advanced illness.[8] When no reversible cause is found, delirium may announce impending death, but, contrary to recent thinking, duration can be prolonged (as in the case history). A similar situation is found in elderly persons with cognitive compromise, when life is not at risk, and where acutely occurring symptoms can persist for a very long time.[14]

No focal signs are required for the diagnosis of delirium. Some neurological signs can be valued, such as the pathological reflexes: palmo-mental, snout, grasping, and

Table 22–3. **Aid to the Screening and Correction of Delirium Etiologies or Contributory Factors**

Toxic factors	Bedside screen of medication profile Urine or blood drug screening
Sepsis	Temperature Blood/urine and other cultures for infection screen Leukocyte count Urinalysis
Glucose oxydative brain deficiency	Pulse oxymetry Red cell count Blood gases and acid base balance Blood glucose
Electrolyte imbalances Renal failure Liver failure	Serum electrolytes (Na, K, CL, Mg, Ca) Urea, creatinine, creatinine clearance Liver function tests Ammonia
CNS vascular infections or structural lesion	DIC screening and coagulation profile CSF examination: blood, glucose, proteins, lymphocytes l eukocytes, malignant cells, culture Brain CT or MRI
Cofactor deficiency malnutrition	B12 levels Administer B1 1g/day°
Endocrine dysfunction	Thyroid hormone and TSH Adrenal function
Paraneoplastic limbic encephalitis	Anti-neuronal auto-antibodies

° The determination of B1 levels is problematic; our practice is to give supplementary B1 to every patient with poor nutritional status

glabella reflex and the presence of tremors, asterixis, and myoclonus that are characteristic of toxic metabolic deliria.

Differential Diagnosis

The most important differential diagnoses of delirium are dementia and psychosis. The clinical picture of dementia can be very similar to delirium with a widespread failure of higher cerebral functions. The classic distinction between dementia and delirium is, for delirium, an acute onset and derangement of consciousness level ('clouding of consciousness' in the ICD-10) and, for dementia, a more chronic process sparing consciousness, at least in the initial phase, and for a period that typically can be very long.

Dementia poses specific clinical difficulties. Many elderly patients have a prolonged course after episodes of delirium, with incomplete reversibility of symptoms and functional compromise. The pathogenesis of dementia is associated with failure of cortical activity and cholinergic transmission that are thought also to be compromised in delirium. The observation that dementia or cognitive compromise is an important risk factor for developing delirium is consistent with this hypothesis.

An acute behavioral change with altered cognition and attention can be also the result of a psychosis. Often the patient has an history of psychiatric disease but he or she could present for the first time with a dramatic bizarre course ('poussez delirant' in the French literature). A patient with psychiatric illness with complicated medical problems or terminal disease can develop delirium, and the differential diagnosis

will be challenging. Toxicity with amphetamines or amphetamine-type street drugs often
can mimic personality disorders and psychiatric reactions. Secondary mental changes may
present as depressive attitudes and symptoms
in elderly persons with systemic medical illness, but psychiatric consultation may then
suggest a diagnosis of delirium.[15]

Subjective Components

Delirium impacts significantly on a patient's
affect. Fluctuations of severity, with lucid
phases, may allow awareness of further mental
changes, generating anxiety, anguish, and fear.
In children this can manifest as fear of going
asleep or refusal to take sedation. Emotional
reactions can include apathy, depression,
perplexity (when the clinical situation is perceived as worsening), and cognitive compromise (feared as part of an inevitable grim
course). Severe affective changes are not
common, however, and the possibility that
delirium can facilitate suicidal thoughts or acts
is merely hypothetical.[16]

The quality of the delirium subjective
experience is not easy to predict and depends
on the patient's personality and previous
experiences.[17] Paranoid ideation can be present (imprisonment, homicide, jealousy), and
themes related to the severity of actual disease
(death, torture, kidnapping) are common.
Most, or at least many, of the illusional or
delusional interpretations of the medical
environment reported by acutely confused
patients, had very hostile qualities. One
patient perceived physicians around the bed
as ghosts, and therapies as attempted poisoning; another patient recalled being with a
friend (also a patient) in a concentration
camp, where they were held, bald (as indeed
they were, due to chemotherapy), and people
(physicians and nurses) were coming to laugh
at them and torture them.

In delirium following a liver transplant, the
relationship with the donor and donor's family
is often represented. One patient hallucinated
that the donor came to him to request restitu-
tion of the organ—a very negative experience.
Another patient had a vision of a kaleidosco-
pically colored forest inhabited by fantastic
flora and fauna; on recall he found it a very
positive and interesting experience that he
connected with an earlier curiosity about the
effect of hallucinogenic drugs, popular among
his peers (that he had never tried). How the
meaning and the psychological impact of
delirium at the end of life is influenced by
specific medical, psychological, existential, or
spiritual issues is unknown, since clinical
observations and studies are very limited.[18,19]

Monitoring and Assessment Tools

The high prevalence of delirium in patients
with terminal illness is enough to recommend
the routine use of instruments for the
screening of cognitive function in patients
admitted to palliative care programs[7] enabling
early diagnosis and facilitating staff and family
communication.

The Mini-Mental State Examination
(MMSE)[20] is the most popular tool for a quick
assessment of cognitive functions, but is not
specific for delirium. For this reason we
recommend, in addition, the use of the
Delirium Rating Scale (DRS)[21] or the Memorial Delirium Assessment Scale (MDAS).[22]
Both have been studied in advanced cancer
patients[23] and are helpful in documenting
fluctuations in mental function (as demonstrated by the case presented). It is important
that nursing staff are familiar with at least one
screening tool and with the principles of
assessment, but no screening tool can substitute for clinical diagnosis.

The assessment of graphical abilities
(spontaneous sentence writing, copying a
design such as a clock or geometrical figure) is
a very sensitive tool to evaluate early nonspecific changes of mental function and to
monitor therapy outcomes.[24] Two items of the
MMSE test graphic abilities, but this is not
specifically required by the MDAS or DRS.
The EEG, already mentioned as a diagnostic
tool, may have a potential role in monitoring
the course of delirium.

Causes; Predisposing and Precipitating Factors

No list of potential delirium etiologies will be
comprehensive. Causes of delirium can
be classified in a few main classes (see also
Table 22–3).

PRIMARY CNS DISEASES

Right-sided cerebral vascular lesions have been associated with delirium.[25] Whether brain vascular lesions will cause delirium probably depends on the previous cognitive state and not on the side or site of the lesion itself.[26] Epilepsy may cause an altered mental status and mimic delirium in postictal states. Non-convulsive status epilepticus should be considered more often in patients with advanced disease.[27,28] Only a more widespread use of EEG in palliative care facilities, would reveal this etiology.[29,30]

Metastases to the brain and meninges can present with changes in cognition and delirium or can predispose to the onset of delirium.[31,32] The first sign of CNS metastases may be the development of delirium, in combination with the effect of psychotropic drugs which were well tolerated beforehand.[33]

SYSTEMIC DISEASES

Electrolyte imbalances and multi-organ failure are very common in terminal illness. As in the case presented, the sum of many slight abnormalities of homeostasis is more often found than a single well-defined pathology. Hypoxia has been found to be associated with irreversible deliria in advanced cancer patients in one recent series.[8]

Vitamin deficiency, especially thiamine, is relevant to delirium in the elderly and in patients admitted to hospice with poor nutritional status.[34] Improved hydration may prevent toxic deliria in terminal disease by maintaining renal function and preventing the accumulation of drug metabolites.[35,36]

EXOGENOUS INTOXICATION AND DRUG WITHDRAWAL

Drugs are a very frequent cause of delirium. The enhanced sensitivity to their toxic effects of patients with cognitive impairment, older age, systemic illness, metabolic abnormalities, and structural brain lesions is of crucial importance in palliative care. Drugs with central anticholinergic effects are the most likely to precipitate toxic deliria. Tricyclic antidepressants are responsible for 10%–15% of confusional states in the general population and of 35% of cases in the elderly.[37]

A Multifactorial Model

A multifactorial model for the development of delirium in the elderly, hospitalized patient shows that predictive baseline factors (already present at admission) modify the susceptibility of patients to precipitating factors. Baseline vulnerability factors are age, cognitive impairment, visual impairment, and severity of disease. High baseline vulnerability means that relatively mild precipitating factors such as the use of psychotropic drugs and other iatrogenic events may precipitate delirium.[38,39] The role of cortical atrophy disclosed at MRI in the case reported can only be inferred, as well as the potential central toxicity of the long-term IV 5-FU.

Other studies add infections and electrolyte and renal function abnormalities as vulnerability factors.[40,41] All these factors are frequently encountered in palliative care patients.

A multifactorial model implies that it may not be possible to establish an etiology in classic terms for many delirious episodes occurring in patients with severe systemic disorders and significant risk factors.[42]

Reversibility and Prognosis

Delirium is usually perceived as a transient and brief clinical condition, but in a study of elderly patients, the average duration of an episode was longer than two weeks.[43] In acutely hospitalized, elderly patients, resolution of symptoms was often incomplete—only 4% experiencing resolution of all new symptoms before hospital discharge, and 21 and 18% with persisting symptoms for three and six months, respectively.[14]

Delirium may be substantially less transient than currently believed, and persistent irreversible delirium can characterize 'a way of dying', with an intermediate to long course and fluctuating phases. However, in one study of terminal patients, 50% of the delirium episodes were reversible or at least amenable to improvement[7,8] when dehydration and drug toxicity were involved, whereas hypoxia due to pulmonary disease was associated with irreversible cases.[8]

The mortality associated with delirium varies. Delirium is not associated with higher mortality in the hospitalized elderly after comorbities are taken into account,[44] but it identifies those patients at risk for worse outcome in terms of prolonged hospitalization, loss of independent community living, and future cognitive debility.[45]

The prognostic impact of delirium changes in more selected populations. Delirium was associated with a worse prognosis in cancer patients admitted to a tertiary cancer center,[46] and it was independently associated with shorter survival in palliative care programs.[9] Several clinical findings can be used to establish a prognosis in the advanced phases of cancer, such as anorexia, dyspnea, performance status, and granulocyte and lymphocyte count.[9,42,47] Some of these factors were present in the case history (anorexia, poor performance, low lymphocyte rate).

TREATMENT

Interventions aim first at correcting infectious, toxic, and metabolic causes or risk factors (Table 22–4). Simultaneous symptomatic management is often required in both reversible and irreversible cases and employs non-pharmacological and pharmacological therapies.

Environmental Intervention

A calm, quiet environment facilitates potential recovery and helps the patient to reorient to time and space (with a visible clock, calendar, or well-known object from the patient's house), plus good light. Systematic reorientation and a risk-modifying protocol can reduce the incidence of delirium among elderly hospitalized patients.[39] The presence of family members can be very important.

Communication with Patient and Family

Close collaboration with the family is fundamental, with special attention to communication between patient and the family. Change in usual behavior and an apparent communication barrier is very stressful to family members and they need to be informed about delirium, its relationship to disease conditions, its potential for reversibility and short-term prognosis, the fluctuations of cognitive function, and the role of therapies.

The goals of care need to be shared, the level of patient suffering assessed and explained. There is a tendency to overemphasize suffering when delirium complicates assessment,[48] and family members may seek disproportionate interventions for relieving what they interpret as suffering or pain. Requests may swing from withdrawal of medication to increased sedation. Such requests are often compounded by personal problems in facing suffering and death.

It is common to blame opioid medications for mental changes caused by the complex interaction of several factors. Previous experience with opioids, and erroneous medical beliefs, can lead relatives to feel guilty about administering therapies that are seen to be related to mental changes. But the etiology often cannot be established and the decision to use drugs that may contribute to delirium is based on the priority of providing symptom control and comfort care.

It is important to demonstrate empathy with the patient by asking simple questions ('Do you feel confused?'). While consciousness level fluctuates, the patient needs to be reassured. Employ more direct non-verbal communication skills rather than logic and rational communication. Communication should focus more on affective aspects than on cognition and try to distract from delusional experiences and interpretations.

Pharmacological Therapy

Agitated delirium often requires pharmacological treatment to control behaviors that could result in harm for the patient and others, and to treat hallucinations or delusions that may contribute to patient suffering. The treatment of hypoactive deliria is more debatable and will depend on individual clinical judgement.

First choice drug is haloperidol[49,50] since it has lower sedating potency and less anticholinergic and cardiovascular effects than other neuroleptics. Table 22–5 gives guidelines for the use of haloperidol and alternative drugs. These guidelines are general and should be adapted to each individual clinical

Table 22–4. **Drugs that have been Associated with Delirium**

Psychotropics	Barbiturates
	Benzodiazepines
	Bromides
	Chloral hydrate
	Chlorpromazine
	Lithium
	Neuroleptics
	Paraldehyde
	Tricyclic antidepressants
	SSRIs
	Zolpidem
Anticholinergic medications	Scopolamine
	Atropine
	Hyoscine
	Biperidene
	Triesifenidile
	Hyoscine butylbromide
Analgesics	Opioids
	NSAIDs (rare)
	Aspirin
Antihistamines	Prometazine
	Marzine
	Hydroxizine
Cardiovascular therapies	Digitalis
Immunosuppressants or medications with immunologic activity	Steroids
	Interferons and interleukins
	Tacrolimus
	Cyclosporin
Antibiotics and antivirals	Ciprofloxacin
	Acyclovir
	Gancyclovir
Antisecretory medications	H2-antagonists (cimetidine, ranitidine, famotidine)
	Omeprazole
Neurologic therapies	Anticonvulsants
	Levodopa
Chemotherapy drugs	Methotrexate (high doses)
	Cisplatin
	Vincristine
	Procarbazine
	Asparaginase
	Cytosine arabinoside
	5-fluorouracil
	Ifosfamide
	Tamoxifen (very rare)
	Etoposide (high doses)
	Nitrosurea (high doses or arterial route)

Table 22–5. **Pharmacological Therapy of Delirium**

Haloperidol OS	0.5–5 mg every 8/12 hours; a dose of 2 mg/day can be efficacious in mild cases. EKG monitoring is recommended.
Haloperidol SC, IM or EV	0.5–2 mg per dose, titrating dose to clinical effect, hour by hour. IV infusion 0.2–1 mg with careful titration to clinical effect can be used in difficult cases. EKG monitoring is recommended.
Chlorpromazine OS, IM or EV	12.5–50 mg every 8/12 hours. More sedating, anticholinergic, and hypotensive effects
Clozapine OS	12.5–50 mg at night (monitoring of blood cell count is needed). Very sedative; has less extrapyramidal effects than other neuroleptics.
Risperidon OS	From 0.5–1 mg/day up to 2–4 mg/day. In the elderly has less extrapyramidal effects.
Lorazepam OS, SL or EV	0.5–2 mg every 4/8 hours if sedating anxiolitic effects required.
Midazolam SC or EV	20–100 mg 24/hour IV or SC continuous infusion for sedation in refractory cases. 3–5 mg IV priming dose if rapid sedation is required. Start IV infusion with 1 mg/hour, dose should be frequently titrated to effect.
Promazine OS, IM or EV	50 mg every 8/12 hours. Antihistamine very sedative; useful if sedation desired.

case. Haloperidol has been used via IV infusion, although it is not licensed for that route of administration.[49] Very high IV doses up to 1200 mg per day have been safely administered; in our experience therapeutic effects are seen at doses of 2–5 mg/day. Difficult cases may require higher doses or sedation with other drugs. Careful titration of the dose at the bedside is the most important recommendation to improve outcome. *ECG* allows monitoring of prolongation of the Q-T interval that can occasionally occur. *Torsade de pointe* has been described with haloperidol, administered via IV and oral route.[51,52] Droperidol and chlorpromazine have more sedative effects. Recently, risperidone, clozapine, and olanzapine have been used.

Benzodiazepines can worsen delirium, especially in the elderly[50] and are avoided in hepatic encephalopathy. They are first choice drugs for the treatment of delirium due to alcohol withdrawal. Benzodiazepines may be added when anxiolytic and sedative effects are desirable or in cases unresponsive to neuroleptic medications.

Delirium in cancer patients with terminal disease often requires use of more than a single drug. In one series only 20% of cases could be managed by haloperidol alone.[53] When sedation is the goal of therapy or there are severe symptoms such as pain, hemorrhage, or dyspnea, the combination of an opioid with a neuroleptic and an antihistamine such as promethazine can be particularly effective.

SUMMARY

This chapter is a short summary of the numerous, intriguing areas of research and clinical knowledge that go under the heading of delirium. Lipowski's unrivalled book on delirium was published in 1990,[42] and since then hundreds of papers have been published addressing this clinical problem from the perspective of pathophysiology, definition, risk factors, epidemiology, and assessment. The contributions of several specialties is fundamental as most cases of delirium are seen in a clinical context that may lack neurological and psychiatric input; while it is absolutely necessary that palliative care specialists are sophisticated experts in diagnosing and managing delirium.[54] Management of delirium at the end of life is certainly one important aspect of palliative care that overlaps with the need of appropriate management of delirium in general. In critically ill patients, therapeutic strategies to manage delirium are poorly defined and a special effort in pharmacological research is needed to improve patients' care.

REFERENCES

1. Mesulam M–M. Attention, confusional states, and neglect. In: Mesulam M–M, ed. Principles of Behavioral Neurology. Contemporary Neurology Series. F.A. Davis, Philadelphia, 1985:125–168.
2. Plum F, Posner JB. The Diagnosis of Stupor and Coma. F.A. Davis, Philadelphia, 1980.
3. Adams RD, Victor M. Principles of Neurology, 6th Ed. McGraw–Hill, New York, 1997.
4. Engel GL, Romano J. Delirium: a syndrome of cerebral insufficiency. J Chronic Diseases 1959;9: 260–277.
5. Perry E, Walker M, Grace J, et al. Acetylcholine in mind: a neurotrasmitter correlate of consciousness. Trends Neurosci 1999;22:273–280.
6. Trzepacz PT. Update on the neuropathogenesis of delirium. Dement Geriatr Cogn Disord 1999;10: 330–334.
7. Gagnon P, Allard P, Masse B, et al. Delirium in terminal cancer: a prospective study using daily screening, early diagnosis and continuous monitoring. J Pain Symptom Manage 2000;19:412–426.
8. Lawlor PG, Gagnon B, Mancini IL, et al. Occurrence, causes and outcome of delirium in patients with advanced cancer. Arch Intern Med 2000;160: 786–794.
9. Caraceni A, Nanni O, Maltoni M, et al. The impact of delirium on the short-term prognosis of advanced cancer patients. Cancer 2000;89:1145–1149.
10. Inouye SK, van Dyck CH, Alessi CA, et al. Clarifying confusion: the confusion assessment method. A new method for detection of delirium. Ann Intern Med 1990;113:941–948.
11. Albert MS, Levkoff SE, Reilly CR, et al. The delirium symptom interview: an interview for the detection of delirium symtoms in hospitalized patients. J Geriatr Psychiatry Neurol 1992;5:14–21.
12. Young GB, Leung LS, Campbell V, et al. The electroencephalogram in metabolic/toxic coma. Am J EEG Technol 1992;32:243–259.
13. Jacobson SA, Leuchter AF, Walter DO. Conventional and quantitative EEG in the diagnosis of delirium among the elderly. J Neurol Neurosurg Psychiatry 1993;56:153–158.
14. Levkoff SE, Evans DA, Lipzin B, et al. Delirium. The occurence and persistence of symptoms among elderly hospitalized patients. Arch Intern Med 1992;152:334–340.
15. Farrell KR, Ganzini L. Misdiagnosing delirium as depression in medically ill elderly patients. Arch Intern Med 1995;155:2459–2464.
16. Breitbart W. Suicide in the cancer patient. Oncology 1987;1:49–54.
17. Wolf HG, Curran D. Nature of delirium and allied states. The disergastic reaction. Arch Neurol Psychiatry 1935;33:1175–1215.
18. Massie MJ, Holland JC, Glass E. Delirium in terminally ill cancer patients. American Journal of Psychiatry 1983;140:1048–1050.
19. Kubler–Ross E. On Death and Dying. Macmillan, New York, 1969.
20. Folstein M, Folstein S, McHugh P. Mini-mental state. J Psychiatr Res 1975;12:189–198.
21. Trzepacz PT, Baker RW, Greenhouse J. A symptom rating scale for delirium. Psychiatry Res 1988;23: 89–97.
22. Breitbart W, Rosenfeld B, Roth A, et al. The Memorial Delirium Assessment Scale. J Pain Symptom Manage 1997;13:128–137.
23. Grassi L, Caraceni A, Beltrami E, et al. Assessing delirium in cancer patients the Italian versions of the Delirium Rating Scale and the Memorial Delirium Assessment Scale. J Pain Symptom Manage 2001;21:59–68.
24. Macleod AD, Whitehead LE. Dysgraphia in terminal delirium. Palliat Med 1997;11:127–132.
25. Mesulam MM, Waxman SG, Geschwind N, et al. Acute confusional state with right cerebral artery infarction. J Neurol Neurosurg Psychiatry 1976;39:84–89.
26. Henon H, Lebert F, Durieu I, et al. Confusional state in stroke. Relation to preexisting dementia, patient characteristics and outcome. Stroke 1999;30:773–779.
27. Dexter DDJ, Westmoreland BF, Cascino TL. Complex partial status epilepticus in a patient with leptomemninegeal carcinomatosis. Neurology 1990;40:858–859.
28. Wengs WJ, Talwar D, Bernard J. Ifosfamide-induced nonconvulsive status epilepticus. Arch Neurol 1993;50:1104–1105.
29. Engel JJ, Ludwig BI, Fetell M. Prolonged partial complex status epilepticus: EEG and behavioral observations. Neurology 1978;28:863–869.
30. Towne AR, Waterhouse EJ, Boggs JG, et al. Prevalence of non-convulsive status epilepticus in comatose patients. Neurology 2000;54:340–345.
31. Posner JB. Neurologic complications of cancer. F.A. Davis, Philadelphia, 1995.
32. Weitzener MA, Olofson SM, Forman AD. Patients with malignant meningitis presenting with neuropsychiatric manifestations. Cancer 1995;76: 1804–1808.
33. Caraceni A, Martini C, De Conno F, et al. Organic brain syndromes and opioid administration for cancer pain. J Pain Symptom Manage 1994;9:527–533.
34. Barbato M, Rodriguez PJ. Thiamine deficiency in patients admitted to a palliative care unit. Pall Medicine 1994;8:320–324.
35. Bruera E, Franco JJ, Maltoni M, et al. Changing pattern of agitated impaired mental status in patients with advanced cancer: association with cognitive monitoring, hydration and opioid rotation. J Pain Sympt Manage 1995;10:287–291.
36. Burke AL. Palliative care: an update on 'terminal restlessness'. Med J Aust 1997;166:39–42.
37. Hollister LE. Psychotherapeutic drugs. In: Levenson JA, ed. Neuropsychiatric Side Effects of Drugs in the Elderly. Raven Press, New York, 1979.

38. Inouye SK, Charpentier PA. Precipitating factors for delirium in hospitalized elderly persons. Predictive model and interrelationship with baseline vulnerability. JAMA 1996;275:852–857.

39. Inouye SK, Bogardus ST, Charpentier PA, et al. A multicomponent intervention to prevent delirium in hospitalized older patients. N Engl J Med 1999;340:669–676.

40. Francis J, Martin D, Kapoor WN. A prospective study of delirium in hospitalized elderly. JAMA 1990;263:1097–1101.

41. Schor JD, Levkoff SE, Lipsitz LA, et al. Risk factors for delirium in hospitalized elderly. JAMA 1992;267:827–831.

42. Lipowski ZJ. Etiology, Delirium: Acute Confusional States. Oxford University Press, New York, 1990: 109–140.

43. Koponen HJ, Riekkinen PJ. A prospective study of delirium in elderly patients admitted to a psychiatric hospital. Psychol Med 1993;23:103–109.

44. Francis J, Kapoor WN. Prognosis after hospital discharge of older medical patients with delirium. J Am Geriatr Soc 1992;40:601–606.

45. Pompei P, Foreman M, Rudberg MA, et al. Delirium in hospitalized older persons: outcomes and predictors. J Am Geriatr Soc 1994;42:809–815.

46. Tuma R, DeAngelis LM. Altered mental status in patients with cancer. Arch Neurol 2000;57:1727–1731.

47. Maltoni M, Nanni O, Pirovano M. Successful validation of the palliative prognostic score in terminally ill cancer patients. J Pain Symptom Manage 1999;17:240–247.

48. Morita T, Tsunoda J, Inoue S, et al. The palliative prognostic index: a scoring system for survival prediction of terminally ill cancer patients. Support Care Cancer 1999;7:128–133.

49. Association AP. Practice guideline for the treatment of patients with delirium. Am J Psychiatry 1999;156:1–20.

50. Breitbart W, Marotta R, Platt MM, et al. A double-blind trial of haloperidol, chlorpromazine and lorazepam in the treatment of delirium in hospitalized AIDS patients. Am J Psychiatry 1996;153:231–237.

51. Wilt JL, Minnema AM, Johnson RF, et al. Torsade de pointes associated with the use of intravenous haloperidol. Ann Intern Med 1993;119:391–394.

52. Jackson T, Ditmanson L, Phibbs B. Torsade de pointes and low-dose oral haloperidol. Arch Intern Med 1997;157:2013–2015.

53. Stiefel F, Fainsinger R, Bruera E. Acute confusional states in patients with advanced cancer. J Pain Symptom Manage 1992;7:94–98.

54. Caraceni A, Grassi L. Acute confusional states in palliative medicine. Oxford University Press, Oxford, 2003.

Chapter 23

Respiratory Symptoms

Gian Domenico Borasio
D. Kaub–Wittemer

DEFINITION AND PATHOPHYSIOLOGY OF DYSPNEA
Definition
Pathophysiology
ASSESSMENT
History and Examination
Sleep and Respiratory Muscle Weakness in Neuromuscular Patients
Scales
Tests of Respiratory Muscle Strength
Blood Gas Analysis

Overnight Oximetry and Polysomnography
Assessment of Related Constructs
NON-PHARMACOLOGICAL TREATMENT
PHARMACOLOGICAL TREATMENT
Dyspnea
Death Rattle
Cough
VENTILATION
Non-Invasive Ventilation
Tracheostomy Ventilation

Dyspnea is a frequent symptom in neurologic disorders, especially neuromuscular disease. Careful assessment of the underlying cause is paramount. Like pain, 'total dyspnea' includes physical, psychosocial, and spiritual aspects. Drug and non-drug measures are equally important in the management of dyspnea. In neuromuscular patients, non-invasive ventilation is an excellent palliative measure for symptoms of chronic hypoventilation, while invasive ventilation should be restricted to selected cases. Other respiratory symptoms that can be efficiently palliated through appropriate medication include death rattle and cough. Management options for thick mucous secretions in patients with diaphragmatic weakness are still insufficient and further research is required.

CASE HISTORY

Anna, aged 41, was admitted to hospital because of increasing weakness in her right hand as well as muscle cramps in both legs and 'muscle twitching'. She was diagnosed with amyotrophic lateral sclerosis (ALS). After several months of progressive weakness, she developed a right foot drop. During the following months, her limb weakness grew progressively worse, necessitating the use of a wheelchair. Her husband reported a slightly slurred speech.

By this time Anna was still working as a management director of a large company. She was married and had two children, aged six and eight. A nanny looked after the children during the daytime. Her husband was also working in a full-time job as a bank manager. The family was financially independent.

During the course of the disease, Anna became severely disabled because of generalized weakness. She experienced no intellectual deterioration or sensory problems. Later on, difficulty in swallowing required the insertion of a gastrostomy (PEG) tube for feeding. The need for hospice and nursing services for her home care increased and she had to stop working.

Around three years after disease onset, sleep disturbances, daytime fatigue, and thick mucous secretions appeared and severely hampered Anna's quality of life. Dyspneic bouts on exertion led to panic attacks, which were well controlled by sublingual lorazepam. At this point, the patient and her husband were informed about respiratory failure in ALS. Aspects of mechanical ventilation and medical treatment of dyspnea, as well as the terminal phase, were brought up for discussion. Anna wished to be ventilated for as long as possible to see her kids growing up.

Her husband and the day-care team built up a 24-hour home-care system, so that the husband, as the primary caregiver, could go on working to guarantee the family's income. Over six months the patient used non-invasive nocturnal positive-pressure ventilation via a mask, which effectively reduced the symptoms of chronic hypoventilation. Mild dyspnea during the day was relieved with low-dose morphine. With increasing bulbar weakness, the mask fitting decreased and invasive ventilation via tracheostomy became necessary. Advance directives including the issue of discontinuation of invasive ventilation and medication in the terminal phase were set up. For a further three years, Anna lived with a full-time ventilator, communicating via a computer. The family reported a good quality of life. Husband and children were supported by a psychologist.

When the disease progressed to the point where a locked-in syndrome became imminent, Anna expressed the wish to discontinue ventilation. She received morphine and midazolam for comfort, and died peacefully in the presence of her family after the ventilator was stopped.

DEFINITION AND PATHOPHYSIOLOGY OF DYSPNEA

Definition

Dyspnea has been described as an 'unpleasant awareness of difficulty in breathing' or 'subjective experience of breathing discomfort'. It may occur in patients with neurologic disorders, particularly patients with neuromuscular disease (e.g. ALS; see Chapter 8). Almost all patients with ALS will suffer from symptoms of chronic hypoventilation and dyspnea during the course of their disease. Nearly 90% of all patients with Parkinson's disease show a loss of lung volume, which correlates with disease severity.[1] In the terminal phase of patients with space-occupying lesions

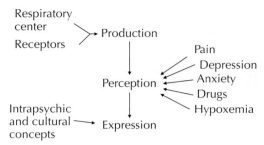

Figure 23–1. Factors which modulate dyspnea.

of the brain, particularly infratentorial lesions, disordered breathing can appear due to direct involvement of the medulla and brain stem.

Dyspnea should not be confused with tachypnea (increased breathing frequency caused by elevated metabolic rate, e.g. fever), hyperpnea (increased ventilation due to metabolic acidosis), orthopnea (inability to lie down because of increase in breathlessness, e.g. in cardiac disease), or hyperventilation (psychogenic increase in respiration).

It is important to think of dyspnea in terms of 'total breathlessness', which includes physical, psychological, social, cultural, environmental, and spiritual aspects (e.g. fear of death and dying). Both the perception and the expression of dyspnea are modulated by these factors (Fig. 23–1), which have to be taken into account for assessment and treatment.

Pathophysiology

The exact pathophysiology of dyspnea is still a matter of controversy.[2] A proposed unifying theory suggests that dyspnea results from a mismatch between central respiratory motor activity and afferent information from peripheral receptors.[3]

The respiratory center of the medulla oblongata in the brain stem (consisting of several discrete neuronal clusters, see Figure 23–2) controls breathing through the innervation of the lungs, the airways, and skeletal and diaphragmatic muscles. Efferent signals activate the respiratory muscles that expand the chest walls, inflate the lungs, and produce ventilation.

Chemical stimuli in the blood and mechanical stimuli in the lungs influence volume and pattern of breathing through specific receptors (Figure 23–3). Changes in pCO_2 and pO_2 are sensed by central chemoreceptors in the medulla and peripheral chemoreceptors in the carotid and aortic bodies. Signals from these receptors are transmitted back to the respiratory center, which adjusts breathing to maintain blood gas and acid base homeostasis. Pulmonary stretch receptors in the bronchi and diaphragm are activated when the lung expands. The juxtapulmonary capillary receptors (J-receptors) respond to changes in pulmonary interstitial and capillary pressure. Muscle spindles and tendon organs in the respiratory muscles relay information on muscle tension to the respiratory center and the cortex.

Clinically, dyspnea occurs when the load on the respiratory muscle pump exceeds capacity. This can arise due to an increased load placed upon normal respiratory muscles (conditions causing chest wall restriction such as kyphoscoliosis, or reduced upper airway diameter arising from vocal cord abnormalities such as in multi-system atrophy) or a reduced capacity (conditions causing respiratory muscle weakness, such as neuromuscular disorders). Respiratory drive can be augmented by psychological (wakefulness, anxiety, anger), metabolic (fever, acidosis, hypoxia/hypercapnia), and physical factors (lung distortion/deflation).

Due to the prominence of the symptom of dyspnea in neuromuscular disease, much of this chapter will focus on the treatment of respiratory symptoms in these patients, although the general principles of drug and non-drug treatment may be applied to all types of dyspnea with intractable cause. In any neurologic patient who develops dyspnea, unrelated treatable causes such as infection, pre-existent pulmonary disease, cardiac failure, and anemia should be considered and sought for.

ASSESSMENT

History and Examination

In the majority of cases, dyspnea will occur initially on exertion, but where mobility is limited by the underlying neurologic disorder, other symptoms such as a weak voice, poor cough, or orthopnea may predominate. In most cases, symptoms occur insidiously, but an acute presentation can be precipitated by, for example, aspiration pneumonia. Symptoms of respiratory insufficiency are mostly unspecific, and develop with different intensity in the individual patient (Table 23–1).

Patients with diaphragm weakness will often complain of orthopnea because assuming a recumbent position displaces the abdominal contents into the thorax. However, orthopnea is not a universal finding. Some neuromuscular

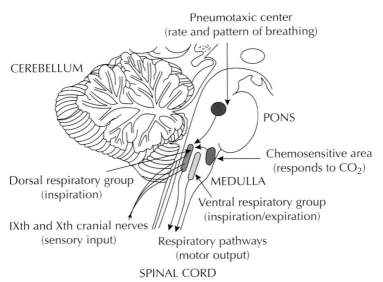

Figure 23–2. Components of the central 'respiratory center'.

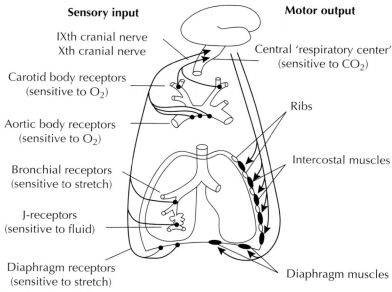

Figure 23–3. Central and peripheral regulation of breathing.

Table 23–1. Symptoms of Chronic Hypoventilation

- Difficulty falling asleep, disturbed sleep, nightmares
- Daytime fatigue and sleepiness, concentration problems
- Morning headache
- Nervousness, tremor, increased sweating, tachycardia
- Depression, anxiety
- Tachypnea, dyspnea, phonation difficulties
- Visible efforts of auxiliary respiratory muscles
- Reduced appetite, weight loss, recurrent gastritis
- Recurrent or chronic upper respiratory tract infections
- Cyanosis, edema
- Vision disturbances, dizziness, syncope
- Diffuse pain in head, neck, and extremities

muscle weakness is profound and, at this stage, most patients are in hypercapnic ventilatory failure.

The signs of respiratory muscle weakness are subtle. Diaphragm weakness can cause paradoxical (inward) movement of the abdomen on inspiration. As diaphragm weakness becomes profound, use of the accessory muscles of respiration (sternocleidomastoids, scalenes, trapezii, and abdominals), becomes prominent. With severe generalized weakness, chest wall movement becomes obviously reduced.

Careful physical examination is of paramount importance in the assessment of neurologic patients with dyspnea. In particular, non-neurological conditions that may contribute to the symptom need to be excluded (e.g. infection, pulmonary disease, cardiac or renal failure, thoracic deformities, hepatomegaly, and anemia).

patients find that they are more breathless on sitting up (platypnea), possibly due to severe abdominal muscle weakness leading to downward displacement of the diaphragm to a disadvantageous position.

As weakness progresses and becomes severe, the volume of speech declines and cough and sneeze become audibly weaker. Dyspnea at rest occurs when respiratory

Sleep and Respiratory Muscle Weakness in Neuromuscular Patients

In neuromuscular patients, alveolar hypoventilation primarily occurs during sleep when the degree of respiratory muscle weakness is not sufficient to cause daytime blood gas derangement or dyspnea.[4,5] As weakness progresses, episodes of hypoventilation occur throughout sleep and cause repeated arousals and sleep fragmentation. This manifests as daytime sleepiness, nightmares, lack of concentration, mood disturbance, and loss of appetite. In many instances, patients will not recognize that frequent awakening is due to respiratory muscle weakness and complain of 'dry mouth' or urinary problems. In other patients, it is the partner or family who is aware of restless and disturbed sleep, periods of apnea at night, or an apparent change of personality or behavior. Eventually, hypoventilation leads to nocturnal hypercapnia and morning headaches, difficulty concentrating, and lethargy.

It should be emphasized that the symptoms of nocturnal hypoventilation arise insidiously, often without daytime dyspnea. Frequently, the hypersomnolence, lack of appetite, and personality change can be wrongly attributed to depression. It is, therefore, important that patients are regularly questioned about sleep disturbance and, if present, appropriate investigations instituted.

Scales

The use of a visual analog scale for dyspnea, similar to that used for the assessment of pain, is simple and straightforward, but only useful for intra-individual comparisons. To look at differences between patients or patient groups, the revised Borg category scale has proven useful.[6] For audit purposes, the dyspnea scale from the Support Team Assessment Schedule (STAS) comprises seven points (0–6) and looks at intensity of the symptom, frequency, and interference with activity.[7] The assessment is performed by a staff member. No specific scale for neurogenic dyspnea has so far been developed.

Tests of Respiratory Muscle Strength

A number of investigations can be used to evaluate respiratory muscle strength.[8] A useful screening test for patients with suspected neuromuscular weakness is the vital capacity (VC) test, performed in the upright and supine positions. Diaphragm weakness is suggested by a greater than 25% fall in VC on assuming a supine position.[9] A normal supine VC makes significant inspiratory muscle weakness unlikely. ALS patients often have difficulty achieving an adequate seal around the mouthpiece causing an underestimation of VC.

Level of ability to cough is the measurement of the cough peak flow, both unassisted and after manual insufflation, which can be achieved using an anesthetic bag and mask.[10] An abnormal result, despite adequate insufflation, indicates an abnormality of the upper airway precluding the adequate glottic closure required for effective cough.

Blood Gas Analysis

Analysis of arterial blood gas tensions is useful and can be done easily on ear lobe samples. However, in the initial stages of respiratory muscle weakness, daytime blood gases are usually normal or show only mild hypoxia. As weakness progresses, daytime hypercapnia occurs. Most ALS patients have normal lungs and, by the time the blood gases show substantial daytime hypoxia in addition to hypercapnia, respiratory muscle weakness is profound and the prognosis is likely to be limited to months or weeks. In neuromuscular disease, it is uncommon to see severe hypoxia in the absence of hypercapnia, and in this case a lung parenchymal cause such as pneumonia or pulmonary embolus should be sought.

Overnight Oximetry and Polysomnography

Most episodes of nocturnal hypoventilation in neuromuscular patients cause significant oxygen desaturation, which leads to arousal and sleep fragmentation. Many pulse oximeters can now store at least eight hours of information and patients can be given the machines to use at home, overnight, to identify desaturations. If the oximetry yields equivocal results, transcutaneous pCO_2 measurements or polysomnography may be helpful where available.[11]

Assessment of Related Constructs

When assessing a complex multifactorial symptom such as dyspnea, the impact of the symptom on daily life and its relationship to concurrent symptoms need to be addressed. Anxiety and pain are known to increase dyspnea and, conversely, dyspneic patients show greater levels of distress from other somatic complaints. The perception of dyspnea may be modulated by hypoxemia and by concomitant drug treatment. Relevant questions include: How much is the patient bothered by the symptom? How much is the family bothered? What is the impact of dyspnea on the patient's quality of life? What are the other elements which influence the patient's quality of life? This information will be required to determine the goals of care, which will lead all subsequent decisions.

NON-PHARMACOLOGICAL TREATMENT

The importance of the non-drug approach to dyspnea treatment in palliative care is highlighted by the premise that 'the emotional experience of breathlessness cannot be separated from its physical experience'.[12] In most cases, dyspnea is accompanied by anxiety, which in turn may increase dyspnea and lead to a vicious cycle resulting in panic attacks. Reassurance and explanation to the patient and relatives, and the calm presence of staff members, are invaluable.

When managing the dyspneic patient, communication with the patient and family is particularly important. It should be emphasized that the patient will not 'choke to death'.[13] Patients and families may benefit from knowing that somnolence related to hypercapnia will probably occur if the dyspnea is associated with declining pulmonary function (as in ALS) and that this will eventually lead to a peaceful death in sleep.

Where respiratory muscle weakness predominates, positioning in an upright position reduces the load on the diaphragm and eases breathing. A fan or a current of fresh air are often perceived as helpful, possibly due to stimulation of mechanoreceptors on the face. Adequate space should be available around the patient.

In pulmonary disease, improvements in dyspnea and anxiety have been shown following distraction interventions such as music during exercise. Other cognitive-behavioral approaches such as relaxation techniques and guided imagery may also be helpful. The effects of physical therapy and breathing retraining exercises vary considerably between patients and are often short-lived, but worth trying.

A standardized approach to non-drug treatment of dyspnea has been tested recently in a multicenter study with favorable results.[14] This nurse-led intervention focuses on helping patients engage with the fear engendered by breathlessness, addressing negative feelings and introducing coping strategies such as activity pacing, breathing retraining, and relaxation techniques, as well as helping patients find meaning in their suffering. In addition, family members are trained in developing supportive skills. The success of this study emphasizes the importance of the non-drug approach in the palliative treatment of dyspnea.

PHARMACOLOGICAL TREATMENT

Dyspnea

A variety of treatments may be considered for the management of dyspnea (Table 23–2). Opioids are widely accepted as the mainstay approach. Oral opioids are commonly used in the clinical situation. In one study of patients with far advanced cancer, 5 mg of parenteral morphine reduced dyspnea and did not cause respiratory depression.[15] This finding has been confirmed in two recent controlled trials,[16,17] thus disproving the myth that morphine administration to dyspneic patients is tantamount to active euthanasia. In the opioid-naïve patient, a starting dose of morphine 2.5–5 mg orally every 4 hours, or the equivalent dose of another opioid, ensures safety and can be rapidly titrated to optimize effects. In patients who are already receiving opioids for pain, the starting dose is typically 25–50% higher than the baseline dose. In urgent situations, repeated boluses of morphine at short intervals, such as 1.5 mg every 10 minutes in the opioid-naïve patient, may be required.[18] Clinical experience shows that

Table 23–2. **Dyspnea Therapy**

1. *Treat reversible causes if present*
   e.g. bronchospasm, heart failure, pneumonia, lung edema due to hyperhydration

2. *Non-pharmacological measures*
   Explanation, reassurance, positioning, breathing exercises, relaxation techniques, calm presence of family, cool draft/fan, physical therapy, space

3. *Intermittent dyspnea*
   Relieve anxiety: lorazepam (0.5–2.5 mg s.l.) or diazepam (2.5–5 mg rectally)
   Use opioids (e.g. morphine) starting with 2.5–5 mg p.o. or 1–2 mg s.c. every 4 hours in the opioid-naïve patient or 25–50% of baseline dose in opioid-treated patients, and titrating as needed; controlled-release preparations are less effective
   If severe: midazolam 5 mg s.c. or 2.5 mg i.v. slowly (i.v. administration carries a higher risk of respiratory depression)

4. *Constant dyspnea*
   Opioids (e.g. morphine); starting dosage as above
   Diazepam or midazolam 2.5–5 mg, mainly as add-on nocté
   In the terminal phase: continuous parenteral infusion of morphine and midazolam may be necessary (the drugs can be mixed together in one syringe)

5. *Oxygen*
   Only if clinically manifest hypoxia is present
   Side effects: respiratory depression, restricts patient's mobility, psychological dependency, may prevent discharge home

controlled-release morphine preparations are often less effective for dyspnea treatment.

Nebulized morphine[19] has also been employed for dyspnea, but controlled studies suggest that it is not better than nebulized saline[20] and may produce side effects.[21] Additional studies are needed before this approach can be recommended as standard practice. Recent data from cancer patients indicate a possible role for nebulized fentanyl[22] and nebulized furosemide;[23] confirmation in larger trials is awaited.

In the terminal phase of patients with brain tumors or other space-occupying lesions, disordered breathing often occurs. Since patients are usually unconscious at this stage, it is assumed that these changes in breathing pattern, which generally appear a few hours before death, do not reflect a subjectively perceived breathlessness. However, they can impart considerable distress to the relatives and require prior explanation, especially in the outpatient setting. If necessary, parenteral morphine may be titrated carefully until labored breathing subsides, in order to relieve the anxiety of the family.

Benzodiazepines also are used frequently in the management of dyspnea, despite the lack of well-controlled studies in neurologic patients. A dose of 25 mg diazepam has been shown to have a negative effect on exercise tolerance and blood gases, but a single 5 mg dose in chronic obstructive airway disease patients improved sleep duration without worsening nocturnal hypoxemia.[24] Lorazepam and midazolam both may be useful in the treatment of terminal dyspnea.[25] For dyspneic bouts that usually have a pronounced anxiety component, sublingual lorazepam (0.5–2.5 mg) is the drug of choice.

The role of oxygen is controversial. It is often applied indiscriminately to all dyspneic patients, despite serious side effects (dry mouth, psychological dependency, reduced mobility). Although oxygen should not be applied on a routine basis, it has been shown to significantly reduce dyspnea in a double-blind, crossover study, provided there is proven hypoxia.[16] In patients with weakness of respiratory muscles and chronic hypercapnia, oxygen administered during sleep may lead to hypoventilation and even respiratory arrest.

Table 23–3. **Therapy for Death Rattle**

1. Explain to family
2. Stop hyperhydration
3. Gentle aspiration and lateral placement
4. 10–20 mg N-butyl-scopolamine s.c. (no central effect)
5. Alternatively, hyoscine (scopolamine base or hydrobromide) or atropine 0.5–1 mg s.c. or i.m. every 2–4 hours; if atropine or hyoscine is used, add anxiolytic (e.g. lorazepam)
6. If necessary, add midazolam 5 mg s.c.

Other strategies have been used to manage dyspnea. Promethazine has been shown to reduce dyspnea in patients with chronic lung disease, but no studies in neurologic patients are available. Some surveys suggest that acupuncture may be effective against dyspnea.[25,26] No benefit has been shown with nebulized lignocaine.[28]

Death Rattle

A disturbing noise, called death rattle, occurs in about half of all dying patients and may contribute significantly to the distress of family members.[29] Death rattle may be caused by salivary and/or bronchial secretions.[30] In patients with brain tumors, this symptom may be relatively prevalent and require aggressive therapy.[29,30] The usual approach to treatment involves the administration of an anticholinergic drug combined with additional measures, like suction. Hyoscine (scopolamine), atropine, and glycopyrrolate are used. Atropine may be centrally excitatory, which can be controlled by benzodiazepines. In a prospective study, good symptom control was achieved in 71% of patients (see Table 23–3).[29] Especially in comatose patients, noisy tachypnea, with a respiratory rate of 30–50/minute, may also give the impression of severe distress. Parenteral morphine titrated to a rate of respiration of 10–15/minute may be useful.[31]

Cough

Two types of cough-related problems need to be distinguished: ineffective cough in neuromuscular patients due to weakness, which can contribute to the accumulation of thick mucous secretions, and chronic cough due to central or peripheral triggering of the cough reflex.

INEFFECTIVE COUGH AND THICK MUCOUS SECRETIONS

This is one of the most harrowing symptoms in neuromuscular disorders such as ALS. Late-stage ALS patients often suffer greatly because of thick mucous secretions blocking the upper airways, which result from a combination of diminished fluid intake and reduced coughing pressure, as well as chronic upper respiratory tract infections damaging the transporting ability of the mucosal hair cells.

A normal cough requires the patient to inspire an adequate volume of air, which is then held behind the closed vocal cords while the contracting expiratory muscles build up a large intra-thoracic pressure. The vocal cords then open suddenly to release the air as a cough. Weakness of the expiratory muscles frequently coexists with inspiratory muscle weakness and neuromuscular patients often complain of an ineffective cough.

The expiratory pressure can be augmented by assisted coughing techniques,[31] in which the patient or carer provides a manual abdominal thrust as the patient coughs. This technique can be extended by providing inspiratory support or manual insufflation using a bag and mask prior to the cough.[31] If this cannot adequately clear secretions, then a mechanical insufflator-exsufflator (In-Exsufflator, J.H. Emerson Co., Cambridge, MA; www.jhemerson.com) can be used.[31,32]

Several attempts at treating thick mucous secretions have been tried, albeit none in a controlled fashion. The nebulization of saline or an adrenergic bronchodilator such as terbutaline can improve the effectiveness of cough by loosening mucus or stimulating ciliary movement.[33] Physical therapy with vibration massage may also be helpful, especially in the initial stages. Drugs which claim to reduce the viscosity of mucus have usually been found to be lacking in effectiveness.[34] N-acetylcysteine is helpful only in a minority of cases, because it requires a large fluid intake and basically dilutes the secretions, resulting in a higher secretion volume that does not necessarily ameliorate the problem if the coughing effort is insufficient. Suction may become necessary, but is usually not fully effective unless performed via a tracheostomy.

Other treatments which have shown benefit in an uncontrolled survey include dark grape juice, papaya enzymes, sugar-free citrus lozenges, grape seed oil, and betablockers.[35] Reduction of alcohol and caffeine, substitution of dairy products, moistening of the air, and steam inhalation may be helpful. It should be noted that the inhalation of anticholinergic drugs, such as hyoscine compounds, or the use of oral nabilone, may reduce ciliary motion and thus thicken mucus. A satisfactory palliative therapy for thick mucous secretions is still not available and more research is needed in this area.

CHRONIC COUGH

Cough is a normal protective mechanism, but if it becomes chronic it can cause great suffering to patients and caregivers. Chronic cough can be exhausting and lead to anxiety, vomiting, pain, and even rib fractures.

Cough can arise through excessive bronchial secretions, by aspiration of foreign material, or through abnormal stimulation of receptors in the airway (e.g. by ACE inhibitors). Aspiration of gastric contents or saliva may cause nocturnal cough. Respiratory infections may produce excess sputum and trigger the cough reflex. Cough may be wet or dry (i.e. non-productive).

The first aim of treatment, where possible, is elimination of the underlying cause (e.g. antibiotics for infection). If smoking is the likely cause, three to four weeks or longer are needed to obtain antitussive effect from stopping it. This should be balanced against the patient's life expectancy and quality. Non-drug measures such as positioning of the patient (e.g. lying on the same side as a pleural effusion), postural drainage, and physiotherapy can be helpful.

In most cases oral cough suppressants are sufficient for relief of cough. The most effective agents are opioids.[34] Codeine or dihydrocodeine are the drugs of first choice. Hydrocodone (3×5–10 mg, add laxatives) may help in refractory cases.[36] Dextromethorphan hydrobromide, which is often incorporated in cough mixtures, is structurally related to opioids and has a central cough suppressant action with few or no analgesic and sedative effects.

Nebulized local anesthetics (lignocaine or bupivacaine) are particularly helpful when irritation of the pharynx or airways is the cause of cough, but duration of the effect is short (20–30 minutes), and they may induce bronchospasm. If nocturnal aspiration of saliva is the cause of cough (as in patients with bulbar symptoms due to ALS or MS), lateral positioning of the patient to allow drooling outside the oral cavity and drugs for reduction of salivary secretions (hyoscine hydrobromide s.c. or transdermal, or glycopyrronium bromide) are recommended.

VENTILATION

Non-Invasive Ventilation

Non-invasive ventilation has been used to correct the physiological abnormalities and symptoms arising from nocturnal hypoventilation in a wide variety of neuromuscular and chest wall diseases[37] and in many disorders such as kyphoscoliosis and the late sequelae of polio. Non-invasive intermittent positive pressure ventilation (NIPPV) via a nasal or naso-facial mask is now standard practice.

A number of non-invasive forms of ventilation have been successfully used to treat respiratory failure in ALS patients[38] and several reports have shown that NIPPV is associated with increased survival[38,39] and relieves symptoms of sleep disturbance, reduces breathlessness and morning headache, improves appetite, and makes the voice louder.[40,41] However, wide differences exist in the uptake of ventilation among ALS patients.[42] In the United Kingdom, the majority of ALS patients are not offered NIPPV. By contrast, the recently published recommendations by the Quality Standards Subcommittee of the American Academy of Neurology propose the use of NIPPV for symptomatic relief of hypoventilation in ALS.[43] This difference may in part be due to financial considerations, but the major cause of reluctance to offer NIPPV appears to be related to the inevitable progressive loss of function with prolonged survival and the belief that quality of life will eventually be so poor that the benefits of any initial improvements are lost. Studies on patients with neuromuscular diseases using long-term ventilation, however, do not support this assumption. Simonds et al.[44] reported SF-36 data on Duchenne muscular dystrophy patients using long-term NIPPV (3–72 months). As might be expected, the domain covering physical function was reduced, but domains covering mental health, role limitation due to physical and emotional factors, and social function did not differ from age-matched controls. Moss and co-workers[45] reported the views of 50 ALS patients on long-term mechanical ventilation (43 on tracheostomy ventilation (TV) and seven on NIPPV). The majority were satisfied with their lives and would choose ventilation again (80% of those on TV, 100% on NIPPV), particularly those who were living at home rather than in an institution, and who had made the decision to go onto mechanical ventilation themselves rather than starting it as an emergency without prior discussion. This, and a previous study,[40] emphasized the huge burdens that caring for a TV patient at home place on the family. Non-invasive techniques of ventilation are reported to be preferable to TV both by patients and caregivers.[46]

TYPES OF NON-INVASIVE VENTILATION

Non-invasive methods of ventilation either apply negative pressure to the thorax or abdomen, effectively sucking out the chest wall, or positive pressure to the airway, pushing in air. The first negative pressure ventilator was the tank ventilator (the 'iron lung'), which required the patient to be enclosed in a cabinet. Negative pressure devices, which enclose only the chest and/or abdomen (cuirass, pneumojacket, intermittent abdominal pressure ventilator, pneumobelt), are more portable and have been used extensively by ALS patients for both nocturnal and continuous ventilation. However, there are a number of disadvantages. As negative pressure is applied to the thorax, it can intensify or precipitate upper airway collapse and obstructive apnea due to bulbar insufficiency. Pressure from the devices can cause chest wall discomfort, and may cause skin ulceration if used continuously.

Most ALS patients are treated with positive pressure ventilation, in which ventilation is delivered via a nasal mask of the type used to treat obstructive sleep apnea. Many positive pressure ventilators exist, which are suitable for home use. They can either deliver an intermittent positive inspiratory pressure or bi-level positive pressure in which different levels of positive pressure are delivered in inspiration and expiration. It is essential that the ventilator used can be programed with a back-up rate capable of achieving adequate ventilation during apnea or hypoventilation. Most can be 'triggered' by the patient to deliver extra breaths if required.

BULBAR PATIENTS

Inability to protect the upper airway is generally regarded as a relative contraindication to the use of NIPPV. Bulbar ALS patients can have abnormalities of the upper airway and are at increased risk from aspiration if impaired swallowing leads to pooling of saliva. However, aspiration with NIPPV has not been an important problem in our clinical practice, even in bulbar patients.

Bulbar ALS patients may find that NIPPV does not relieve their symptoms. In a further study,[39] about two-thirds of patients who were unable to tolerate NIPPV had moderate or severe bulbar symptoms, although 30% of patients with significant bulbar symptoms did tolerate the treatment. In our experience, a small number of bulbar patients are intolerant of NIPPV and in these cases the patients complained of intermittent episodes of breathlessness and had abnormal flow volume loops and uncoordinated movement of the vocal cords on endoscopy. If the patient's swallowing is severely impaired, we would advocate gastrostomy. If the patient does not tolerate NIPPV, it is important to discuss the advantages and disadvantages of proceeding to TV.

GOALS AND LIMITATIONS OF NON-INVASIVE VENTILATION

There are no generally accepted criteria for initiation of NIPPV in neuromuscular disease. NIPPV is primarily aimed at the palliation of symptoms rather than prolongation of life.[11] A selection of patients is based on the symptoms shown in Table 23–1. Studies on prophylactic NIPPV in patients with Duchenne's muscular dystrophy without signs or symptoms of hypoventilation have shown no survival advantage, and patients did not tolerate the treatment well.[47]

However, even for patients meeting our criteria, NIPPV is not universally indicated or appropriate. When discussing NIPPV, patients and carers need to be aware of the burden that this treatment can place on the family, the limits of social service provision, and the fact that it may prolong survival in the face of increasing disability. Patients should understand that the symptoms of breathlessness can be palliated with drugs such as benzodiazepines and opioids, although NIPPV is clearly superior to these in the treatment of symptoms of nocturnal hypoventilation. NIPPV does not preclude the use of these drugs. Although discussion about the progressive nature of respiratory muscle weakness and ventilator dependency may cause anxiety in both the patient and healthcare worker, most patients wish to have detailed information and prefer to participate actively in decisions about their care.[48] In addition, it is our practice to refer all patients (with their consent) to local hospice services. This includes those who accept and those who decline NIPPV. The respiratory and hospice services should be seen as part of the multidisciplinary approach to the care of these patients.

Tracheostomy Ventilation

If progression of respiratory muscle weakness or bulbar symptoms limit NIPPV, the initiation of TV needs to be discussed. TV is usually initiated as a life-prolonging treatment, often in an emergency situation without prior consent. A voluntary ending of TV, even if requested by a competent patient, is still a problem for many physicians. If patients are informed in advance on the course of the terminal phase and the available treatments for dyspnea, the majority of ALS patients refuse TV.[49]

When discussing this option, patients and caregivers should be made aware of the added burden that a TV entails, especially for caregivers. Tracheostomies have to be regularly suctioned, can be detrimental to swallowing,

thereby precipitating the need for a gastrostomy, and although speaking tubes are available, they require a degree of respiratory muscle strength to generate speech which patients frequently cannot achieve. In general, patients prefer to remain on non-invasive methods of ventilation for as long as possible. However, TV may be an important option and lead to good quality of life for patient and family in selected cases.[50]

REFERENCES

1. Mehta AD, Wright WB, Kirby BJ. Ventilatory function in Parkinson's disease. Br Med J 1978;280:1456.
2. Ripamonti C, Bruera E. Dyspnea: pathophysiology and assessment. J Pain Symptom Manage 1997;13:220–232.
3. American Thoracic Society. Dyspnea—mechanisms, assessment, and management. A consensus statement. Am J Respir Crit Care Med 1999;159:321–340.
4. Gay PC, Westbrook PR, Daube JR, Litchy WJ, Windebank AJ, Iverson R. Effects of alterations in pulmonary function and sleep variables on survival in patients with amyotrophic lateral sclerosis. Mayo Clin Proc 1991;66:686–694.
5. Fergerson KA, Strong MJ, Ahmad D, George CFP. Sleep-disordered breathing in amyotrophic lateral sclerosis. Chest 1996;110:664–669.
6. Mahler DA, Rosiello RA, Harver A, Lentine T, McGovern JF, Daubenspeck JA. Comparison of clinical dyspnea ratings and psychophysical measurements of respiratory sensation in obstructive airway disease. Am Rev Respir Dis 1991;135:1229–1233.
7. Higginson I, McCarthy M. Measuring symptoms in terminal cancer: are pain and dyspnea controlled?. J R Soc Med 1989;82:264–267.
8. Polkey MI, Green M, Moxham J. Measurement of respiratory muscle strength. Thorax 1995;50:1131–1135.
9. Allen S, Hunt B, Green M. Fall in vital capacity with posture. Br J Dis Chest 1985;79:267–271.
10. Bach JR, ed. Pulmonary rehabilitation. The Obstructive and Paralytic Conditions. Hanley and Belfus Inc., Philadelphia, 1995: 312–313.
11. Lyall R, Moxham J, Leigh N. Dyspnea. In: Oliver D, Borasio GD, Walsh D, eds. Palliative Care in Amyotrophic Lateral Sclerosis. Oxford University Press, Oxford, 2000:43–56.
12. Corner J, Meinir K, Bredin M, Plant H, Bailey C. Cancer nursing practice development: understanding breathlessness. J Clin Nurs 2001;10:103–108.
13. Neudert CH, Oliver D, Wasner M, Borasio GD. The course of the terminal phase in patients with amyotrophic lateral sclerosis. J Neurol 2001;248:612–616.
14. Krishnasamy M, Corner J, Bredin M, Plant H, Bailey C. Cancer nursing practice development: understanding breathlessness. J Clin Nurs 2001;10:103–108.
15. Bruera E, Macmillan K, MacDonald RN. Effects of morphine on dyspnea of terminal cancer patients.

Journal of Pain and Symptom Management 1990;5:341–344.

16. Bruera E, de Stoutz N, Velasco–Leiva A, Schoeller T, Hanson J. Effects of oxygen on dyspnea in hypoxemic terminal-cancer patients. Lancet 1993;342:13–14.

17. Mazzocato C, Buclin T, Rapin CH. The effects of morphine on dyspnea and ventilatory function in elderly patients with advanced cancer: a randomized double-blind controlled trial. Ann Oncol 1999;10:1511–1514.

18. Kumar KS, Rajagopal MR, Naseema AM. Intravenous morphine for emergency treatment of cancer pain. Palliat Med 2000;14:183–188.

19. Zeppetella G. Nebulized morphine in the palliation of dyspnea. Palliat Med 1997;11:267–275.

20. Noseda A, Carpiaux JP, Markstein C, Meyvaert A, de Maertelaer V. Disabling dyspnea in patients with advanced disease: lack of effect of nebulized morphine. Eur Respir J 1997;10:1079–1083.

21. Lang E, Jedeikin R. Acute respiratory depression as a complication of nebulized morphine. Can J Anaesth 1998;45:60–62.

22. Coyne PJ, Viswanathan R, Smith TJ. Nebulized fentanyl citrate improves patients' perception of breathing, respiratory rate, and oxygen saturation in dyspnea. J Pain Symptom Manage 2002;23:157–160.

23. Shimoyama N, Shimoyama M. Nebulized furosemide as a novel treatment for dyspnea in terminal cancer patients. J Pain Symptom Manage 2002;23:73–76.

24. Woodcock A, Gross E, Geddes D. Drug treatment of breathlessness: contrasting effects of diazepam and promethazine in pink puffers. Br Med J 1981;283:343–346.

25. Mc Namara P, Minton M, Twycross R. Use of midazolam in palliative care. Palliat Med 1991;5:244–249.

26. Filshie J, Penn K, Ashley S, Davis C. Acupuncture for the relief of cancer-related breathlessness. Palliat Med 1996;10:145–150.

27. Pan CX, Morrison RS, Ness J, Fugh–Berman A, Leipzig RM. Complementary and alternative medicine in the management of pain, dyspnea, and nausea and vomiting near the end of life. A systematic review. J Pain Symptom Manage 2000;20:374–387.

28. Wilcock A, Corcoran R, Tattersfield AE. Safety and efficacy of nebulized lignocaine in patients with cancer and breathlessness. Palliat Med 1994;8:35–38.

29. Morita T, Tsunoda J, Inoue S, Chihara S. Risk factors for death rattle in terminally ill cancer patients: a prospective exploratory study. Palliat Med 2000;14:19–23.

30. Bennett MI. Death rattle: an audit of hyoscine (scopolamine) use and review of management. J Pain Symptom Manage 1996;12:229–233.

31. Bach JR. Update and perspective on noninvasive respiratory muscle aids. Part 2: The expiratory aids. Chest 1994;105:1538–1544.

32. Bach JR, Smith WH, Michaels J, et al. Airway secretion clearance by mechanical exsufflaton for postpoliomyelitis ventilator assisted individuals. Arch Phys Med Rehabil 1993;74:170–177.

33. Sutton PP, Gemmell HG, Innes N, et al. Use of nebulized saline and nebulized terbutaline as an adjunct to chest physiotherapy. Thorax 1998;43:57–60.

34. Fuller RW, Jackson DM. Physiology and treatment of cough. Thorax 1990;45:425–430.

35. Foulsom, M. Secretion management in motor neuron disease. Proceedings of the 10th International Symposium on ALS/MND. International Alliance of ALS/MND Associations, Vancouver, 1999.

36. Homsi J, Walsh D, Nelson KA, et al. A phase II study of hydrocodone for cough in advanced cancer. Am J Hosp Palliat Care 2002;19:49–56.

37. Bach JR, Alba AS. Management of chronic alveolar hypoventilation by nasal ventilation. Chest 1990;97:52–57.

38. Bach JR. Amyotrophic lateral sclerosis: predictors for prolongation of life by non-invasive respiratory aids. Arch Phys Med Rehabil 1995;76:828–832.

39. Aboussouan LS, Khan SU, Meeker DP, Stelmach K, Mitsumoto H. Effect of non-invasive positive pressure ventilation on survival in amyotrophic lateral sclerosis. Ann Intern Med 1999;127:450–453.

40. Moss AH, Casey P, Stocking CB, Roos RP, Brooks BR, Seigler M. Home ventilation for amyotrophic lateral sclerosis patients: outcomes, costs and patient, family and physician attitudes. Neurology 1993;43:438–443.

41. Schlamp V, Karg O, Abel A, Schlotter B, Wasner M, Borasio GD. Non-invasive intermittent home mechanical ventilation as a palliative treatment in amyotrophic lateral sclerosis. Nervenarzt 1998;69:1074–1082.

42. Borasio GD, Gelinas DF, Yanagisawa N. Mechanical ventilation in amyotrophic lateral sclerosis: a cross-cultural perspective. J Neurol 1998;245(Suppl. 2):S7–S12.

43. Miller RG, Rosenberg JA, Gelinas DF, et al. Practice parameters: the care of the patient with amyotrophic lateral sclerosis (an evidence based review) Report of the quality standards subcommittee of the American Academy of Neurology. Neurology 1999;52:1311–1323.

44. Simonds A, Muntoni F, Heather S, Fielding S. Impact of nasal ventilation on survival in hypercapnic Duchenne muscular dystrophy. Thorax 1998;53:949–952.

45. Moss AH, Oppenheimer EA, Casey P, et al. Patients with amyotrophic lateral sclerosis receiving long-term mechanical ventilation. Advance care planning and outcomes. Chest 1996;110:249–255.

46. Bach JR. A comparison of long-term ventilatory support alternatives from the perspective of the patient and care-giver. Chest 1993;104:1702–1706.

47. Raphael J, Chevret S, Chastang C, Bouvet F. Randomized trial of preventative nasal ventilation in Duchenne muscular dystrophy. Lancet 1994;343:1600–1604.

48. Silverstein M, Stocking C, Antel J, Beckwith J, Roos R, Seigler M. Amyotrophic lateral sclerosis and life-sustaining therapy: patients' desires for information, participation in decision making and life sustaining therapy. Mayo Clin Proc 1991;66:906–913.

49. Gelinas DF, O'Connor P, Miller RG. Quality of life for ventilator-dependent ALS patients and their caregivers. J Neurol Sci 1998;160(Suppl. 1):S134–S136.

50. Gelinas DF. Amyotrophic lateral sclerosis and invasive ventilation. In: Oliver D, Borasio GD, Walsh D, eds. Palliative Care in Amyotrophic Lateral Sclerosis. Oxford University Press, Oxford, 2000:56–62.

Chapter 24

Bowel Symptoms

Nigel P. Sykes

CONSTIPATION
Background
Pathophysiology
Assessment
Prophylaxis
Non-Drug Treatment of Constipation
Laxative Therapy

DIARRHEA
Pathophysiology
Assessment
Management
FECAL INCONTINENCE
SUMMARY

CASE HISTORY

Constipation in palliative care is a *symptom*, not a disease, and is, therefore, defined by the patient rather than the physician. In the assessment of bowel function, it is important not to be misled by the 'diarrhea' resulting from fecal impaction; rectal examination reveals most cases of impaction.

Good general symptom control is important in the prophylaxis of constipation, as it will maximize physical activity and food and fluid intake. However, too much dietary fiber may not be tolerated, and fiber alone is unlikely to resolve severe constipation.

When prescribing laxatives, cost and patient preference should be taken into account. For other than mild constipation, a combination of stimulant and softening laxatives may be preferable to either category used alone. The most common causes of diarrhea are laxative excess and intestinal infections.

Diarrhea has to be distinguished from fecal impaction with overflow. Supportive measures in the management of diarrhea are hydration (usually possible orally or via a gastrostomy tube) and provision of electrolytes and carbohydrates. The most effective antidiarrheal agents are opioids, of which loperamide has the most evidence for efficacy and codeine is the cheapest.

Diarrhea that is persistent or accompanied by toxicity may benefit from antibiotic treatment.

A 60-year-old woman was referred to a palliative care unit with a seven-year history of a gradual global loss of function that had begun with problems in balancing. A diagnosis of multiple system atrophy had been made. She now found it difficult to move without help and had some dysphagia and speech deterioration due to bulbar impairment. Mentation was not affected. Catheterization had been carried out for urinary incontinence but the sensation of the need to defecate was retained, although she was often unable to do so.

A laxative combination of magnesium hydroxide/ liquid paraffin mixture and senna was being used. However, she tended not to be able to open her bowels for several days at a time and then, in response to titration of her laxatives, to have an urgent bowel movement resulting in incontinence and, on two occasions, rectal prolapse. It was decided to maintain her on a softening laxative alone and to precipitate defecation by use of rectal interventions when appropriate support was available. Trials established that she preferred the use of mini-enemas to that of stimulant suppositories for this purpose.

Initially, stimulation of a bowel movement was attempted each day. Although this was largely successful, the patient eventually felt that as her habit in health had been to open her bowels on alternate days she would rather maintain this pattern now, and so the frequency of rectal interventions was halved. In this way continence was largely achieved and further episodes of rectal prolapse avoided.

Discussion

This case illustrates the individual approach that is necessary in the management of constipation in any advanced illness. Appropriately, an attempt was made to provide a balance of softening and peristalsis-stimulating laxatives in order to secure easy bowel opening. Unfortunately, the patient's immobility, and probably a degree of anal sphincter impairment, meant that it was difficult in practice to steer a middle path between constipation and an urgency of defecation that resulted in incontinence.

The response was to use oral laxatives simply to soften the stool and so avoid colic. Timing of defecation was achieved by use of rectal measures to provide direct stimulation of stool expulsion together with some local stool softening and lubrication. This could, in theory, have been accomplished either by suppositories containing a peristaltic stimulant or by a variety of proprietary enema preparations. The patient herself preferred the subjective effect of an enema. Despite some evidence that in these circumstances daily rectal intervention provides better results in terms of continence, she preferred an alternate day approach, and this was agreed. The issue here is that in the context of concurrent disease, constipation has importance as a symptom rather than as another disease entity. It is treated in order to improve the patient's comfort. Hence, it is for the patient, with professional support, to define when they are constipated, when that constipation has been relieved, and what treatment is least burdensome for them.

CONSTIPATION

Background

Constipation is common across a range of neurological diseases.[1] A prevalence of 54% has been reported in multiple sclerosis (MS)[2] and 65%–86% in advanced amyotrophic lateral sclerosis (ALS). These figures are not widely removed from those found in hospitalized elderly people[3] or in cancer palliative care patients who are not taking opioid analgesics.[4] The importance of the condition lies in the distress it causes as a symptom, which in some surveys has been more troublesome than pain.

Therefore, it is appropriate that constipation is treated as a symptom, and defined by each person for themselves. Objective criteria have been suggested and widely accepted in gastroenterology, in particular an average of less than three stools per week, or the existence of straining during at least 25% of defecations, but many people who would not meet these criteria nevertheless consider themselves to be constipated.[5] The range of normal bowel function is very wide and what matters is the deviation from what the individual considers normal for themselves rather than a deviation from a population average.

Pathophysiology

In neurological disease constipation may be due either to the neurological damage itself, or may result non-specifically from being chronically ill or from the drugs used for symptom control. These factors may, of course, occur in combination and, occasionally, there has been a history of idiopathic constipation predating the current condition.

Neural control of intestinal activity is mediated via the myenteric nerve plexus which lies between the circular and longitudinal muscle layers. This, and the less dense submucosal plexus, are linked to the central nervous system (CNS) by both sympathetic and parasympathetic systems. Animal studies provide evidence that the sympathetic system exerts an inhibitory influence on colonic contractility. In man, the megacolon of Ogilvie's syndrome—a response to severe medical or surgical stress in the elderly—has been attributed to sympathetic effects on the intestine. Interruption of the sympathetic supply to the gut causes no clear pattern of effects, but it has been postulated that reduction in sympathetic input may play a part in the diarrhea that has been reported to occur occasionally after celiac plexus blockade.[6]

However, there is clinical evidence for an excitatory effect of parasympathetic input to the large bowel in humans, as a low spinal transection or interruption of the extrinsic pelvic nerves in man markedly reduces motility, leading to colonic dilation and slowed transit in the descending and distal transverse colon. This excitation is apparently generated at spinal cord level, since a high cord transection produces little change in colonic activity, although such injury does abolish the colonic motility response to food. The sympathetic and para-sympathetic nervous systems are not the only nerve influences on intestinal activity though. There is evidence for the existence of non-adrenergic, non-cholinergic inputs; and the intestine itself has inherent contractile and pacemaking abilities.

Constipation may reflect not only delayed transit of food residues through the bowel but also difficulties in initiating defecation. In MS, both prolonged colonic transit and abnormal-ities of defecation have been found.[7] Normal defecation depends on the ability of upper anal canal receptors to detect the presence of stool, and on the relaxation of the involuntary internal anal sphincter and of puborectalis, which also exerts a sphincter function. These actions are abolished by lower motor neuron lesions to produce loss of rectal sensation, decreased rectal tone, and inability to defe-cate. Upper motor neuron lesions also destroy rectal sensation, but leave intact both reflex relaxation of the internal sphincter and the anocolonic reflex. Hence many patients with high spinal lesions learn to initiate defecation by digital stimulation of the anal canal.

The reasons why chronic illness produces constipation are multiple. Most activity in the large bowel consists of mixing movements, and peristaltic activity to move colonic con-tents distally occurs only a few times a day, triggered by gastric emptying of meals and by general physical activity. As meals become smaller and less frequent, and mobility is reduced, both these triggers will become less effective. There is often reduced intake of fluid as well as food, which results in more complete water absorption from the bowel and consequently a drier, harder stool. Whe-ther constipation is exacerbated by physiolo-gical involvement of disease-induced cytokines in the control of gut motility and secretion remains to be determined.

Among drugs, morphine and other opioids are probably the most important single con-stipating factor which can be isolated, but they operate against a background of widespread constipation arising from debility. Opioids reduce gut peristalsis and rectal sensitivity, increase sphincter tone throughout the bowel, and may increase net water absorption from the gut contents. In addition, any drug with anti-cholinergic effects has constipating potential, as do anticonvulsants and iron.

Assessment

History taking should include an inquiry about constipation and, if it is present, details about the patient's current bowel frequency and need to strain at stool and of how these differ from what has normally been experienced in the past. If there has been a change, a rectal examination is needed, unless there is a clear report of a satisfactory evacuation within the past day or so. The purpose of the examination is to assess the consistency of the stool and, particularly, to uncover the existence of fecal impaction in the rectum which might need local intervention for removal.

A major pitfall in the clinical assessment of bowel function is impaction, which produces overflow of liquid stool past the fecal mass, leading the patient to complain of diarrhea. Any diarrhea which occurs following a prior period of constipation, or is frequent but of small volume, or produces fecal incontinence, should prompt a rectal examination. Ninety-eight percent of impactions are said to occur in the rectum and, therefore, should be picked up by adequate clinical assessment.

Bowel distension from constipation can cause nausea or precipitate urinary incon-tinence in the elderly or debilitated, so the onset of either of these symptoms ought to stimulate enquiry about bowel function.

Occasionally there is doubt as to whether a patient has severe constipation or an obs-tructive ileus. Erect and supine abdominal radiographs are then indicated to help make the distinction, but in general, investigations are not required in the routine assessment of constipation.

Prophylaxis

The pathophysiology of constipation suggests several prophylactic measures such as increas-ing dietary fiber, encouraging oral fluids, and improving mobility. Specialist dietary advice can help in maximizing dietary fiber intake when appetite is declining or dysphagia is increasing. An adequate fluid intake is very important, as dehydration will result in a dry stool that is difficult to expel. Good control of symptoms, physiotherapy, and the provision of appropriate mobility aids will help avoid constipation through facilitating activity. However, in practice, the possibility of making significant changes in these areas diminishes as the disease progresses and disability increases.

Non-Drug Treatment of Constipation

Biofeedback, or behavioral treatment focused on the bowel, has been used with some success in chronic idiopathic constipation. Some of the same physiological abnormalities of defecation found in a proportion of this group, such as paradoxical puborectalis muscle contraction, can also be demonstrated in people with MS.[8] Biofeedback has now been tried in a small number of subjects with MS who were constipated.[9] A beneficial effect was reported in a minority of the patients who were relatively well and were free of relapsing disease, but no improvement was obtained in those whose condition was more advanced and progressive.

Claims are made for a variety of complementary approaches to constipation, but without evidence of usefulness. Abdominal massage has been found to be as effective as laxative therapy in a group of adults with learning difficulties, but at the expense of over 1.5 additional hours of staff time each week.[10]

As a result of the difficulties with prophylaxis or non-drug approaches in the later stages of illness, most people with advanced neurological disease who are constipated will require laxative therapy.

Laxative Therapy

The basic division of laxatives is between *stimulants* and *softeners*. This division seems useful in clinical practice although, in fact, any drug that stimulates peristalsis will accelerate transit, allow less time for water absorption, and so produce a softer stool. Similarly, softening the stool involves increasing its bulk, which will result in increased distension of the

intestinal wall and a consequent stimulation of reflex enteric muscle contraction.

Most trials of laxative drugs have been carried out in idiopathic constipation or in geriatrics rather than in neurology or palliative medicine. The results do not allow a clear recommendation of one agent over another because of the small size of the studies, the number of different preparations, and the various endpoints and conditions involved. However, certain statements can be made:

- Systematic review evidence suggests that any kind of laxative can increase stool frequency by about 1.4 bowel actions per week compared with placebo.[11]
- There is limited experimental evidence that the optimal combination of effectiveness with few adverse effects and low dose is achieved by using a combination of stimulant and softening laxatives rather than either alone.[12]
- Laxative preparations vary significantly in price and physical characteristics. Ready-made combinations tend to be expensive. Given the lack of major differences in efficacy, cost and individual patient acceptability should both be strong influences in prescribing choice.[13]

The aim of laxative therapy is comfortable defecation, not any particular frequency of evacuation. No single laxative dose is adequate for everyone, and many patients are subjected to both rectal interventions and an inadequate oral dose of laxative. The dose needs to be titrated against the response and the advent of adverse effects, remembering the latent period of action of the drug concerned, and should be increased prophylactically if, say, opioids are introduced or their dose is being substantially increased.

ORAL LAXATIVES

Stimulant Laxatives

Examples: senna, bisacodyl, sodium picosulfate, danthron (only available in combination-preparations).

Starting doses: senna 15 mg daily, bisacodyl 10 mg daily, sodium picosulfate 5 mg daily, danthron 50 mg daily.

- Act directly on the myenteric nerves to evoke gut muscle contraction
- Reduce gut water absorption

- Evidence for intestinal damage from these agents is poor
- Can produce marked colic, particularly if not combined with a softening agent
- Onset of action 6 to 12 hours
- Danthron causes red urinary discoloration and perianal rashes

Softening Laxatives

Osmotic Laxatives. Examples: magnesium sulfate, magnesium hydroxide, lactulose, polyethylene glycol (PEG)

Starting doses: magnesium hydroxide or sulfate 2–4 g daily, lactulose 15 ml b.d., PEG one sachet in 125 ml water daily (fecal impaction, 8 sachets in 1 liter of water over 6 hours)

- Magnesium sulfate and hydroxide have stimulant as well as osmotic actions at higher doses. The sulfate is the more potent. They are cheap.
- Magnesium sulfate used alone can help resistant constipation. There is a risk of hypermagnesemia with chronic use.
- Lactulose—is expensive; needed in large volumes if used alone in marked constipation; causes flatulence in around 20% of users
- PEG has been reported to be effective as an oral treatment for fecal impaction and in particular, in a small study, to be of benefit for constipation associated with Parkinson's disease and multiple systems atrophy.[14] However, it may have to be taken in substantial volumes (500–1000 ml per day), which can prove unacceptable to frailer patients.

Surfactant Laxatives. Examples: docusate sodium, poloxamer (available only in combination with danthron)

Starting dose: docusate sodium 300 mg daily

- These drugs increase water penetration of the stool
- Evidence for laxative efficacy is limited

Lubricant Laxative. Example: Liquid paraffin

Starting dose: 10 ml daily

- Chronic paraffin use can cause fat-soluble vitamin deficiencies, has been associated with anal fecal leakage, and has been reported to have caused a bezoar. None of these adverse effects has been linked with the emulsion of liquid paraffin with magnesium hydroxide, which is currently the most common form in which it is used in the United Kingdom
- Inexpensive

Bulking Agents. Examples: bran, methylcellulose, ispaghula

Starting doses: bran 8 g daily, others 3–4 g daily

- Bulking agents are 'normalizers' rather than true laxatives: they will soften a hard stool but make firmer a loose one.
- Increase stool bulk partly by providing material that resists bacterial breakdown and hence remains in the gut, and partly by providing a substrate for bacterial growth and gas production.
- Effective in mild constipation, but probably not in severe constipation.
- Need to be taken with ample water (at least 200–300 ml); this and their consistency are unacceptable to many ill patients.
- If taken with inadequate water, a viscous mass may result, which can cause intestinal tract obstruction.

Rectal Laxatives

Most patients prefer oral laxatives to rectal, whose use should accordingly be minimized by optimizing laxative treatment by mouth. There is, however, a particular role for enemas and suppositories in the relief of fecal impaction and in bowel management in patients whose neurological dysfunction is resulting in fecal incontinence. Evidence to guide their use is scantier even than that for oral laxatives. Anything introduced into the rectum can stimulate defecation via the anocolonic reflex, but among rectal laxatives only bisacodyl suppositories have a pharmacological stimulant action. Glycerine suppositories, and arachis or olive oil enemas, soften and lubricate the stool, as do proprietary mini-enemas, which contain mixtures of surfactants.

DIARRHEA

Diarrhea, defined as the passage of loose stool frequently or with urgency, is much less common in neurological palliative care than constipation. No prevalence figures appear to have been reported other than in spinal injury, where 14% of patients experience diarrhea.[15] This may in part be due to impaired anal sphincter control, so that it becomes much easier to precipitate urgency of defecation and hence a sense of diarrhea.

Pathophysiology

The daily fluid flow through the jejunum is 6–8 liters, only about 1.5 liters of which come from the diet. Virtually all of this fluid is absorbed again in the ileum and colon, to leave only 100–200 ml per day to be excreted in the stools. In particular, the colon absorbs over 90% of the fluid presented to it, and so a small proportional change in net colonic fluid absorption will make a major alteration in fecal consistency. Such a change can occur through four principal mechanisms:

1. Increased osmolality of intestinal contents, resulting in osmotic flow of water into the gut. The disaccharide-containing elixirs, which form the basis of some liquid medications, can cause diarrhea in this way.
2. Increased electrolyte (and hence fluid) secretion in response to luminal factors. These factors may be hormones, such as vasoactive intestinal polypeptide (VIP), bacterial toxins as in *E. coli* diarrhea, or detergents. This last category includes not only some laxatives but also bile acids and fatty acids. Damage to the spinal cord or to the autonomic or myenteric nervous systems may cause changes in intestinal motility which, instead of themselves accounting for the change in stool consistency and frequency, may do so by altering the balance of gut flora and reducing bile acid absorption.[16] Bile acid absorption is normally nearly complete by a process of active uptake of conjugated bile acids in the terminal ileum. This process can be impaired by acceleration of ileal transit, reducing the time available for absorption. Bacterial overgrowth results in deconjugation of bile acids and, again, impaired absorption. Excess bile acids in the gut lumen stimulate secretion and so can precipitate diarrhea. If bile acid loss exceeds the ability of the liver to synthesize sufficient replacement, there will then be a relative lack of bile acids, which will reduce fat absorption and cause steatorrhea through the presence of excessive amounts of fatty acids.
3. Diminished fluid absorption, either through mucosal damage or reduction of mucosal area as a result of intestinal resection.
4. Increased motor activity resulting in accelerated transit and reduced exposure of luminal contents to the absorptive mucosa.

Although studies are lacking, it is probable that, in common with cancer palliative care, the most common causes of diarrhea in neurological patients are an excess of laxatives and the type of intestinal infection that can strike any member of the population. Laxative diarrhea particularly occurs when doses have been increased to clear a backlog of constipated stool. The diarrhea normally settles within 24–48 hours if laxatives are temporarily stopped, after which they should be reinstated at a lower dose. Iatrogenic diarrhea also may be caused by a variety of drugs other than laxatives, including antibiotics, NSAIDs, cytotoxics, diuretics, and antacids.

Intestinal infections may be viral, but in ill patients are probably also more likely to be bacterial or from the overgrowth of candida. *Clostridium difficile*, pathogenic *Escherischia coli* or *salmonella* occur, but so do anaerobes which are more difficult to isolate.

Assessment

The fundamental distinction is between diarrhea and the leakage of liquid stool past a fecal impaction. Most impactions are rectal and will be revealed by rectal examination. A history of 'diarrhea' occurring after a period of constipation and characterized more by incontinence than urgency is suggestive. Pale, offensive-smelling, buoyant stools reflect fat malabsorption. In the community, any diarrhea lasting more than about 72 hours merits a stool specimen for culture and antimicrobial sensitivities, although in hospital different rules may apply.[17]

If in doubt about the nature of the diarrhea, the stool osmolality and sodium and potassium concentrations can be measured. The anion gap (the difference between the stool osmolality and double the sum of the cation concentrations) is over 50 mmol/1 in osmotic diarrhea because of the presence of an additional non-absorbed solute, such as a disaccharide from a medicinal elixir. An anion gap of below 50 mmol/1 shows secretory diarrhea, resulting from active secretion of fluid and electrolytes.

Management

Occasionally, rehydration and electrolyte replacement might be needed intravenously but, in the absence of dysphagia, encouragement of oral (and increase in gastrostomy) fluid intake, especially fruit juices and salty soups, is usually sufficient. A carbohydrate source, such as biscuits, bread, or pasta, should also be provided.

Specific treatments are available for a number of types of diarrhea, but no type of diarrhea is specific for neurological disease. If the person with diarrhea is otherwise well, it is reasonable to use a general antidiarrheal drug. The most effective and palatable are the opioids.

- In man, approximate equivalent antidiarrheal doses are 200 mg/day of codeine, 10 mg/day of diphenoxylate, and 4 mg/day of loperamide.[18]
- Trials show loperamide to be superior in effectiveness and adverse effects to either diphenoxylate or codeine.[19] However, codeine is cheaper and, idiosyncratically, may sometimes work better and be well tolerated.

Several alternative general antidiarrheals exist:

- Bulk-forming agents (e.g. psyllium, methylcellulose) can be used since, as discussed in the section on laxatives, they are stool normalizers, which absorb water to form a gelatinous mass and so thicken a loose stool just as they loosen a hard stool.
- Adsorbents such as kaolin have little evidence for efficacy.
- Bismuth subsalicylate is a mucosal prostaglandin inhibitor that also has antibacterial properties and has been shown to reduce acute infective diarrhea. However, it blackens not only the stool but also the tongue, can produce salicylate toxicity, and is less effective than loperamide.[20]

Other than in dysentery with fever and blood and mucus in the stools, or in known shigellosis, there is no evidence that use of an antidiarrheal will prolong illness or delay excretion of the pathogen. On the other hand, there is quite clear evidence that ciprofloxacin will shorten the period of diarrhea and hasten the clearance of pathogens when given empirically to those with acute community-acquired diarrhea producing more than four fluid stools a day for over three days and signs of toxicity.[21]

Where diarrhea is suspected to be due to bacterial overgrowth as a result of neurological damage causing alteration of intestinal transit, co-trimoxazole has been found to improve symptoms.[12] Metronidazole is an alternative with greater activity against anaerobes. This approach may prove more helpful than trying to treat the secondary manifestations of steatorrhea or chologenic diarrhea, even though both have specific treatments.

Steatorrhea can be diagnosed clinically and pancreatic supplementation can be given, but this may involve either swallowing a significant number of capsules or having food altered by sprinkling the capsule contents on top of it. The positive diagnosis of chologenic diarrhea requires tests involving the use of radioactive tracers and, therefore, specialist facilities, and its specific treatment, cholestyramine, is unpalatable. Where diarrhea is persistent and otherwise unexplained, an empirical trial of an antibiotic can be worthwhile. An alternative method of management where the diarrhea relapses is the use of calcium carbonate, which has been found to produce significant improvement in diarrhea characterized by malabsorption of bile acids and fatty acids after small bowel resection.[22] Calcium produces insoluble complexes with free bile acids and insoluble soaps with fatty acids.

FECAL INCONTINENCE

Incontinence of feces is liable to occur when the spinal cord is damaged by demyelination, tumor, or injury. Twenty-nine percent of MS patients[2] and sixty-six percent of spinal injury patients[11] have been reported to experience some degree of fecal incontinence. Conversely, fecal incontinence is uncommon in ALS. Injury above the T12 level produces a reflex neurogenic bowel in which anal sphincter tone is preserved but, without input from higher centers, defecation occurs automatically once or twice a day in response to rectal distension. Injury below this level abolishes both higher control and local reflex activity so that a stool continually seeps past a flaccid anal sphincter.

Fecal incontinence is a considerable handicap to morale, and success in avoiding such episodes has been reported from tailored programs of bowel management.[23] These involve initial clearance of constipation, followed by maintenance of a soft stool by a combination of laxatives appropriate to the individual, as well as by attention to the diet and fluid intake. A consistent timing for a daily bowel action is then determined based on the person's previous pattern. An alternative is to aim for a bowel action every second or third day, but there is evidence that a higher success rate is achieved by the daily approach.[24] Having assured a suitable posture and adequate privacy, a bisacodyl suppository or a mini-enema is administered and defecation is normally stimulated within approximately 30 minutes. Careful liaison between nurse, patient, and family is required, together with persistence. One to five weeks is the usual time required for achievement of continence.

SUMMARY

Constipation and diarrhea are conditions that understandably lack professional appeal for many nurses and, particularly, physicians. Nevertheless, they cause deep distress to patients. Although severe diarrhea can be harmful to patients with advanced neurological disease, the significance of constipation generally lies in its impact as a symptom. Healthy people, as well as those who are ill, vary markedly in bowel habits and, hence, how they define constipation. It is, therefore, patient satisfaction that is the aim of management, just as with the relief of any other symptom. This is not always easy to achieve, but it is important for the caring team to work with patients to minimize the burden of treatment and any further loss of dignity.

REFERENCES

1. Johanson JF, Sonnenberrg A, Koch TR, McCarty DJ. Association of constipation with neurologic diseases. Digestive Diseases and Sciences 1992;37:179–186.
2. Hennessey A, Robertson NP, Swingler R, Compston DA. Urinary, fecal and sexual dysfunction in patients with multiple sclerosis. Journal of Neurology 1999;246:1027–1032.
3. Wigzell FW. The health of nonagenarians. Gerontologia Clinica 1969;11:137–144.
4. Sykes NP. The relationship between opioid use and laxative use in terminally ill cancer patients. Palliative Medicine 1998;12:375–382.
5. Herz MJ, Kahan E, Zalevski S, Aframian R, Kuznitz D, Reichman S. Constipation: a different entity for patients and doctors. Family Practice 1996;13:156–159.
6. Dean AP, Reed WD. Diarrhea—an unrecognized hazard of celiac plexus block. Australia and New Zealand Journal of Medicine 1991;21:47–48.
7. Weber J, Grise P, Roquebert M, et al. Radiopaque markers transit and anorectal manometry in 16 patients with multiple sclerosis and urinary bladder dysfunction.
8. Chia YW, Gill KP, Jameson JS, et al. Paradoxical puborectalis contraction is a feature of constipation in patients with multiple sclerosis. Journal of Neurology, Neurosurgery and Psychiatry 1996;60:31–35.
9. Wiesel PH, Norton C, Roy AJ, Storrie JB, Bowers J, Kamm MA. Gut focused behavioral treatment (biofeedback) for constipation and fecal incontinence in multiple sclerosis. Journal of Neurology, Neurosurgery and Psychiatry 2000;69:240–243.
10. Emly M, Cooper S, Vail A. Colonic motility in profoundly disabled people: a comparison of massage and laxative therapy in the management of constipation. Physiotherapy 1998;84:178–183.
11. Petticrew M, Watt I, Sheldon T. Systematic review of the effectiveness of laxatives in the elderly. Health Technology Assessment 1997;1:1–52.
12. Sykes NP. A volunteer model for the comparison of laxatives in opioid-induced constipation. Journal of Pain and Symptom Management 1997;11:363–369.
13. NHS Center for Reviews and Dissemination. Effectiveness of laxatives in adults. Effective Health Care 2001;7(1):1–12.
14. Eichhorn TE, Oertel WH. Macrogol 3350/electrolyte improves constipation in Parkinson's disease and multiple system atrophy. Movement Disorders 2001;16:1176–1177.
15. Glickman S, Kamm MA. Bowel dysfunction in spinal cord-injury patients. Lancet 1996;347:1651–1653.
16. Feurle GE. Pathophysiology of diarrhea in patients with familial amyloid neuropathy. Digestion 1987;36:13–17.
17. Wood M. When stool cultures from adult inpatients are appropriate. Lancet 2001;357:901–902.
18. Twycross RG, Lack SA. Diarrhea. In: Control of Alimentary Symptoms in Far Advanced Cancer. Churchill Livingstone, London, 1986:208–229.
19. Palmer KR, Corbett CL, Holdsworth CD. Double-blind cross-over study comparing loperamide, codeine and diphenoxylate in the treatment of chronic diarrhea. Gastroenterology 1980;79:1272–1275.
20. Johnson PC, Ericsson CD, Dupont HL, Morgan DR, Bitsura JA, Wood LV. Comparison of loperamide with bismuth subsalicylate for the treatment of acute travelers' diarrhea. Journal of the American Medical Association 1986;255:757–760.
21. Gorbach SL. Treating diarrhea. British Medical Journal 1997;314:1776–1777.

22. Steinbach G, Lupton J, Reddy BS, Lee JJ, Kral JG, Holt PR. Calcium carbonate treatment of diarrhea in intestinal bypass patients. European Journal of Gastroenterology and Hepatology 1996;8:559–562.

23. Beddar SAM, Holden–Bennett L, McCormick AM. Development and evaluation of a protocol to manage fecal incontinence in the patient with cancer. Journal of Palliative Care 1997;13(2):27–38.

24. Munchiando J, Kendall K. Comparison of the effectiveness of two bowel programs for CVA patients. Rehabilitation Nursing 1993;18(3):168–172.

Chapter 25

Urological Symptoms

Darshan K. Shah
Gopal H. Badlani

In order to best manage a neurologically impaired patient, it is important to consider the patient's age, sex, level of lesion, and degree of ambulation, manual dexterity, and independence. The concerns of the urologist are primarily the preservation of the upper urinary tract or renal function and avoidance of urinary tract infection. This translates to ensuring adequate bladder storage and emptying at low intravesical pressures. The patient's concern, conversely, has to do with social mores such as preservation of continence. The patient needs a solution that is both socially acceptable and easily adopted.

CASE HISTORY

A 38-year-old quadriplegic male presented to the emergency department with complaints of right shoulder pain and cold sweats. The patient had previously suffered a C5 injury at age 17, secondary to a sports accident. Urological history revealed recurrent urinary tract infections over the past several months. Urine culture was positive for *E. coli* and serum creatinine was 1.3 mg/dl. Screening sonographic findings of bilateral hydronephrosis and bladder wall thickening were confirmed on CT. The patient was on terazosin (alpha-blocker) to reduce bladder outlet resistance. Immediate management with passive bladder drainage via an indwelling catheter, in addition to intravenous antibiotics, was initiated.

Discussion

The treatment choice in this patient would be based on urodynamic (UDS) findings and the cause of bilateral hydronephrosis. UDS revealed bladder overactivity (detrusor hyperreflexia) (DH) with no sensory perception of filling or voiding. During voiding, the bladder neck opened synergistically on fluoroscopy whereas the external sphincter remained closed (detrusor external sphincter dyssynergia or DESD). The resulting high bladder pressures precipitated autonomic dysreflexia (syndrome of uncontrolled hypertension, cold sweats). No vesicoureteral reflux was seen on fluoroscopy.

The treatment for a patient diagnosed with DH with DESD can be challenging. Bladder outlet obstruction (BOO) caused by DESD in a paraplegic spinal cord injury patient would be treated with anticholinergic therapy and intermittent self catheterization. A cervical spinal cord quadriplegic patient, however, requires a passive drainage system at persistently low pressures. We chose to place a Urolume endourethral stent across the external sphincter to relieve outlet obstruction (as opposed to performing an external sphincterotomy).

Chronic bladder outlet obstruction can result in bladder wall thickening and subsequent bilateral ureterovesical junction (UVJ) obstruction and hydronephrosis. Persistent hydronephrosis despite urethral catheterization would imply such an outcome. In such a patient, supravesical urinary diversion with ileal conduit is required.

Preservation of upper urinary tracts is the primary goal in these patients. This is achieved by ensuring a low pressure reservoir and appropriate emptying.

INTRODUCTION

In Western societies a large proportion of those who die after the age of 65 years suffer from complex neurological disorders such as Alzheimer's or cerebrovascular accident, which are synonymous with aging,[1] and only 23% of deaths in this age group are due to cancer. Palliative care in the neurologically impaired patient entails attention to quality of life and personal dignity. These are frequently compromised by urological manifestations of neurological disease. A balance must be sought between the patient's and family's wishes for social continence and the urological goal of renal function preservation.

Voiding dysfunction may result from medications, cognitive changes, physical impairments, or neurological etiologies.

VOIDING DYSFUNCTIONS ASSOCIATED WITH COMMON NEUROLOGICAL DISORDERS

The lower urinary tract in adults is a system of interrelated structures that function together for low-pressure bladder filling, low-pressure urinary storage, and total continence, with periodic voluntary urine expulsion at low pressure (see Table 25–1).

Voiding dysfunction in the neurologically impaired usually involves difficulty with emptying or storage. Symptoms secondary to emptying dysfunction include difficulty initiating a stream, decreased force of stream, strain to void, hesitancy, or intermittency in urine flow. Storage problems include urinary frequency, urgency, and nocturia with or without urinary incontinence. Lower abdominal and pelvic pain may coexist with these symptoms. The patient with a neurogenic bladder may present with signs and symptoms of urinary tract decompensation such as incomplete bladder emptying or urinary retention, renal insufficiency, and recurrent urinary tract infections in the absence of any symptoms due to sensory loss.

Table 25–1. Common Urodynamic Findings and Urological Manifestations Depending on Site of Lesion

Site of Lesion	Common Urodynamic Findings	Symptoms
Suprapontine	Bladder overactivity	Frequency, urgency, urge incontinence
Suprasacral (Infrapontine)	Bladder overactivity with detrusor sphincter dyssynergia	Loss of volitional voiding; incontinence; poor emptying
Sacral or peripheral	Bladder under-activity; acontractile with normal compliance; acontractile with decreased compliance (anterior horn injury)	Poor emptying; overflow incontinence

Suprapontine Lesions

Cerebrovascular disease, head injuries, Parkinson's disease, or multiple sclerosis can cause a suprapontine lesion, leading to detrusor hyperreflexia without detrusor sphincter dyssynergia. Associated conditions such as prostate obstruction, poor cognition, or the effect of medications may further alter the type of voiding dysfunction.

Cerebrovascular Accidents

Early presentation after a cerebrovascular accident (CVA) commonly includes acute urinary retention with detrusor areflexia that is poorly understood and often referred to as cerebral shock.[2] The size, location, and extent of the CVA may have a profound effect on micturition. However, acute urinary retention may not necessarily be a result of the CVA but be related to inability to communicate a need to void, impaired consciousness, temporary over-distension of the bladder, and restricted mobility.[3]

The later symptoms of bladder dysfunction after an established CVA include frequency, urgency, and urge incontinence.[4,5] Various series have reported that 49% to 60% of patients are incontinent one week post-CVA.[4,6] In the inpatient rehabilitation setting, a 33% incidence of incontinence during the first three months post-CVA has been reported,[6] but the problem significantly improves in the majority of patients.[4,6] Detrusor hyperreflexia (uninhibited bladder contraction) is the most common urodynamic finding following a stroke, occurring in 70% to 90%,[4,7] but patients rarely develop true detrusor sphincter dyssynergia (see Chapter 2).[4]

Parkinson's Disease

37% to 72% of patients with Parkinson's disease have symptoms of bladder dysfunction. Among these patients, detrusor hyperreflexia (frequency, urgency, urge incontinence) is present in 72–90%, bladder outlet obstruction in 23%, and a combination of the two in 20% of patients. Detrusor hyperreflexia occurs due to loss of inhibitory input from the basal ganglia on the micturition reflexes; however, detrusor overactivity can be secondary to bladder outlet obstruction. In the male an electromyography study of the external sphincter reveals bradykinesia but not true detrusor sphincter dyssynergia. The majority of patients have normal sphincter function.[8] Females with Parkinsonism may present with urinary retention due to the anticholinergic side effects of pharmacological treatment of the disease (see Chapter 5).

Multiple Sclerosis

Detrusor external sphincter dyssynergia is commonly seen in patients with spinal cord involvement secondary to multiple sclerosis (15%–20%).[9] It can also lead to urological complications such as vesicoureteral reflux, hydronephrosis, urolithiasis, and sepsis.[10] Suprapontine lesions cause loss of voluntary control and usually manifest as detrusor hyperreflexia causing urgency, frequency, and urge incontinence. These patients are usually incontinent but are at little risk of developing complications unless they have other urological abnormalities. Neurologic lesions that interfere with the sacral reflex arcs are less common, causing various combinations of detrusor areflexia, intrinsic sphincter deficiency, and paralysis of the striated urethral sphincter (see Chapter 3).[11]

Suprasacral Spinal Cord Lesions

Most common suprasacral spinal cord lesions occur secondary to spinal cord trauma. Transverse myelitis, multiple sclerosis, and metastatic or primary spinal cord tumor also cause suprasacral spinal cord lesions and voiding dysfunction from detrusor hyperreflexia with detrusor sphincter dyssynergia. During spinal shock or in the case of a partial lesion, this typical pattern of voiding dysfunction may not be seen.[12] Injury results in the initial phase of spinal shock; the bladder is areflexic, resulting in urinary retention. Usually, reflex bladder activity returns within 2–12 weeks, but sometimes not for 6–12 months. Most peripheral somatic reflexes of the sacral cord segment, including the anal and bulbocavernosus, may never disappear, or if they do, may return within minutes or hours after the injury.[13] As sphincter tone remains near normal in this phase, overflow incontinence occurs when the bladder is overdistended. This stage last for 6–12 weeks in complete suprasacral lesions.[14] In the next phase of recovery following spinal trauma, reflex activity returns. Generally, detrusor contractility returns if the distal spinal cord is intact, but it is isolated from higher central control. The strength and duration of this involuntary contraction commonly increases, producing involuntary voiding, usually with incomplete bladder emptying due to detrusor sphincter dyssynergia.

The eventual pattern of voiding dysfunction depends upon the type and level of injury. Kaplan et al. reviewed 489 consecutive patients with spinal cord lesions of varying causes, and described three main patterns of voiding dysfunction.[12] With incomplete spinal cord injury, detrusor hyperreflexia with synergistic external sphincter functions is seen; complete thoracic or cervical level lesion results in detrusor hyperreflexia with detrusor external sphincter dyssynergia; and following sacral and lower lumbar injury, detrusor areflexia is seen. The correlation is not absolute, and clinical neurological examination alone is not adequate to predict urological dysfunction. A urodynamic evaluation is necessary for accurate diagnosis.[12]

Sacral Lesions

Sacral cord or root injury, lumber disc herniation, tumor, myelodysplasia, arteriovenous malformation, lumbar stenosis, and an inflammatory process may cause sacral lesions, resulting in a highly compliant acontractile bladder, particularly with a posterior horn lesion. In patients with partial injuries, and anterior horn lesions, areflexia may be accompanied by decreased bladder compliance, resulting in progressive increases in intravesical pressure with filling. The exact mechanism by which sacral parasympathetic decentralization of the bladder causes decreased compliance in unknown.[15] The external sphincter remains unaffected as pelvic nerve innervation to the bladder usually arises one segment higher than the pudendal nerve innervation of the sphincter.[16]

Peripheral Lesions

Diabetes mellitus causing peripheral neuropathy is the most common peripheral lesion resulting in voiding dysfunction. Chronic alcoholism, paraneoplastic syndromes, and pelvic surgery may also lead to peripheral neuropathy and voiding dysfunction. In diabetes-induced sensory neuropathy, urodynamic findings include decreased bladder sensation, chronic bladder overdistension, and increased post-void residual volume. Bladder decompensation may result from overdistention secondary to a decreased sensation of fullness.[17,18]

EVALUATION OF URINARY DYSFUNCTION IN THE NEUROLOGICALLY IMPAIRED PATIENT

For the initial management, the neurologist, internist, and physiotherapist have key roles; the urologist is consulted, in most cases, only after the patient is transferred from an intensive care unit or an acute care facility to a rehabilitation unit.

Patient History

A thorough patient history is required to identify the neurological diagnosis, cognitive deficits, and associated medical problems. The lack of specificity and sensitivity for many urodynamic tests heightens the reliance on history to differentiate disorders, determine etiology, and plan therapy. Other than history, evaluation in a neurologically impaired patient should include voiding diary, physical examination (including neurological examination), urine analysis and culture, renal function, endoscopy, and urodynamic study. Symptoms related to other organs that receive similar somatic and autonomic innervation are especially important. A temporal correlation between the triad of bladder, bowel, and sexual dysfunction should alert the clinician to the possibility of a neurogenic etiology. The clinician should ascertain two things when obtaining a history: first, what is bothering the patient or most affecting quality of life; second, what is the possible etiology. In patients who are cognitively impaired, history should be gathered from family members, nurses, and from the patient's fluid balance chart.

The urological history should focus initially on the patient's voiding complaints (i.e. failure to store, failure to empty, or both). Significant *past* history which may affect *present* voiding dysfunction includes diabetes, CVA, hypertension, use of diuretics, and major surgical procedures such as previous transurethral resection of the prostate (TURP) or surgery for stress incontinence or pelvic surgery. Reversible or transient causes of urinary incontinence should be sought and treated.

A *voiding diary* provides objective documentation of symptoms. A diary can assess daytime urinary frequency, incontinence, and voided volumes. The voiding diary is also important in monitoring therapy.

Physical Examination

Specific attention should be given to mobility, visual acuity, hand coordination, and mental status of the patient in addition to pelvic floor assessment in women and digital rectal examination for prostatic evaluation in men. In elderly postmenopausal women, the urethral and vaginal introitus should be examined for atrophic changes suggestive of estrogen deficiency.

Sensory Examination

This should be done to determine the level of injury. Injury above T6 level makes the patient prone to autonomic dysreflexia. Sacral sensation evaluates the afferent limb of the sacral micturition center (pudendal nerve). Loss of pinprick and light touch sensation in the hands and feet is suggestive of peripheral neuropathy.

Motor Examination

This helps to establish the level and completeness of the neurogenic lesion. Upper and lower limb spasticity, sitting, standing, and ambulating needs to be evaluated. Hand function is assessed to determine ability to undress or possibility to perform intermittent self-catheterization. Decreased or absent anal sphincter tone suggests a sacral or peripheral nerve lesion, whereas increased tone suggests a suprasacral lesion. Voluntary contraction of the anal sphincter tests sacral innervation, suprasacral integrity, and ability to understand commands. Cutaneous reflexes helpful to the neuro-urological examination are cremasteric (L1–L2) and bulbocavernosus (S2–S4), and absence of these cutaneous reflexes suggests pyramidal tract disease or a peripheral lesion.

Evaluation of the upper urinary tract should be done if there is any suggestion of upper tract involvement such as an episode of fever or hematuria. Tests designed to evaluate the upper tract include a renal ultrasound, intravenous urography, quantitative renal scan, and 24-hour urine creatinine clearance.[19]

It is important to have a clear understanding of the patient's signs and symptoms, but one should not initiate treatment based on symptoms alone. Symptoms often correlate poorly with the actual voiding problem. Resnick and Yalla found, in the geriatric female population, that presenting symptoms were predictive of the urodynamic diagnosis in only 55% of those with pure urge incontinence.[20] Katz and Blaivas, in a prospective study of more the 400 patients, found that the clinical assessment based on symptoms did not correlate with the objective urodynamic findings in 45% of patients thought to have storage problems, in 25% believed to have emptying problems, and 54% of those believed to have storage and emptying problems.[21]

Urodynamic Study

The most useful urodynamic study is cystometry, which should be done as a screening test with post-void residual urine volume measurement. Complex urodynamic testing, when required, should be performed with fluoroscopy and measurement of several other parameters, including the Valsalva leak point pressure. Electromyography is only included if detrusor sphincter dyssynergia is suspected.

There are several technical difficulties in performing urodynamic testing in the neurologically impaired. Studies are tailored to individuals rather than applying an identical template to each individual. Often elderly patients have decreased mobility and are unable to stand or use the uroflowmetry machine. In such cases only a supine study may be possible. Every attempt is made to encourage voiding before the study because post-void residual urine volume is an important measure in the neurologically impaired patient. Using the rectal pressure balloon is often mandatory to detect straining and for performing the Valsalva maneuver during cystometry. Despite these problems, Resnick et al. have demonstrated that it is feasible to perform a complex urodynamic study in frail elderly patients.[3]

TREATMENT STRATEGIES

The primary aim of any intervention is to establish an adequate storage at low intravesical pressure. McGuire and co-workers have clearly shown that upper tract deterioration is apt to occur when storage, even though adequate in term of continence, occurs at sustained intravesical pressures of greater than 40 cm H_2O.[22]

When treating patients with voiding dysfunction, a perfect result may not be achieved, and a flexible approach to therapy must be adopted. Any decision must take into account the wishes of an informed patient and the practicality of each proposed solution, especially in those patients with neurologic disease.[23] Patient factors such as prognosis of underlying disease, limiting factors such as inability to perform certain tasks, mental status, motivation, desire to remain catheter- or appliance-free, desire to avoid surgery, sexual activity status, reliability, educability, psychosocial environment, economic resources, and age should be taken into consideration before deciding upon any therapy. The simplest, least destructive and most reversible form of therapy that can satisfy the goals of treatment should be tried first.

Obstruction or Retention in Men

During the period of active neurological injury and urinary retention, *clean intermittent catheterization* every 4 to 6 hours may be a useful minimally invasive therapy. As spontaneous voiding returns and post-void residual urine volume is consistently less than 100 ml, clean intermittent catheterization may be discontinued. It is also an extremely effective

method of treating an adult or child whose bladder fails to empty, especially when efforts to increase intravesical pressure or decrease outlet resistance have been unsuccessful. In patients with inadequate urine storage because of involuntary bladder contraction, decreased compliance, or stress incontinence, self-catheterization may also be useful if the dysfunction can be converted solely or primarily to one of retention by pharmacological or surgical means.[24] When clean intermittent catheterization is not feasible, an indwelling Foley catheter may be inserted and changed monthly.

Crede's maneuver, external compression, and Valsalva manual compression of the bladder can be effective in patients with decreased bladder pressure who can generate a pressure greater than 50 cm H_2O with this maneuver, and whose outlet resistance is low.[24] A similar increase in intravesical pressure is achieved by abdominal straining. The greatest likelihood of success with this therapy is in patients with an areflexic and hypo-contractile bladder and some outlet denervation. The most frequent misuse of this form of management is in patients with a decentralized or denervated bladder and decreased compliance during the filling phase, developing silent upper tract deterioration with minimum filling.

For documented bladder outlet obstruction, new medical and surgical therapies are becoming available. Long-acting *α1-blockers*, as terazosin or doxazosin, are started once the patient is medically stable.[3]

Some *temporary prostatic stents or catheters* currently under trial have a narrow lumen and are prone to clot occlusion in patients receiving anticoagulants. The 'ContiCath' (under trial and not currently available) bridges the space from the bladder neck, through the prostate, and ends proximal to the external sphincter, and may be used for as long as 30 days. It permits voiding with much less discomfort and there are very few contraindications to its use. However, in a multicenter prospective study of 24 patients with non-neurogenic retention lasting greater than one week or neurogenic retention, only three patients voided after 'ContiCath' insertion. Stents rely on active drainage, such that detrusor function is essential, and they are not useful for retention secondary to detrusor failure. In high-risk patients a permanent prostatic stent may be placed. The 'UroLume', much like a temporary stent, may be placed using local anesthesia with minimal patient discomfort. It is epithelized from 6–8 weeks.[3] It may be used in patients receiving anti-platelet therapy and, with caution, in those on warfarin. The 'UroLume' stent sphincter prosthesis is an attractive treatment modality for spinal cord injured men, especially those with hope of recovery or who refuse destructive and irreversible urological surgeries.[25]

Less invasive endoscopic procedures, such as transurethral microwave thermotherapy, transurethral needle ablation, and holmium or indigo laser prostatectomy, may prove useful in high-risk cases of bladder outlet obstruction secondary to begnign prostatic hyperplasia (BPH) [3].

The urologist should refrain from performing transurethral prostatic resection for 6 to 12 months after a stroke because incontinence and morbidity may be increased. Lum and Marshall identified several variables associated with an unsatisfactory prostatectomy outcome in 50% or more of patients.[3] Variables most closely correlated with poor clinical outcome (higher incidence of urinary incontinence) were patient age older than 70 years, worsening neurological symptoms, a cerebrovascular accident that was bilateral or involved the non-dominant hemisphere, absent associated urinary symptoms, and surgery within one year of a cerebrovascular accident.

In *Parkinsonian patients*, subcutaneous apomorphine (a dopamine D1 and D2 agonist) can elicit voiding.[26] Similarly, the dopamine agonist pergolide (Permax) has been shown to facilitate voiding in Parkinsonian patients. Recently, it has been shown that sublingual apomorphine triggers a voiding reflex in spinal cord injured patients.[27] In the patient with Parkinsonism and bladder outlet obstruction secondary to BPH, frequency and urgency does not respond predictably to TURP, which may make the condition worse. Use of a temporary prostatic stent may help predict response to bladder outlet resistance reduction surgery.

Retention in Women

Until recently, women with urinary retention secondary to detrusor hyporeflexia had only the options of clean intermittent catheterization or an indwelling Foley catheter. Although clean intermittent catheterization offers excellent long-term management, its use in neurologically impaired patients is often restricted by their inability to perform this procedure. Indwelling Foley catheters have the disadvantages of infection and discomfort.

Pharmacological Therapy for Detrusor Hyperreflexia or Areflexia[28]

Because a detrusor contraction depends on stimulation of the parasympathetic post-ganglionic muscarinic receptors by acetylcholine or acetylcholine-like neurotransmitters, bethanechol chloride has been used to improve bladder emptying. Although attractive from a physiological and pharmacological standpoint, clinical efficacy has not been demonstrated in most trials.[29] To our knowledge no study has specifically addressed its use for detrusor hyporeflexia or areflexia in neurologically impaired patients, nor have we found bethanechol useful for treating detrusor hyporeflexia or areflexia after a cerebrovascular accident. There is anecdotal evidence of the efficacy of other oral cholinergic agonists, including the dopamine antagonist metoclopramide and the synthetic benzamide, cisapride, in improving bladder contractility, but formal clinical studies are lacking.[30,31]

Intermittent catheterization is the most effective means of attaining a catheter-free state in patients with acute spinal cord lesion.

Management of Nocturia

Managing nocturnal polyuria in the elderly often focuses on the daytime mobilization of edema from the lower extremities. When the patient reclines during sleep, these fluids mobilize naturally and increase night-time urine output. Current treatment for nocturnal polyuria includes evening fluid restriction, mid- to late afternoon or early evening diuretics, compressive stockings, afternoon sleep or leg elevation, imipramine, anti-diuretic hormone, and nasal continuous positive airway pressure.[3,32]

When using fluid restriction or diuretics, the urologist or primary care physician should follow the patient closely for signs and symptoms of hypokalemia and dehydration. Oral or intranasal antidiuretic hormone has been useful with few side effects in the elderly. However, close monitoring of serum electrolytes for hyponatremia is mandatory and this medication should not be given in patients with a history of congestive heart failure or hypertension.[32] In some patients with obstructive sleep apnea, nocturnal polyuria is mediated by plasma atrial natriuretic peptide. Using continuous positive airway pressure considerably decreases nocturia.

Nocturnal detrusor overactivity results in decreased bladder capacity. These patients often have underlying detrusor instability, bladder outlet obstruction, sensory urgency, infection, or malignancy. Treating the underlying urological disorder may be expected to improve bladder capacity and decrease nocturia. In mixed nocturia, the predominant cause of nocturnal polyuria or detrusor overactivity may be treated first, and the case may then be re-evaluated. Another approach is that of Weiss and Blaivas, who recommended the initial treatment of the nocturnal polyuria component of mixed nocturia because the measures are non-invasive.[32]

Incontinence

The urologist's goal in incontinence is to restore a socially acceptable level of urinary continence while minimizing the risk of infection. Patients with detrusor hyperreflexia may be treated with timed voiding, concomitant fluid restriction, and anticholinergic drugs such as oxybutynin, tolterodine, dicyclomine hydrochloride, and hyoscyamine sulfate. However, outlet obstruction in men and detrusor hyperactivity with impaired contractility[33] in men and women may result in urinary retention with the injudicious use of anticholinergic medication.

Tolterodine[34] is our first choice for relieving detrusor hyperreflexia in patients with neurologic disease. This agent, approved by the United States Food and Drug Administration in 1998, binds less to cholinergic receptors in the salivary glands than traditional drugs of this class. Therefore, patients are bothered

less by dry mouth and fewer discontinue therapy secondary to adverse effects. Traditionally, as many as 43% of patients on oxybutynin terminate its use secondary to dry mouth. Appell reported on 1120 patients randomized to 2 mg tolterodine twice daily, 5 mg oxybutynin 3 times daily, or placebo.[35] When adverse effects, dose decreases, and discontinuation were considered, tolterodine was more efficacious than oxybutynin.

The traditional medication, oxybutynin, is now available in a once-daily, controlled-release formulation. In a multicenter, placebo-controlled study, patients on the long-acting product reported fewer problems with moderate or severe dry mouth.[3] To our knowledge, its efficacy in neuropathy and cerebrovascular accident is not known. Cognitive impairment, at least theoretically, was possible with oxybutynin when compared to tolterodine. In women with detrusor hyperreflexia and stress urinary incontinence, oral medications such as imipramine or phenylpropanolamine hydrochloride with guaifenesin, are available, which increase bladder outlet resistance. However, their use may be limited in hypertension.

If medical and behavioral therapy fails in patients with urethral incontinence, a few minimally invasive procedures are available that provide fair to excellent improvement. It is imperative that detrusor dysfunction should be addressed before treating urethral incontinence. Newer and refashioned procedures may be performed using local anesthesia for stress incontinence of types II (urethral hypermobility) and/or III (intrinsic sphincter deficiency). They include periurethral or transurethral collagen injection with a 20%–30% five-year success rate; the 'Urosurge' device, which is an investigational self-detachable balloon system that is placed at the bladder neck under endoscopic guidance to create an effect similar to that of collagen therapy; and a pubo-vaginal sling, with or without bone anchors, using autologous rectus fascia or fascia lata, allogenic donor cadaver fascia, or synthetic polypropylene or polytetrafluoroethylene.[3,36,37] These pubo-vaginal sling procedures were historically reserved for patients with type III stress urinary incontinence or those with failed anti-incontinence surgery. More recently, the pubo-vaginal sling procedure has been performed with minimal tension on the sling, and new onset incontinence and permanent urinary retention necessitating urethrolysis have been decreased to 3% and 2%, respectively. Compared with autologous tissue, cadaveric or synthetic material decreases operative time, postoperative pain, and cost without sacrificing patient outcome or increasing morbidity. The success and complication rates associated with polypropylene with bone anchors have been excellent in this patient population.[3]

Another new therapy for stress urinary incontinence is tension-free vaginal tape. In a multicenter trial of 131 patients, the one-year cure rate was 91%, 7% of patients improved, while only 2% had failure.[38] All patients received local anesthetic and mean operative time was 28 minutes (range 19–41 minutes). Of the patients, 90% were discharged home within 24 hours without an indwelling catheter and only four patients needed catheterization for three or more days. In high-risk patients, tension-free vaginal tape may become the preferred means of treating each type of stress urinary incontinence.

Nursing Care

Sometimes all that is necessary for successful incontinence therapy in the neurologically impaired patient is simple behavioral modification, such as fluid restriction and a timed voiding schedule, as are determined by a voiding diary. Many patients with dementia, who no longer have socially appropriate behavior, also benefit substantially from a prompted voiding schedule. Gelber et al. reported that 37% of severely handicapped (aphasia, dementia, or immobility), incontinent patients had a normally functioning bladder, and even these debilitated patients benefited from prompted voiding and fluid restriction.[3] The drawback is the labor-intensive nature of this method of management, which is most effective in a home environment with one-to-one patient attention.

There is a wide assortment of absorbent, containment, and protective products available on the market. Before discussing specific products, it is important to assess the patient's needs and the characteristics of each product.[39] Consider the patient's size, mobility, self-care skills, finances, and motivations. *Absorbent products* like pad and pant systems have become popular and consist of disposable pads held in place by lightweight reusable briefs. *Compression devices* such as a penile clamp may be an alternative for keeping the patient dry. The clamp should be removed every four hours so that the bladder can be emptied and the penile shaft inspected for swelling and irritation. If possible, the clamp should be kept off during the night. *External collection devices* that attach to a leg or bedside drainage bag are available for both men and women. Regardless of which brand of device is chosen, the principles of application remain the same. The penile skin must be clean and dry before application. Shaving the pubic hairs is not recommended, as it can cause irritation. Trimming pubic hair with scissors is preferable. In the uncircumcised patient, the foreskin must never be retracted during application because paraphimosis can occur. Care should be taken to fit the patient properly. Excoriation, necrosis, or gangrene can result from a tight-fitting sheath. Regardless of the manufacturer's claims to long-wearing time ability, condom catheters must be changed daily to clean and inspect the skin properly.

External collecting devices for the female patient are not practical in most cases. Regardless of which product is chosen, scrupulous skin care is necessary to prevent breakdown, as dermatological complications increase morbidity and mortality, particularly in the elderly.[40] Between the pad or device changes, the skin should be cleaned with soap and water or disposable wet wipes. Irritation and rashes must be dealt with immediately. A variety of water-soluble moisturizing creams and lotions are available, as well as barrier creams and salves that are water soluble.

SUMMARY

Urological manifestation, especially incontinence, can be a significant factor in the care of a neurologically impaired individual. Treatment assessment and objective evaluation is helpful in successful management of most patients. Renal function preservation is the primary objective of the urologist, whereas the patient wishes volitional voiding with social continence.

REFERENCES

1. Olshansky SJ, Ault AB. The fourth stage of the epidemiologic transition: the age of delayed degenerative disease. Milbank Q 1986;64:355–391.
2. Hald T, Bradley WE. The Urinary Bladder: Neurology and Urodynamics.: Williams and Wilkins, Baltimore, MD, 1982:48–51.
3. Marincovic S, Badlani G. Voiding and sexual dysfunction after cerebrovascular dysfunction. J Urol 2001;165(2):359–370.
4. Arunabh MB, Badlani G. Urologic problems in cerebrovascular accidents. Problems Urol 1993;7:41–53.
5. Barer DH. Continence after stroke: Useful predictor or goal of therapy? Age Ageing 1989;18:183–191.
6. Linsenmeyer TA. Characterization of voiding dysfunction following recent cerebrovascular accident. Arch Phys Med Rehabil 1990;71:778–791.
7. Linsenmeyer TA. Urodynamic findings in patients with urinary incontinence after cerebrovascular accident. Neuro Rehabil 1992;2(2):23–26.
8. Pavlakis AJ, Siroky MB, Goldstein I, Krane RJ. Neurourologic findings in Parkinson's disease. J Urol 1983;129:80–83.
9. Blaivas JG, Barbalias GA. Detrusor external sphincter dyssynergia in men with multiple sclerosis: an ominous urologic condition. J Urol 1984;131:91–94.
10. Anderson JT, Bradley WE. Abnormalities of detrusor and sphincter function in multiple sclerosis. Br J Urol 1976;48:193–197.
11. Gonor SE, Carroll DJ, Metcalfe JB. Vesical dysfunction in multiple sclerosis. Urology 1985;25:429–431.
12. Kaplan SA, Chancellor MB, Blaivas J. Bladder and sphincter behavior in patients with spinal cord lesion. J Urol 1991;146:113–117.
13. Sullivan M, Yalla S. Spinal cord injury and other forms of myeloneuropathies. Problem Urol 1992;6:643–650.
14. Wein A, Rovner ES. Adult voiding dysfunction secondary to neurologic disease or injury. In: Ball T, Jr, ed. AUA Update Series. Vol. XVIII. AUA Office of Education, Houston, Texas, 1999:42–48.
15. Sharr MM, Garfield JC, Jenkins JD. Lumbar spondylosis and neuropatic bladder investigations of 73 patients with chronic urinary symptoms Br Med J 1976;1(6011):695–697.
16. Sislow JG, Mayo ME. Reduction in human bladder wall compliance following decentralization. J Urol 1990;144:945–947.
17. Appell RA, Whiteside HV. Diabetes and other peripheral neuropathies affecting lower urinary tract function. In: Krane RJ, Siroky MG, ed. Clinical Neuro-urology, 2nd Ed. Little, Brown & Co., Boston, 1991:965–973.
18. Bradly WE. Autonomic neuropathy and the genitourinary system J Urol 1978;119:299–302.
19. Rao KG, Hackler RH, Woodlief RM, Ozer MN, Fields WR. Real time renal sonography in spinal cord injury patients: Prospective comparison with excretory urography. J Urol 1986;135:72–77.
20. Resnick NM, Yalla SV. Management of urinary incontinence in the elderly. N Eng J Med 1985;313:800–805.
21. Katz GP, Blaivas J. A diagnostic dilemma: when urodynamic finding differ from the clinical impression. J Urol 1983;129:1170–1174.
22. McGuire EJ, Woodside JR, Borden TA, Weiss RM. The prognostic value of urodynamic testing in myelodysplastic patients. J Urol 1981;126:205–209.
23. Steers W, Barrett D, Wein A. Voiding dysfunction: diagnosis, classification, and management. In: Gillenwater J, Grayhack JT, Howards SS, Mitchell ME, eds. Adult and Pediatric Urology, 4th Ed. Lippincott Williams & Wilkins, 2002.
24. Wein AJ, Raezer DM, Benson GS. Management of neurogenic bladder dysfunction in the adult. Urology 1976;8:432–440.
25. Chancelllor MB, Bennett C, Simoneau AR, et al. Long-term follow-up of the north American multicentrer Urolume trial for the treatment of external detrusor sphincter dyssynergia. J Urol 1999;161:1545–1550.
26. Christmas TJ, Kempster PA, Chapple CR, et al. Role of subcutaneous apomorphine in the treatment of Parkinsonian voiding dysfunction. Lancet 1998;2:1451.
27. Steers WD. Effect of sublingual apomorphine on bladder function in patients with spinal cord injury (abstract). J Urol 2000;163(Suppl):39.
28. Zderic SA, Levin RM, Wein AJ. Voiding function: relevant anatomy, physiology, pharmacology and molecular aspects. In: Gillenwater JY, Howards J, Grayhack J, et al., eds. Adult and Pediatric Urology, 3rd Ed. Chicago: Mosby, Chicago, 1996:1159.
29. Finkbeiner AE. Is bethanechol chloride clinically effective in promoting bladder emptying? A literature review. J Urol 1985;134:443–447.
30. Nestler JE, Stratton MA, Hakim CA. Effect of metoclopramide on diabetic neurogenic bladder. Clin Pharmacol 1983;2:83–88.
31. Carone R, Vercelli D, Bertapelle P. Effects of cisapride on anorectal and vesicourethral function in spinal cord injured patients. Paraplegia 1993;31:125–131.
32. Weiss JP, Blaivas JG. Nocturia. J Urol 2000;163:5–15.
33. Resnick NM, Yalla SV. Detrusor hyperactivity with impaired contractile function. An unrecognized but common cause of incontinence in elderly patients. JAMA 1987;257:3076–3081.
34. Abrams P, Freeman R, Anderstrom C, et al. Tolterodine, a new antimuscarinic agent: as effective but better tolerated than oxybutynin in patients with an overactive bladder. Br J Urol 1998;81:801.
35. Appell RA. Clinical efficacy and safety of tolterodine in the treatment of overactive bladder: a pooled analysis. Urology 1997;50(Suppl):90.
36. Marinkovic S, Mian H, Evankovich M, et al. Burch versus the pubovaginal sling. Int Urogynecol J 1998;8:260–267.
37. Wright EJ, Iselin CE, Webster GD. Pubovaginal sling using cadaveric allograft fascia lata for the treatment of intrinsic sphincter deficiency. J Urol 1998;159(Suppl):214, abstract 828.
38. Ulmsten U, Falconer C, Johnson P, et al. A multicenter study of tension-free vaginal tape (TVT) for surgical treatment of stress urinary incontinence. Int Urogynecol J 1998;9:210–213.
39. Faller N, Jeter KF. ABCs of product selection. Urol Nursing 1992;12:53–54.
40. Hogstel MO. Nursing care of the older adult. John Wiley & Sons, New York, 1981:116–129.

Chapter 26

Psychiatric Symptoms

Alexandre Berney
Friedrich Stiefel

INTRODUCTION
MAJOR PSYCHIATRIC DISORDERS
Major Depression
Anxiety Disorders
Adjustment Disorders

Other Psychiatric Disorders
**GENERAL ASPECTS: COPING, DEFENSES,
  AND ADAPTATION**
SUMMARY

This chapter focuses on the main diagnostic and treatment issues related to patients presenting with psychiatric symptoms in the palliative care setting. Specific pharmacological treatments and general aspects such as coping, defenses, and communication skills are discussed. A supportive attitude towards the patient's own efforts to cope with a severe illness, as well as a proactive attitude, intended to integrate major biographical and contextual aspects in the patient's treatment plan are proposed here.

CASE HISTORY

Anthony, a 52-year-old, very active and successful manager of an international company was diagnosed with a sporadic form of amyotrophic lateral sclerosis (ALS) one year ago. At that time, he presented with fatigue, fasciculation, cramps, and atrophy of the arm and hand. During the first months following the diagnosis he seemed to cope well, increased his professional activities, and showed no signs of emotional or behavioral disturbances. On several occasions, he was reluctant to meet the physician together with his family in order to discuss the medical situation. He mentioned only that his daughter was just about to marry and that his wife was very much involved in her professional career and that he didn't want to discuss his problems with the family. Progressively he became less talkative, irritable, and had

recurrent thoughts related to the fear of becoming a burden. He ruminated about a statement from his physician that 'there is not much I can do for you' and stated that he would like to precipitate the fatal evolution of his disease to which the neurologist had once referred. At work he complained of fatigue and weakness, and a lack of motivation. He also reported anxious states, sometimes lasting several hours. When he spoke of anxiety to his physician and complained of insomnia, inability to concentrate, and the feelings of hopelessness and worthlessness, it was suggested he consult a psychiatrist. He refused this and asked the neurologist about assistance in suicide should he feel unable to stand his situation any longer.

Discussion

The case illustrates a major challenge of neurological palliative care: the integration of biographical and contextual aspects of a patient in the treatment plan in order to assist him to adapt to the advancing disease. How to take into account, in the treatment plan, of this patient's identity as an 'independent chief executive' when he is facing a slowly progressive disease leading to dependence and loss of control? How to challenge his way of coping when he is apparently doing well, though his distraction by an increased workload may be the first sign of an inability to adapt to the disease? How to relate to the family and to negotiate their changing roles? How to suggest that accepting help is not a sign of weakness or that 'dignity' is an inner state unrelated to physical condition? How to monitor the patient's psychological state by asking the necessary questions in a respectful way? How to evaluate and diagnose depression without referral to a psychiatrist which may be perceived by the patient as his being abandoned and becoming a 'psychiatric case'? And finally, how can the patient's request for physician-assisted suicide be explored and decoded in order to respond to his underlying fear of dependency and his need for control?

INTRODUCTION

For severely ill patients with advanced disease, the psychological and social aspects become most important and the role of the treating staff cannot be limited to medical and nursing interventions. Appropriate care requires knowledge, communication skills, empathy, and the sensitivity and ability to integrate the patient's life narrative within treatment. Such an integrated and global approach—a cornerstone of palliative care—may be considered by some as 'mission impossible'. There are of course limits (another cornerstone of palliative care) in our ability to take care of patients; however, if we try at least to pursue a global and integrated approach, we will achieve the possible, which is far more important than 'reaching for the impossible'.[1]

Integration of all important aspects in the treatment, based on the biopsychosocial model of disease, certainly depends on both the patient and the palliative care specialist. But even qualities such as empathy, communication skills, and the sensitivity for important biographical elements and contextual factors can be enhanced by pre- and postgraduate training, regular participation in supervision and Balint groups, and communication skills training. A most effective contribution is the inclusion of a consultation–liaison psychiatrist in the palliative care team.

This chapter focuses on the major psychiatric disturbances in neurological palliative care and ends with some general thoughts on adaptation to disease.

MAJOR PSYCHIATRIC DISORDERS

Major Depression

IMPORTANCE

Depression is frequent both in palliative care and neurological disease. Stroke,[2] Parkinson's disease, and ALS patients have a 20% prevalence of major depression, approximately two times higher than in the general population;[3] and major depression is diagnosed in up to 25% of the terminally ill.[4] The etiology is often mixed, due to psychological (e.g. ineffective coping, conflicts), genetic (e.g. family history of depression), or organic (e.g. structural changes of the CNS) causes and external stressors (e.g. chronic pain, loss of professional identity).[5]

DIAGNOSIS

Under-detection and under-treatment of depression is well documented for somatic patients and for neurological and palliative care patients.[6–8] The most important cause for this is that a diagnosis can only be established by asking the patient about the affective core symptoms of depression, and physicians unfortunately often fear that such questions may be intrusive, time-consuming, and difficult to manage. However, clinical and scientific evidence show that patients feel relieved and understood when they are invited to express their emotions.[9]

The diagnosis of major depression is based on the presence of depressed mood (dysphoria) and/or the loss of interest or pleasure (anhedonia) for at least two weeks, and on the presence of at least four (three if the patient is experiencing both dysphoria and anhedonia) of the symptoms listed in Table 26–1. Physical and cognitive symptoms of depression are less reliable in the palliative care setting since they can be caused by the disease or its treatments. Nevertheless, criteria such as those proposed in standard classifications like the Diagnostic and Statistical Manual of Mental Disorders (DSM-IV)[10] are valid and can be applied for neurological patients. Specific organic pseudodepressive manifestations due to a CNS disease such as pathological crying, facial akinesia, catastrophic reactions, loss of psychic

Table 26–1. DSM-IV Criteria of a Major Depressive Episode

Five symptoms present for two weeks with at least one of the criteria in A:

A	Depressed mood°
	Anhedonia°
B	Weight loss or gain
	Insomnia or hypersomnia
	Agitation or motor retardation
	Fatigue or loss of energy
	Depreciation or guilt feelings°
	Concentration difficulties
	Death wishes or suicidal thoughts°

° Most reliable symptoms in palliative care

self-activation, and apathy may at times render depression more difficult to diagnose in neurological patients.[11]

TREATMENT

In non-cancer populations less than a quarter of patients diagnosed as depressed receive effective treatment.[6] It is possible that in neurological palliative care the rate of effective treatment is even lower. Treatment requires a combined approach of antidepressant drugs and empathic support of the patient. Palliative care physicians should be able to offer such a combined treatment, if necessary with the help of other team members, such as nurses and social workers.[12] In complex cases, in patients with psychiatric comorbidities (e.g. anxiety disorders, alcohol abuse), in treatment-resistant depressive states, and where a risk of suicide is suspected, a psychiatrist should be consulted. Response rate for a first treatment with any antidepressant reaches 60% to 85%. Regulation of sleep is frequently the earliest sign of improvement, while amelioration of affective symptoms may progress only over weeks.

Since the efficacy of different agents are very similar, the choice of a specific agent is based on its potential adverse effects and the concomitant somatic morbidity (see [13,14] for review). In general, the newer antidepressants, such as the selective serotonin re-uptake inhibitors (SSRIs) or mirtazepine, are better tolerated, have less side effects (most often transient sleep disturbance and nausea), and are therefore first choice medications in palliative care. In patients with renal insufficiency, doses should range between one-third and two-thirds of the usual dosage; in cardiovascular disease tricyclics should be avoided; in liver insufficiency drugs with short half-lives are preferable.

Failure of response to a first trial of an antidepressant treatment given for 4–6 weeks with a standard dosage should be discussed with a psychiatrist; several strategies with a similar success rate of about 50% can then be advocated. Sudden interruption of antidepressant treatment (especially of the SSRIs) can cause withdrawal symptoms with anxiety, malaise, or recurrence of depressive mood. In patients with a short life expectancy, psychostimulants (e.g. methylphenidate) may be an alternative to antidepressants, since their therapeutic effect may be achieved within days.[15] Psychostimulants may be of special interest to those neurological patients for whom an amelioration of attention, concentration, and sedation is desired.

Any antidepressant treatment requires monitoring of adverse and therapeutic effects and clear information provided to the patient about its risks and benefits and the delay in treatment response. The family should be instructed to seek a balance between protecting the patient from stressors without isolating him, and stimulating him without putting too much pressure on him.

Anxiety Disorders

IMPORTANCE

Anxiety is frequent in medically ill patients, but rarely qualifies as a psychiatric disorder, such as generalized anxiety, phobias, or panic disorder. However, it is a mistake to deduce that anxiety is therefore normal in palliative care and that there is no further need to evaluate anxious states.[16] Few studies examined the prevalence of anxious symptoms in the terminal stage of neurological disease, but the available data show a high proportion of patients experiencing anxiety, for instance about 30% in end-stage ALS[17,18] or 40% in Parkinson's disease, often associated with depression.[11]

DIAGNOSIS

Anxiety may be a symptom of depression, delirium, adjustment disorders, pain, isolation, dyspnea, or fear of death. As with depression, the main diagnostic and therapeutic tool remains the dialog with the patient and his significant others.[19] If an organic cause is suspected, medical examinations, diagnostic workup, and cognitive testing may be necessary to identify an organic cause or to rule out an acute confusional state. Unlike depression, it is less important to achieve an exact diagnosis to classify the anxiety disorder, since treatment remains essentially the same, except for cases where anxiety is of organic origin (including delirium) or part of a major depression. More important is the indication for treatment, which is at times difficult to establish. Some criteria to differentiate pathologic from normal anxiety (and therefore indications for treatment) are summarized in Table 26–2.

TREATMENT

The treating physician should focus on the reasons underlying the anxious state to clarify possible misconceptions or unrealistic anticipations and facilitate the therapeutic expression of anxious feelings. If such supportive interventions fail, non-pharmacological, non-verbal approaches such as relaxation may be helpful. Both benzodiazepines and low-dose neuroleptics are effective and safe in bringing rapid relief to a patient suffering from anxious mood or refractory insomnia (see[20] for review) and are indicated in patients who have limited verbal expression, poor insight, and who do not respond to non-verbal interventions. Intermediate-acting benzodiazepines without active metabolites (e.g. lorazepam) are the first choice in palliative care, since terminally ill patients are at risk of accumulation of long-acting drugs. Short-acting drugs on the other hand may cause rebound and withdrawal phenomena. Risks of abuse, dependence, or withdrawal are minimal in this population. In the elderly, benzodiazepines can induce paradoxical excitement or delirium, and low-dose neuroleptics (e.g. haloperidol) may be a better choice. Low-dose neuroleptics (e.g. haloperidol 3 × 1 mg, levomepromazine 3 × 6.5 mg or thioridazine 3 × 10–30 mg) are helpful also in patients

Table 26–2. Criteria to Differentiate Normal from Pathological Anxiety

	Normal	Pathological
Intensity	Low	high
Duration	Transitory	persistent
Origin	Related to stressors	Not related to stressors
Functional impact	Low	Impaired relationships, thinking, and coping

who suffer from very intense symptoms and who feel literally invaded and overwhelmed by anxiety.

Adjustment Disorders

IMPORTANCE

In a mixed cohort of cancer patients of whom about 50% had psychiatric disorders, adjustment disorders accounted for a large majority (68%) of all diagnoses.[4] Adjustment disorders (AD) are states of subjective distress and emotional disturbance interfering with social functioning and performance. The symptomatology of AD does not reach the intensity of major psychiatric disorders, but is more intense and of longer duration than normal stress reactions (which usually resolve within days) and more stable than grief associated with loss (which is characterized by intervals in which the patient experiences the normal range of emotions). Any stressors challenging human adaptation may initiate AD: pain, medical procedures, hospitalization, conflicts and losses, disability, or approaching death. Despite the high prevalence of AD, there is no empirical research providing information on its most effective treatment or natural course.

DIAGNOSIS

A diagnosis of AD should be considered in patients who experience a disproportionate reaction to a stressor with anxious and depressed symptoms or behavioral disturbances such as agitation or agression. Beside anxious and depressed feelings, manifestations include an inability to cope, loss of control, or significant impairment in social or occupational functioning (see Table 26–3 for differential diagnosis with major depression). AD should be also differentiated from posttraumatic stress disorder, which occurs as a delayed response to a life-threatening or very stressful event with repeated reliving of the trauma in intrusive memories, dreams, and nightmares, and avoidance of reminiscent activities and situations.

Self-administered instruments for anxiety and depression like the Beck's Depression Inventory (BDI), the General Health Questionnaire (GHQ), or the Hospital Anxiety and Depression Scale (HADS) may help to screen for AD. The determination of an optimal cut-off point is an ongoing debate and the few available studies report a sensitivity and specificity of about 75% for the HADS in identifying adjustment disorders.[9]

TREATMENT

Since there is a lack of scientific evidence with regard to the treatment of ADs, the following suggestions are based on our clinical experience. Non-pharmacological approaches are first line of treatment. Providing adequate information on diagnosis, prognosis, and treatment is the first step in helping patients cope with a severe illness; comprehension of this information may be distorted by concomitant intellectual and psychological factors and may need to be evaluated and repeated over time. Counseling is a special intervention to provide support, facilitate emotional expression, and encourage coping. Effective counseling can be provided by specialized nurses. Psychodynamic psychotherapeutic interventions for AD are based on the development of a trusting relationship in which comprehension of the experience is enhanced by the perception of links between the present feelings and older, at times unconscious, feelings, as well as biographical circumstances.

Psychodynamic interventions are provided by psychologists and psychiatrists with a psychotherapeutic background; from our point of view these interventions are most effective for the treatment of AD.[21] Cognitive therapy is problem-focused and tries to identify maladaptive thoughts and irrational beliefs, which are then confronted with reason and reality. Behavioral therapies employ conditioning techniques based on precise observation of

Table 26–3. Differential Diagnosis of Major Depression (MD) and Adjustment Disorder (AD)

	AD	MD
No. of symptoms	<5	>5
Intensity	+ +	+ + +
Permanence	No	Yes
Functional impact	Yes	Yes

behavior and the use of directive methods (desensibilization, stepwise confrontation) to change behavior. Cognitive-behavioral interventions are provided by a specialized therapist and, clinically, seem to be effective.

Few psychotropic medications have been tested in AD, but clinical experience supports their value in palliative care. The role of antidepressants for AD with depressed mood is debated, but anxiolytics are generally recognized to be of benefit in patients with anxious mood.[20] For patients with difficulties in applying relaxation techniques, benzodiazepines are effective for rapid symptom relief. In severely ill patients with numerous stressors, a complete remission of AD may not always be achieved despite adequate efforts; psychopharmacological treatment should have been adequately tried before accepting the patient's distressing symptoms as intractable.

Other Psychiatric Disorders

Delirium or acute confusional state is a common complication of neurological disease and is covered elsewhere in this book (see Chapter 22). The main diagnostic criterion of delirium is the presence of disturbed consciousness and cognition (not present in major depression, anxiety, and adjustment disorders or acute stress reactions), its acute onset (unlike dementia), and the suspicion of an organic causal factor. Delirium and *dementia*, which is also covered in another chapter (see Chapter 6), often remain unrecognized, misdiagnosed, or diagnosed with a considerable delay when the patient is agitated or manifestly disorganized and a psychiatric intervention becomes necessary.

Psychosis, defined as the presence of delusions and/or hallucinations, may be part of an acute confusional state. Another psychotic state frequently observed in patients without disturbed consciousness—the *organic hallucinosis*—is most frequently due to alcohol withdrawal or active drinking. Given the fact that organic hallucinosis may last for weeks or months, neuroleptics (e.g. haloperidol, risperidone, olanzapine) are the treatment of choice if the underlying cause cannot be identified and treated.[22,23] In Parkinson's disease patients, clozapine 12.5–100 mg a day is preferred to avoid extrapyramidal side effects (see Chapter 5).

Psychotic states in patients with psychiatric disorders of the *schizophrenic spectrum* are rare in palliative care and can be diagnosed with a careful anamnesis from the patient or his significant others. *Mania* is characterized by inflated self-esteem, decreased need for sleep, distractibility, flights of ideas, hyperactivity, and, at times, aggressiveness and can present with or without psychotic symptoms. Mania is also rare in palliative care and often is due to a recurrence of primary bipolar disorder or is secondary to medications, stroke, HIV encephalopathy, and other brain lesions. To ensure an exact diagnosis and adequate treatment, a psychiatric consultation should be requested; in agitated patients, sedating neuroleptics are indicated until psychiatric and medical evaluation can take place.

Difficult patients are frequently individuals with *personality disorders*, defined as a pattern of enduring traits with an impact on most of the individual's personal and social interactions. For instance, *antisocial personality* disorder is characterized by a disregard for, and violation of, the rights of others. *Borderline personality* disorder consists of a pattern of instability in interpersonal relationships, self-image, and affects and marked impulsivity. Patients with *narcissistic personality* disorder present with grandiosity, need for admiration, and lack of empathy. Even health-care professionals who are used to coping with difficult situations may feel helpless when confronted with patients with personality disorders. The consulting psychiatrist can sometimes be very helpful by searching, with the patient, for the sources of his behavior (often due to anxiety), by clarifying that some but not all of his needs can realistically be met, by enhancing his perception of control,

and by setting firm limits on conscious and unconscious manipulative behavior. It is important when confronting the patient to acknowledge the reality of the stresses he experiences in order to avoid a breakdown of his defenses.[24,25]

Personality disorders are not easy to diagnose and the consulting psychiatrist can help by explaining the psychopathology of the patient to the staff, decreasing negative attitudes towards the patient. Such information often cools down the 'heated interpersonal atmosphere' and has an indirect positive effect on the patient's behavior. In addition, the psychiatrist may spell out the limited therapeutic possibilities and the notion of a 'palliative psychiatric situation', which often makes the accompaniment of the patient less stressful.

GENERAL ASPECTS: COPING, DEFENSES, AND ADAPTATION

Severely ill patients with advanced disease face a variety of stressors such as physical symptoms, social and financial problems, uncertainty, and changes in close relationships. Coping with these stressors is influenced by different factors, including the patient's biography, contextual factors, and personality traits. Coping may be defined as what one does about a problem in order to bring about relief, reward, quiescence, and equilibrium.[26] A variety of coping strategies have been identified, which can be classified into active and passive strategies (see examples in Table 26–4). It might be difficult to relate the individual coping strategies to a specific outcome, but it seems that the strategies which are more passive (such as wishful thinking) are less adaptive in the long run.

Table 26–4. **Examples of Coping Strategies**

Active	Passive
Seek information	Submit to the inevitable
Share concern	Withdraw into isolation
Try to forget, distract	Blame someone, something
Confront, take actions	Wishful thinking, wait and see

Coping strategies are conscious, but defense mechanisms, such as denial, are not conscious. In patients with advanced disease, defenses play a regulatory role for the preservation of psychic equilibrium and protect from painful emotions or threatening thoughts. Rationalization, (partial) denial, or projection are frequently observed defense mechanisms in palliative care patients. Some examples are:

- Partial denial: 'I know that this is a fatal disease, but I am pretty sure that for me it will take a much more favorable course than predicted by medicine.'
- Isolation of affect: 'I know very well that I will be dying within the next few weeks, but I do not feel sad or angry about it.'
- Projection: 'I'm fine, but all these other ill patients, they must have a hard time.'

Defense mechanisms have also been classified as mature and immature. This is not helpful in the palliative care setting, where these mechanisms should not be challenged but observed as a source of information, illustrating the vulnerability of a patient.

Adaptation is related to coping and to defense mechanisms, but also depends on a variety of other factors, such as social support, biographical circumstances, personality traits, individual resources, or physical threats, such as enduring symptoms. Repeated and inadequate or inefficient efforts for adaptation may be an important source for exhaustion, depressive symptoms, anxiety disorders, or behavioral disturbances. It is therefore important that palliative care professionals repeatedly evaluate their patients' adaptive efforts and assist them in their individual efforts to adapt to a severe and incurable disease.

SUMMARY

Psychiatric symptoms are very common and still under-recognized in the palliative care setting. Lack of clearly established diagnostic and therapeutic procedures, uncertainties surrounding psychosocial issues, and lack of effective communication underlie this unsatisfactory situation. It is our hope that this chapter will be of some help to neurologists and palliative care specialists in detection and treatment, as well as educational aspects towards this complex topic.

REFERENCES

1. Stiefel F, Guex P. Palliative and supportive care: at the frontier of medical omnipotence. Ann Oncol 1996;7:135–138.
2. Ghika–Schmid F, Bogousslavsky J. Affective disorders following stroke. Eur Neurol 1997; 38:75–81.
3. Fogel BS, Schiffer RB, Rao SM. Synopsis of Neuropsychiatry. Lippincott Williams and Wilkins, New York, 2000.
4. Derogatis LR, Morrow G, Fetting J, et al. The prevalence and severity of psychiatric disorders among cancer patients. JAMA 1983;249:751–757.
5. Ozer MN. Management of persons with chronic neurologic illness. Butterworth–Heinemann, Boston, 2000.
6. Lloyd–Williams M, Friedman T, Rudd N. A survey of antidepressant prescribing in the terminally ill. Palliat Med 1999;13:243–248.
7. Chochinov HM, Breitbart W. Handbook of Psychiatry in Palliative Medicine. Oxford University Press, New York, 2000.
8. Doyle D, Hanks GW, MacDonaldN, eds. Oxford Textbook of palliative medicine, 2nd Ed. Oxford University Press, New York, 1998.
9. Razavi D, Stiefel F. Common psychiatric disorders in cancer patients. I. Adjustment disorders and depressive disorders. Journal of Supportive Care in Cancer 1994;2:223–232.
10. American Psychiatric Association. Diagnostic and Statistical Manual of Mental Disorders, 4th Ed. American Psychiatric Press, Washington DC, 1994.
11. Lauterbach EC. Psychiatric Management in Neurological Disease. American Psychiatric Press, Washington DC, .
12. Stiefel F. Psychosocial aspects of cancer pain. Support Care Cancer 1993;1:130–134.
13. Berney A, Stiefel F, Mazzocato C, Buclin T. Psychopharmacology in supportive care of cancer: a review for the clinician. III. Antidepressants. Journal of Supportive Care in Cancer 2000;8:277–285.
14. Stiefel F, Di Trill, Berney A, Olarte JN, Razavi D, the EAPC Research Steering Committee. Depression in palliative care: a pragmatic report from the Expert Working Group of the European Association for Palliative Care. Journal of Supportive Care in Cancer 2001; 9:477–488.
15. Bruera E, Miller MJ, Macmillan K, et al. Neuropsychological effects of methylphenidate in patients receiving a continuous infusion of narcotics for cancer pain. Pain 1992;48:163–168.
16. Razavi D, Stiefel F. Psychiatric disorders in cancer patients. In: Klastersky J, Schimpff SC, Senn HJ, eds. Supportive Care in Cancer. A Handbook for Oncologists. 2nd Ed. revised and expanded. Marcel Decker, Inc., New York, 1999.
17. Voltz R, Borasio GD. Palliative therapy in the terminal stage of neurological disease. J Neurol 1997;244(suppl 4):2–10.
18. Borasio GD, Voltz R. Palliative care in amyotrophic lateral sclerosis. J Neurol 1997;244 (suppl 4):11–17.
19. Stiefel F, Razavi D. Common psychiatric disorders in cancer patients. II. Anxiety and confusional states. Journal of Supportive Care in Cancer 1994;2(4):233–237.

20. Stiefel F, Berney A, Mazzocato C. Psychopharmacology in supportive care of cancer: a review for the clinician. I. Benzodiazepines. Journal of Supportive Care in Cancer 1999;7:379–385.
21. Guex P, Stiefel F, Rousselle I. Psychotherapy with patients with cancer. Psychotherapy Review 2000; 2:269–275.
22. Mazzocato C, Stiefel F, Buclin T, Berney A. Psychopharmacology in supportive care of cancer: a review for the clinician. II. Neuroleptics. Journal of Supportive Care in Cancer 2000;8:89–97.
23. Stiefel F, Holland J. Delirium in cancer patients. International Psychogeriatrics 1991;3:333–338.
24. Haan N. Coping and Defending: Processes of Self-Environment Organization. Academic Press, New York, 1977.
25. Groves JE. Difficult patients. In: Cassem NH, Stern TA, Rosenbaum JF, Jellinek MS, eds. Handbook of General Hospital Psychiatry, 4th Ed. Mosby Year Books Inc., 1997:337–366.
26. Weisman A. Coping with Cancer. McGraw–Hill, New York, 1979.

PART **4**

OTHER PROBLEMS WITH ADVANCED ILLNESS

Chapter 27

Neurological Emergencies

Janet Hardy
Donal Martin

Spinal cord compression (SCC) has the potential to impair, suddenly and drastically, the quality of life, not only of a patient but also their relatives and/or carers. The devastating effects of SCC and the speed at which irreversible neurological damage occurs defines this condition as a true oncological emergency. The outcome of treatment, as measured by the degree of residual neurological impairment, is dependent on the time from first development of symptoms to the start of treatment. In many instances, patients are left with marked impairment in performance status and neurological function. This has profound implications for palliative care services that are often called upon to provide the ongoing care for these patients.

Raised intracranial pressure (ICP) is a common complication of both metastatic and primary brain disease. It is characterized by specific clinical features and can present as an oncological emergency because of the risk of seizures and loss of consciousness. The symptoms are often difficult to manage

in the absence of any specific treatment of the underlying condition and can present a major challenge to those providing the palliative care of these patients.

Status epilepticus is an oncological, neurological, and palliative care emergency with the potential to cause enormous distress unless properly managed. The cornerstone of good palliative management lies in an early decision as to level of treatment undertaken. Full or 'extended' emergency care can only be given in a center with appropriate intensive care facilities

There are a number of clinical situations in which the speed of delivery of treatment will significantly effect outcome. These are known as emergencies. In general, the more rapid the diagnosis and intervention, the better the outcome. In the palliative care setting, it may not be possible, appropriate, or reasonable to deliver active treatment in these cases. It is essential, however, to know how to palliate symptoms rapidly in emergency situations.

283

SPINAL CORD COMPRESSION

CASE HISTORY

The elderly wife of a 72-year-old man suffering from carcinoma of the prostate requests a home visit by his physician after he has a fall. The patient, who had been previously ambulant, gives a two-week history of midline lumbar back pain, difficulty in micturition, and recalls episodes of his legs 'giving way'. Clinical examination reveals local lumbar spine tenderness, reduced lower limb power (3/5), lower limb hyperreflexia, and equivocal plantar reflexes. There is abnormal sensation to the level of the umbilicus and an enlarged bladder is palpable. The physician prescribes corticosteroids, opioid analgesia, and arranges hospital admission.

Plain X-rays of the spine prove unremarkable, but MRI shows widespread vertebral disease with compression of the spinal cord at the level of the lower thoracic vertebrae. Urgent radiotherapy is given over the next 10 days and steroids are gradually withdrawn following completion of treatment. The patient requires urethral catheterization and attempts at removing the urinary catheter are unsuccessful. Analgesia is achieved but constipation becomes a difficult symptom to control and he develops a sacral pressure sore. There is little improvement in lower limb power.

The patient remains chairbound despite regular physiotherapy. He requires the assistance of two to transfer from chair to bed and full nursing care for personal hygiene. After a home assessment by an occupational therapist in consultation with patient and family, a multidisciplinary decision is made to refer the patient for nursing home care.

Introduction

Spinal cord compression (SCC) is an oncological emergency that has the potential to reduce performance status dramatically and to affect quality of life profoundly.[1] The reversibility of neurological deficit depends on the magnitude, rate, and duration of compression.[2] It is imperative, therefore, to treat this condition as an emergency. SCC has an incidence of 5% in cancer sufferers but larger numbers are thought to have asymptomatic epidural metastatic spread.[3] Tumors of the breast, lung, and prostate account for 60% of cases.[4] With improving survival rates in patients with cancer, the symptomatic incidence is expected to rise in the future.

Pathophysiology

The most common cause of SCC in malignant disease, is compression of the dural sac, spinal cord, and/or cauda equina by extradural tumor. Less often, compression may be due to leptomeningeal or intramedullary disease. Other causes of SCC must be considered however (e.g. epidural abscess, hemorrhage, and disc herniation).

SCC may be secondary to metastatic or primary malignant disease. It may originate from spinal parenchyma metastases or laterally from vertebral foramina invasion, but anterior cord compression from metastatic growth and expansion of the vertebral body is the most common mechanism.

Presentation

SCC often occurs at multiple levels[1] but most frequently at the level of the thoracic spine.[5] Patients commonly present with bilateral 'band'-like pain extending around the chest from the back, that may be followed up days to months later by limb weakness. Thoracic spine secondaries are more often associated with primary cancers of the breast and lung.[6] Lumbosacral spinal metastases are more common with colon and pelvic primary tumors. Here, nerve roots have a longer course in a wider spinal canal and compression therefore may well present with radicular pain rather than weakness.[5] Cauda equina compression can present with low back pain, leg weakness, perianal 'saddle' anesthesia, urinary retention, and paresthesia in the legs or buttocks.

As back pain is a common symptom of malignancy, the possibility of SCC can easily be overlooked. Pain secondary to SCC is typically focal and mid vertebral or radicular, aching, and unremitting. It may also be aggravated on lying down, moving, sneezing, or neck flexion.

Whilst the development of motor symptoms increases the probability of a diagnosis of

SCC, it reduces the likelihood of functional recovery and shortens survival expectation.[1] Weakness may present with difficulty in climbing stairs or rising from a sitting position. A patient will often be reported to have 'gone off their legs'. The loss of power is associated with increased reflexes and limb tone. Plantar reflexes may be up-going. Altered sensation and paresthesia can also occur in keeping with the level of compression. Proprioception loss may produce ataxia. Signs of autonomic dysfunction (i.e. constipation and urinary retention) occur late in the development of SCC.

Investigations

A sensitive and specific investigation is important for early detection and for establishing a diagnosis. Plain radiographs detect vertebral body involvement by tumor in 85% of cases,[7] but are not sufficient to make a diagnosis of SCC. Magnetic resonance imaging (MRI) is the investigation of choice. MRI is non-invasive, produces a better soft tissue image, is more efficient in the detection of bone instability than myelography, and identifies significantly more patients with multiple sites of compression.[8] MRI has been shown to improve radiotherapy field targeting[9] but can be uncomfortable and claustrophobic to some patients and may be prohibited by the presence of metal objects or prosthesis. At present, myelography is used only if MRI is contraindicated. This investigation involves a risk of cerebrospinal fluid leak, infection, and bleeding.

Treatment

The main aims of treatment of SCC are:
- Prevention of neurological deterioration
- Preservation or recovery of function and performance status
- Pain control
- Prevention of local disease progression
- Maintenance of spinal stability

CORTICOSTEROIDS

There is a general consensus of opinion that steroids should be commenced on first suspicion of SCC. The primary intention is to stabilize or improve neurological deficits whilst awaiting definitive treatment.

The choice of steroid dosage regimen (i.e. 'high' dose dexamethasone 96 mg/day versus 'moderate' dose 16 mg/day) is controversial. One study of good methodological quality has compared high-dose dexamethasone plus radiotherapy with no steroids and radiotherapy. A greater number of patients were ambulatory post-treatment in the steroid arm.[10] Higher doses of steroids give a higher incidence of rapid analgesia[11] but significantly more side effects[4], and have been associated with fatality. Other studies have failed to show a difference in outcome between high- and moderate-dose dexamethasone.[12,13] There is fair evidence that steroids do not have to be given to those patients with asymptomatic SCC undergoing radiotherapy.[14]

All regimens should include a system of steroid dose reduction when definitive treatment is completed. When using moderate doses of dexamethasone (16 mg/day), this could take the form of a 2–4 mg/day dose reduction every four days.

SURGERY

Neurosurgical decompression may be considered for patients with low-volume or single-site disease and good performance status.[1] Indications for a surgical opinion include unknown diagnosis, spinal instability, radio-resistant tumors, or spinal compression by bone. Vertebral body resection (VBR) and spinal stabilization effectively removes the tumor and is the superior procedure for those with a reasonable life expectancy and performance score. However, VBR incurs a higher complication rate than laminectomy (a temporary measure for relieving posterior lesions causing anterior spinal pressure).[15] The evidence to guide practice in this area remains poor. One study of factors affecting survival of surgical patients has suggested that patients with two or more of the following—limb strength less than or equal to 3/5; lung or colon cancer; multiple vertebral disease—should *not* be considered for surgery.[16]

RADIOTHERAPY

Radiotherapy is the mainstay of treatment for malignant SCC. Doses vary between centers, but are most often within the range 8 Gy in 1 fraction[15] (for analgesia) to 30 Gy in 10 fractions over two weeks. Total dosage is limited by spinal cord tolerance, but may be altered to account for the radiosensitivity of the tumor. For example, lymphoma, breast, and testicular tumors tend to respond better than more radioresistant tumors such as melanoma. There is little evidence to suggest that total doses higher than 30 Gy improve functional outcome for the common primary cancers.[8]

CHEMOTHERAPY

Combination chemotherapy has been used to control metastatic SCC in those patients unsuitable for surgery or radiotherapy and/or those with highly chemosensitive tumors such as lymphoma and small cell cancers.

Continuing Care

Pre-treatment ambulatory and performance status are significant predictors of both treatment response and survival. Unfortunately, as so many patients present with advanced SCC, the realistic goal of treatment is often the prevention of further neurological deterioration rather than an improvement in neurological status. In one study, only 20% of symptomatic patients showed neurological improvement following treatment with radiotherapy, although at least 50% failed to deteriorate (which may in itself reflect a treatment response).[1]

SCC is most often a complication of advanced metastatic disease and the development of SCC is a poor prognostic factor with a median survival from treatment of less than three months.[1] Survivors of SCC have a 45% chance of developing relapse or new site spinal disease within the following three years.[8]

However, a significant proportion of patients will live for many months following the development of SCC, and will require intensive rehabilitation and ongoing care. The symptoms encountered include reduced mobility, constipation, urinary retention, pressure sores, pain, and major depression.[17] Patients will often be chair or bedbound. They are likely to need long-term catheterization. Daily assistance will be required in washing, feeding, and toileting. Symptom control needs will demand regular attention.

Discharge to home will necessitate substantial input from community services. Major renovations are often required to make a home wheelchair and hoist compatible. Long-term community placement is often difficult to obtain, especially for younger patients. The devastating and often sudden loss of mobility and the patient's total dependency can have a profound affect on families and carers who will need to be offered both practical and emotional support.

STATUS EPILEPTICUS

CASE HISTORY

A 62-year-old insulin-dependent diabetic male with a history of renal cell carcinoma presented following a right-sided tonic clonic fit lasting 10 minutes which left him with a residual right-sided weakness. A cerebral CT scan revealed a single metastasis which was excised via a frontal craniotomy. Prior to, and following surgery, he continued to have focal as well as generalized tonic clonic seizures. He was unable to tolerate phenytoin and was commenced on sodium valproate. The focal seizures involving the right arm became more frequent, often lasting for hours at a time. The patient remained conscious throughout but was very distressed by the constant jerking which he attempted to control with the other arm.

Carbamazepine was introduced and steroids were avoided because of the history of diabetes. A subsequent CT revealed progressive cerebral disease for which he underwent whole brain radiotherapy. Following the radiotherapy he continued to suffer from almost continuous seizure activity in the right arm. A diagnosis of epilepsia partialis continua was confirmed by a neurologist who advised the addition of clobazepam and to continue increasing the dose of both sodium valproate and carbamazepine. The fits were eventually controlled but the patient remained very drowsy, confused, and agitated and had frequent falls.

He was highly dependent on nursing staff for daily cares and his wife became very concerned about her ability to look after her husband at home. An intensive community 'support package' was arranged with the help of the district nurse, his physician, the hospital outpatient clinic, and the local hospice community team.

Introduction

A fit or convulsion is probably one of the most distressing ways that a cerebral neoplasm or metastatic spread can manifest. The event itself can leave behind it a wake of acute despair and dread of future physical, psychological, and social morbidity in both patients and carers. Fears of fit recurrence and of a loss of cognitive function or sanity can come to dominate daily life. Patients and their relatives may be left preoccupied with existential thoughts or death anxiety.[18] It is therefore imperative that the physician has a clearly defined plan of diagnostic investigation and management to deal with such emergency situations.[19,20]

Definition and Classification

Although controversy exists in the definition of this phenomenon,[21] most would broadly agree with a definition including the following parameters: 'status epilepticus is any epileptic seizure(s) lasting longer than 30 minutes without recovery of consciousness. Fits may be convulsive or non-convulsive, generalized or partial in nature.'

The types of status epilepticus most often encountered by palliative medicine physicians are: tonic clonic, epilepsia partialis continua (EPC), and complex partial non-convulsive status epilepticus. EPC originates in the cerebral cortex and leads to clonic jerking of distal muscle groups for weeks or even months. Complex partial non-convulsive status epilepticus may present as a confusional state without obvious fitting.

Etiology

Status epilepticus in palliative care will most commonly result from a primary brain tumor or metastatic spread to meningeal or parenchymal brain tissue. Other possible non-tumor causes are:

- Primary brain tumor or metastases
- Cerebral infarction, bleeds, or infections
- Metabolic conditions e.g. hyper- or hypoglycemia, hyponatremia, hyopmagnesia, or hypoxia
- Iatrogenic factors e.g. inappropriate dose reduction of antiepileptic agents, radiation therapy, chemotherapy (including the anti-metabolites, alkylators,[33] vinca alkaloids), opioids,[34] phenothiazines, some penicillin-based antibiotics and contrast medium.[35]
- Alcohol abuse or withdrawal

Alcohol abuse or withdrawal can be an easily overlooked cause within a palliative care setting.[22]

Pathophysiology

Convulsive status epilepticus presents as epileptic activity increasing in frequency with tonic clonic convulsions merging into continuous motor activity. This stage will eventually lead to electro-mechanical dissociation and, if untreated, culminate in death.

Physiologically, status epilepticus can be divided into two phases:[23]

1. The compensatory phase (lasting approximately 30 minutes)

During this time compensatory mechanisms protect the fitting brain by increasing cerebral blood flow and metabolism. Subsequent to this, lactate levels may rise, cardiac function increases, hypertension and hypergylcemia occur. Autonomic activation may cause hyperpyrexia and vomiting.

2. The decompensatory phase

During this phase, long-term cerebral damage occurs as compensatory mechanisms fail. Cerebral blood flow and metabolism are reduced in response to systemic hypotension. The patient will become hypoxic. Cerebral edema may develop in response to an imbalance between raised intracranial pressure and systemic hypotension.

Acidosis (both metabolic and respiratory), hypoglycemia, hypokalemia, and hyponatremia may develop. Renal failure can be aggravated by acute tubular necrosis, hyperuricemia, and rhabdomyolysis due to repeated convulsive activity. Cardiac dysrhythmias may also occur. Brain damage from areas of neuronal necrosis, including the hippocampus, will result in loss of cognitive function.

Treatment

Status epilepticus offers a particular challenge to palliative care physicians. The management will depend on the patient's diagnosis, age, performance status, and prognosis and whether a full recovery could be expected. A good knowledge of the patient's and/or carers wishes can be invaluable in formulating management plans for unpredicted events. The decision should be made early on in the convulsive activity as to whether the patient should be transferred from a 'low-tech' medical environment (e.g. hospice or home) to a 'high-tech' facility (e.g. hospital intensive care unit). The intensity of treatment, investigations, and monitoring that can be done will depend entirely on the chosen facility.

Comprehensive emergency treatment of status epilepticus in a hospital setting is outlined in Table 27–1. Extended management involves cardiac and electroencephalograph monitoring when following the treatment plan. Intensive treatment therefore necessitates transfer to an intensive care unit with facilities for intubation, ventilation, anesthesia, and management of renal, hepatic, cardiac, and metabolic complications.

Whatever the setting of care, a state of status epilepticus will always be distressing to both the patient and his or her carers. In all cases, after ensuring safe positioning and a patent airway, it is appropriate to palliate fitting or convulsive activity using fast-acting benzodiazepines in the first instance. Intravenous diazepam may be used but lozazepam has a longer duration of antiepileptic action.[24] Clonazepam can also be used as an alternative. Absorption from an intramuscular injection or from a rectal suppository is relatively slow. Therefore, these are not ideal routes of drug delivery but may provide the only practical solution in an emergency situation. Blood glucose levels should be checked as fitting secondary to hypoglycemia can easily be reversed. Similarly, parenteral thiamine should be considered if alcohol abuse is suspected.

Should the decision be made for the patient to remain in a place with fewer technological facilities, and benzodiazepines have failed to control the situation, an intramuscular injection of phenobarbitone may be given, followed by a subcutaneous infusion over 24 hours (Table 27–2).[25]

Other agents that may be employed against resistant seizures are shown in Table 27–2. Midazolam is a fast-acting benzodiazepine

Table 27–1. Emergency Treatment of Status Epilepticus

As the neurological damage sustained is dependent on the duration of the fit, it is important to monitor time as fitting continues.[36]

Time 0 minutes
- Maintain an airway, give oxygen by mask or nasal prongs
- Monitor ECG
- Achieve IV access, maintain patency by normal saline drip
- If hypoglycemia is suspected or recorded give 50 mls of 50% dextrose and 100 mg of thiamine
- Send blood for laboratory testing (hematology, renal and hepatic function, glucose, calcium and magnesium, anticonvulsant drug levels)
- Monitor oxygen saturation by oximetry or arterial gas levels as appropriate

Time 10 minutes
- Diazepam 0.2 mg/kg IV up to 20 mg given at a rate no faster than 5 mg/minute
or
- Lorazepam 0.1 mg/kg IV at a rate of 2 mg/minute up to a total dose of 4 mg

Time 20–30 minutes
(Status is now becoming established and has failed to respond to short-term measures)
- Phenytoin 15 mg/kg IV given at a rate no faster than 50 mg/minute; total dosage 1000 mg over 20 minutes in average adult
(Fosphenytoin, a prodrug of phenytoin, which can be given faster with fewer local side effects, may be used as an alternative)
Monitor ECG and blood pressure
or
- Phenobarbital IV 10 mg/kg at < 30 mg/minute for adults

Time 60+ minutes
(Anesthesia is generally now required)
- Propofol 2 mg/kg IV bolus, followed by an infusion of 5–10 mg/kg/hour gradually reduced to 1–3 mg/kg/hr over 12 hours
or
- Thiopental 100–250 mg IV bolus over 20 seconds followed by 50 mg boluses every 2–3minutes until fits are controlled; then give as a continuous infusion of 3–5 mg/kg/hour, and slowly withdraw 12 hours after fits stop

which can be given by intramuscular or buccal routes. Its activity is prolonged in liver disease.[26]

Propofol is an intravenous anesthetic agent which permits rapid control of depth of sedation and has been successfully used in the treatment of status epilepticus.[27] It has been used in a hospice setting,[28] but has the disadvantage of requiring venous access and close monitoring.

It is advisable to try to avoid or discontinue all phenothiazine sedatives (e.g. haloperidol, levomepromazine [now 'methotrimeprazine']) because of the theoretical risk of lowering the epileptic threshold. In all cases, the continued use of benzodiazepines should be avoided if they are only giving short-term control as these agents can precipitate hypotensive or respiratory collapse. It is thought that benzodiazepines may have a therapeutic 'ceiling' after which the GABA inhibitory system is maximally induced and further increase in dosage has minimal effect.[29]

It is important to be aware of non-convulsive status epilepticus as a differential diagnosis for a confused individual. Appropriate antiepileptic treatment may therefore benefit the altered mental state.[30] Similarly, it is mandatory to follow up any episode of status epilepticus with antiepileptic therapy,[6] as the event itself may induce epileptogenic lesions within the brain leading to further risk of fitting.

Prognosis

Mortality following a first episode of status epilepticus is approximately 10% in adults,

and epilepsy is thought to recur in over 13% of cases.[31] Most patients die from the underlying condition and morbidity is mainly sustained during the phase of decompensation. One study has shown the main predictors of fatality to be age, duration of status before commencement of treatment, and CNS infection.[32]

Support for Carers and Family

Regular communication with relatives and carers will be essential at all stages. The relatives of patients with recurrent epileptiform attacks must have clear instructions as to what to do in the case of fitting and of whom to contact in an emergency. Issues such as resuscitation and prognosis need to be addressed so that informed decisions can be made regarding the appropriateness or intensity of further treatment.

Summary

Status epilepticus is an oncological, neurological, and palliative care emergency with the potential to cause enormous distress unless properly managed. The cornerstone of good palliative management lies in an early decision as to the level of treatment undertaken. Full or 'extended' emergency care can only be given in a center with appropriate intensive care facilities.

Table 27–2. Treatment of Status Epilepticus in the Absence of Intensive Care Facilities

• *Benzodiazepines*		Diazepam 10–20 mg IV at a rate of 5 mg per minute or 10–20 mg per rectum
	or	Lorazepam 4 mg by slow IV injection
	or	Clonazepam 1 mg by slow IV injection

Midazolam is a fast-acting benzodiazepine which can be used for maintenance treatment once control has been achieved. It can be delivered by subcutaneous, intramuscular, or buccal routes. The usual subcutaneous dosage is 10–15 mg stat followed by 50–200 mg over 24 hours.

• *Phenobarbitone*: when benzodiazepines have failed to give control consider phenobarbitone 200 mg by deep intramuscular injection followed by a subcutaneous infusion of 600–2400 mg over 24 hour[25]

• *Propofol*: 100–200 mg IV bolus followed by 5–70 mg/hour IV (see text)

RAISED INTRACRANIAL PRESSURE

CASE HISTORY

A 34-year-old mother of three small children presented with carcinoma of the left breast and bone metastases. Her initial treatment consisted of mastectomy with axillary clearance followed by post-operative radiotherapy to the chest wall. While receiving adjuvant chemotherapy she was found to have bone metastases. She was given radiotherapy to the thoracic spine and ovaries and was commenced on tamoxifen.

Two years later, she presented with early morning headaches, vomiting, and left-sided facial hypersensitivity. A cerebral CT confirmed the presence of cerebellar metastases. She underwent whole brain irradiation but, by this time, she had developed unsteadiness of gait and poor co-ordination.

The patient remained reasonably well at home until three months later when she re-presented with increasing headaches and nausea. An initial cerebral CT scan showed no evidence of progression and she was managed symptomatically with analgesia and antiemetics. Readmission was necessary as she was too ill to be cared for at home with worsening of early morning headaches, nausea and vomiting, double and blurred vision, and unsteady gait, leading to frequent falls. Corticosteroids relieved her symptoms to some extent but a repeat CT scan revealed a new midline cerebellar lesion causing obstructive hydrocephalus, mass effect, and risk of 'coning'.

After prolonged discussion with the patient and her partner the largest of the cerebellar metastases was surgically removed. The post-operative course was difficult and complicated by dizziness on any movement, deafness, nausea and vomiting, and a left-sided weakness. The patient was confined to bed and became very withdrawn and regretted the decision to proceed with surgery. There was slow improvement and two months later she was discharged to her local hospice, in order to be near her family. Five months following surgery she remained significantly handicapped, but discharge home was considered.

Introduction

Raised intracranial pressure (ICP) is a pressure greater than 25 mm Hg, when measured by an intraparenchymal monitor placed in the right frontal brain via a small burr hole.[37] Normally, ICP varies rhythmically with pulse and respiration. When ICP is raised, large 'plateau' waves of pressure build up.[38] 'Cerebral perfusion pressure' (mean arterial pressure (MAP) minus ICP) is the main factor controlling cerebral blood flow. 'Autoregulation' via cerebral vasoconstriction or vasodilatation normally provides a balance between MAP and ICP, thereby maintaining cerebral blood flow. An increase in ICP not matched by an increase in MAP will therefore result in anoxic brain damage.

Raised ICP can be due to a variety of causes—primary brain tumor, metastatic spread, cerebral bleeds, infarction, abscess, trauma, meningitis, and any pathology whereby normal flow of cerebrospinal fluid is blocked. In everyday practice, this state is reflected by a characteristic clinical picture:

- Morning headaches (aggravated by cough or strain)
- Nausea and vomiting
- Transient loss of vision with papilledema
- False localizing signs (e.g. sixth nerve lateral rectus palsy, ipsilateral pyramidal limb signs due to midline cerebral shift)
- Intellectual or personality changes

The onset may be relatively slow (brain metastases) or acute (cerebral hemorrhage or herniation). A lowering of level of consciousness is a serious prognostic factor and may indicate the brain stem being forced through the foramen magnum or 'coning'. This condition will culminate in death if not treated.

Treatment

Treatment should take into account age, performance score, neurological condition, tumor type, extent of systemic illness, expected quantity and quality of life outcome, and patient's wishes. Supportive care only, may be totally appropriate.[39] Thought should be given to the impact of any treatment on the quality of time remaining to the patient. Difficult decisions about active treatment are best made with multidisciplinary help. If active management is then decided upon, rehabilitation should be an integral part of care.

SPECIFIC ANTI-CANCER THERAPY

Surgery, radiotherapy, and antibiotics may all be appropriate to correct the underlying problem in specific patients—even those with widespread metastatic disease if the performance status is good and the expected outcome favorable.

SUPPORTIVE CARE

Headaches should be treated according to standard WHO guidelines. It is often said that opioids are contraindicated in cases of raised ICP because of the risk of respiratory depression causing hypercapnia leading to a spiral of reflex vasodilation, a further increase in ICP, and increased headache. We have not found this to be a problem in routine practice. Similarly, nausea and vomiting need to be treated aggressively with standard antiemetics. There is no evidence that any one antiemetic is better than any other in this condition. In theory, phenothiazine antipsychotics (e.g. haloperidol) should be avoided because of the possible risk of fit exacerbation.[40]

CORTICOSTEROIDS

These provide the mainstay of palliation in raised ICP as they can dramatically improve neurological deficits associated with brain edema. The mechanism of their action is not yet fully understood and may be multifactorial.[41] Clinical improvement can be seen before any reduction in ICP. It has been postulated that corticosteroids initially reduce the size of 'plateau' pressure waves, encourage regional cerebral blood flow, and improve tissue compliance.[42] Dexamethasone is prescribed as the steroid of choice because of its relative potency and minimal salt-retaining properties. The usual doses of dexamethasone prescribed (16–24 mg/day) are arbitrarily based and cautious downwards titration for individual maintenance dosing is advised.

Steroids have significant side effects in the longer term and should be steadily reduced to the lowest dose that controls symptoms.[43] If steroids are not, or no longer controlling neurological deficits, they should be discontinued.

The side effects of steroids can be particularly distressing in children (e.g. voracious appetite, massive weight gain, behavioral changes). In children with primary brain tumors, attempts are often made to avoid steroids if at all possible, whilst treating symptoms aggressively with antiemetics and analgesia, as above.[44]

MANITOL

The use of a hyperosmolar solution (mannitol 20% solution, 1.5–2 g/kg IV over 15–20 minutes) to reverse the osmotic gradient and drive fluid from brain to blood is thought to produce a short-term effect.[45] Mannitol has been associated with acute oliguric renal failure—possibly by renal vasoconstriction[46]—and it is advisable to monitor the osmolal gap if repeat infusions are needed.[47] Other complications include: electrolyte and fluid imbalance, cardiopulmonary edema, and even a rebound increase in vasogenic cerebral edema.[48] However, some workers have used mannitol infusions very successfully in the home setting on an 'as required' basis to palliate the symptoms of raised ICP without complication.

HYPERVENTILATION

Patients in intensive care may be ventilated to a PCO2 of 25–20 mm Hg. This induces vasoconstriction, a reduction in cerebral blood volume, and reduction in ICP.

Support of Patient and Family

In palliative care, raised ICP is most commonly seen in patients with primary brain tumors or cerebral metastases. By the time of referral, most patients will have already undergone surgery or radiotherapy or will have been deemed unfit for such treatment. The emphasis must then be on the control of symptoms and the support of the patient and his/her family. The family will have to face the inevitable progression of disease and deterioration of neurological functioning. It is likely that at some stage steroids will cease to be effective. Neurological deficits may well be complicated by side effects of long-term steroid use (proximal myopathy, Cushingoid habitus, skin thinning, edema). There may have been a dramatic change in body image following steroid use and cranial radiotherapy (e.g. obesity, hair loss).

Patients will become more and more dependent; it may become impossible for them to be cared for at home, necessitating hospital or hospice admission. Home care will require mobilization of community services that must be tailored to the specific needs of the patient and his/her family.

Death from Raised ICP

The dying process is likely to be heralded by a gradual reduction in level of consciousness but may be complicated by fitting and agitation. When the patient can no longer take medications by mouth, most essential drugs such as analgesics, antiepileptics, antiemetics, and benzodiazepines can be delivered by the subcutaneous or rectal routes. There is controversy over the abrupt discontinuation of steroids in dying patients as this may exacerbate terminal restlessness. The authors prefer to continue to wean the dose by giving a single daily subcutaneous dose.

REFERENCES

1. Cowap J, Hardy JR, A'Hern R. Outcome of malignant spinal cord compression at a cancer centre: Implications for palliative care services. J Pain Symptom Manage 2000;19(4):257–264.
2. Tarlow IM, Klinger H, Vitale S. Spinal cord compression studies. 1: Experimental techniques to produce acute and gradual compression. Arch Neurol Psychiatry 1954;71:271.
3. Ruckdeschel JC, Harper GR, et al. Early detection and treatment of spinal cord metastases ; the role of myelography. Ann Neurol 1986;20:696–702.
4. Loblaw DA, Lapierre NJ. Emergency treatment of malignant extradural spinal cord compression; an evidence based guideline. J Clin Oncol 1998; 16(4):1613–1624.
5. Helweg–Larsen S, Sorensen PS. Symptoms and signs in metastatic spinal cord compression: a study of progression from first symptom until diagnosis in 153 patients. Eur J Cancer 1994: 3;396–398.
6. Quinn JA, DeAngelis L. Neurologic emergencies in the cancer patient. Seminars in Oncology 2000; 27(3):311–321.
7. Ingham J, Beveridge MB, Cooney N. The management of spinal cord compression in patients with advanced malignancy. J Pain Symptom Manage 1993;8(1):1–6.
8. Huddart RA, Rajan B, Law M, Meyer L, Dearnaley DP. Spinal cord compression in prostate cancer: treatment outcome and prognostic factors. Radio & Oncol 1997;44 3):229–236.
9. Cook AM, Lau TN, Tomlinson MJ, et al. Magnetic resonance imaging of the whole spine in suspected malignant spinal cord compression; Impact on management. Clin Oncol 1998; 10(1):39–43.
10. Sorensen S, Helweg–Laren S, Mouridsen H, Hansen HH. Effect of high-dose dexamethasone in carcinomatous metastatic spinal cord compression treated with radiotherapy; a randomised trial. Eur J Cancer 1994;30A(1):22–27.
11. Turner S, Maroszeky B, Timms I, et al. Malignant spinal cord compression; a prospective evaluation. J Radiat Oncol Biol Phys 1993;26(10):141–146.
12. Vecht CJ, Haaxama–Reiche H, van Putten WL, de Visser M, Vries EP, Twijnstra A. Initial bolus of conventional versus high-dose dexamethasone in metastatic spinal cord compression. Neurol 1989;39(9):1255–1257.
13. Heimdal K, Hirechberg H, Slettebo H, et al. High incidence of serious side effects of dexamethasone treatment in patients with epidural spinal cord compression. J Neuro-Oncol 1992;12(2):141–144.
14. Maranzano E, Latini P, Beneventi S, et al. Radiotherapy without steroids in selected metastatic cord compression. Phase II trial. Am J Clin Oncol 1996;19(2):179–183.
15. Barton R, Brazil L, Brada M. In: Slevin M, Tate T, eds. Cancer. How Worthwhile is Non-Curative Treatment? Springer–Verlag, 1998:168–169.
16. Sioutos PJ, Arbitt E, Meshulam CF, Galicich JH. Spinal metastases from solid tumours. Analysis of factors survival. Cancer 1995;76(8):1453–1459.
17. Stiefel FC, Breibart W, Holland JC. Corticosteroids in cancer. Neuropsychiatric complications. Cancer Invest 1989;7:479–491.
18. Adelbratt S, Strang P. Death anxiety in brain tumour patients and their spouses. Palliative Medicine 2000;14:499–507.
19. Reuber M, Hattingh L, et al. Epileptological emergencies in accident and emergency; a survey of St James's University Hospital, Leeds. Seizure 2000;9(3):216–220.
20. Recommendations of the Epilepsy Foundation of America's Working Group on Status Epilepticus. JAMA 1993;270(7):854–859.
21. Coeytaux A, Jallon P. The difficulty of defining and classifying status epilepticus. Neurophysiologie Clinique 2000;30(3);133–138.
22. Pilke A, Partinen M. Status epilepticus and alcohol abuse: an analysis of 82 status epilepticus admissions. Acta Neurologica Scandinavica 1984;70(6):443–450.
23. Shorvon S. Handbook of Epilepsy Treatment. Blackwell Science Ltd. 2000;184–185.
24. Goldbloom AL. The use of Lorazepam in the management of seizures. Pediatric Rev 1990; 12:31.
25. Stirling LC, Kurowska A, Tookman A. The use of phenobarbitone in the management of agitation and seizures at the end of life. J Pain Symptom Manage 1999;17:363–368.
26. Hanley DF, Pozo M. Treatment of status epilepticus with midazolam in the critical care setting. Int J Clin Practice 2000;54(1):30–5.
27. Kuisma M, Roine RO. Propofol in prehospital treatment of status epilepticus. Epilepsia 1995;36(12):1241–1245.
28. Moyle J. The use of propofol in palliative medicine. J Pain Symptom Manage 1995;10(8): 643–646.

29. Edwards A, Gerrard G. The management of cerebral metastases. Eur J Palliat Care 1998;5 (1):7–10.

30. Drislane FW. Non-convulsive status epilepticus in patients with cancer. Clin Neurol Neurosurgery 1994;96(4):314–318.

31. Fountain NB. Status epilepticus: risk factors and complications. Epilepsia 2000;41(Suppl 2): S23–S30.

32. Sagduyu A, Tarlaci S, Sirin H. Generalised tonic-clonic status epilepticus: causes, treatment, complications and predictors. J Neurol 1998;245(10):640–646.

33. Bhardwaj A, Badesha PS. Ifosfamide-induced non-convulsive status epilepticus. Ann Pharmacotherapy 1995;29(12):1237–1239.

34. Bertran F, Denise P, et al. Nonconvulsive status epilepticus; the role of morphine and its antagonist. Neurophysiologie Clinique 2000;30(2):109–112.

35. Avrahami E, Cohn DF. Epilepsy in patients with brain metastases triggered by intravenous contrast medium. Clin Radiol 1989;40(4):422–423.

36. Towne AR, Pellock JM. Determinants of mortality in status epilepticus. Epilepsia 1994;35: 27–34.

37. Grant I, Andrews P. ABC of intensive care. BMJ 1999;319:110–113.

38. Richardson A, Hilde TAH, et al. Long term intracranial-pressure monitoring by means of a modified subdural pressure transducer. Lancet 1970;2(7675):687–690.

39. Carencini A, Martini C. Neurological problems. In: Doyle D, Hanks GW, MacDonaldN, eds. Oxford Textbook of palliative medicine, 2nd Ed. Oxford University Press, New York, 1998: 727–729:

40. Batey SR. Schizophrenic disorders, In: DiPiro JT, Talbert RL, Hayes PE, et al., eds. Pharmacotherapy: A Pathophysiologic Approach. Elsevier, New York, 1989.

41. Weissman DE. Glucocorticoid treatment for brain metastases and epidural spinal cord compression: a Review. J Clin Oncol 1988;6(3):543–551.

42. Kirkham S. The palliation of cerebral tumours with high dose dexamethasone. Palliative medicine 1988;2:27–33.

43. Hardy J. Corticosteroids in palliative care. Eur J Palliat Care 1998;5(2):46–50.

44. Glaser AW, Buxton N, Walker D. Corticosteroids in the management of central nervous system tumours. Archives Disease Childhood 1997;76:76–78.

45. Silver P, Nimkoff L, et al. The effect of mannitol on intracranial pressure in relation to serum osmolality in a cat model of cerebral oedema. Intensive Care Medicine 1996;22(5):434–438.

46. Suzuki K, Miki M, et al. Acute renal failure following mannitol infusion. Acta Urologica Japonica 1993;39(8):721–724.

47. Doorman HR, Sondheimer JH, et al. Mannitol induced acute renal failure. Medicine 1990;69 (3):153–159.

48. Kaufman AM, Cardoso ER. Aggravation of vasogenic cerebral oedema by multiple-dose mannitol. J Neurosurgery 1992;77(4):584–589.

Pressure Ulcers

Paul W. Walker

Important considerations for the management of pressure ulcers include the goals of treatment, patient preferences, expected outcomes, and both the benefits and burdens of treatment. The dogma that all pressure ulcers are caused by poor quality care and that all patients should undergo treatment directed at healing these lesions is not substantiated. Although pressure ulcers can usually be prevented, it must remembered that, in high-risk patients, even the most exemplary care may not prevent their development. In patients with advanced disease it should be acknowledged that repositioning, debridement, dressing changes, and nutritional interventions can cause significant discomfort with no resulting benefit. For select patients, the goal of providing comfort through the use of analgesic drugs, and the selection of appropriate support surfaces and dressings, may be considered the most desirable approach to management.

CASE HISTORY

A 24-year-old man with advanced melanoma presented to the palliative care service for management of lower extremity pain and muscle cramping. Clinical findings compatible with evolving paraplegia were apparent on physical examination and investigations revealed leptomeningeal disease involving the cauda equina. While his pain came under good control with the use of opioids and a muscle relaxant, his progressive paraplegia led the

palliative care team to consider his risk for pressure ulceration. An early stage II pressure ulcer was found when observing the sacral area on physical examination that day. The patient denied any pain over this area, as he had decreased sensation due to the cauda equina syndrome. The patient was counseled concerning the need to avoid pressure at this area and that the semi-Fowler position he most favored would be a contributing factor. It was suggested that he considered positions in which he leaned to one or the other side, as well as sitting upright in a chair. A enterostomal therapy nurse was consulted and a hydrocolloid dressing was applied after cleansing of the wound with normal saline. Discussion ensued with the nursing staff to ensure he had a pressure-reducing mattress on his bed. He was later discharged to home.

In follow-up one week later, examination revealed that the ulcer had progressed and was now stage III. No evidence of infection was present but yellow necrotic slough was evident within the wound. The enterostomal therapy nurse suggested an enzymatic debridement utilizing an ointment containing papain to be used until the necrotic material was removed. It was arranged that he would try to ingest several cans each day of a high-protein/calorie supplement, containing vitamins and minerals, that was to his taste. Following this, the wound was to be considered for vacuum-assisted closure which would be provided in his local hospital.

On follow-up two weeks later he returned with a much smaller wound bed that appeared clean, and the vacuum-assisted device had been removed. With the assistance of his parents, who were taking an active role in caring for him, attention had been given to keeping the pressure off the ulcer area, to nutritional supplementation, and to proper wound care, with follow-up visits by the enterostomal therapy nurse. His wound now appeared to be a healing stage III ulcer of approximately 3 cm diameter with a healthy base of granulation tissue.

Following this visit his disease became refractory to anti-neoplastic treatment and he deteriorated, secondary to the development of multiple distant metastases. He elected to return to his home town for hospice care and it is expected that his pressure ulcer will never completely heal within his short life expectancy. The palliative team and enterostomal therapy nurse considered this management successful, as the treatment employed allowed for improvement in the patient's sacral ulcer and prevented the situation from escalating to a serious stage IV ulcer or the development of infectious complications. Had his cancer not progressed, it was expected that his ulcer would have completely healed.

INTRODUCTION

Pressure ulcers are lesions that occur in patients who are often debilitated, elderly, or have neurological injury such as spinal cord injury. Common clinical parlance includes a variety of terms for these lesions—bedsore, decubitus ulcer, skin breakdown, and pressure sore. The term preferred by researchers in the literature is 'pressure ulcer'. This is a better term as it clearly indicates the primary cause of these lesions. A definition used by the Agency for Health Care Research and Quality (previously the Agency for Health Care Policy and Research) is: 'any lesion caused by unrelieved pressure resulting in damage of underlying tissue'.[1] This statement implies that these ulcers occur when tissue is compressed between an external surface and a bony prominence resulting in ischemia and eventually necrosis. Spinal cord injury is the classic condition where pressure ulcers are a major focus of care. Other neurological conditions that result in decreased sensation or mobility may also predispose the patient to having pressure ulcers.

SPINAL CORD INJURY AND PRESSURE ULCERS

In the United States there are an estimated 200,000 spinal cord injured patients. The annual incidence of pressure ulcer formation in these individuals is between 23%–30%. However, up to 85% of spinal cord injured patients develop a pressure ulcer at some point in their life. Treatment for new spinal cord injured patients who develop pressure ulcers costs 66 million dollars each year for initial hospitalization and rehabilitation. More than 70% of spinal injured patients with pressure ulcers will have multiple pressure ulcers. Among the spinal cord injured, 7%–8% will die of complications of pressure ulcers.[2]

PATHOPHYSIOLOGY

Pressure ulcers occur when there is disruption of the normal protective mechanism that prevents tissue pressure damage. This has been explained by Chicarilli:

> The key factors that provide for avoidance of pressure ulcerations include the sensory input of discomfort followed by voluntary motor execution to alter one's position and alleviate the noxious stimulus. These actions are such an integral part of our daily living that we accept then as second nature. We continually alter compressive weight bearing forces by shifting our weight while standing or sitting and adjusting our position when lying down, mitigating their injurious nature. It is only when the conscious and subconscious safeguards become impaired that the destructive consequences of unmitigated pressure become evident.[3]

Neurological diseases that cause impaired sensory feedback or lost of mobility impair this protective mechanism and may result in pressure ulcer formation.

Extrinsic and Intrinsic Factors

Physical forces that act on body tissue to cause injury are termed extrinsic factors. Pressure produced by the patient's body weight is the critical factor in the development of pressure ulcers. This is reflected in the aphorism 'no pressure, no ulcer'. Other physical forces that can cause injury include friction, shear, and maceration. Friction occurs when the skin surface is dragged across the bedding. Shearing commonly occurs when the head of the bed is elevated resulting in the patient sliding downward while the skin remains in a relatively fixed position. This causes deformation of the vasculature of the tissue and impedes perfusion. Maceration of the skin is caused by moisture which is usually due to urinary or fecal incontinence or by profuse sweating. This results in weakening of the normal skin barrier.

Other factors, that are intrinsic to the patient, are known to increase the risk of developing pressure ulcers. Most importantly are conditions that limit spontaneous movement and thereby interfere with the essential protective mechanism described above. Medical conditions that reduce tissue oxygenation such as peripheral vascular disease, diabetes, dehydration, smoking, and anemia are known intrinsic risk factors. Advanced age causes deleterious changes in the skin resulting in decreased numbers of the elastic fibers and dermal blood vessels as well as reduced epidermal proliferation. Aged skin is therefore less resilient and has a decreased rate of healing. A further important intrinsic factor in the development of pressure ulcers is that of malnutrition.

The damage that occurs to tissues undergoing pressure ulceration is due to ischemia. When this tissue becomes trapped between a support surface and a bony prominence pressure is exerted that can exceed normal capillary filling pressure. This leads to capillary collapse and cessation of profusion. Normally, body tissues can tolerate brief periods of ischemia, but once this threshold is exceeded, hypoxia ensues, with a cascade of damaging events occurring including acidosis, vessel leakage, hemorrhage, and accumulation of toxic cellular waste. With cell death occurring, tissue necrosis follows and this can become a locus for a further complicating process, that of infection.

This mechanical process causes pressure closest to the bony prominence where the most severe tissue deformation occurs. This is where the necrosis begins. A cone of tissue destruction then forms, that is largest in the area adjacent to bone and extends outward to a smaller area closer to the skin surface. What is seen at physical examination is therefore only the 'tip of the iceberg', with the larger area of tissue damage lying deep under the skin. It is often not appreciated clinically that this tissue damage occurs first in the deep muscle and subcutaneous tissue before it extends to the skin. This cone of tissue damage is the reason extensive undermining is seen in advanced pressure ulcers. This type of lesion is most often seen in the pelvic region because of the bony prominences of the sacrum, the ischium, and the greater trochanter. Areas where superficial 'skin breakdown' occurs include the bony prominences of the heels, malleoli, fibular heads, knees, elbows, spinous processes, and scapulae. At these sites friction may play a significant role and cause more superficial injury.

The diagnosis of a pressure ulcer is usually not difficult. The lesion is found to be in a dependent position over a bony prominence that is sustaining pressure, in a patient who has lost some of the protective mechanism of spontaneous movement. However, other differential diagnoses should be considered, especially in ulcers of the extremities where venous, arterial, neuropathic, and neoplastic ulcers must be ruled out.

PREVENTION

It is important to identify patients at risk for development of pressure ulcers so that preventive measures can be instituted. Prevention represents the optimum level of wound care for debilitated patients by proactively preventing the formation of these lesions. To this end risk assessment tools have been developed for screening of at-risk populations. The Norton scale, established in 1962 and based on 250 geriatric patients, was one of the first scales developed. It accurately predicts pressure ulcer formation in orthopedic patients, but its use in other patients is less successful. The Braden scale was developed in 1987, based on 199 patients. It evaluates six domains: sensory perception, moisture, activity, mobility, nutrition, and friction/shear. Several studies showed accurate prediction. However, validation studies did not confirm these results.[2] Other risk assessment scales for pressure ulcers have been proposed in the literature but none have been proven effective in the spinal cord injured population.[2] In fact, recent studies have proposed that present risk assessment tools may have limitations. It appears that predicting pressure ulcer formation is complex and that institution of preventive measures does not always prevent ulcer formation in all patients.

Byrne and Salzberg, in a literature review, found more than 200 risk factors for pressure ulcers described in the literature.[2] They have listed risk factors according to various features such as: physical, nutritional, movement, socio-economic, psychological, and medication. In their assessment of the major risk factors, several were named most significant including: completeness of the spinal cord injury, urinary incontinence, advanced age, tobacco use, impaired cognitive function, residing in a nursing home or hospital, and malnutrition. Nutrition has been stressed as one of the most important risk factors in the development of pressure ulcers. Physician assessment of nutritional status, however, has not been shown to be a good predictor. The use of objective nutritional indicators has been recommended and the literature supports hypoalbunemia, (levels below 3.5 gm/dl) and anemia (hematocrit below 36% or hemoglobin less than 12 gm/dl) as important indicators of malnutrition that may predispose to pressure ulcer formation. The use of nutritional supplements has been shown to increase hematocrit and albumin levels in spinal cord injured patients and increase the rate of pressure ulcer healing.[2]

In spinal cord injured patients that utilize a wheelchair, instrumentation is available that can assess pressures over the seating area. This is advisable, as this information can be used to customize a seat cushion so that high pressure areas can be minimized. Teaching strategies such as pressure-relieving maneuvers, proper posture, and transference of weight is important. Such proper habits can prevent the formation of lesions. In addition, including the family in the care and training will help in developing a strong support team for successful management.

For patients with neurological illnesses, that are bedbound, many types of pressure-reducing support surfaces or mattresses exist (Table 28–1). Any patient deemed at risk

Table 28–1. **Support Surfaces Used for Pressure Reduction**

Static

- *Foam mattress overlay*: thick foam slab with a textured surface designed to be placed on top of the standard hospital mattress to reduce pressure by enveloping the body. Its effectiveness is influenced by its thickness, density, and stiffness (e.g. Geo-Matt, Clinizert, Ultra-Foam).
- *Static air or water mattress*: a vinyl mattress or overlay composed of interconnected compartments filled with air or water to distribute pressure uniformly over the support surface to create a flotation effect (e.g. Roho).

Dynamic

- *Alternating air mattress*: a mattress or overlay with interconnecting air cells that cyclically inflate and deflate to produce alternating high- and low-pressure intervals. Cells with large depth and diameter produce greater pressure relief over the body (e.g. Dyna-Care, Sof-Care).
- *Low air loss bed*: a series of interconnected woven fabric air pillows that allow some air to escape through the support surface. The pillows can be variably inflated to adjust the level of pressure relief (e.g. Flexicair, KinAir).
- *Air fluidized bed*: a high rate of air flow is used to fluidize fine particulate material (such as sand) to produce a support medium that has characteristics similar to a liquid (e.g. Clinatron, Fluid-Air).

Source: adapted from Bergstrom et al.[1]

for pressure ulcer development should be considered for one of these surfaces. Knowledge of positioning the patient is also important. It is not recommended to place the patient in the lateral decubitus position with the trochanters bearing weight. Unfortunately, elevating the head of the bed, which many patients do to watch television and partake in meals, results in increased friction and shear forces. The head of the bed should therefore be kept at the lowest degree of elevation consistent with care and not raised for prolonged periods.

The use of 'donut' or ring-type devices is contraindicated. To the unknowing they may appear to be a logical approach to avoid pressure over at risk areas. However, these devices are contraindicated because they impair circulation, causing venous congestion and edema, and cause new pressure areas. Repositioning or 'turning' a patient is a successful nursing strategy that alters the weight-bearing surfaces. This allows alternate skin surfaces to carry the brunt of the body's pressure, much as the protective mechanism of normal spontaneous movement does in a healthy individual. If feasible, it is recommended that the patient should be turned at least every two hours.

It is essential to take measures to protect the skin in patients who are at risk for pressure ulcers. It is important to avoid maceration of the skin. This may be accomplished through the use of absorbent garments and attention to skin cleanliness. Catheterization may be required in some cases. Protective dressings and ointments that act as moisture barriers for the skin may be helpful. In cleaning the skin, care should be taken not to use harsh chemicals or to traumatize the skin with vigorous washing and excessive drying. Massage over the bony prominences should be avoided, as there is no evidence that it encourages blood flow in these areas and it has been suggested that it may cause deep tissue trauma. It is important to avoid friction on the skin when the patient is being transferred. To this end the use of a life sheet or trapeze can be helpful.

STAGING

Clinical staging of pressure ulcers provides a common language to describe the severity of these lesions. It is based on the level of tissue destruction observed from the 'outside looking in'. However, it is important to remember that the process of necrosis occurs from the 'inside out', with the exception of damage due to friction and shear forces, as previously described. Unfortunately, the staging of pressure ulcers has the potential to confuse caregivers about the mechanism or extent of injury. Two provisos are required for the use of this staging system. First, it is not possible to stage a pressure ulcer until the eschar is removed. Second, in darkly pigmented skin the diagnosis of stage I pressure ulcers may be difficult.[1]

- *Stage I*. This stage consists of non-blanchable erythema of intact skin—the heralding lesion of skin ulceration.

- *Stage II*. This stage is characterized by partial-thickness skin loss, involving epidermis, dermis, or both. The ulcer is superficial and presents as an abrasion, shallow crater, or blister.
- *Stage III*. The third stage is characterized by full-thickness skin loss, involving damage to or necrosis of subcutaneous tissue that may extend down to, but not through, the underlying fascia. The ulcer presents clinically as a deep crater, with or without undermining of adjacent tissue.
- *Stage IV*. In this final stage, full-thickness skin loss occurs, with extensive destruction, tissue necrosis, or damage to muscle, bone, or supporting structures (e.g. tendon, joint capsule). Undermining and sinus tracts also may be associated with stage IV pressure ulcers.

Assessment of the pressure ulcer patient should include not only pressure ulcer staging but also a comprehensive assessment of the patient, including a complete history and physical examination and full delineation of clinical problems. Attention to the patient's nutritional status is essential. It is also important to be aware of psychosocial issues including the patient's understanding of the problem, motivation, plans, and needs.[1]

TREATMENT

When a pressure ulcer is diagnosed an initial assessment and development of a treatment plan is required (Fig. 28–1). It has been recommended that wound care teams be developed to educate the patients, family, and caregivers about the ways to prevent and treat pressure ulcers. The main areas in pressure ulcer treatment include management of tissue loads, ulcer care, and nutritional support.

Management of Tissue Loads

A central premise for healing pressure ulcers is that complete relief of pressure to the injured area should be provided. Attention to positioning the patient is critical. Avoidance of the position that has caused the pressure ulcer (usually the patient's favorite position) may be required. For bedbound individuals, several

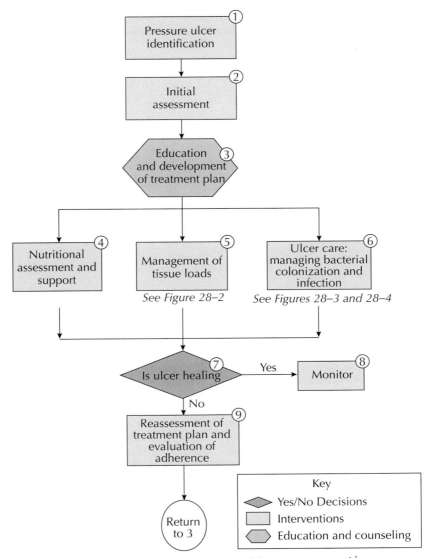

Figure 28–1. Management of Pressure Ulcers: Overview. Adapted from Bergstrom et al.[1]

pillows or foam wedges may be useful for making adjustments to their position. Many specialized beds and mattresses have been designed to lessen the pressure applied over bony prominences.[4] They can be divided in two major categories: static surfaces and dynamic surfaces (see Table 28–1). Chiefly, these support surfaces achieve their goal by increasing the surface area of weight dispersion. Other benefits may include decreased heat accumulation, low moisture retention, and shear force reduction (Table 28–2).

Determining which of these various support surfaces may be most appropriate can be challenging. The assistance of an algorithm is helpful (Fig. 28–2).

Ulcer Care

Local care of the ulcer consists of debridement, wound cleansing, dressings, and adjuvant therapies. Debridement of necrotic tissue is essential to reduce the risk of infection

Table 28-2. **Characteristics of Support Surfaces**

| Performance Characteristics | SUPPORT DEVICES | | | | | |
	Air Fluidized	Low Air Loss	Alternating Air	Static Flotation (Air or Water)	Foam Mattress	Standard Mattress
Increased support area	Yes	Yes	Yes	Yes	Yes	No
Low moisture retention	Yes	Yes	No	No	No	No
Reduced heat accumulation	Yes	Yes	No	No	No	No
Shear reduction	Yes	?	Yes	Yes	No	No
Pressure reduction	Yes	Yes	Yes	Yes	Yes	No
Dynamic	Yes	Yes	Yes	No	No	No
Cost per day	High	High	Moderate	Low	Low	Low

Source: from Bergstrom et al.[1]

and allow wound healing (Fig. 28–3). Four methods are available:

1. **Sharp or surgical debridement**. This is the most rapid treatment and is recommended, especially for infection, large necrotic areas, or thick eschar.
2. **Mechanical debridement**. This includes hydrotherapy, wound irrigation, dextranomers, and the archaic technique of wet-to-dry dressing changes. A simple method of providing the correct pressure for ulcer irrigation is to inject fluid from a 35 ml syringe through a 19 gauge needle or angiocatheter. The pressure produced by this is effective for removing necrotic tissue, but does not increase the risk for infection by driving bacteria into the wound.
3. **Enzymatic debridement**. Collagenase, papin, or other enzymes may be applied to the necrotic areas for a slower form of debridement. This may be useful if sharp debridement is not tolerated and the ulcer is not infected.
4. **Autolytic debridement**. This allows digestion of the necrotic tissues by enzymes normally present in wound fluid. This is a slow process and is not appropriate for infected ulcers.

After the wound has been debrided, regular wound cleaning is recommended at each dressing change by irrigating the ulcer using a 35 ml syringe and a 19 gauge angiocatheter or needle. Saline solution is recommended

for irrigation because other antiseptics and cleansers have various degrees of toxicity to fibroblasts and leukocytes.[1]

Wound dressings are required to keep the ulcer tissue moist and the surrounding skin dry and intact. An important principle of wound management is to maintain a moist wound environment which promotes the migration of fibroblasts and epithelial cells. The presence of many growth factors in the serous exudate speeds healing. No differences were found in pressure ulcer healing in five controlled trials comparing various types of moist wound dressings.[5–9] Physicians therefore may choose the most appropriate moist wound dressing for the situation. It is often helpful to consult a enterostomal therapy nurse who is familiar with care of wounds and knowledgeable in dressing selection and local wound care. Moist saline gauge dressings are inexpensive but require frequent changes to keep them from drying out and, therefore, more intensive nursing care. More expensive dressings that require less frequent changes include hydrocoloids, foams, hydrogels, and alginates. Semi-permeable film dressings (Tegaderm™, Opsite™) may be used to treat stage I ulcers.

Hydrocolloid dressings (DuoDerm™ and other brands) are self-adhesive and promote autolysis, angiogenesis, and granulation. They are designed to remain in place for 5–7 days. However, one study revealed an average duration of only 3.5 days.[10] Both film and

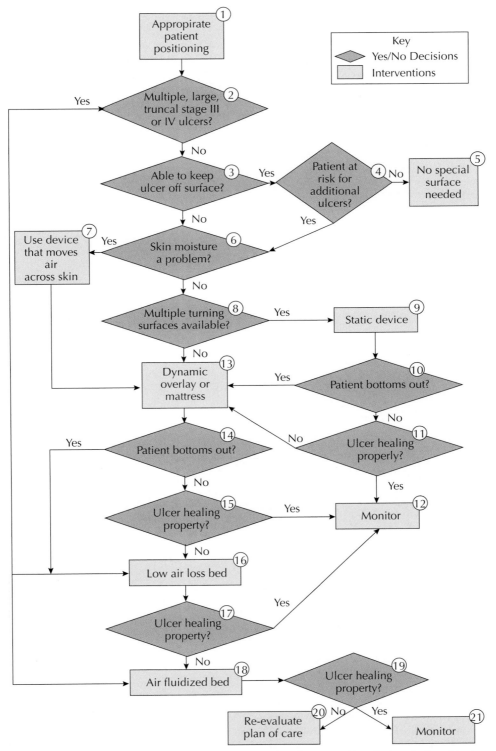

'Bottoming out' refers to an inadequate mattress overlay determined by placing the hand (palm up) under the mattress and detecting a <1 inch thickness under the involved area.

Figure 28–2. Management of Tissue Loads. Adapted from Bergstrom et al.[1]

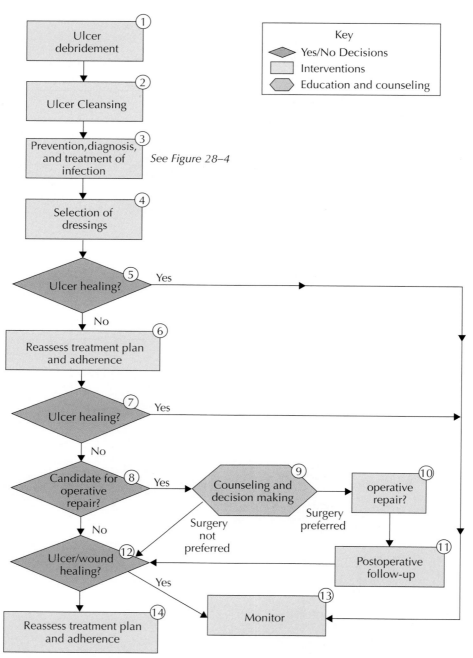

Figure 28–3. Ulcer Care. Adapted from Bergstrom et al.[1]

hydrocolloid dressings may not remain intact over the anal area. Edges of hydrocolloid dressings placed over the sacral or perianal regions often roll because of the patient's changing position. The technique of 'window paneing' or taping down the edges of the dressing may help prevent this. Hydrocolloid dresssings may not adhere to highly exudative wounds. In these situations, absorbent wound dressings such as alginates, forms, or hydrogels may be a better choice. It is important to avoid maceration of the surrounding skin by wound exudate as this leads to further susceptibility to injury. Alternatively, care must be taken that the use of highly absorbent dressings, such as alginates, does not lead to wound desiccation.

A variety of adjunctive therapies exist. In clinical trials, electrotherapy has been documented to enhance healing rates. It is recommended for treatment of stage III and IV pressure ulcers that have not responded to conventional therapy and for refractory stage II ulcers.[1] Presently this treatment appears to be limited to a small number of research centers and may be under-utilized. The use of growth factors to assist wound healing has been controversial.[11] The topical gel formation of recombinant human platelet-derived growth factor, becaplermin, has been approved by the Food and Drug Administration in the United States for treatment of diabetic neuropathic ulcers. Earlier studies utilizing this agent for the treatment of pressure ulcers were not successful.[12] However, in a recent controlled trial the incidence of complete healing was significantly better in the group treated with daily bercaplermin gel of 100 or 300 mg/g compared to the placebo group.[13] Due to its high cost it may be best utilized for healing of small ulcers.

It is unclear whether estrogen plays a role in wound healing.[11] In a small clinical trial, estrogen replacement therapy of three month's duration significantly reversed age-related delays in wound healing.[14] It has been recommended that these findings need to be substantiated by larger studies.[11] Vacuum-assisted closure is a popular recent development in which a polyvinyl foam connected to negative pressure of 125 mm Hg is inserted into a deep wound and covered by film dressing. It is believed to decrease chronic edema and exudate, increase blood flow, decrease wound dimension, and enhance the formation of granulation tissue.[15] Anecdotal and case series reports have been published in support of this technique. However, it has not been evaluated by controlled clinical trials.[11,16]

Treatments with ultrasound, infrared, ultraviolet, and low-energy laser are not recommended because of lack of controlled clinical trials and inadequate data relating to pressure ulcers.[1] The use of topical opioids to treat painful ulcers of various causes has been reported in case series.[17,18] Controlled clinical trials are required to more carefully evaluate this method of providing analgesia for wound pain. If adjuvant therapy for wound healing is utilized, attention to the basic principles of ulcer treatment must still be maintained.

Infection

High levels of bacterial colonization may prevent pressure ulcers from healing. Lesions in the pelvic region are at particular risk because of fecal incontinence leading to increased levels of bacterial colonization. Even without fecal contamination, all ulcers are colonized by skin bacteria. Therefore, the common practice of swabbing the ulcer for bacterial culture is not helpful in determining if infection is present because all ulcers, both colonized and infected, will grow organisms. To obtain a meaningful culture, the Center for Disease Control and Prevention in the United States recommends a subcutaneous injection of sterile fluid at the ulcer margin, followed by aspiration and culture of this fluid.[19]

An algorithm may assist in a rational approach to managing pressure ulcer infections (Fig 28–4). Pressure ulcer infections commonly are polymicrobial, with gram-negative, gram-positive, and anerobic organisms. Evidence is present to support the use of topical antibiotics.[20] The use of a broad spectrum topical agent such as silver sulfadiazine would therefore be appropriate. When evidence of more severe spreading infection is present, such as cellulitis, bacteremia, or osteomyelitis, systemic antibiotics are then recommended. It is important that empiric systemic antibiotic coverage be administered until blood culture results are available to guide therapy. In sepsis related to pressure ulcers, *Staphylococcus aureus*, gram-negative bacilli, and *Bacteroides fragilis* are commonly cultured. Mortality in this situation is particularly high, approaching 50% or more. Osteomyelitis may be particularly difficult to diagnose and has been associated with 26% of non-healing pressure ulcers.

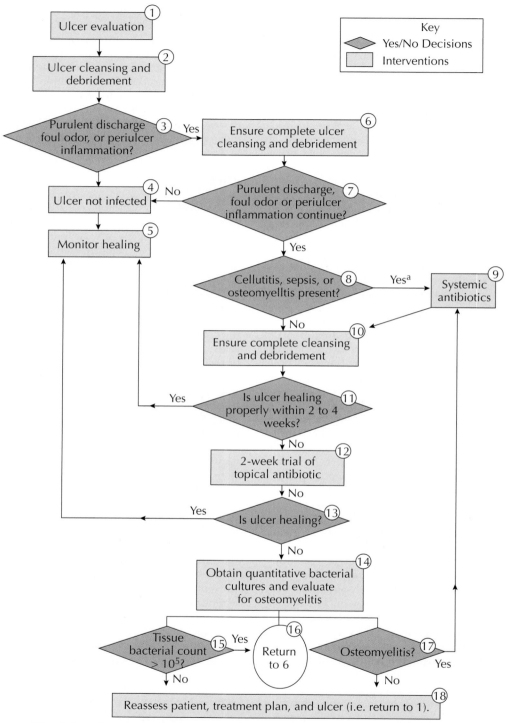

^{a}Suspicion of sepsis requires urgent medical evaluation and treatment. Treatment of sepsis is not discussed in this guideline.

Figure 28–4. Managing Bacterial Colonization and Infection. Adapted from Bergstrom et al.[1]

Operative Repair

Surgical repair may be considered for non-infected stage III and IV pressure ulcers that do not improve with optimal therapy. Musculocutaneous flaps have classically been considered the best treatment for paraplegic patients. Skin grafting and skin flaps are alternative procedures. Musculocutaneous flaps are considered advantageous because they aid in the treatment of osteomylitis by improving blood flow and providing a barrier to infection. Patients must be carefully selected for these procedures. A musculocutaneous flap procedure can result in blood loss of up to 1500 ml and require anesthesia for 1–3 hours.[1] Candidates for this procedure are required to be medically stable, have good nutritional status, have appropriate goals, an expectation for a good rehabilitative outcome, and lowered risk for ulcer recurrence.

NUTRITION

As previously mentioned, poor nutrition is an established risk factor for pressure ulcers. The severity of malnutrition has been correlated with the stage of pressure ulcer development. Breslow et al.,[21] in a non-randomized trial in malnourished nursing home patients, found that a high protein and calorie intake (up to 40 kcal/kg/day) accelerated pressure healing. The assistance of a dietician in developing a nutritional strategy is often helpful as each case is unique and requires individualization.

There is little evidence regarding the use of vitamin and mineral supplements. Taylor et al.,[22] in a small controlled study, found that patients receiving 500 mg of vitamin C twice a day, exhibited improved pressure ulcer healing. It is recommended that if vitamin and mineral deficiencies are suspected, supplementation with high potency vitamin and mineral supplements containing vitamin C and zinc is appropriate.[23]

SUMMARY

The management of pressure ulcers includes setting goals of treatment, listening to patient preferences, and considering expected outcomes, as well as the benefits and burdens of treatment. The dogma that all pressure ulcers are caused by poor quality care and that all patients should undergo treatment directed at healing these lesions is not substantiated. Although pressure ulcers can usually be prevented, it must remembered that, in high-risk patients, even the most exemplary care may not prevent their development. In patients with advanced disease it should be acknowledged that repositioning, debridement, dressing changes, and nutritional interventions can cause significant discomfort with no resulting benefit. For selected patients, the goal of providing comfort through the use of analgesic drugs, and the selection of appropriate support surfaces and dressings may be considered the most desirable approach to management.

REFERENCES

1. Bergstrom N. Treatment of Pressure Ulcers. Clinical Practice Guideline, No. 15. U.S. Department of Health and Human Services. Public Health Service, Agency for Health Care Policy and Research, Rockville, MD, December 1994.
2. Byrne DW, Salzberg CA. Major risk factors for pressure ulcers in the spinal cord disabled: a literature review. Spinal Cord 1996;34:255–263.
3. Chicarilli AN. Pressure sores in the elderly. In: Katlic MR, ed. Geriatric Surgery, Comprehensive Care of the Elderly Patient. Urban & Schwarzenberg, Baltimore, 1990:549–587.
4. Cullum N, Deeks J, Sheldon TA, et al. Beds, Mattresses, and cushions for pressure sore prevention and treatment. Cochrane Database Syst Rev 2000:2CD001735.
5. Alm A. Care of pressure sores: a controlled study of the use of a hydrocolloid dressing compared with wet saline gauze compresses. Acta Dermatol Venereol (Stockholm) 1989;149(suppl):1–10.
6. Colwell JC, et al. A comparison of the efficacy and cost-effectiveness of two methods of managing pressure ulcers. Decubitus 1992;6:28–36.
7. Neill KM. Pressure sore response to a new hydrocolloid dressing. Wounds 1989;1:173–185.
8. Oleske DM. A randomized clinical trial of two dressing methods for the treatment of low-grade pressure ulcers. J Enterostomal Ther 1986;13:90–98.
9. Xakellis GC. Hydrocolloid versus saline gauze dressings in treating pressure ulcers: a cost-effectiveness analysis. Arch Phys Med Rehab 1992;73:463–469.
10. Yarkony GM. Pressure sore management: efficacy of a moisture reactive occlusive dressing. Arch Phys Med Rehab 1984;65:597–600.
11. Bello YM. Recent advances in wound healing. JAMA 2000;283:716–718.
12. Mustoe TA. A phase II study to evaluate recombinant platelet-derived growth factor-BB in the treatment of stage 3 and 4 pressure ulcers. Arch Surg 1994;129:213–219.

13. Rees RS. Becaplermin gel in the treatment of pressure ulcers: a phase II randomized, double-blind, placebo-controlled study. Wound Repair Regener 1999;7:141–147.
14. Ashcroft GS. Estrogen accelerates cutaneous wound healing associated with an increase in TGF-B1 levels. Nature Med 1997;3:1209–1215.
15. Argenta LC. Vacuum-assisted closure: a new method for wound control and treatment: clinical experience. Ann Plast Surg 1997;38:563–576; discussion 577.
16. Ford CN, Reinhard ER, Yeh D, et al. Interim analysis of a prospective, randomized trial of vacuum-assisted closure versus the healthpoint system in the management of pressure ulcers. Ann Plast Surg 2002;55–61.
17. Twillman RK. Treatment of painful skin ulcers with topical opioids. J Pain Sympt Manag 1999;17:288–292.
18. Krajnik M. Potential uses of topical opioids in palliative care—report of 6 cases. Pain 1999;80:121–125.
19. Garner JS. CDC definitions for nosocomial infections, 1988. Am J Infec Control 1988;16:128–140.
20. Kucan JO. Comparison of silver sulfadiazine, povidone-iodine and physiologic saline in the treatment of chronic pressure ulcers. J Am Geriat Doc 1981;29:232–235.
21. Breslow RA. The importance of dietary protein in healing pressure ulcers. J Am Geriatr Soc 1993;41:357–362.
22. Taylor TV. Ascorbic acid supplementation in the treatment of pressure sores. Lancet 1974;2:544–546.
23. Houston S, Haggard J, Williford J, et al. Adverse effects of large-dose zinc supplementation in an institutionalized older population with pressure ulcers. J Am Geriatr Soc 2001;49:1130–1131.

Chapter 29

Stomatitis

Paul Rousseau

INTRODUCTION
ETIOLOGY AND PATHOPHYSIOLOGY
CLINICAL FEATURES

PREVENTION
TREATMENT
MANAGEMENT OF XEROSTOMIA

Stomatitis is a painful and debilitating oral mucosal inflammation that reduces quality of life and precipitates and/or contributes to malnutrition, dehydration, an inability to communicate, and depression. The most significant risk factors for stomatitis are pre-existing oral or dental disease;[1-3] medication use; infection; malnutrition; xerostomia; age older than 65 years or younger than 20 years; self-care deficits; exposure to additional oral stressors such as alcohol and tobacco;[1,2] and sensitization to dyes. However, preventive measures are available to help preclude the development of stomatitis, including regular oral care and non-alcohol mouthwashes, but once oral inflammation is present, various treatment options provide efficacious and definitive therapy while assuaging painful discomfort and improving quality of life.

CASE HISTORY

Mr D is a 50-year-old male with advanced multiple sclerosis who is routinely admitted to the hospital for intravenous methylprednisolone for symptomatic flares of his disease. One week after receiving five days of intravenous methylprednisolone, Mr D noticed a sore throat which he attributed to a minor viral infection. However, after three days of increasing oral discomfort, he was unable to eat and was barely able to drink two glasses of water a day. After five days of a painful throat, he became confused and his wife was concerned that he was getting dehydrated and scheduled an appointment with his family physician.

Upon examination, diffuse mucosal erythema was noted throughout the oral cavity without any observable discrete lesions. A preliminary diagnosis of a viral stomatitis versus aphthous stomatitis was made, and a generic non-alcoholic mouthwash was prescribed. After three days, the oral pain was significantly worse, and Mr D returned to his physician. Examination still revealed diffuse erythema. However, his physician wondered about an atypical fungal stomatitis secondary to prior methylprednisolone use, and prescribed nystatin, 5 ml four times daily to swish and swallow. Within three days, Mr D was feeling better and able to eat and drink, the mucosal erythema was abating, and the diagnosis of fungal stomatitis was clinically confirmed.

INTRODUCTION

Stomatitis is an inflammation, infection, or ulceration of the mucosa of the oral cavity, and is frequently confused and used interchangeably with the term mucositis, which refers to a generalized inflammation of the mucosa of the gastrointestinal tract anywhere from the mouth to the anus.[1,4] The prevalence of stomatitis among neurological patients is unknown. However, medication use, poor nutrition, and changes in respiratory function and oral hygiene that frequently accompany end-stage neurological disorders ostensibly promote the development of stomatitis. In addition, chemotherapy, increasingly used as a therapeutic intervention with multiple sclerosis, may also play a role in the development of stomatitis, dependent upon the agent used (i.e. mitoxantrone).

Stomatitis can unquestionably influence quality of life and adversely affect a patient's overall comfort level by causing pain, reducing the ability to savor and enjoy the taste of food, and restricting the ability to communicate with friends and loved ones. Consequently, it is not a benign nuisance to be ignored and relegated to derisory neglect and ineffectual therapies, but rather a complex and problematical symptom mandating immediate and efficacious treatment.

ETIOLOGY AND PATHOPHYSIOLOGY

The most significant risk factor for stomatitis is pre-existing oral or dental disease including caries, gingivitis, broken teeth, faulty restorations, ill-fitting prosthodontic appliances, inadequate oral hygiene, and any dental factor that may locally compromise or disrupt oral mucosal integrity.[1-3] Other risk factors include chemotherapy; radiotherapy to the oral cavity; medication use such as corticosteroids, antibiotics, anticholinergic agents, and morphine; infection; malnutrition; and xerostomia due to medications, radiation, mouth breathing, and oxygen use.[4] Generalized risk factors not directly related to neurological disease include age older than 65 years or younger than 20 years, self-care deficits, exposure to additional oral stressors such as alcohol and tobacco,[1,5] and sensitization to dyes in food and lipstick and ingredients in toothpaste and denture cleaning products (Table 29–1).

The pathophysiology of stomatitis varies, dependent upon the underlying etiology, but basically involves disruption of the rapidly proliferating stratified squamous non-keratinizing epithelium that lines the oral cavity from the mucocutaneous junction of the lip to the oropharynx, including the buccal and labial mucosa, ventral and lateral tongue, soft palate, and floor of the mouth.[1,5] Accordingly, stomatitis may be physiologically caused by direct mucosal injury, interference with cell growth, maturation, replication, decreased mucosal blood flow with ischemia, or impaired

Table 29–1. Risk Factors for the Development of Stomatitis

Pre-existing oral/dental disease
  Caries
  Gingivitis
  Broken teeth
  Faulty restorations
  Ill-fitting prosthodontic appliances
  Inadequate oral hygiene

Chemotherapy
  Mitoxantrone

Medication use
  Corticosteroids
  Antibiotics
  Anticholinergic agents
  Morphine

Infection

Malnutrition

Xerostomia
  Medications
  Mouth breathing
  Oxygen use
  Buccal infections
  Dehydration
  Autoimmune disorders

Age >65 years or <20 years

Self-care deficits

Exposure to oral stressors
  Alcohol
  Tobacco

Sensitization to dyes and ingredients in toothpaste and denture cleaning products

immune response and protein synthesis with secondary infection and inflammation.[6] In addition, when oral mucosa is exposed to continuous oral breathing or nasal oxygen flow, intermittent suctioning, or the absence of oral intake for over five hours, mucosal deterioration and stomatitis may occur secondary to xerostomia and mucosal trauma.[7]

CLINICAL FEATURES

The main symptom of stomatitis is pain, which when severe, may prevent eating or drinking as well as cause an inability to take oral medications. The pain may be described as burning, aching, or throbbing, and while the discomfort may be well localized with a discrete lesion, it may also be generalized and associated with dysphagia and/or odynophagia. Other signs and symptoms may also include halitosis, bleeding from the mouth,[4] and nausea and vomiting, and, if treatment is delayed or the inflammation severe, depression, dehydration, and malnutrition.

On physical examination, the lips may be dry, fissured, and bloody, with varying degrees of erythema, excoriation, ulceration, mucosal bleeding,[1,4,8,9] and xerostomia of the oral mucosa. If an infectious etiology is considered, the precipitating organism will determine the physical presentation:

- Fungal stomatitis, such as that caused by *Candida albicans* and related species, generally produces small white plaques on inflamed erythematous mucosa with frequent tongue involvement. However, candidiasis may also present as diffuse mucosal erythema without white plaques (atrophic candidiasis). Another form of erythematous candidiasis is chronic atrophic stomatitis, also known as denture stomatitis, and is marked by erythematous lesions limited to denture-covered mucosa.[10]
- Denture stomatitis may occur in 50% of upper complete denture wearers and is reportedly more common among women and older age groups. However, while *Candida* may be a causative factor, the underlying etiology is often multifactorial and frequently unknown.[11,12]
- Bacterial stomatitis generally produces localized gray or brown lesions with pseudomembranous formation, and is usually caused by streptococci and Gram-negative organisms, the latter more prevalent among immunocompromised patients.[13]
- Viral stomatitis produces vesicular and ulcerated lesions that can be exceptionally painful, particularly when caused by herpes simplex. The herpetic lesions can be observed on the lips and perioral area (keratinized as well as non-keratinized epithelium), with ulcerations frequently developing a yellow pseudomembrane.[4] Both herpes simplex virus type 1 and 2

can cause stomatitis. However, differentiating the herpes virus is inconsequential as treatment is the same for both types.
- Epstein–Barr virus can also cause stomatitis. However, it is asymptomatic and characterized by vertically corrugated hyperkeratotic lesions usually found on the lateral border of the tongue. Although Epstein–Barr can be confused with candidiasis, the lesions do not wipe off with gauze similar to *Candida* plaques, and also, unlike *Candida*, they are not painful and require no treatment.[10]
- Aphthous ulcers, also known as canker sores, are frequent causes of recurrent stomatitis, and are commonly localized, painful, shallow, and round to oval ulcer(s) covered by a gray to tan fibromembranous slough surrounded by an erythematous halo.[14,15] The etiology of aphthous ulcers is unknown, but may be related to genetics, food hypersensitivities, stress, menstruation, trauma, smoking, infection, and immune dysregulation.[15]

Although stomatitis can be clinically graded, its value is questionable in neurological disease (grading is primarily used with chemotherapy and radiotherapy). However, if utilized, the grading assessment should include physical evaluation of the mucous membranes for color, intactness, evidence of ulceration, bleeding, or infection, and functional assessment of the patient's ability to eat and drink.[11] If a grading classification is used, the system originally developed by Capizzi et al. is recommended:[11,16]

Grade I. Erythema of oral mucosa; patients able to eat and to drink fluids

Grade II. Isolated small ulcerations or white patches; patients able to eat and to drink fluids

Grade III. Confluent ulceration or white patches covering >25% of oral mucosa; patients only able to drink fluids

Grade IV. Hemorrhagic ulceration; ulceration covering >50% of oral mucosa; patients unable to eat or to drink fluids

PREVENTION

Patients with end-stage neurological disease should receive a program of regular oral care in an effort to deter the development of oral complications, including stomatitis. Promoting oral health involves meticulous oral care, including routine dental visits; regular brushing or cleansing of dentures, daily flossing, and use of non-alcohol antibacterial mouthwashes (some mouthwashes contain up to 27% alcohol); and good nutrition and fluid intake.

Obviously, with end-stage neurological disease, comprehensive and fastidious oral care may not be possible, in which case brushing with a soft-bristle toothbrush and/or the use of a non-alcohol antibacterial mouthwash should be utilized to dislodge food particles that may serve as a source of caries, gingivitis, and infection. Four inexpensive antibacterial mouthwashes can be made by mixing simple ingredients, including:

- Sodium bicarbonate in water (1 teaspoon in a cup of water)[17]
- Hydrogen peroxide and water in a ratio of 1:4 (although hydrogen peroxide may reportedly impair granulation tissue)[13]
- Salt and sodium bicarbonate ($\frac{1}{2}$ − 1 teaspoon of each in a liter of water)[18]
- Simple saline rinses prepared by adding 1 teaspoon of salt to a liter of warm water[4,19]

Although chlorhexidine has also been found useful to inhibit bacterial and fungal growth, particularly in immunocompromised patients,[1] others suggest antiseptics have not been found to have any advantage over saline rinses and regular brushing.[19] If chlorhexidine is used, patients and families should be aware that staining of teeth and changes in taste may occur, the latter potentially deleterious to nutritional intake.[20] Lemon-glycerin swabs are another product frequently used for oral hygiene, but they reportedly decalcify teeth, acidify the oral pH, reduce the buffering capacity of saliva, inactivate salivary amylase, and dry oral tissues, and as such, should not be utilized for routine oral care.[1]

TREATMENT

Once stomatitis has developed, the mainstay of therapy is to systematically correct any underlying etiology, treat infections, manage pain, and regularly irrigate/rinse the oral cavity with a non-alcohol mouthwash. Correcting underlying causes includes a three-step approach:

1. Reviewing medication use for drugs that can cause xerostomia, reduce immune function, promote infection, and reduce appetite
2. Providing and supplementing nutrition and hydration if possible and in accord with the patient's advance directives, including the placement of a percutaneous endoscopic gastrostomy
3. Repairing dental caries, broken teeth, and faulty or ill-fitting dental appliances

If an infectious etiology is evident, aggressive treatment with specific antimicrobial therapy should be instituted if the underlying organism is known (Table 29–2). Fungal stomatitis is ideally treated with an agent such as oral ketoconazole. If nausea and vomiting develops, or the patient is taking a concomitant antacid (ketoconazole requires gastric acid to be adequately absorbed), fluconazole or itraconazole are alternative antifungals.[17] If the patient is unable to swallow pills, clotrimazole lozenges may be dissolved in the mouth four to five times a day.[12] However, if xerostomia is present, the lozenges may cause further mucosal trauma and should be used cautiously. Two oral suspensions are available—itraconazole and nystatin. Itraconazole is used in the same dose as the pill form. Nystatin is much more cost-effective and equally efficacious and may also be administered as a frozen treat that can be licked and sucked to provide antifungal medication and a soothing coolness to inflamed mucosa.[12]

Bacterial stomatitis should be treated based upon suspected or identified organisms, but should include oral antibiotic coverage for streptococci and gram-negative bacteria if therapy is empiric. Chlorhexidine mouthwashes (15 ml swish and spit two times daily) may be synergistic with antibiotics and help alleviate bacterial contagions, but once again, patients and families must be advised that it may stain teeth and alter taste perception.

Herpes stomatitis treatment may involve povidone–iodine mouthwashes, oral acyclovir, or famciclovir, and, for severe infections, intravenous acyclovir. Acyclovir cream may also be applied to herpetic lesions on the lips, but should not be used in the oral cavity as it has little intra-oral efficacy.[21]

Table 29–2. **Treatment of Infectious and Aphthous Stomatitis**

Fungal

  Ketoconazole 200 mg tablet daily for 7–10 days
  Fluconazole 100 mg tablet daily for 7–10 days
  Itraconazole 100–200 mg tablet daily for 7–10 days
  Itraconazole 100–200 mg oral suspension daily for 7–10 days
  Nystatin 5 ml (500,000 units) of oral suspension four times daily for 7–10 days[1]
  Clotrimazole 10 mg lozenge five times daily

Bacterial

  Antibiotics[2]
  Chlorhexidine 15 ml swish and spit 2–4 times daily for 7–10 days
  Povidone–iodine 5 ml swish and spit once or twice daily

Herpes[3]

  Acyclovir 200 mg tablet five times daily for 7–10 days (may use intravenous acyclovir 5 mg/kg every
    eight hours for seven days for severe infections)
  Famciclovir 500 mg tablet every eight hours for seven days

Aphthous

  Carboxymethylcellulose mucosal protective paste (i.e. Orabase[R] with or without 0.1% triamcinolone)
  Tetracycline 250 mg oral suspension swished and swallowed four times daily for 7–10 days
  Chlorhexidine 15 ml swish and spit four times daily for 7–10 days
  Dexamethasone 5 ml (0.5 mg/ml) oral suspension swish and spit after meals and at bedtime for five days
  Prednisone 40 mg tablet daily tapered over 10 days
  Dexamethasone 8 mg tablet tapered over 10 days

---

[1] May freeze and administer as a frozen treat to suck on
[2] If organisms not identified, provide antibiotic coverage for streptococci, and if immunosupression is present, provide antibiotic coverage for gram-negative organisms
[3] Adjust dosage of antiherpetic agents when renal insufficiency is present

Aphthous ulcers require empiric treatment that may include the use of a carboxymethylcellulose mucosal protective paste (Orabase[R] with or without 0.1% triamcinolone), and, in more extensive cases, tetracycline oral suspension, 250 mg swished for 2–5 minutes then swallowed four times daily for 10 days. Another option is rinsing with 15 ml of chlorhexidine for 30 seconds two times daily for 7–10 days. For severe cases, topical and systemic corticosteroid therapy may be necessary. Dexamethasone elixir swished and then expectorated after meals and at bedtime for five days, or 8 mg of oral dexamethasone or 40 mg of oral prednisone tapered over 10 days are recommended regimens.[21]

Pain management is imperative to quality of life in palliative neurological diseases. Mild to moderate pain can usually be controlled with mouthwashes containing an anesthetic with or without coating agents; one such concoction combines equal amounts of viscous lidocaine, diphenhydramine, and magnesium hydroxide, while another also includes nystatin in the medication mixture. If an anesthetic or anesthetic-containing product is utilized, the patient should swish and spit and not swallow, as the gag reflex may already be diminished by underlying neurological disease and worsened or abolished by the anesthetizing agent, potentiating the risk for choking and aspiration. If pain is severe, opioid analgesics should be prescribed.[4] However, clinicians should keep in mind that morphine can cause and/or contribute to xerostomia.[22] Nevertheless, this should not preclude or deter the use of opioids in severe pain, including but not limited to morphine, oxycodone, hydromorphone, methadone, and fentanyl.

Finally, patients should be encouraged to regularly rinse/irrigate the oral cavity using a non-alcohol mouthwash three to four times a day. Saline rinses are cheap and readily available. However, if crusted debris is evident, a saline and sodium bicarbonate mixture should be used.[4]

MANAGEMENT OF XEROSTOMIA

Xerostomia can be a significant problem for chronically ill patients and contribute to stomatitis, warranting an aggressive approach to diagnosis and treatment. The prevalence of xerostomia among end-stage neurological disease is unknown, although numerous causes have been identified, including mouth breathing, continuous oxygen use, surgery to the oral cavity, chemotherapy, buccal infections, dehydration, autoimmune disorders, and medications (Table 29–3).[23] Aside from being a causal factor for stomatitis and periodontal disease, xerostomia also promotes intolerance to dental prostheses, impairs taste, and provokes difficult mastication and swallowing, all of which exacerbate anorexia and malnutrition and contribute to a poor quality of life.

The management of xerostomia involves several strategies, most of which are readily incorporated into a daily oral regimen. Recommended measures include:

- good oral hygiene
- frequent sips of water
- sucking on ice cubes, frozen tonic water, or frozen pieces of pineapple
- use of smooth, sugarless candy and sugarless gum
- use of saliva substitutes (although sips of cold water are reportedly as effective as saliva substitutes)[24]

Table 29–3. Medications Capable of Causing Xerostomia

Sedatives/hypnotics
Antipsychotics
Anticonvulsants
Tricyclic antidepressants
Beta blockers
Morphine
Diuretics
Antihistamines
Anticholinergics

- humidified air[12] avoidance of caffeine-containing beverages and alcohol-containing mouthwashes
- in severe cases, a trial of the sialagogue pilocarpine 2.5–10 mg three times daily[23]

The most common side effects observed with pilocarpine include hyperhidrosis, rhinorrhea, increased lacrimation, diarrhea, dyspepsia, asthenia, urinary urgency, dizziness, nausea, and chills. However, such side effects are more common with doses greater than 5 mg three times daily.[25–27]

REFERENCES

1. Dose AM. The symptom experience of mucositis, stomatitis, and xerostomia. Semin Oncol Nurs 1995;11:248–255.
2. Sonis ST, Woods PD, White BA. Pretreatment Oral Assessment. Journal of the National Cancer Institute Monograph 9. National Cancer Institute, Bethesda. 1990:29–32.
3. Peterson DE. Oral toxicity of chemotherapeutic agents. Semin Oncol 1992;19:478–491.
4. Woodruff R. Palliative Medicine, 3rd Ed. Oxford University Press, Oxford, 1999:151.
5. Sonis S, Clark J. Prevention and management of oral mucositis induced by antineoplastic therapy. Oncology 1991;5:10–11.
6. Rider CA. Oral mucositis: a complication of radiotherapy. New York State Dent J 1990;56:37–39.
7. Dewalt EM, Haines AK. The effects of specified stressors on healthy oral mucosa. Nurs Res 1969;18:22–27.
8. Carl W. Oral complications of local and systemic cancer treatment. Curr Opin Oncol 1995;7:320–324.
9. Krishnasamy M. Oral problems in advanced cancer. Eur J Cancer Care 1995;4:173–177.
10. MacDonald N. Palliative Medicine. Oxford University Press, Oxford, 1998:143.
11. Wilson J. The aetiology, diagnosis and management of denture stomatitis. Br Dent J 1998;185:380–384.
12. Ventafridda V, Ripamonte C, Sbanotto A, De Conno F. Mouth care. In: Doyle D, Hanks GWC, MacDonald N, eds. Oxford Textbook of Palliative Medicine, 2nd Ed. Oxford University Press, Oxford, 1998:691–707.
13. Wilkes GM. Potential toxicities and nursing management. In: Barton–Burke M, Wilkes GM, Ingwerson K, eds. Cancer Chemotherapy: A Nursing Process Approach, 3rd Ed. Jones & Bartlett, Sudbury, MA, 2001:110–117.
14. Rogers RS. Recurrent aphthous stomatitis: clinical characteristics and associated disorders. Semin Cut Med Surg 1997;16:278–283.
15. Woo SB, Sonis ST. Recurrent aphthous ulcers: a review and diagnosis. Jam Dent Assoc 1996;127:1202–1211.
16. Capizzi RL, DeConti RC, Marsh JC, et al. Methotrexate therapy of head and neck

cancer: Improvement in therapeutic index by the use of leucovorin rescue. Cancer Res 1970;30:1783.

17. Abrahm JL. A Physician's Guide to Pain and Symptom Management in Cancer Patients. Johns Hopkins University Press, Baltimore, 2000:286–289.

18. Chambers MS, Toth BB, Martin JW, et al. Oral and dental management of the cancer patient: prevention and treatment of complications. Support Care Cancer 1995;3:168–175.

19. Rogers RS. Recurrent aphthous stomatitis: clinical characteristics and associated systemic disorders. Semin Cutan Med Surg 1997;16:278–283.

20. Woo SB, Sonis ST. Recurrent aphthous ulcers: a review of diagnosis and treatment. J Am Dent Assoc 1996;127:1202–1211.

21. The Merck Manual, 17th Ed. Merck Research Laboratories, Whitehouse Station, NJ. 1999:755–757.

22. White ID, Hoskin PJ, Hanks GWC, et al. Morphine and dryness of the mouth. Br Med J 1989;298:1222.

23. Rousseau PC. Nonpain symptom management in terminal care. Clin Geriatr Med 1996;12:313–327.

24. Regnard C, Allport S, Stephenson L. Mouth care, skin care, and lymphoedema. Br Med J 1997; 315:1002–1005.

25. Rieke JW, Hafermann MD, Johnson JT, et al. Oral pilocarpine for radiation-induced xerostomia: Integrated efficacy and safety results from two prospective randomized clinical trials. Int J Radiat Oncol Biol Phys 1995;31:661–669.

26. Johnson JT, Ferretti GA, Nethery WJ, et al. Oral pilocarpine for post-irradiation xerostomia in patients with head and neck cancer. N Engl J Med 1993;329:390–395.

27. Fox PC, van der Ven PF, Baum BJ, et al. Pilocarpine for the treatment of xerostomia associated with salivary gland dysfunction. Oral Surg Oral Med Oral Pathol 1986;61:243–248.

Chapter 30

Managing the Dying Patient

Nigel P. Sykes

RECOGNITION OF DYING
RESPIRATORY SYMPTOMS
Breathlessness
Retained Secretions
CHOKING AND ASPIRATION

RESTLESSNESS AND AGITATION
SUPPORTING THE FAMILY
SUPPORTING THE PROFESSIONALS
SUMMARY

In the final days of life, patients may develop new symptoms that require relief, and their families and friends need information and support to help them through an experience that is likely to be unfamiliar and possibly frightening. The key symptom areas that require careful attention as death approaches are respiratory problems, pain, and restlessness or agitation.

Oxygen should not be the automatic response to breathlessness, and both dyspnea and cough can be eased by the use of opioids and benzodiazepines in carefully titrated doses. Choking is a common symptom in bulbar impairment but is not a cause of death. Anticholinergic drugs are helpful in the relief of noisy respiration caused by retained secretions, but it is also important to provide adequate explanations for the patient's family and friends.

Myoclonus must be distinguished from agitated restlessness, as the implications for choice of medication are different. It may be appropriate to use sedatives for restlessness but the aim is the relief of distress, not the achievement of a particular level of sedation.

Families and carers are the ones who have to go on living. Care should be taken to discover their needs for information and support, and provide for them. Death is also stressful for professional staff who, if they are to continue to be effective, require appropriate training and the opportunity to share feelings about the care they have given. These are key ways in

which to build and maintain the properly functioning multiprofessional team that optimal care at the end of life requires.

CASE HISTORY

A 62-year-old man was referred to the palliative care service with a two-year history of bulbar onset amyotrophic lateral sclerosis (ALS). He now had no diaphragmatic or lower intercostal muscle function and was troubled by breathlessness on mild exertion. He had repeatedly refused insertion of a gastrostomy feeding tube. A trial of non-invasive ventilation (NIPPV) had been made, but ventilation had not been tolerated. Dyspnea was alleviated by a combination of morphine 7.5 mg four hourly and diazepam 4 mg b.d. Drooling and sensations of choking were improved by application of a hyoscine hydrobromide transdermal patch.

As oral medication became too difficult to swallow reliably, he was transferred to a subcutaneous infusion of diamorphine 15 mg/24 hours, combined with midazolam 10 mg/24 hours. His respiratory distress worsened and, despite the hyoscine, he developed noisy breathing due to secretions retained in the airways, to the great distress of his family. Addition of a second hyoscine patch produced temporary improvement in the respiratory noise.

By now he was barely conscious, but the apparent effort of breathing was reduced by titration of the diamorphine to 25 mg/24 hours and the midazolam to 20 mg/24 hours. A modest quietening of respiration was achieved by replacing the hyoscine patch with glycopyrronium bromide 1.2 mg/24 hours added to the subcutaneous infusion. He died peacefully two days later.

Discussion

This case illustrates characteristic problems of the last days of life, although in the case of ALS, death can also be sudden or can be postponed indefinitely by the introduction of tracheostomy ventilation where this is practicable and acceptable. The therapeutic interventions used will be discussed later in this chapter, but a critical part of the care of this man was communication with his family. Good end-of-life care not only benefits the patient but also those whose lives continue, their attitudes towards death and dying shaped by what they have witnessed. Their ability to grieve normally, to relate to health-care workers in the future in the context of life-threatening illness, and, ultimately, to face their own deaths will be strongly influenced by what they have witnessed and understood of this person's dying. Thus, the care that is offered to the patient must also include those who are close to him. For them, palliative care is a public health measure.

RECOGNITION OF DYING

Driven by financial considerations, attempts have been made to define signs that prognosis is less than six months in a number of neurological conditions.[1] The symptoms associated with end-stage disease have been examined more closely in cancer than in neurological conditions, as malignancy has

been the main focus of specialist palliative care. Good information exists for ALS, but is incomplete elsewhere.[2] Table 30–1 shows the principal symptoms found in late ALS, Multiple Sclerosis (MS), and dementia.

However, these and many other symptoms can be present for weeks or even months, and do not indicate that the person is actually dying. The signs that death is near as a result of progressive illness are identified through anecdote and experience. Because of their more continuous contact with patients, nurses may be more perceptive about the imminence of death than physicians. The trajectory of dying varies between individuals and to some extent between diseases, as 58% of ALS patients have been reported to die within 24 hours of a change in condition first being noticed.[3] Characteristically, however, some warning signs can be perceived, and it has been suggested that death is likely to occur within a few days when the ill person is:[4]

- Profoundly weak
- Essentially bedbound
- Drowsy for extended periods
- Disorientated with respect to time, with a severely limited attention span
- Increasingly uninterested in food and drink
- Finding it difficult to swallow medication (where there had been no previous dysphagia)

All these signs and symptoms have been identified principally in groups of cancer patients, but from observation, many of them apply also to people dying of neurological conditions. Indeed, studies of dying patients involving a range of different terminal

Table 30–1. **Prevalence of Symptoms in Selected Late-stage Neurological Diseases (adapted from**[2]**)**

ALS	MS	Dementia
Weakness (100%)	Cognitive impairment (65%)	Dyspnea (70%)
Immobility (100%)	Pain (25%–50%)	Pain (59%)
Constipation (65%–86%)	Spasticity	Pyrexia (42%)
Pain (57%–75%)	Ataxia	
Impaired speech (77%)		
Insomnia (48%–64%)		
Dyspnea (47%–50%)		
Drooling (38%–45%)		

Table 30–2. **Symptoms in the Last 48 Hours of Life**

Noisy and moist breathing	56%
Pain	51%
Restlessness and agitation	42%
Urinary incontinence	32%
Dypnea	22%
Urinary retention	21%
Nausea and vomiting	14%
Sweating	14%
Jerking, twitching, or plucking	12%
Confusion	9%

Figures derived from a series of 200 palliative care patients (Lichter I, Hunt E. The last 48 hours of life. Journal of Palliative Care, 1990;6(4):7–15)

conditions have demonstrated much in common between the various groups (Table 30–2).[3] The characteristics of individual conditions may increase the likelihood of certain symptoms. For instance, dyspnea, which increases in prevalence as death approaches regardless of specific lung injury, becomes more prominent in the final stages of ALS, where the usual cause of death is respiratory failure.[5] Nonetheless, it is clear that whatever the nature of the disease, the key symptom areas that are likely to require careful attention at the very end of life are respiratory problems, pain, and restlessness or agitation.

RESPIRATORY SYMPTOMS

Respiratory symptoms encompass not only breathlessness but also choking sensations and the noisy breathing caused by retained airway secretions.

Breathlessness

Breathlessness tends to increase in prevalence and severity as death approaches, irrespective of whether lung damage is present. It is not amenable to resolution in the way that pain often is, but a significant degree of relief may be obtainable.[6] ALS and Duchenne's muscular dystrophy (DMD) are particularly likely to produce breathlessness in the terminal phase because of increasing respiratory muscle weakness, but this pattern may be modified

greatly by the use of ventilation—either invasive ventilation with a tracheostomy or non-invasive ventilation (NIPPV).

Some 25% of cases of tracheostomy ventilation in ALS are commenced in an emergency as a response to acute respiratory failure.[7] This is far from the ideal way in which to initiate ventilation as, without having had the ability to express choice, the patient finds him or herself in a situation in which they face a steady progression towards a locked-in state or otherwise must decide to have their life ended by ventilator withdrawal. Their family are faced with an ongoing burden of care extending into extreme dependence, with possible financial liabilities as well. Up to a third of tracheostomy ventilated ALS patients' carers consider their own quality of life to be worse than that of the patient.[8] This course of events should be avoidable if an accessible team with palliative care expertise is available in the community.

As ALS and DMD progress, NIPPV use extends to become 24-hour, or nearly so. It is claimed that with full use of aids to assisted coughing, NIPPV can provide long-term effective relief in these conditions.[9] Ultimately, progression to tracheostomy ventilation would be needed because of the extent of loss of respiratory muscle function. If this is not wanted, or if cough maintenance whilst using NIPPV is not sufficient, a respiratory crisis supervenes characterized by breathlessness and retained secretions. This is the most acute form of a symptom combination frequently met with at the end of life.

The aim of treatment is to reduce awareness of breathing, not to reduce ventilatory drive. Sometimes in practice the one cannot be achieved without the other, but the objective should always be clear in the clinician's mind. Ideally, the respiratory rate should be 15–20 per minute, but the need is to relieve distress.

In the dying person, the principal agents for the relief of breathlessness are opioids and benzodiazepines. Subcutaneous morphine, at a dose of 5 mg, has been found to be more effective than placebo in reducing breathlessness in terminally ill patients, without precipitating respiratory depression.[10] The effect can be maintained by a continuous subcutaneous infusion of morphine using a portable syringe driver. The initial opioid dose used for dyspnea depends on that previously used for pain (if any) and should be titrated against response. In controlled trials, administration of morphine by nebulizer has been no more effective for breathlessness than nebulized saline.[11]

Anxiety often accompanies and exacerbates breathlessness, making the use of the benzodiazepines, as muscle-relaxant anxiolytics, logical, and helpful. Lorazepam is rapidly effective for anxiety and breathlessness by the sublingual route, although it has not been subjected to controlled trials. Similarly, midazolam, which is usually given subcutaneously (but in a crisis can, with care, be given intravenously), has found a firm role in the palliation of dyspnea in terminal illness.[12] These drugs complement the action of opioids and can be used in combination with them. Indeed, midazolam mixes well with morphine in a single syringe for subcutaneous infusion. Again, dose should be titrated against response and, to begin with, small individual doses (2.5 mg) of midazolam given every 10–20 minutes can establish prompt symptom control and indicate the likely 12- or 24-hour dose requirement for administration by infusion.

Oxygen should not be an automatic response to breathlessness, as many terminally ill people with dyspnea are not hypoxic and the oxygen apparatus can be an unwelcome intrusion of intensive medicine into a family's companionship with a dying relative. If hypoxia is present, oxygen is appropriate and helpful.

Life is very rarely shortened by the competent use of analgesia, but it may be so by attempts to control severely breathlessness in a person with very poor chest function. Ethically, there is no objection to making the attempt as long as the physician does not intend to cause death by this treatment.[13] However, it should be made clear to those close to the patient, how critically ill he or she is and how, as a result, there is a risk that any efforts to ease distress might truncate their already brief life expectancy.

Retained Secretions

About half of dying patients develop the 'death rattle'. This is noise caused by the bubbling of air through secretions in the upper airways that the person is now too weak to clear by coughing. It is commonly said to be far more distressing to those at the bedside than to the sick person. The basis for this view is the frequent observation of a tranquil expression on the face of an unconscious patient exhibiting the death rattle, when at other times the same person has worn an expression of distress which has been relieved by, for instance, additional analgesia. Primary brain tumors have been reported to be an independent risk factor for the occurrence of death rattle.[14]

Retained secretions are managed by the use of suction and anticholinergic drugs. Unless carefully applied, suction can be damaging to the buccal mucosa and can cause distress through pain, coughing, or gagging. It is not, therefore, the mainstay of the management of death rattle. The anticholinergics used are hyoscine hydrobromide (scopolamine), hyoscine butylbromide, and glycopyrronium bromide. Hyoscine hydrobromide is available not only as an injection but also as a sublingual tablet or a transdermal patch. Hyoscine butylbromide has an oral formulation but is poorly absorbed by mouth; it is usually given by subcutaneous injection. Glycopyrronium is prepared as an injection, but any of the anticholinergic injectable preparations can also be given via a gastrostomy. Atropine is little used because of its tendency to cause excitation.

All these agents reduce oral and airway secretions, increase bronchodilation, and are antispasmodic. However, hyoscine hydrobromide crosses the blood–brain barrier and, although usually sedative, can cause paradoxical excitation. Glycopyrronium is said to have at least twice the drying potency of hyoscine hydrobromide. Anticholinergics are reported to be successful in relieving death rattle in around 30%–50% of cases, but because of the lack of standardized measures it is difficult to compare studies.

It has been proposed that the very partial success rates are due to the existence of two types of death rattle: type 1 results from the presence of airway secretions, but type 2 is caused by the presence of infective exudates.[15] Type 1 might be expected to respond to an antisecretory drug but type 2 would not. This is plausible but has not been experimentally tested. Clinically, it is probable that a mixture of the two mechanisms is common. It has not been shown that antibiotics are effective for death rattle.

As no drug can dry up secretions that are already present, anticholinergics are best started at the first sign of noisy breathing. Individual subcutaneous injections may be adequate, but all the agents mentioned combine satisfactorily with opioids or midazolam for continuous infusion. Transdermal hyoscine hydrobromide has been reported to be useful for retained secretions.[16] It is likely that anticholinergics are used more often and for longer in death rattle than their success can justify, so that staff can be seen to be trying to control a very evident symptom.

The fundamental aspect of management is explanation to family and friends at the bedside concerning the origin of the noise and a realistic estimate of how much can be done about it. This should be accompanied by reassurance that the sound is probably not disturbing to the patient and guidance as to how to tell if the ill person is comfortable or is in distress.

CHOKING AND ASPIRATION

In bulbar ALS, and other conditions giving rise to dysphagia, sensations of choking as a result of the lodging of food particles or thick secretions in the upper airway can be troublesome. As well as being uncomfortable, the feeling of choking is frightening, as it threatens asphyxiation. The risks of choking increase as the disease progresses and hence it is a natural fear this will be the mode of death. Unfortunately, this impression has been reinforced through the media. However, in a study of the end-of-life care of 124 people with ALS, only one was thought to have died in this way, and even then postmortem examination showed that in fact the airways were unobstructed.[17] Both patients and families need to receive the clear message that choking episodes are alarming but not fatal.

Aspiration of secretions may contribute to the chest infection that is almost universal in those who die after an identifiable terminal phase. As already noted, such infections probably contribute to the irreversible component of the death rattle. If this appears to be contributing to a patient's restlessness at this extreme end of life, the most effective response

is to lessen the awareness of breathing through the use of appropriate doses of opioids and sedatives.

RESTLESSNESS AND AGITATION

Agitation and restlessness are words often associated when discussing the care of a dying person. Restlessness is an unfocused motor disturbance which, if sufficiently severe, can amount to agitation. It is distinct from, although may be accompanied by, myoclonus. Myoclonic jerking is co-ordinated but sporadic contraction of particular muscle groups, usually involving the limbs, that can occur in clear consciousness. It can be caused by drugs, particularly opioids and phenothoiazines, and its onset in a person near the end of life may indicate rising drug plasma levels as a result of deteriorating renal function.

Restlessness characteristically occurs in association with reduced consciousness and may reflect a progressive delirium. Some impairment of consciousness is usual prior to death from progressive disease, although its duration may be brief. Mental impairment is common with advanced MS, has a raised incidence in Parkinson's disease, and is now recognized to occur in up to 20% of people with ALS, particularly in association with bulbar impairment. Stroke, cerebral tumors, and progressive supranuclear palsy also frequently give rise to changes in conscious level.

The importance of restlessness and agitation is that they imply to carers the presence of distress, even if it is often hard to establish whether this perception is actually true. The first part of the management is to look for reversible causes such as urinary retention, fecal loading, or hypoxia, whose relief might resolve the restlessness. A further factor can be nicotine withdrawal in a patient who is no longer able to smoke, in which case a transdermal nicotine patch can be helpful.

It is claimed that the occurrence of delirium can be reduced by the maintenance of hydration and the switching of opioids, such as the switch from morphine to hydromorphone.[18] However, it seems that most dying patients do not have significant electrolyte disturbances, even if they do not receive supplementary fluids, suggesting that the body compensates for a degree of dehydration. It has also been suggested that some dehydration at this time might be helpful in reducing such symptoms as death rattle and urinary incontinence, although no clear link has been found between hydration and the likelihood of retained airways secretions. Additional fluids may exacerbate peripheral edema where this is present.

Restlessness and agitated delirium are among the most common reasons for the use of sedation in palliative care, although the figures vary from country to country, presumably reflecting the involvement of cultural factors.[19] It is important that sedation does not become an automatic response to restlessness and agitation. As well as the reversible factors noted above, some patients in this situation settle if they sense the companionship of someone sitting with them. It has been noted that marked agitation appears more common in people who have previously had difficulty in acknowledging that their illness will cause their death. For these people calming fear and instilling a feeling of safety are important aims in end-of-life care.

On the other hand, severe illness may prevent someone being accessible to reason or consolation, and restlessness may be the result of the global deterioration of the body's systems and therefore be irreversible. In these circumstances, sedation is the only practicable way of relieving distress. But it is vital to understand that the aim of sedation is not to induce sleep but rather, simply, to relieve the signs of distress. The dose of sedative drug is titrated upward against response in the same way that morphine doses are titrated against pain relief. As soon as adequate relief is judged to have been achieved dose escalation ceases. The right dose is that which just settles the restlessness or agitation—not any higher dose or one that has been pre-decided irrespective of the patient's needs. Otherwise it can legitimately be said that sedation in the dying is simply covert euthanasia. There is evidence that sedation used in this way for palliation is not associated with life shortening.[20] Communication with relatives, and between members of the caring staff, is essential before and throughout this process. The aims and methods of treatment must be understood by all concerned and a consistent approach adopted by the caring team as to the use of medication.

The principal sedating drugs used in palliative care are haloperidol, levomepromazine, and midazolam. Of these, the first two also have use as antiemetics, if that is a consideration, but can contribute to myoclonus and may lower the fit threshold. Midazolam, an injectable benzodiazepine, is a muscle relaxant and is antiepileptic. It is now widely used for control of restlessness and agitation at the end of life.[8] As required, subcutaneous doses of 2.5 mg may be sufficient, but if these are needed regularly more even control can be achieved by incorporating the doses over a 12- or 24-hour period into a subcutaneous infusion. If further 'as required' doses are needed, these can also be incorporated into the infusion until it is sufficient without the addition of any extra medication. Midazolam can be combined in a syringe with other palliative care drugs without significant loss of effect, but for volume reasons it becomes inconvenient to use doses above 100–150 mg/24 hours.

If midazolam is insufficiently effective there is sometimes a better response to levomepromazine or a combination of the two, but where neither provides adequate symptom control, phenobarbital or propafol can be used. Both are highly sedative and antiepileptic. Phenobarbital is miscible with diamorphine but not with other commonly used drugs in palliative care, and is usually given from a second syringe driver. Single doses of 100–300 mg subcutaneously can be followed by subcutaneous continuous infusions of 600–3000 mg/24 hours according to response.[21]

Propafol is given as a 10 mg/ml solution by intravenous infusion. It has an extremely rapid onset of action (about 30 seconds) and a brief duration of effect (5 minutes). In principle it is possible to tailor the dose very exactly to the level of sedation required by adjusting the infusion rate. Excessive sedation can be diminished easily by turning off the infusion for two or three minutes.[22] In practice it remains virtually impossible to achieve the ideal state of a patient who is calm yet conscious.

SUPPORTING THE FAMILY

By family is meant those who are closest and most significant for the patient, whether they be relatives or friends. It is important, although not always easy, to identify who these are. This is not accomplished simply by obtaining details of the next of kin. A great help is to construct a genogram, or family tree, which allows the professional team to see at a glance who constitutes the family, where they are, and what other difficulties the family might be enduring at the moment.[23] Around the edge of the genogram should be listed particular friends and 'significant others' including, sometimes, pets. Ideally this be done well before the terminal phase of the illness.

Being close to someone with a terminal illness is enormously stressful. The family may be at greater risk of depression and social isolation than the patient. The progressive functional deterioration is apparent to all, but family members may not recognize how this links with shortening of the prognosis. In ALS and DMD they may not realise that death can be sudden. When the end of life is considered, thoughts may be colored by unfounded apprehension about symptoms such as suffocation, choking, and pain. A family's need for accurate information is at least as great as that of the patient.

Without guidance as to what to expect as the patient deteriorates, and how they can gain urgent help in a crisis, an acute episode such as choking or breathlessness can be terrifying not only to the patient but also the family. Involvement of a multiprofessional team, with 24-hour availability, can allow the making of informed choices about aspects of management and be a resource for advice and practical help in an emergency.

Such a team can also facilitate the continuing care of the patient at home, where most terminally ill people wish to be. As life becomes more difficult the proportion wishing to stay at home diminishes, but still remains about 50%.[24] Despite assistance from community nursing services, the brunt of home care is borne by the family. Respite admissions to a hospice, hospital, or nursing home can help carers to recuperate and resume their task. Alternatively, additional respite nursing help may be available for limited periods. However, for a significant number of families there comes a point when they feel they can no longer look after the patient at home. In this the patient may agree, or there may be divergence. A particular

precipitant is the onset of confusion, not uncommon in patients with advanced neurological disease. For instance, families of people with brain tumors may feel that the person they have known and loved for so many years has changed character and has become a stranger—sometimes a frightening and unpleasant one.

Even if all are in agreement that admission is needed, family members may still be left with a sense of failure and of guilt that they have let their relative down. This may be especially marked if the ill person dies soon after they have been admitted, leading to feelings that 'if only we had kept going that little bit longer we could have looked after him to the end'. It is important for their response in bereavement that families receive reassurance about the quality of their caring efforts prior to the admission, and the appropriateness of seeking inpatient care. It is also important that there are the facilities and encouragement to enable them to remain with the patient as death approaches, if that would be helpful to them.

For some families it is important that their relative does not die in their home, because of the memories that would leave for the future. Any service caring for terminally ill patients at home needs, if at all possible, to have conversations with patient and family about the preferred place of death. This will facilitate discussion and understanding, if not always agreement, in the case of differences. Plans can be made so that admission does not occur as an acute event in response to the distress of a family who have never been able to reveal their concerns about end-of-life care of their relative. Even when death does take place in a hospice or other inpatient unit, usually at least 80% of the patient's last year of life will have been spent at home, and afterwards the perception of families is that they have indeed cared for the person themselves.[23]

Most bereaved people do not need specific bereavement care: they will work through the feelings of loss (experienced by every individual at some point) by themselves, with the support of their own network of family and friends. For a minority, perhaps up to 25%, their adjustment can be helped by specialist bereavement support. This is increasingly widely available, and in Britain can be accessed through Cruse Bereavement Care, the local hospice/specialist palliative care provider, or social services department.

SUPPORTING THE PROFESSIONALS

The professionals looking after someone dying of a neurological disease may have known that person for a long time. Where there has been a progressive loss of function, a sense of helplessness and failure can be engendered in carers, compounded if there are also difficulties in communication. This leads to feelings of frustration and de-skilling that can result in avoidance of the patient by carers unless the problem is recognized.

To some extent these tensions are eased in the terminal phase, as the end comes into sight. Afterwards, however, staff memories of the case may be influenced by feelings that persist from earlier stages of care. These factors risk leaving a residue of distress which might impair professionals' ability to look after dying patients in the future. The situation is worsened by the relative rarity of some neurological conditions which means that staff can find it difficult to gain and maintain confidence in their expertise in caring for those with the same conditions.

Therefore it can be helpful if there is both a program of staff education covering the management of end-of-life symptoms, and also the opportunity for staff, as a multiprofessional group, to meet and share views on how the care of a particular patient went. This session may well identify ways in which care could be improved in the future, but should in addition be a chance for congratulation on the ways in which things have gone well. It should be a managerial responsibility to identify staff members who have particular problems resulting from the experience of care and, without imparting a sense of inadequacy, enable them to talk through the important issues confidentially, either within their organization or with an independent counselor.

SUMMARY

The very end of life provides some of the most powerful memories for those who are left behind, and so how palliative care is provided at this time is crucial. The future attitudes of the patient's family and friends towards severe illness in themselves or others, and towards death itself (which in the developed world today is rare for anyone below advanced middle age) will be moulded by this experience. Good symptom control and good communication with the patient (as long as this is possible) and with the family have direct benefit to the person who is dying. However, they also constitute a public health measure for those who are bereaved, helping or hindering their adjustment to loss and shaping their future attitudes to severe illness and to health care.

REFERENCES

1. Standards and Accreditation Committee. Medical Guidelines for Determining Prognosis in Selected Non-cancer Diseases. National Hospice Organisation, Arlington, 1996.
2. Voltz R, Borasio GD. Palliative therapy in the terminal stage of neurological disease. Journal of Neurology 1997;244(Suppl. 4):S2–S10.
3. O'Brien T, Kelly M, Saunders C. Motor neuron disease: a hospice perspective. British Medical Journal 1992;304:471–473.
4. Twycross R, Lichter I. The Terminal Phase. In: Doyle D, Hanks GWC, MacDonald N, eds. Oxford Textbook of Palliative Medicine, 2nd edition. Oxford: Oxford University Press, 1999:977–992.
5. Leigh PN, Ray–Chaudhuri K. Motor neuron disease. Journal of Neurology, Neurosurgery and Psychiatry 1994;57:886–896.
6. Higginson I, McCarthy M. Measuring symptoms in terminal cancer: are pain and dyspnoea controlled? Journal of the Royal Society of Medicine 1989;82:264–267.
7. Oppenheimer EA. Decision-making in the respiratory care of amyotrophic lateral sclerosis: should home mechanical ventilation be used? Palliative Medicine 1993;7:49–64.
8. Kaub–Wittener D, von Steinbuchel N, Wasner M, Borasio GD. A Cross-sectional Study on the Quality of Life of Ventilated ALS Patients and Their Caregivers in Germany. Proceedings of the 9th International Symposium on ALS/MND. International Alliance of ALS/MND Associations, Munich, 1998.
9. Bach JR. Prevention of morbidity and mortality with use of physical medicine aids. In: Bach JR, ed. Pulmonary Rehabilitation: the Obstructive and Paralytic Conditions. Philadelphia: Hanley and Belfus, Philadelphia, 1995:303–329.
10. Bruera E, Macmillan K, Pither J, MacDonald RN. Effects of morphine on dyspnea of terminal cancer patients. Journal of Pain and Symptom Management 1990;5:341–344.

11. Davis CL, Penn K, A'Hern R, Daniels J, Slevin M. Single dose randomised controlled trial of nebulised morphine in patients with cancer related breathlessness. Palliative Medicine 1996;10:64.

12. McNamara P, Minton M, Twycross RG. Use of midazolam in palliative care. Palliative Medicine 1991;5:244–249.

13. Latimer EJ. Ethical decision-making in the care of the dying and its applications to clinical practice. Journal of Pain and Symptom Management 1991;6:329–336.

14. Morita T, Tsunoda J, Inoue S, Chihara S. Risk factors for death rattle in terminally ill cancer patients: a prospective exploratory study. Palliative Medicine 2000;14:19–23.

15. Bennett M. Death rattle: an audit of hyoscine (scopolamine) use and review of management. Journal of Pain and Symptom Management 1996;12:229–233.

16. Dawson HR. The use of transdermal scopolamine in the control of death rattle. Journal of Palliative Care 1985;5(1):31–33.

17. O'Brien T, Kelly M, Saunders C. Motor neurone disease: a hospice perspective. British Medical Journal 1992;304:471–473.

18. Fainsinger R, Tapper M, Bruera E. A perspective on the management of delirium in terminally ill patients on a palliative care unit. Journal of Palliative Care 1993;9:4–8.

19. Fainsinger R, Waller A, Bercovici M, et al. A multicentre international study of sedation for uncontrolled symptoms in terminally ill patients. Palliative Medicine 2000;14:257–265.

20. Morita T, Tsunoda J, Inoue S, Chihara S. Effects of high dose opioids and sedatives on survival in terminally ill cancer patients. Journal of Pain and Symptom Management 2001;21:282–289.

21. Stirling LC, Kurowska A, Tookman A. The use of phenobarbitone in the management of agitation and seizures at the end of life. Journal of Pain and Symptom Management 1999;17:363–368.

22. Moyle J. The use of propafol in palliative medicine. Journal of Pain and Symptom Management 1995;10:643–646.

23. McGoldrick M, Gerson R. Genograms in Family Assessment. Norton, New York, 1985.

24. Hinton J. Which patients with terminal cancer are admitted from home care? Palliative Medicine 1994;8:197–210.

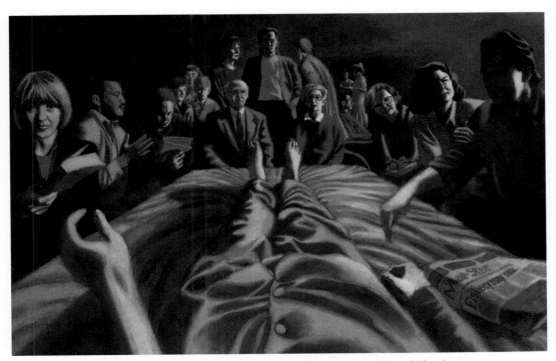

Plate 4 'Visitors' by Robert Pope, 1989. (Acrylic on canvas, 81.3×121.9 cm)

PART 5

ETHICAL ISSUES

Chapter 31

Personal Identity and Palliative Care

Carlo A. Defanti

THE CONCEPTS OF PERSON AND PERSONAL IDENTITY
BRAIN DISEASES, PERSONS, AND PERSONAL IDENTITY
DECISION MAKING AND PERSONAL IDENTITY

This chapter explores the issue of personal identity and its possible alterations due to brain diseases. Impairment of cognition and other higher nervous functions can be severe enough to alter the personality of affected people to such a degree that the question of their personal identity is raised. Even though this philosophical problem may appear to be far removed from the reality of hospital wards, in fact it is relevant for the clinical decision-making process, especially during the advanced stages of dementia, in, for instance, challenging the authority of advance directives for health care. Moreover, personal identity and its preservation can and should be a therapeutic goal for palliative care of demented people.

CASE HISTORY

Sybil is a 54-year-old woman, with advanced Alzheimer's disease. She is cared for in her apartment by an attendant. Her apartment has locks to keep her from slipping out at night and wandering in the park. She tells visitors that she is reading mysteries, but in fact she cannot read at all. Most of the time she sits in a chair, humming to herself and rocking back and forth. She cannot recognize relatives or friends and is unable to store new memories. Sometimes she appears not to recognize herself when looking in the mirror. Friends say that she is

PERSONAL IDENTITY AS A THERAPEUTIC TARGET IN THE CARE OF DEMENTED PEOPLE
CONCLUSION: DEMENTIA AND PALLIATIVE CARE

no longer herself. Nevertheless, according to one of them 'despite her illness Sybil is undeniably one of the happiest people I have ever known'.

Now imagine that some years earlier Sybil had written an advance directive refusing life-sustaining treatment, including cardio-pulmonary resuscitation (CPR) in case of cardiac arrest. Currently, Sybil is well, but if she were to develop pneumonia or sepsis and has a cardiac arrest, what should be done? Probably CPR could save her life and allow her to return to her previous life, a rather good one (although diminished) according to her friend's account. Given that she appears happy, it seems that CPR would be in her best interest, but obviously it conflicts with her prior directives. Should these directives remain valid now that Sybil has so changed that many friends say she has become a different person? Is there a risk that following her prior directives imposes on her a decision made by a different person that is contrary to her present interests?

Discussion

One may wonder why, in a book on palliative care in neurology, a chapter is devoted to such abstract philosophical concepts as person and personal identity. There are several reasons.

Many acute or chronic neurological diseases lead to cognitive dysfunction. Cognitive impairment can be severe enough to alter the personality of affected people to such a degree that relatives or friends of the patients wonder *if these individuals still are the same persons they once knew* (as in Sybil's case). The marked change in cognitive function raises the question of the personal identity of their relative or friend.

Cases like these raise difficult moral dilemmas. The problem is the authority of an advance directive executed by a person prior to a disease or accident producing severe brain damage and compromising personal identity, as in Sybil's case. Should such a directive retain its authority after the person has changed?

Personal identity and its preservation should be a therapeutic goal for palliative care, as the discussion of dementia care will show.

THE CONCEPTS OF PERSON AND PERSONAL IDENTITY

The concept of *person* is one of the most controversial topics in philosophy and bioethics. It is useful to introduce some simple distinctions among the different meanings the term conveys in common usage. Mostly, *person* is used in a descriptive sense as synonymous with *human being*, but it may carry other meanings. Philosophical analysis identifies at least two other meanings: an *ontological* meaning (i.e. the answer to the question 'what does it mean to be a person?') and a *normative* meaning (a person is a center of responsibility and is entitled with rights). There is no logical connection between these two different facets of the concept of person; in fact they can be dissociated. For instance, the term *person* can be applied in a general sense not only to human beings but to associations and corporations.

The ontological sense is the most controversial. The classic definition proposed by Boetius and subsequently endorsed by Thomas Aquinas, was *rationalis naturae individua substantia* (individual substance of rational nature). Locke,[1] to whom we are indebted for having started the modern debate on the concepts of person and personal identity, asked 'what *person* stood for' and gave this answer: 'a thinking intelligent being, that has reason and reflection, and can consider itself as itself, the same thinking thing, in different times and places'.

If we look for the minimal, common features of contemporary views of what person is, we can sort out the *capacities for conscious experiences and for purposive agency*.[2] But even this minimalist definition leaves out some human beings, like the newborn, the severely retarded, and the permanently unconscious. From a medical perspective, the rigorous distinction between the different meanings of *person* was not as important in the past when death eliminated all the aspects of persons almost simultaneously. But today, owing to the progress of medical technology, the different aspects of *person* may be dissociated, as happens in the persistent vegetative state (PVS), a clinical condition in which affected human beings survive as bodies, but arguably no longer are *persons*.

Now let us analyse the concept of *personal identity* (PI) in greater depth. We are used to thinking of PI as an obvious fact; one not requiring reflection. Then we meet a woman we have not seen for several decades. After this long interval her physical features have changed, sometimes to such a degree that she is hardly recognizable. How do we recognize her? Usually personal recognition occurs through memory. We speak with her about our common past life and immediately recognition occurs (in this case we are resorting to a *psychological criterion of PI*). But the task is much more difficult when the individual does not or cannot co-operate, or worse, is dead ('is this corpse the corpse of X?'). In the latter instance the forensic task is based on indirect evidence such as narratives of witnesses (*social criterion of PI*), finger prints, or, more recently, sophisticated tools like DNA analysis (*physical criterion of PI*).

The problem of PI is not new. In the 17th century, Locke first proposed *continuity of memory* as the criterion of PI. Much more recently, in the 1960s and 70s, the problem of PI was revived in the English philosophical literature. Contemporary scientific and technological developments have re-ignited the debate—principally the study of patients with split brains,[3] the practice of organ transplantations, and the science of artificial intelligence.

Most contemporary discussants frame the problem of PI as a problem of relationships among different *person stages*. One can think of a person, not as a static entity, but as a process or as a series of events (*a chain of person stages*) that pertain to the same person. If we call X and Y two different person stages, occurring respectively at times T1 and T2, the question if a relation of PI subsists between X and Y can be reformulated: 'How can we state that Y at time T2 is identical with X at T1?'

The prerequisite to answering this question is to make a distinction between two meanings of the term *identity*: qualitative identity (that is the relation between two entities that are qualitatively identical), and numerical identity (the relation between two entities that, observed in different times—even though qualitatively non-identical—are the same entity). Only the latter is relevant to the discussion about PI. After this premise, one can write: 'Y at T2 is identical to X at T1 if, and only if, Y at T2 is continuous with X at T1' (formulation A).

In principle, the main criteria of re-identification are the *physical* and the *psychological*. A formulation of the physical criterion could be: 'All that is needed to re-identify Y in T2 with X in T1 is the physical continuity of its body' (formulation B). However, this formulation is subject to several objections. For instance, the development of organ transplantation showed that the continuity of the body as a whole is not a necessary condition; only the continuity of the brain is required. Imagine the science fiction scenario in which brain transplantation is possible. Whereas the transplantation of a thoracic or abdominal organ from X to Y does not undermine Y's PI, a hypothetical transplantation of X's brain to Y would change Y's PI. In fact, it would be more accurate to say that Y's body is being transplanted on X's brain, than the opposite. The resulting person would have Y's body, but the ideas, the personality, and the memory of X.

Daily experience with neurological patients shows that even large destructive lesions of the brain are compatible with the conservation of PI. If this observation is true, even formulation B must be changed. Following arguments of the philosopher Parfit,[4] who has worked through the theory of PI and simplifying its arguments, we could say that the necessary condition is not the continuity of body, but that of the brain or, as he says, of 'enough of the brain to be the brain of a living person'.

The formulation now becomes: 'Y today is the same person as X in the past times if and only if a sufficient part of X's brain continues to exist and is now Y's brain' (formulation B1). However, the case of a permanently unconscious (e.g. PVS) patient defeats B1, because patients in this condition are alive but have neither consciousness nor memory. So we need to add to B1 that X's brain must retain the capacity to support mental states. But is this enough? It isn't, because even so corrected, B1 fails if we think of the patients whose brain has been damaged to such a degree that memories of the past are more or less completely erased (as may happen, for instance, in Alzheimer's patients). It follows that B1 must be further revised, adding two conditions: that the brain has the capacity to support mental states and that the recollections of the original person are at least partly preserved.

So, we arrive at 'Y today is the same person as X in the past times if and only if a sufficient part of X's brain continues to exist, has the capacity to support mental states, and if its recollections are at least in part identical with those of X' (formulation B2).

It is easy to see that the physical criterion, after so many corrections, is rather close to the psychological criterion. The latter, first proposed by Locke, could be simply formulated as: 'Y at T1 is the same person as Y at T2 if and only if Y is psychologically continuous with X.'

The psychological criterion, expressed in its pure form, without reference to the body/brain, is open to many objections. A first criticism was put forward in Locke's time by Butler,[5] who argued that the simple continuity of memory cannot be a criterion of PI insofar as it presupposes it. Besides, there are other empirical difficulties that suggest the rejection of a purely mental criterion and the acceptance, at least provisionally, of formulation B2. Parfit has also refined the concept of continuity: he makes a distinction between *connectedness*, defined as the persistence of direct psychological connections between X and Y, and *continuity*, a broader condition meaning the persistence of overlapping chains of direct connections. According to Parfit, only *continuity* captures what is important in the relation between person stages. Besides, continuity can be thought of as embracing not only memories, but other mental events, like intentions. Adding the difficulties noted above of other logical problems pertaining to the concept of PI (such as those rising from the study of split-brain patients), Parfit's conclusion is that it is more suitable to speak of *personal survival* than of *personal identity*. What really matters is not identity, but continuity. At the same time he emphasizes that *continuity*, and hence personal survival, is not a property of an all-or-nothing type, but is a matter of degree.

This theory appears to loosen existing links between different person stages and questions the common belief in our own identity as a deep, further fact beyond its manifestations. The links existing inside one's life become weaker and personal continuity is understood not as an absolute property but only as a matter of degree. This conclusion has remarkable ethical consequences. When we explore the borders of life, that is when we raise questions such as 'when do human beings become persons?' and 'when do they cease to be persons?'. The gradualist concept tells us that there is no 'natural' border. The choice of a border is in some ways conventional. On the other hand, conventional does not necessarily mean arbitrary; moral considerations can and must lead us to making choices.

The philosophical debate on the concepts of person and of PI remains open and it is unlikely that a consensus will be achieved. Parfit's gradualist view has been harshly criticized by many thinkers, especially by those who are religion-oriented. They question his deliberately *reductionist approach* to the topic and worry about the destruction of some essential idea underlying our society and grounding morality itself. I shall not develop this discussion any further, but fresh ideas are welcome in this field, especially to try to anticipate novel, unforeseen situations created by contemporary technological medicine.

BRAIN DISEASES, PERSONS, AND PERSONAL IDENTITY

Now, let us try to translate these theoretical speculations into the language of neurology, asking ourselves whether some brain diseases can undermine PI and, if so, which diseases. Some neurological conditions already have been considered in the discussion of the philosophy of PI, but now I shall consider them more analytically.

A hallmark of Alzheimer's disease (offered as the paradigm of dementing diseases) is the impairment of *autobiographic memory* (ABM). The status of this kind of memory is disputed among neuropsychologists. According to Tulving's[5] hypothesis of two independent memory systems, *episodic* and *semantic* memory, it would seem that ABM should be ascribed to the first system, because by definition it consists of pieces of context-dependent, individually experienced information. Other scholars maintain that the frequent retrieval (and the resulting public or private narrative) of a relatively small number of significant events change the status of these recollections, giving to this kind of memory a stability closer to that of semantic memory. In any case it is reasonable to speculate that ABM, being one of the most relevant sources in the array of talking and self-portraiting activities,[6] contributes powerfully to the continuity of one's self-identity.

ABM is invariably compromised in Alzheimer's disease, though in various degrees. In the late stages of the disease it is completely lost; the patient does not recognize his/her relatives any more and, finally, does not recognize him/herself in the mirror. In advanced cases, psychological continuity is obviously broken and, so, PI. This raises another difficult question. Because continuity is a matter of degree, at which level of continuity is it sensible to establish the threshold of the loss of PI? In other words, which degree of continuity is needed for declaring that Sybil is still surviving as herself? Beyond this threshold, one might speak of another individual, different from her. Of course a host of problems would arise. Who is this individual? Is she a person or not? What are her rights?

PVS can be either an end stage of dementia or, more commonly, an outcome of an acute brain injury. Consciousness is abolished in PVS; the individual lacks any mental life. According to the theory, the original person does not exist any more and no 'successor person' is left. Some bioethicists argue that, for this reason, PVS is ontologically equivalent to brain death—the so-called theory of cortical death.[7] Sometimes the brain injury falls short of causing PVS. After a prolonged coma and a transient vegetative state, the patient recovers some contacts with the environment, obeying simple orders and uttering some sounds—but does not regain self-consciousness. This condition has been termed the *minimally conscious state* in which continuity of the person is broken and PI is absent as well.

Some *focal brain lesions* can alter the patient's personality profoundly. The most common focal lesion is the frontal lobe syndrome due to brain tumors. Character and behavior may change to such a degree that relatives and friends remark that the person is no longer him/herself. Nevertheless, in the theoretical framework sketched above, these patients, even when their personality is severely disrupted, retain PI, since continuity of their memory is preserved.

A special case of focal brain lesion is *pure amnestic (Korsakoff) syndrome*. In this condition there is no global deterioration of cognition, but long-term and short-term memories are severely impaired. Patients cannot store new memories and their life history is in some way interrupted at the time of the brain insult. Nevertheless, in spite of their extremely severe disability, their ABM is generally spared and psychological continuity (and consequently PI) is preserved.

Another rare but theoretically interesting case is the *split-brain syndrome*—the neuropsychological disorder resulting from surgical section of the corpus callosum. It is well known that in the experimental setting these patients show evidence of two separate streams of mental events in the disconnected hemispheres. In a strict sense, the split-brain patient loses his/her PI, because it is logically impossible that previous whole-brain person stages can be continuous with separate and independent right and left hemispheric functions. Nevertheless, the observed behavior of the patient is fairly normal, as external information reaches both hemispheres and, even if the hemispheres no longer can directly communicate through the corpus callosum, they can do so 'from the outside', observing the actions of each other. Thus, though the split-brain condition is theoretically incompatible with a preservation of PI, continuity or personal survival in Parfit's sense is spared.

Summarizing, we can say that PI disappears in the late stage of dementia and is lost in PVS and in the minimally conscious state. But in other severe, debilitating diseases like Korsakoff's syndrome and frontal lobe syndrome, PI is not threatened. In the split-brain patient, personal survival, if not PI, is the rule.

DECISION MAKING AND PERSONAL IDENTITY

One may ask whether loss of PI coincides with loss of *competence*—a much more familiar concept for both clinicians and ethicists. Should this be the case, the above discussion would be without any practical importance. But the answer is that it is not so; loss of PI usually occurs in Alzheimer's much later than the loss of general competence and even later than the loss of more limited, task-specific competencies.

Let us try to pinpoint the moment when the affected individual loses his/her PI. Philosophers Buchanan and Brock suggest, for practical reasons, to choose a low threshold,[8] specifically the same threshold at which the individual loses his/her person status. They argue that, if we consider loss of PI occurring simultaneously with loss of personhood, we can avoid a big difficulty—that of admitting that the original person is no longer there. But now there is a 'successor self' whose social status is undefined as well as his/her moral rights.

Consider again the case of Sybil who, years ago, executed a living will refusing life-sustaining treatments, should she need them after having lost her competence. Suppose now that Sybil has just reached the moment when her PI is lost. If the 'successor' (let us call her Sybil 2), even though severely disabled, were still a person, the advance directive issued by Sybil would lack any power over Sybil 2, a different person, unless we are ready to justify a relationship of *slavery* between Sybil 2 and Sybil, the latter requiring the former to honor her directives. Buchanan and Brock argue that this way of framing the argument would be greatly disturbing to society and would yield no apparent advantage to anyone.

But choosing a low threshold provides a way to solve this problem. One can speak of loss of personal continuity only in the late stages of dementia, when the original person is no longer there and only a surviving non-person is left.

We need no novel name for the surviving individual and the validity of Sybil's advance directives would not be compromised. This is not to say that this surviving non-person has no rights and does not deserve protection and guardianship (she must be protected against suffering), but simply that she has no right to autonomy of her own and that Sybil's previous decisions do not lose their validity.

This proposal, though reasonable, is open to objections. First, there is no consensus about the definition of person. According to the minimalist definition ('a person has some capacity for conscious experiences and for purposive agency'), this coincidence is not assured, whereas it could be by a stronger definition (adding to the former 'a person has the capacity to perceive herself as a single self conscious individual persisting through time'). Second, it would be difficult to operationalize the criteria for the loss of personhood and of PI. Third, one might argue that the story of Sybil shows that, even though her autobiographical memory is lost and so is her psychological continuity, she is conscious, lives a rather peaceful life, and seems able to appreciate it (i.e. she appears to fulfil the minimalist criterion for personhood). Despite whether we decide to give her a new name, we should protect her actual interests (to live a rather good life) against those of Sybil, thus discounting Sybil's advance directives.

Thus, we are left with unsolved questions. Whereas in principle the theory of PI could help us to more finely attune our approach to the changing situation of the demented patient, its practical application is fraught with doubts.

The identical problem was addressed by Dworkin,[9] an influential legal philosopher, starting from a case study of Margo, originally reported by Firlik[10] and almost identical to Sybil's case. Discussing the conflict between Margo's advance directive and her actual interests, Dworkin discards the theory of PI, taking Margo's identity for granted, and tackles the problem in the conceptual framework of the so-called *principlist* bioethics[11]—the standard account of bioethics as ruled by a set of principles. According to this account, we face an obvious conflict between Margo's right to autonomy (which demands each endeavor of resuscitation be refrained from) and the principle of beneficence (remember that Margo is not suffering at all; she appears to be happy instead). The principle of beneficence tells us to act in the best interests of the patient. Cardiopulmonary resuscitation seems to be in her best interest, inasmuch as it may bring her back to her previous, happy condition. But the principle of respect of autonomy commands us, on the contrary, to honor her previous directives and so to let her die if her heart stops.

Dworkin argues at length about the different options and the conflict of principles. He opposes an *evidentiary* (or *consequentialist*) view of autonomy, according to which autonomy is the overriding principle simply because each person generally knows what is in his/her own interests better than anyone else, and favors a strong *integrity* view of autonomy. He maintains that the value of autonomy does not lie in its ability to bring about good consequences, but derives from the capacity it protects—the capacity to express one's own character (values, commitments, convictions, and critical as well as experiential interest) in the life one lives. The integrity view of autonomy means that anyone has the right to be the author of his/her own story and to decide even against their own future interests—a clear but controversial position.

Both Brock's and Dworkin's proposals stem from principlist bioethics. The difficulties that this approach leaves unsolved have prompted some thinkers to attempt to escape from this conceptual framework and to attack the predominance of the autonomy principle, so strongly defended by Dworkin. Attempts have been made in many directions, but most of them favor adding more weight to the social circumstances in which decisions are taken, stressing the community rather than the individual, often with reference to the communitarian political philosophies.[12,13]

One of the most interesting views is *narrative ethics*, which is connected to the problem of PI. The starting point of narrative ethics can be found in a statement of MacIntyre:

> Man is in his actions and practice, as well as in his fictions, essentially a story-telling animal...But the key question for men is not about their own authorship; I can only answer the question 'What am I to do?' if I can answer the prior question 'Of what story or stories do I find myself a part?'

The basic tenets of narrative ethics are:

- Identity is not static, but a narrative, a story we constantly tell during our lives
- Social relationships ('the story of which we are a part') prevail over the individual
- It is a story told from the patient's perspective, in contrast with principlist bioethics, that is oriented more to duties of physicians and caregivers

The dynamic process of *constructing one's own identity* is well captured by this perspective, together with the social texture in which this construction occurs. A typical move of narrative ethicists, when confronted with an ethical dilemma such as Margo's case, would be to abandon the analytical description of the pros and cons of different options (either beneficence or autonomy-oriented) and to try to read the situation in her social context (an information typically lacking in Dworkin's account) and to discover the main threads of Margo's story. The hard decisions about executing or ignoring her advance directives should be taken only after due consideration of Margo's story and of her hypothetical, reconstructed point of view.

What conclusions can we draw from this discussion? First, loss of PI—not coupled with loss or severe clouding of consciousness—occurs only in dementia. Actually this phenomenon is peculiar to it and is not seen in any other disease. No doubt clinicians see many patients with delirium or unconsciousness, but because these conditions are acute and transient, and lead to either recovery or death, they do not raise the problem of PI.

Second, in the usually progressive course of dementia, some morally important steps occur, generally in this order:

1. Loss of general competence (e.g. the competence to issue an advance directive)
2. Loss of task-specific competences (e.g. the capacity to consent to or refuse a particular treatment)
3. Loss of PI and, simultaneously or not,
4. Loss of personhood

Consequently, with regard to advance directives and their validity, one could speak of a sequence of 'time windows'. A first time window follows the loss of general competence, during which the patient is no longer able to issue a living will but can give his/her consent to treatments or other procedures.

A second time window is seen when the patient is no longer able to take part in the decision-making process but unquestionably remains the same person he/she used to be. A third time window occurs after the loss of PI, and can be conceptualized differently: either the patient, although severely compromised, is still a person, and hence a different person, to whom advance directives cannot apply, or he/she is no longer a person. In the latter case advance directives would retain their validity.

Third, current ideas and practices concerning advance directives are still valid, both legally and morally, except perhaps during the third time window, if loss of PI and loss of person status can be separated. Since no consensus has been reached on this problem, Buchanan's suggestion to make them coincide seems acceptable. However, some cases such those of Sybil and Margo, prompt us to consider possible exceptions to the doctrine of strong autonomy, without necessarily falling back into beneficent paternalism.

Finally, since impairment of PI is such a foreseeable phenomenon in the course of dementia, it deserves special attention by the caregivers as it would seem, from some experiences to be related in the next paragraph, that it can be contrasted with some success.

PERSONAL IDENTITY AS A THERAPEUTIC TARGET IN THE CARE OF DEMENTED PEOPLE

The experiences of those who care for demented people have stimulated a profound revolution of the philosophy of care. I quote the recent contribution of two psychologists, Cheston and Bender,[14] who put forward a severe criticism of the *canonical medical model of dementia* and propose an *alternative, psychological model*. From this model they develop a person-focused approach to the care of demented patients, as follows:

- Dementia needs to be understood as an interaction between psychological and neurological influences
- The main focus of dementia care must be on the person living with the illness, alongside an awareness of the needs of caregivers

- The impact of the process of dementia is experienced in terms of a threat to the person's view of him/herself as a coherent unity; this threat to a person's identity precipitates a range of behaviors whose function is to assert the individual's identity
- To understand the behavior of persons living with dementia we also need to understand their fears and the way in which they assert their own identity
- Without such an understanding of the emotional and identity needs of dementia sufferers we may misinterpret the behaviors that arise when these needs are not met as simply resulting from neurological damage

The person-focused approach to dementia sees the problem of self-identity as the hardest predicament with which demented people are confronted. This awareness has not only theoretical importance but also practical consequences. The organization of services for people with dementia should acknowledge this reality. Several therapeutic approaches have been developed for helping people cope with a threat to their own identity (e.g. reminescence therapy, psychotherapy groups centered upon narratives of the past life of participants). Obviously, the way PI is understood by social psychologists like Cheston and Bender is very different from the philosophical perspective of Parfit. Whereas the latter is based both on scientific data and on the logical aspects of the relation between person stages, social psychologists start their analysis from the empirical fact that, since birth, all of us have lived in a network of interpersonal and social relationships. Acquiring a PI for each of us is a lengthy, life-long process, through which we construct an identity for ourselves. This identity does not rise in isolation but always in dialogue with others (a social, constructionist view of PI).

CONCLUSION: DEMENTIA AND PALLIATIVE CARE

In this book that provides a comprehensive account of palliative care in neurology, a question of practical importance is: should the care of demented people be a task of palliative medicine and, in particular, of the nascent discipline of palliative neurology? Because dementia is a progressive, debilitating neurological illness, eventually leading to death and unresponsive to curative treatments, it seems to be a disease deserving palliative care—not only in the late stages when patients are close to death. In most communities, neurologists are involved more often in the early stages when the diagnosis is made. Palliative care specialists are seldom consulted until the final days of illness. Most demented people are cared for by geriatricians, primary care physicians, nurses, and lay caregivers. This may be a workable arrangement but, even if demented patients are cared for outside departments of neurology and palliative care units, I believe that dementia care falls, at least theoretically, within the scope of palliative neurology.

REFERENCES

1. Locke J. Essay Concerning Human Unterstanding. London, 1690.
2. Brock DW. Life and Death. Cambridge University Press, Cambridge, 1993.
3. Sperry RW. Hemisphere Deconnection and Unity in Conscious Awareness. Am Psychol 1968;23:723–733.
4. Parfit D. Reasons and Persons. Clarendon Press, London, 1984.
5. Tulving E. Episodic and semantic memory. In: Tulving E, Donaldson W, eds. Organisation of Memory. Academic Press, New York, 1972.
6. Fitzgerald GM. Autobiographical memory: a developmental perspective. In: Rubin DC, ed. Autobiographical Memory. Cambridge University Press, Cambridge, 1986.
7. Green M, Wikler D. Brain death and personal identity. Philosophy and Public Affairs 1980; 9:105–133.
8. Buchanan A, Brock D. Deciding for others. Cambridge University Press, Cambridge, 1989.
9. Dworkin R. Life's Dominion. HarperCollins, London, 1993.
10. Firlik AD. Margo's logo. JAMA 1991; 265: 201.
11. Beauchamp TL, Childress JF. Principles of Biomedical Ethics, 5th Ed. Oxford University Press, New York, 2001.
12. MacIntyre A. After Virtue: a Study in Moral Theory. Notre Dame University Press, Notre Dame, 1981.
13. Taylor C. Sources of Self. Cambridge University Press, Cambridge, 1989.
14. Cheston R, Bender M. Understanding Dementia. Jessica Kingsley Publisher, London, 1999.

Chapter 32

Food and Hydration

Janet Hardy
Helen White
Louise Henry
David Oliver

INTRODUCTION
ASSESSMENT
TREATMENT OF ANY REVERSIBLE CAUSE
 AND ANY ASSOCIATED SYMPTOMS
ARTIFICIALLY PROVIDED NUTRITION
 AND HYDRATION
Enteral Tube Feeding
Parenteral Nutrition

Practical Considerations
FOOD IN THE TERMINAL PHASE
ETHICAL DILEMMAS AND DECISION
 MAKING
HYDRATION IN THE TERMINAL PHASE
HYPODERMOCLYSIS
SUMMARY

While most patients with neurological disease will have functional gastrointestinal tracts, they will often have difficulty in taking food and fluids by mouth. This may be because of an impaired ability to swallow or because of a lack of desire to eat. The provision of food and fluids may be essential to maintain life in some patients. In the other extreme, the continued delivery of food and fluids may be inappropriate or even deleterious in those patients with very advanced stage disease. The issue of nutrition in patients with neurological disease is fraught with moral and ethical dilemmas. The involvement of a multiprofessional team is crucial to ensure best practice and optimum patient care. Every case must be treated on an individual basis and the patient and his/her family must be involved in all decision-making processes.

CASE HISTORY

Mrs S, a 63-year-old married lady with three children, had been found to have a glioblastoma multiforme in March 2000. She had been treated with radiotherapy and dexamethasone and had been continued on a maintenance dose but, when this was reduced, her mental state deteriorated.

In September 2000 she became less well, with increasing weakness and evidence of dysphagia and dysarthria. On occasion, she became disorientated. The dose of dexamethasone was increased from 4 mg daily to 8 mg daily, but she continued to become more confused and increasingly drowsy. Her oral intake of fluids reduced and on occasion she coughed and spluttered when taking fluids. An assessment by a speech and language therapist confirmed that the continuation of oral intake was becoming more difficult and there was an increasing risk of aspiration.

On 20th September she was very drowsy and requiring benzodiazepines to control the increasing confusion. Her husband and son approached the nursing staff to demand intravenous fluids as she was taking so little by mouth. A family discussion was held, including her husband, son, and two daughters, with the multidisciplinary team. Her husband remained very concerned that parenteral fluids were essential but her daughters realized that their mother was imminently dying and further intervention was probably inappropriate. It was agreed that a subcutaneous infusion of 500 ml normal saline over 24 hours would be given initially to ensure her comfort and allay Mr S's fears. Two days later Mrs S was unrousable and Mr S

335

and his family asked for the infusion to be stopped and a continuous subcutaneous infusion of morphine, midazolam, and glycopyrronium was commenced to control her symptoms of headache, agitation, and increasing respiratory secretions. She died peacefully 20 hours later with her family with her.

INTRODUCTION

Many people with neurological disease develop problems with their intake of food. This may be because of a direct effect on eating or swallowing or the reduction in the desire for food, either acute (such as following a cerebrovascular accident) or chronic and progressive (such as with motor neurone disease). Careful assessment and differentiation of the cause of the reduction in feeding is essential before any treatment or advice is given.

The common reasons for a reduced intake of food are:

- Lack of desire to eat—dementia, anorexia, severe depression
- Reduced ability to eat—with altered movement of the arms or hands
- Tremor
- Paralysis
- Profound weakness
- Excess drowsiness
- Dysphagia
- Neurological causes (see Table 32–1)
- Mucosal inflammation
- Following radiotherapy or chemotherapy
- Infection—candidiasis, herpes simplex, cytomegalo virus (CMV) infection

Table 32–1. Dysphagia Secondary to Neurological Dysfunction

- Upper motor neurone damage (tumor or infection, postoperative)
- Lower motor neuron damage (motor neuron disease, multiple sclerosis, cranial nerve palsy)
- Motor or sensory cranial nerve palsy (base of skull tumor, leptomeningeal infiltration, brain stem metastases)
- Cerebellar damage (infarction, surgery, tumor, paraneoplastic)
- Neuromuscular dysfunction (myasthenic–myopathic syndrome, Parkinson's disease)

ASSESSMENT

There is the need for a careful assessment involving a multidisciplinary team, with input from a speech and language therapist, a physiotherapist, dietitians, medical and nursing staff, as well as the patient and their carers. Such assessment will include:

- A dietary history
- Neurological examination
- Careful assessment of arm and hand movement
- Swallowing assessment
- General examination—including a psychological assessment

Input from a specialist speech and language therapist, with expertise in swallowing difficulties is essential. Their initial subjective 'bedside' assessment may well indicate the need for specific diagnostic procedures such as videofluoroscopy (modified barium swallow). This will demonstrate swallowing efficiency and identify the cause of any aspiration. Other screening procedures include fiberoptic endoscopy (to visualize the pharynx and larynx before and after a swallow) and cervical auscultation (the sound of swallowing in relation to respiration can aid in diagnosis).[1] Once the cause, level, and nature of the dysphagia has been determined, the therapist can work with other members of the team to develop a management strategy.

The main aim of any intervention is to assist the patient to swallow safely (i.e. without aspiration) and for as long as possible whilst maintaining adequate hydration and nutrition. Intervention can be in the form of therapeutic procedures (e.g. range of motion exercises focusing on the base of the tongue, teaching a supraglottic swallow thus providing voluntary airway protection) or in the development of compensation techniques such as modifying food consistencies or changing posture when swallowing.[2]

TREATMENT OF ANY REVERSIBLE CAUSE AND ANY ASSOCIATED SYMPTOMS

Dietary advice for patients with a poor appetite secondary to medication, depression,

Table 32–2. **Dietary Advice for Patients with a Poor Appetite**

- Small, frequent snacks, attractively presented are most appealing
- Encourage patient to maximize intake when appetite is at its best (usually in the morning)
- Encourage patient to eat what they fancy, whenever they want
- Eat in surroundings as pleasant as possible (e.g. ensure bed pans, vomit bowls, and other waste receptacles are removed from the eating areas)—ideally, patients should be able to go to a separate dining area/room
- Avoid nagging the patient (and caution carers against this)—it places undue stress on the patient and is likely to be counterproductive
- Patients the should be allowed plenty of time to eat (particularly those patients with tremor and poor manual dexterity)
- Where the patient requires a modified texture diet, ensure food is presented as attractively as possible and is well seasoned
- Careful and tactful help for patients requiring feeding by carers

fatigue, or advanced disease is presented in Table 32–2.

INFECTION

Mucositis secondary to radiotherapy or chemotherapy is usually transient and can be palliated with appropriate analgesia, antacid preparations containing local anesthetic (e.g. mucaine), ulcer-healing drugs (e.g. sucralfate), prostaglandin analogs (e.g. misoprostol), and proton pump inhibitors (e.g. omeprazole).

- Candidiasis, a common cause of mucosal ulceration should be treated with fluconazole or ketoconazole.
- Acyclovir should be used if there is any suggestion that the infection is herpetic.
- Oral ulcers may respond to a tetracycline mouthwash. There is now considerable experience in the use of thalidomide for resistant mouth ulcers in AID/HIV patients.[3]

DRY MOUTH

It is important to maximize the symptomatic management of a dry mouth (e.g. the use of saliva stimulants, artificial saliva sprays) and instigate routine mouth care. If possible, drugs that may be exacerbating xerostomia (e.g. anticholinergics, opioids) should be discontinued. Sucking ice cubes, boiled sweets, and citrus fruits may stimulate saliva flow. Dietary advice for patients with altered taste sensation (ageusia, dysgeusia) is to concentrate on foods that taste most pleasant (many patients tolerate sweet foods better and dislike meat, tea, and coffee) and to experiment with food they would perhaps not normally eat. Herbs, spices, and sauces can disguise some unpleasant tastes.[4]

PSYCHOLOGICAL ASPECTS

In the consideration of the psychological aspects of care it is essential to have a low threshold for using antidepressants and to consider the use of psychostimulants[5] in patients whose poor food intake seems directly related to low mood.

GASTROKINETIC AGENTS

Gastrokinetic agents (e.g. metoclopramide) speed gastric emptying, increase the tone of the lower esophageal sphincter, and co-ordinate antroduodenal contractions. They reduce gastroesophageal reflux, dysmotility dyspepsia, and may be a useful adjunct in some patients.[6]

CORTICOSTEROIDS AND PROGESTOGENS

Corticosteroids and progestogens have both been used as appetite stimulants in cancer patients with the ability but no desire to eat. There is evidence that both can produce a non-fluid weight gain in selected patients.[7] Concern remains as to the toxicity of both agents and of their efficacy in cachexia associated with very advanced malignant disease. Steroids are commonly used in brain tumor patients for the control of symptoms of raised intracranial pressure. Ironically, this can result in added problems of obesity and over-eating in this patient group. This is particularly prevalent in children who not infrequently develop voracious appetites with rapid weight gain and distressing changes in body image when started on steroids.[8] For this reason, many centers prefer to avoid steroids if at all possible when palliating the symptoms of raised intracranial pressure, or to use them sparingly according to strict guidelines.[9] Patients who develop steroid-induced hyperglycemia should be started on oral antidiabetic agents or insulin. Strict dietary control is not appropriate in this group of patients.

ARTIFICIALLY PROVIDED NUTRITION AND HYDRATION

When patients are unable to meet their nutritional requirements via the oral route, it may be appropriate to consider artificially provided nutrition and hydration (ANH). ANH is used in both patients unable to eat (e.g. those with permanent neurological impairment or oropharyngeal dysfunction) and in those that require nutritional support to supplement their oral intake (e.g. malnourished patients undergoing major elective surgical procedures or sustaining severe treatment-related gastrointestinal (GI) toxicity). When considering the provision of ANH, enteral feeding should be always instigated in preference to parenteral feeding unless there are special indications, as discussed below.

Enteral Tube Feeding

Enteral feeding and hydration is indicated in patients with an intact GI tract who require long-term nutritional support. The common indications for enteral feeding are:

- Neurological swallowing disorders with high-risk of aspiration
- Patient unable to chew food
- Patient unable to feed themselves and reluctant to be fed by carer
- Difficulty in achieving adequate intake due to the necessity of following a modified texture diet
- Patient feels hungry but due to dysphagia is unable to eat enough to meet their need

Tube feeding is recognized as a safe, efficient, and cost-effective method of nutritional support.[10] Although there are complications, these are generally less than those associated with parenteral feeding. It can be the route for the provision of all the patient's nutritional and fluid requirements or can supplement oral intake (usually as overnight feeding). Those caring for palliative care patients receiving enteral feeding should be flexible in their approach. The rate or volume of feed given will often have to be modified if the patient develops side effects (e.g. nausea or diarrhea), even if this compromises nutritional needs. If a patient's clinical condition deteriorates, the feeding tube is likely to be used less and less, although it can remain as a useful route for drug administration.

A wide range of commercially produced feeds are available. These should be used in preference to 'homemade' mixtures or milk alone as they are sterile and nutritionally balanced. Administration of the feed can be as boluses, via a pump, or by gravity (which is most practical to the patient and their carers).

Tube feeding can be administered via several routes, each of which is indicated in specific circumstances. The different modes of enteral feeding, along with their indications, contraindications, advantages, and disadvantages are shown in Table 32–3. The common complications and solutions to problems are shown in Table 32–4.

Patients should be informed of the possibility of home feeding.[11] Tube feeding is a relatively simple means of providing ANH for patients at home as long as the infrastructure is in place to support it. Carers can be taught how to use the feeding equipment and community nurses can be called upon to help with setting up and stopping feeds in patients unable to do it themselves. Funding should be secured before discussing the prospect of home enteral feeding. The appropriate means of follow-up and monitoring should be organized prior to discharge from hospital.

Parenteral Nutrition

Intravenous feeding—parenteral nutrition (PN)—will rarely be indicated in patients with neurological disease, as most will have a patent GI tract. However, if enteral feeding is not practicable or is inappropriate, parenteral feeding may be considered.

A peripheral intravenous cannula allows for hydration with isotonic fluids, but cannot be used for nutritional formulas. This requires the placing of a peripheral long line or central

Table 32-3. **Enteral Feeding**

Route of Feeding	Description	Indications	Contraindications	Advantages	Disadvantages
Nasogastric tube	Fine bore polyurethane tube specifically developed for enteral feeding. Can be inserted at the bedside. Ideally chest X-ray to confirm position of tube. Position can also be confirmed by use of pH indicator paper and aspiration of gastric contents. Tubes can remain in situ for >6 months	• Short-term supplementary or complete feeding • Impaired swallow/dysphagia	• Patient requiring long-term feeding (i.e. >6 weeks) • Patient with severely impaired gastric emptying • Patient at high risk of aspiration	• Quick and relatively easy to insert and remove • Cheapest way of delivering enteral feed	• Highly visible • Confirmation of position may be difficult without X-rays • Block more easily than wide bore tubes (and are difficult to unblock; hence may require re-intubation with a new tube) • Will not protect patients from aspiration of feed if feed is regurgitated (patient at high risk of aspiration • Possible increase in the production of oropharyngeal secretions

Continued on following page

Table 32–3— *continued*

Route of Feeding	Description	Indications	Contraindications	Advantages	Disadvantages
Nasoduodenal/ nasojejunal tubes	Longer length tubes usually made from polyurethane or silicone. Often have an end specially designed to stay distal to the pylorus	• Patients who require post-pyloric feeding because of poor gastric emptying or a high risk of feed regurgitation and aspiration • Short-term feeding	• Long-term feeding (> 6 weeks)	• Protects the patient from regurgitation of feed • Relatively cheap, and easy to care for once tubes are placed	• Positioning is problematic and usually requires X-ray or endoscopy • Tubes can migrate back into the stomach • Highly visible • Block easily, as relatively fine small diameter • As feed is delivered into the small intestine, patients may feel bloated/ uncomfortable if large volumes of feed are delivered

| Gastrostomy | Can be inserted surgically or endoscopically (PEG: percutaneous endoscopically placed gastrostomy). Can also be placed radiologically (RIG). Tube is held against the stomach wall both inside and on the surface.

Only those tubes designed specifically for the purpose of feeding should be used | • Where feeding is to be for > 6 weeks
• Neurological disorders, head and neck cancer, cystic fibrosis, and in situations where body image is particularly important to the patient
• Good option for patients requiring home enteral feeding | • Gut ileus, ascites, Crohn's disease, previous extensive gastric surgery, cancer of the stomach
• PEGs are contraindicated in patients where it is not possible to pass an endoscope (e.g. total blockage of the esophagus due to tumor)
• Patients with a high risk of aspiration of feed (e.g. tendency to regurgitate feed or very poor gastric emptying) | • No tubes are visible and therefore aesthetically more acceptable for patients
• Less easily displaced than NG tubes
• Suitable for long-term use | • Patients having tubes surgically placed will require a general anesthetic. Surgical tubes will also need replacement more frequently than other types
• For PEG insertion, need access to endoscopy suite and experienced clinician
• RIG placement will require X-ray guidance
• Gastrostomy feeding is not ideal in patients who are at high risk of aspiration and have a tendency to regurgitate feed
• Possibility of gastrostomy tube site infections
• Removal of PEG tube may require endoscopy |

Continued on following page

Table 32–3— *continued*

Route of Feeding	Description	Indications	Contraindications	Advantages	Disadvantages
Percutaneous endoscopic jejunostomy	Requires the formation of a PEG prior to the passage of a jejunostomy tube	• Patient requiring long-term feeding but with a high risk of feed aspiration/regurgitation	• Patients not suitable for endoscopy • Patients requiring short-term feeding	• Does not require a general anesthetic for jejunostomy tube insertion	• Tubes can migrate back into the stomach • Patients can feel bloated if large volumes of feed are infused at a time • Removal of PEG can be difficult • Possibility of infection at insertion site • Requires access to endoscopy suite and skilled clinician for placement
Jejunostomy	Requires formation of a tract between the jejunum and abdominal surface	• When there is a risk of aspiration of gastric contents or slow gastric function • Long-term feeding where gastrostomy feeding is contraindicated	• Complete ileus; severe inflammatory bowel disease, cancer in the small bowel, obstruction of the colon (e.g. due to cancer or adhesions) • Patients with atonic gut • Patients unable to tolerate general anesthetic	• Suitable for patients with high risk of feed aspiration	• Feed is delivered straight into the jejunum; side effects may include diarrhea and distension, particularly if the feed has been administered very quickly • Requires a general anesthetic for insertion • Possibility of infection at insertion site

venous line. This route of feeding is only appropriate for short periods. It is contra-indicated for more than a few weeks or in the presence of sepsis. There is a relatively high incidence of thrombosis and infection asso-ciated with the use of such lines. PN requires close monitoring of urea and electrolytes, glu-cose, liver function, and nitrogen balance and is much more expensive than enteral nutrition.[12]

Practical Considerations

Successful enteral feeding requires a multi-disciplinary approach. Clear goals need to be set and agreed, and the patient and carers should be fully consulted. There are several practical factors which should be taken into account when designing a feeding regimen. The ethical and moral dilemmas often asso-ciated with tube feeding are discussed below.

1. What is the aim of the feeding?
It is important to decide what is the aim of the enteral feeding. Is it to return the patient's nutritional status to normal levels or is it to prevent any further deterioration in nutri-tional status? This is dependent on the underlying disease state and the treatment (if any) and prognosis.

2. What is the likely time course?
Is it long term or short term? If it is short term, what will happen if the patient con-tinues to require feeding at the end of the 'short term' period?

3. What is the underlying disease state/clinical condition/plan for treatment?
This should determine the aims of feeding and will influence nutrient requirements. The medication taken by the patient and hence any drug nutrient interactions will need to be considered. Amongst other things, feeding will effect fluid balance. Disease state and treat-ment will also influence how much time is available for feeding (e.g. breaks for treat-ment, breaks for physiotherapy).

4. What is the status of the patient's GI tract?
This is influenced by disease, nutritional status, medication, treatment, surgical inter-ventions, etc. Gastric emptying should always be assessed as poor function may lead to aspiration of feed. Gut function also deter-mines which type of feed is required (e.g. whole protein or peptide).

5. What is the patient's nutritional status and current nutritional intake?
This will give some indication of which feeds should be used and whether full supplement-ary feeding is necessary and is helpful in set-ting goals for the nutritional support.

FOOD IN THE TERMINAL PHASE

Eating is one of life's great pleasures and meal times are important occasions for social interaction within family groups. Conversely, weight loss is an easily recognizable sign of advancing disease and is often seen as the harbinger of impending death. The provision of food for a loved one is a fundamental component of basic care and the inability to do so can be devastating to relatives and carers.[13,14]

In reality, the intake of food and fluid diminishes during the terminal phase. Many patients with advanced disease lose the desire to eat, such that feeding can become a daily trial despite the best efforts of those around them. Simple measures can help to some extent (e.g. the presentation of small meals, the avoidance of cooking smells). Patients should be encour-aged to 'graze' through the day and to eat what they want, when they want, rather than at set meal times (see Table 32–3).

Relatives are often concerned that not enough attention is being paid to the amount of food a patient is eating and/or that patients are not weighed regularly. It is usually possi-ble to explain that feeding is not going to prolong life nor will stopping feeding shorten life. Moreover, feeding may well cause added problems (e.g., nausea and vomiting, diarrhea, aspiration pneumonia).

ETHICAL DILEMMAS AND DECISION MAKING

A decision to feed or not to feed a patient is tied up with multiple moral and ethical issues[15,16] (see Chapter 35). In patients with a prognosis of a few days to weeks only, a decision not to feed is not usually difficult, for the reasons as described above. Similarly, for patients with a permanent neurological impairment or a long- or medium-term prog-nosis, ANH preserves nutritional status and is

Table 32–4. Complications of Enteral Feeding

Complication	Possible Causes	Solution
Tube related		
Tube displacement	Patient accidentally/deliberately removes tube	Tape tube securely to patient's nose or cheek. If it is a recurrent problem consider gasrostomy/jejunostomy.
Tube in incorrect position	Position not checked on insertion/dislodgement	Always check NG tube position by aspirating or asculation or X-ray. Monitor tube position regularly.
Tube blockage	Failure to flush feeding tube regularly or promptly. Inadequate flushing (i.e using too small a volume). Administration of medication via the tube.	To avoid this problem, flush tube with 30–50 ml of water before and after feeding or medication. If possible avoid using fine bore tubes for the administration of medication. If medication must be administered via the tube, then ensure it is in liquid form or finely crushed.
		If the tube is blocked try soda water/coke/sodium bicarbonate/spirits/pancreatic enzymes to try and unblock tubes.
Mucosal erosion/sinusitis	Local damage to the nasal area or throat by the feeding tube. Common when wide bore, rigid tubes are used.	Use polyurethane, fine bore NG tubes. Considering changing to a gastrostomy tube, jejunostomy tube.
Leakage of gastric/jejunal fluid at tube site	Incorrect dressing or needless dressing of the wound. Erosion around the stoma site (especially if balloon catheters used).	Ensure that the site of insertion is allowed to heal or is dressed in the appropriate dressing. Avoid using catheters instead of specially designed tubes. Consider a wider bore replacement tube if the problem is persistent.
Infection at insertion site	Incorrect dressing; no antibiotic cover given following insertion; poor technique when handling the tube.	Ensure that appropriate dressings have been used and that the patient understands how to care for the site (e.g wash hands before touching the site); swab wound and prescribe antibiotic.
GI complications		
Aspiration	Regurgitation of feed due to poor gastric emptying. Incorrect placement of the tube.	Give medication to improve gastric emptying (e.g metoclopramide). Check tube placement. Try intermittent feeding. Try transpyloric feeding or jejunostomy feeding. Ensure patient has head at 45°.
Nausea and vomiting	Generally related to disease/treatment (e.g. chemotherapy). Could be due to poor gastric emptying or too rapid infusion of feed.	Ensure appropriate antiemetics have been prescribed. Reduce infusion rate. Change from bolus feeding to intermittent feeding.

Diarrhea	Previous undernutrition and other GI abnormalities	Give anti-diarrheal agent.
	Antibiotic therapy or other medication such as chemotherapy, laxatives.	Discontinue antibiotics if possible.
		Change to an iso–osmolar feed.
	Disease related (e.g pancreatic insufficiency secondary to cystic fibrosis). Gut infection, microbial contamination of feed or equipment.	Reduce infusion rate.
		Ensure that microbiological contamination of feed or equipment is not likely.
		Check to see if the patient is receiving drugs in sorbitol or laxatives.
		Check stool appearance/content to see if malabsorption (e.g due to pancreatic insufficiency). Change to peptide feed and/or give pancreatic enzyme supplements.
		Check for GI infection (send stool sample).
		Try a fiber-containing feed.
Constipation	Inadequate fluid intake. Immobility; use of opioid and other medication causing gastric stasis; excessive use of anti-diarrheal agents; or bowel obstruction.	Check fluid balance.
		Suggest laxatives/bulking agents.
		Encourage patient to be as mobile as possible.
		Check if patient is in bowel obstruction—if yes, then discontinue feed.
		? Try fiber-containing feed.
Abdominal distension	Poor gastric emptying; rapid infusion of feed; constipation or diarrhea.	Reduce rate of infusion; prescribe gastric motility agents; encourage patient to be mobile. Check for constipation or diarrhea.
Metabolic hyperglycemia	Underlying diabetes mellitus or insulin resistance as a result of 'stress response'.	Regular monitoring of blood sugars and appropriate medication (e.g sliding scale insulin)

life-saving.[12] Nutritional support is clearly justified in malnourished patients who can be expected to have a reasonable quality and length of life and whose inability to eat is the principle impediment to normal functioning. Even in patients with a limited prognosis, the decision to instigate ANH is not difficult in those with a reasonable quality of life who are undergoing active treatment, especially those likely to respond to, and benefit from treatment. In some cases, outcome might even be improved, although there is considerable controversy as to whether feeding prolongs survival in cancer patients.[12] It is very important to be clear as to the ultimate goal of feeding in each individual situation.

A decision to feed or not to feed is more difficult in those with a limited prognosis but not in the terminal phase of disease. In these cases, a number of factors must be taken into consideration:

- What are the patient's wishes and those of the carers?
- Are the benefits of feeding likely to outweigh the complications?
- Is the feeding likely to impair or improve quality of life?
- Will it give false hope regarding the chance of recovery?
- Will the presence of feeding tubes detract from issues surrounding an inevitable death?
- Is there a living will or advanced directive to be considered?
- Are there cultural or religious beliefs surrounding feeding? Various cultural issues may need to be taken into consideration.
- Is the patient medically fit for placement of a percutaneous endoscopically placed gastrostomy (PEG) line?
- Are there community facilities that would allow the patient to continue feeding at home or will feeding necessitate a prolonged stay in hospital?
- Will there be satisfactory patient monitoring in the community?

Once feeding is commenced, it is very difficult to stop.

There may be hostility towards the idea of feeding as it is often associated with 'force feeding'. Conversely, some relatives will be very concerned that food is being withheld if a patient is not fed. Some relatives may be under considerable pressure in their community to ensure that feeding continues. In the extreme, they may be concerned that they are condoning assisted suicide by agreeing not to feed.

Although it is desirable to take into consideration the opinion of relatives, carers, and the multidisciplinary team, it is the patient's best interest that is paramount, not that of relatives or carers. Moreover, 'best interest' is not confined to best medical interest but should take into account patient values and preferences when competent, their psychological health, well-being, quality of life, relationship with family or carers, spiritual and religious welfare, and their own financial interests.[17] It is both morally and legally permissible to consider whether or not it would be in the patient's best interest to start feeding or to cease feeding.[18]

A blanket policy to give ANH or not to give ANH is not appropriate. There is no 'correct answer' and every case must be considered on an individual basis.

HYDRATION IN THE TERMINAL PHASE

Outside the palliative care setting, most hospitalized patients will receive intravenous fluids, and many will die with intravenous lines in situ.[19] This remains a very controversial issue. Even within palliative care, there are differences of opinion as to whether fluids in the terminal phase are beneficial for patients or not.[20] One school believes that fluid depletion in non-terminally ill patients can result in symptoms of lethargy, weakness, confusion, and even obtundation, as well as thirst and dry mouth. Electrolyte abnormalities can result in muscle twitching, irritability, and seizures. Renal impairment secondary to dehydration can lead to the accumulation of toxic metabolites of opioids resulting in confusion, myoclonus, and delirium. Fluid deprivation may exacerbate constipation and pressure ulcers on the skin.

On the other hand, an inability or unwillingness to drink is considered by many as a 'normal' part of the dying process and that artificial hydration contributes to the over medicalization of the 'modern death'.[19,21] The process of monitoring an infusion can divert attention from the fact that the patient is dying and support can be denied. Hydration might deter from the quality of life by increasing the need for toileting and catheterization and by the chance of clotting or infection related to feeding lines. Moreover, there is the suggestion that giving fluids can actually be deleterious. A degree of dehydration may reduce pulmonary secretions and therefore the chance of pulmonary edema. A reduction in gut secretions may result in less diarrhea and vomiting. It has also been suggested that pain is improved due to a reduction in peritumoral edema. It is claimed that death secondary to dehydration is not unpleasant [22] and that the associated symptoms can be easily managed by good mouth care and sips of fluid as tolerated.[23]

Much has been written in this area but, in the absence of definitive research, the balance of benefits and burdens remains subjective.[24] A recent systematic review on the effects of fluid status and fluid therapy on the dying was unable to draw any firm conclusions, primarily because of limitations in all studies reviewed.[20] All would be in agreement, however, that the comfort of the patient is paramount. Unfortunately, at the present time, there is no evidence that forgoing hydration reduces comfort in these patients or that providing it contributes to comfort. Every case must be considered individually.

Families and carers must be fully informed of all relevant issues when making any decisions regarding hydration and should be involved in any decision-making process.

HYPODERMOCLYSIS

Up to two liters a day can be delivered subcutaneously via a small cannula.[25] Intravenous access does not have to be found and urea and electrolytes do not have to be monitored. It is said by some to reduce delirium in dying patients by preventing dehydration and, thus, the accumulation of renally excreted toxic metabolites.[26] On the other hand, this method of hydration can rarely be sustained over any prolonged period, can cause unacceptable local swelling, and facilitates avoidance of the primary issue (i.e. whether the giving of fluids is in the patient's best interest or not). Whether hypodermoclysis improves the comfort of dying patients, or whom it might benefit, are questions still to be answered.[15]

SUMMARY

The assessment of a patient with neurological disease, who develops swallowing difficulties, is complex, involving the person him/herself, their family and close carers, and the professionals involved in their care. There is the need to consider each individual person, and there can never be a universal or simple approach that applies for all. With this careful, individualized approach, the most appropriate treatment can be given, but it is essential that the assessment is seen as a continuous process, so that the treatment can be altered as the person's condition changes.

REFERENCES

1. Zenner PM, Losinski DS, Mills RH. Using cervical ausculation in the clinical dysphagia examination in long term care. Dysphagia 1995;10:27–31.
2. Logemann JA. Evaluation and Treatment of Swallowing Disorders. Pro-ed International Publishers, Texas, 1998;156–157.
3. Revuz J, Guillaume JC, Janier M, et al. Crossover study of thalidomide versus placebo in severe recurrent apthous stomatitis. Archives of Dermatology 1990;126:923–927.
4. Gallagher–Alfred C. Nutritional Care of the Terminally Ill. Aspen, Maryland, 1989.
5. Martin D. The use of psychostimulants in terminally ill patients. Eur J Palliat Care 2001;8(6):228–232.
6. Twycross R. The use of prokinetic drugs in palliative care. Eur J Palliat Care 1995;2(4):143–145.
7. Loprinzi CL, Kugler JW, Sloan JA, et al. Randomized comparison of megestrol acetate versus dexamethasone versus fluoxymesterone for the treatment of cancer anorexia/cachexia. J Clin Oncol 1999; 17(10):3299–3306.
8. Glaser AW, Buxton N, Walker D. Corticosteroids in the management of central nervous system tumours. Achives of Disease in Childhood 1997;76:76–78.
9. Hardy J. Corticosteroids in palliative care. Eur J Palliat Care 1998;5(2):46–50.
10. Payne–James J, Enteral nutrition: tubes and techniques of delivery. In: Grimble G, Silk D, eds. Artificial Nutrition Support in Clinical Practice, 2nd Ed. Greenwich Medical Media Ltd, London, 2001; 281–302.
11. Elia M. An international persceptive on artificial nutritional support in the community. Lancet 1995;345:1345–1349.
12. Souba WW. Nutritional support. Drug therapy. New Eng J Med 1997;336(1):41–48.
13. Holden CM. Anorexia in the terminally ill cancer patient: the emotional impact on the patient and the

family. Hospice Journal: Physical, Psychosocial and Pastoral Care of the Dying 1991;7(3):73–84.

14. Hawkins C. Anorexia and anxiety in advanced malignancy: the relative problem. Journal of Human Nutrition and Dietetics 2000;13:113–117.

15. Huang Z–B, Ahronheim JC. Nutrition and hydration in terminally ill patients. Clinics in Geriatric Medicine 2000;16(2):313–325.

16. Bozzetti F (on behalf of the Instituto Nazionale Tumori, Milan, Italy). Guidelines on artificial nutrition versus hydration in terminal cancer patients. Nutrition 1996;12(3):163–167.

17. Department of Health Reference Guide to Consent for Examination or Treatment. *www.doh.gov.uk/consent*

18. Farsides C. PEG feeding, palliative care and ethics. Palliat Care Today 2000;IX(II):25–26.

19. Burge FI, King DB, Willison D. Intravenous fluids and the hospitalized dying: a medical last rite? Can Fam Physician 1990;36:883–886.

20. Viola RA, Wells GA, Peterson J. The effects of fluid status and fluid therapy on the dying: a systematic review. J Palliat Care 1997;13(4):41–52.

21. O'Neill WM. Subcutaneous infusions—a medical last rite (editorial). Palliat Med 1994;8:91–93.

22. Hoefler JM. Making decisions about tube feeding for severely demented patients at the end of life: clinical, legal and ethical considerations. Death Stud 2000;24(3):233–254.

23. Twycross R, Lichter I. The terminal phase. In: Doyle D, Hanks GWC, MacDonald N, eds. Oxford Textbook of Palliative Medicine, 2nd Ed. Oxford University Press, Oxford, 1998:500.

24. Dunphy K, Finlay I, Rathbone G, Gilbert J, Hicks F. Rehydration in palliative and terminal care: if not—why not. Palliat Med 1995;9(3):221–228.

25. Fainsinger RL, MacEachern T, Miller MJ, et al. The use of hypodermoclysis for rehydration in terminally ill cancer patients. J Pain Sympt Management 1994;9(5):298–302.

26. Bruera E, Franco JJ, Maltoni M, et al. Changing pattern of agitated impaired mental status in patients with advanced cancer: association with cognitive monitoring, hydration and opioid rotation. J Pain Symptom Manage 1995;10:287–291.

Chapter 33

Sedation in the Imminently Dying Patient

Raymond Voltz
Kathleen M. Foley

SEDATION IS NOT EUTHANASIA
FREQUENCY OF SEDATION IN
    PALLIATIVE CARE
SEDATION DOES NOT HASTEN DEATH

Sedation in the imminently dying patient is an aspect of aggressive palliative care. It is most commonly a treatment option for refractory symptoms in a dying patient. The indication for sedation is dependent on several factors including the intractable nature of the symptoms, the articulated goals of care for comfort only, and the options for care. Sedation does not hasten death but is a commonly observed aspect of impending death. The goals of treatment, the methods used, and the decision making must be transparent and openly discussed, with guidelines focused on providing comfort and reducing suffering, not hastening death.

CASE HISTORY

A 39-year-old hospital administrator with progressive bilateral lumbosacral plexopathy from metastatic lung cancer began to complain of escalating pain and some dyspnea. The patient was taking 40 mg of oral methadone per day and IV Dilaudid 6 mg per hour with 2 mg rescues every 20 minutes via a PCA pump. He discussed his prognosis with his oncologist who suggested that there were no available Phase I studies. He refused any standard protocols and wanted aggressive palliative care to maintain his quality of life. He remained functional, working at home until he developed acute worsening of his pain, and he was re-admitted.

INDICATIONS FOR SEDATION
CLINICAL MANAGEMENT
SUMMARY

On admission, his rapidly escalating pain required aggressive titration of his pain medication including doubling the dose to obtain some relief. He developed a progressive inferior vena cava occlusion and evolving cauda equina compression, all occurring in his radiated sites. He developed dyspnea and was clearly imminently dying. Increased requirements for analgesia were associated with sedation. Following a patient and family discussion, it was decided that the focus of care should be pain relief and sedation was an acceptable side effect.

Case discussion

This case represents a typical example of palliative care within neurology. In this patient, the disease process is not responsive to curative treatment and is progressing. The paramount goal becomes the achievement of the best possible quality of life. In palliative care, certain assumptions are made (see Chapter 1):[1-4]

1. Patients who are dying are living human beings; there is an ethical imperative to offer care and to provide adequate relief of suffering.
2. Dying patients should not be subject to ineffective primary treatments that are causing distress.
3. All patients have a right to adequate relief of physical and psychological symptoms and to social support.

349

4. All patients have a right to the care that enables them the best possible life in the given circumstances.

5. There is a disease-inherent downward course, which will take place independent of all interventions. It is our obligation to make the patient as comfortable as possible.

Whether sedation in the imminently dying patient is ever necessary, ethical, and distinguishable from active euthanasia has been a recent controversy in the literature. We would like to review this discussion and present the facts showing that sedation is indeed an appropriate palliative care option for an imminently dying neurological patient. The distinction between incurable patients with limited life expectancy and patients who are imminently dying is useful for clinical decision making in palliative care. The main goal of treatment in imminently dying patients is an 'appropriate death'.[2] This includes

1. An adequate relief of physical and psychological symptoms

2. A functional level as high as possible, within the limits of disability, in all stages of the dying process

3. An opportunity to resolve uncompleted life tasks and goals through reconciliation, resolution of conflicts, communication in significant relationships, and pursuit of remaining hopes

4. Yielding of control to others in whom the patient has confidence

In the imminently dying patient, the functional level irreversibly deteriorates. Often, it can only be maintained at the expense of unacceptable patient distress. As clinicians, we have the obligation to optimize comfort until death ensues.

Our case illustrates a situation in which all conventional symptomatic treatment options have failed (to provide analgesia without sedation) and the patient who is imminently dying is suffering. What to do in such a situation is one of the most difficult and controversial decisions in palliative medicine. However, agreement is growing that sedation in the imminently dying patient is indeed an acceptable treatment option. This treatment must be distinguished clearly and sharply from practices of active euthanasia by its intention and its reality.

SEDATION IS NOT EUTHANASIA

Sedation in the imminently dying as proposed by palliative care experts has been conflated with the use of morphine drips as a form of slow euthanasia where the intentions are unclear, without definitive target symptoms, and then, regardless of how symptoms are controlled, the dosage maintained or adjusted upward.[5] Balfour Mount, a founder of palliative medicine, states:

It is precisely because of the apparent subtlety of this distinction in the minds of some colleagues and the public alike that the palliative care approach in these difficult cases must be clarified if the hospice response to euthanasia is to be forcefully and clearly heard. We believe the distinction is critically important, ethically clear, and not at all subtle.[6]

Numerous terms have been used to describe sedation in the imminently dying. They include 'terminal sedation',[7] 'artificial sedation at the end of life',[8] or 'palliative sedation'. Palliative sedation is the term recently proposed by a working group of the European Association of Palliative Care[9] and is defined as 'the intention of inducing and maintaining deep sleep but not deliberately causing death in a very special circumstances'. This definition was the result of deliberation by 50 palliative experts, 36% of whom had more than 15 years of palliative care experience.[10]

Medical decisions can be seen in the four ethical axioms of autonomy, beneficence, non-maleficence, and justice.[11–13] Autonomy regards the patient as a unique person with a right to compassion, gentle truth, and independent decision making. Beneficence tells us to relieve suffering through excellence in physical, psychological, and supportive care, while making all efforts to enhance the patient's quality of life. Non-maleficence asks for clinical vigilance and not to harm the patient. Justice implies allocation of sufficient health-care resources to this aim.[2]

Sedation in the imminently dying recognizes the right of adequate relief of unendurable symptoms and the right of all patients to choose from among appropriate therapeutic options. In pursuing the goal of optimal symptom control, however, consciousness—this highest neurological function may be diminished or lost. Moreover, when the patient dies, it is difficult to know exactly what caused the patient's death: the underlying natural course of the disease or the side effects of the medication? This may be very confusing not only for relatives,[14] but also for health-care professionals.[15,16] Therefore, it is paramount to be absolutely open about the intentions of inducing sedation (to relieve suffering), and to be careful with the dosing of the medication (see above). A U.S. Supreme Court decision argued that sedation in the imminently dying intended for symptom relief was not assisted suicide but appropriate palliative care.[17]

Ethical validity of sedation has been derived from the 'principle of double effect' which distinguishes between the primary therapeutic intent (to relieve suffering) and unavoidable, untoward consequence (the decrease of interactional function).[12,13] The same principle has been used to justify the second potential consequence—an accelerated death. However, the clinical experiences with sedation suggest that there is no correlation between sedation and the timing of death.

Intentionally applying the same drugs (in lethal doses) to cause death is active euthanasia. This action has a clearly different intention.[1,18–24] As in many other decisions in palliative care, it is not the means of treatment which are 'good' or 'bad' in themselves, but it is the intention with which they are used.[11,12] Proponents of active euthanasia and physician-assisted suicide attempted to conflate the differences between these practices and sedation on the grounds that sedation would 'inevitably cause death' and the 'doctrine' of double effect would give the physicians more moral weight than the wishes of the patients.[15]

FREQUENCY OF SEDATION IN PALLIATIVE CARE

By itself, the process of dying is commonly associated with diminished consciousness prior to death. Exact epidemiological data for how patients with neurological illness die is lacking. In general oncology patients, studies have shown that roughly 30% of the patients are able to communicate 24 hours prior to death, 20% at 12 hours, and about 10% at one hour.[25] The necessity to further sedate patients is denied by a few proponents of palliative care, but has been described in several studies in oncology patients.[26–31] Of the 50 palliative care experts studied by Chater et al., 88% thought that sedation was sometimes indicated, and 78%

had themselves taken part in sedation in the last 12 months, 69% with groups of between one and four patients.[10] The only study looking at a subgroup of neurological patients (with amyotrophic lateral sclerosis) shows sedation used with 10%.[32] The most difficult symptoms which tend to precipitate the need for sedation are severe pain (as in our case history), dyspnea, agitated delirium, and persistent vomiting.

The frequency of sedation varies greatly however in these studies—from 10% to 57%. This range may be so broad because of differences of definition between the studies and several heterogeneous factors which influence the amount of suffering, such as underlying disease, type of symptom, cultural background, and amount of knowledge of the patients about their disease.[6–8,33–37] Further studies are needed to better assess and define the clinical role of sedation, especially in neurology patients.

If the occurrence of uncontrolled symptoms could be prevented, this might reduce the need for sedation. It has been proposed—though never formally proven so far—that prophylactic interventions and contingency planning may avoid these situations.[2,38] Contingency planning includes easy access to adequate pharmacotherapy for emergent situations. The specific drugs, doses, and routes of administration should be appropriate to the patient's clinical situation, and all members of the caring team (including family members) must be informed and instructed.[2] This contingency planning should be included in the broader advance care planning for palliative care patients.[38,39] Recently, we conducted a cross-cultural survey of palliative care patients and health-care professionals and compiled a 'checklist' of what decisions to discuss with the patients, and how to procede with advance directives.[40] This discussion, however, should be initiated as early in the course of the disease as possible.

SEDATION DOES NOT HASTEN DEATH

In has been stated in several articles that sedation hastens death, and anecdotal evidence for this is presented.[5,15,16] There are, however, well-designed retrospective studies proving that sedation in the imminently dying does not hasten death. In the study by Ventafridda et al., the survival time of 63 oncological patients in a palliative home care service who needed sedation was compared with 57 non-sedated patients, and no difference found.[29] Similarly, a study looking into survival times after withdrawal of life support in an ICU did not find differences between sedated and non-sedated patients (22 versus 22 patients).[41] Stone and colleagues also did not report differences in 30 versus 85 palliative care patients (survival times 18.6 versus 19.1 days after admission).[30] The average survival time after onset of sedation was 1.3 days. From this it may be concluded that the need for sedation is an indicator of near death, but not its cause.

INDICATIONS FOR SEDATION

The decision to sedate an imminently dying patient is always very difficult for everybody involved. Also, most experienced palliative care experts feel a personal burden in this issue.[10] Although the decision for sedation must be tailored to the individual patient, we do believe that some guidelines for sedation in the imminently dying patient can be set up, and should be set up, because of all the confusion surrounding this topic:[2,34]

1. The patient has a terminal disease, and is imminently dying.
2. All attempts of curative therapies have been exhausted or are not indicated.
3. The symptom is 'refractory' (see below).
4. 'Do not resuscitate' orders are in effect (see below).
5. Patients, all family members, and all members of the team have discussed all of the options.

Such a clinical decision should start with an open discussion between patient, family, and professionals, and a case conference approach is recommended. Neurologists, palliative care specialists, anesthesiologists, neurosurgeons, psychiatrists, nurses, social workers, and other health-care professionals involved should discuss the case. The goal of this discussion should be to clarify the remaining therapeutic options and goals of care. If the above mentioned prerequesites are met, sedation can be proposed to the patient and his family as a group consensus.

A symptom can be viewed as 'refractory' if the clinician perceives that further invasive and non-invasive interventions are:[34,42]

1. Incapable of providing adequate relief
2. Associated with excessive and intolerable morbidity
3. Unlikely to provide relief within a tolerable time frame

Clinicians should not subject the severely distressed patients to therapies that provide inadequate relief or excessive morbidity. At the same time, they should not sacrifice conscious function when viable alternatives remain unexplored. Therefore they must distinguish 'refractory' from 'difficult' symptoms, which could potentially respond within a reasonable time frame to other approaches without excessive adverse effects.[34] Consultation with palliative care specialists are advised before a symptom is considered 'refractory'. The most common symptoms which may be 'refractory' are pain, dyspnea, agitated delirium, and persistent vomiting. Whether otherwise refractory psychological symptoms of depression, anxiety, and existential distress may justify sedation, remains a controversial issue.[34,43]

Sedation should not be initiated until a discussion about cardio-pulmonary resuscitation (CPR) has taken place with the patient or proxy, and there is agreement that CPR is not initiated. CPR in this situation is almost always futile and inconsistent with agreed goals of care.[44]

Another situation (which is especially relevant in neurology) is the withdrawal of respiratory support in a conscious patient (e.g. a patient with amyotropic lateral sclerosis). It has been proposed that sedation before the withdrawal itself gives least distress to the patient. This is now accepted as a standard guideline in neurology.[1,45,46]

Finally, all other changes of management (e.g. restricting fluid intake) which are not entirely justified by the aim of symptom control, must be avoided, as they might be perceived as 'helping to kill'.[15,16]

CLINICAL MANAGEMENT

Sedation in the imminently dying, as reported in these studies, is still an empirical treatment. However, there are several options available which should be individually tailored to the specific clinical situation. As a guideline, the drug of choice is the one which is also effective for the prevalent symptom in the patient. If the patient is already on opiates for pain or dyspnea, one may switch from oral to parenteral administration and attempt to escalate the dose.[47,48] Some patients will benefit from this approach. Some will have inadequate sedation or will develop neuroexcitatory side effects, such as myoclonus or agitated delirium. A second agent, usually a benzodiazepine, can relieve the symptoms in the latter case. Agents with a short half-life (e.g. midazolam (1–3 hours), lorazepam (10–20 hours), or flunitrazepam) are easier to titrate against the symptoms.[49,50]

In catastrophic events in which a rapid induction of sedation is necessary, midazolam (5–10 mg) has been recommended because of its rapid onset of action and its versatility of administration (IV, SC, IM).[51,52] Benzodiazepines have also been described as useful in patients with refractory depression, anxiety disorder, or existential distress.[34] Rarely, benzodiazepines can cause a paradoxical agitation, and an alternative approach is then required. Experienced palliative care experts will use one single drug in only one-third of the patients, two drugs in the second third, and even three drugs in one quarter.[10] Chater et al. found that midazolam was the most widely used drug, followed by methotrimeprazine and other benzodiazepines.[10]

Recently, a new anesthetic drug, propofol, has been described for terminal sedation.[53–55] It has a very short length of action, and it allows the depth of sedation to be easily controlled from minute to minute. The level of sedation follows a change in infusion rate within 5–10 minutes. Usually, the infusion should be initiated at 10 mg/hour and increased by 10 mg/hour every 15–20 minutes, until satisfactory level of sedation is achieved. A later daily increase of dose due to tachyphylaxis may be necessary.[56] In patients with severely reduced hepatic blood flow, caution should be exercised, and administration of the drug should be strictly aseptic.[57,58]

As another alternative for a single-agent approach to sedation, the use of barbiturates has been advocated.[43,59] Barbiturates are symbolically associated with killing, as they are used by the proponents of active euthanasia, in capital punishment, and in suicides.

Barbiturates are by themselves not analgesic, but sedate very well. They are an accepted treatment option for status epilepticus and for patients on ventilatory support. In a series of 17 patients, thiopental (initiated at 20–80 mg/hour, then titrated to an average of 107 mg/hour) was found to be superior to amobarbital sodium due to its shorter half-life.[59] In some patients, the IV dose was lowered (e.g. if a visitor came). In all patients, the systolic blood pressure remained at or above 88 mm Hg immediately prior to death, without a downward trend, also suggesting that the natural process, and not the medication, was the cause of the patient's death.

Whatever medication is chosen, the dose should be escalated slowly, titrating the dose against the symptoms and level of sedation.[2,30] This escalation must be stopped as soon as a steady-state situation is achieved in which there is no indirect indication of distress of the patient (i.e. no restlessness, sweating, tachycardia, or tachypnea). As in other situations in palliative medicine, there is no absolute limit to the doses of medication which may be necessary. A careful observation and frequent re-evaluation of the clinical state of the patient is paramount. Any unindicated escalation of the dose should not occur. Guidelines for titration should be written down to guide dose administration for the caregivers.

Recently, it has been argued that fluids should be substituted automatically while the patient is sedated.[60] However, fluid substitution is a medical procedure—not a basic right—with its own clear indications and contraindications.[12,61] The decision for fluid substitution must be taken on an individual basis, with the intention to avoid anything which might worsen the symptoms (such as fluid overload). Any change in management which is not indicated for symptom control should be avoided as this might be perceived as 'helping to kill'.[15,16] However, usually, parenteral fluid substitution will not be necessary.[61–63]

SUMMARY

To summarize, sedation in the imminently dying patient is a commonly acceptable last treatment option for refractory symptoms in palliative care. The goals of treatment, its indication, and the decision making must be transparent to everybody involved. It is considered an appropriate palliative care option and should not be confused with active euthanasia.

REFERENCES

1. Bernat JL, Goldstein ML, Viste KM Jr. The neurologist and the dying patient. Neurology 1996;46(3):598–599.
2. Cherny NI, Coyle N, Foley KM. Guidelines in the care of the dying cancer patient. Hematol Oncol Clin North Am 1996;10(1):261–286.
3. Council on Scientific Affairs, AMA. Good care of the dying patient. JAMA 1996;275:474–478.
4. The American Academy of Neurology, Ethics, and Humanities Subcommittee. Palliative Care in neurology. Neurology 1996;46:870–872.
5. Billing JA, Block SD. Slow euthanasia. J Pall Care 1996;12(4):21–30.
6. Mount B. Morphine drips, terminal sedation, and slow euthanasia: definitions and facts, not anecdotes. J Palliat Care 1996;12(4):31–37.
7. Caraceni A, Zecca A, Martini C, Gorni G, Galbiati A, DeConno F. Terminal sedation: a retrospective survey of a three-year experience. Eur J Pall Care 2002 (Abstracts of 2nd Congress of the EAPC Research Network):4.
8. Müller–Busch HC, Andres I, Jehser T. Artificial sedation at the end of life and patient's will. Eur J Pall Care 2002 (Abstracts of 2nd Congress of the EAPC Research Network):4.
9. Poullain F, Pourchet S. Palliative sedation. Working Group of the EAPC. Eur J Pall Care 2002 (Abstracts of 2nd Congress of the EAPC Research Network):3.
10. Chater S, Viola R, Paterson J, Jarvis V. Sedation for intractable distress in the dying—a survey of experts. Palliat Med. 1998;12(4):255–269.
11. Beauchamp TL, Childress JF. Principles of Biomedical Ethics, 4th Ed. Oxford University Press, New York, 1994.
12. Bernat JL. Ethical Issues in Neurology. Butterworth–Heinemann, Boston, 1994.
13. Latimer EJ. Ethical decision-making in the care of the dying and its applications to clinical practice. J Pain Symptom Manage 1991;6(5):329–336.
14. Walker Campi C. When dying is as hard as birth. The New York Times, Jan 5 1998:A19.
15. Quill TE, Dresser R, Brock DW. The rule of double effect—a critique of its role in end-of-life decision making. New Engl J Med 1997;337:1768–1771.
16. Quill TE, Lo B, Brock DW. Palliative options of last resort—a comparison of voluntary stopping eating and drinking, terminal sedation, physician-assisted suicide, and voluntary active euthanasia. JAMA 1997;278:2099–2104.
17. Burt RA. The Supreme Court speaks. Not assisted suicide but a constitutional right to palliative care. New Engl J Med 1997;337:1234–1236.
18. Bernat JL. Physician-assisted suicide should not be legalized. Arch Neurol 1996;53(11):1183–1184.
19. Foley KM. Competent care for the dying instead of physician-assisted suicide. N Engl J Med 1997;336(1):54–58.
20. Krakauer EL, Penson RT, Truog RD, King LA, Chabner BA, Lynch TJ. Sedation for intractable distress of a dying patient: acute palliative care and the principle of double effect. Oncologist 2000;5:53–62.
21. Moulin DE, Latimer EJ, Macdonald N, et al. Statement on euthanasia and physician-assisted suicide. J Pall Care 1994;10(2):80–81.
22. Sulmasy DP, Pellegrino ED. The role of double effect: clearing up the double talk. Arch Int Med 1999;159:545–550.
23. Wein S. Sedation in the imminently dying patient. Oncology (April) 2000:585–601.
24. Wanzer SH, Federman DD, Adelstein SJ, et al. The physician's responsibility toward hopelessly ill patients. A second look. N Engl J Med 1989;320(13):844–849.
25. Ingham JM, Layman–Goldstein M, Derby S, et al. The characteristics of the dying process in cancer patients in a hospice center. Proc Annu Meet Am Soc Clin Oncol 1994;13:172.
26. Enck RE. Drug-induced terminal sedation for symptom control. Am J Hosp Palliat Care 1991;8(5):3–5.
27. Fainsinger R, Miller MJ, Bruera E, Hanson J, Maceachern T. Symptom control during the last week of life on a palliative care unit. J Palliat Care 1991;7(1):5–11.
28. Lichter I, Hunt E. The last 48 hours of life. J Palliat Care 1990;6(4):7–15.
29. Ventafridda V, Ripamonti C, De Conno F, Tamburini M, Cassileth BR. Symptom prevalence and control during cancer patients' last days of life. J Palliat Care 1990;6(3):7–11.
30. Stone P, Phillips C, Spruyt O, Waight C. A comparison of the use of sedatives in a hospital support team and in a hospice. Palliat Med 1997;11(2):140–144.
31. Fainsinger RL, Waller A, Bercovici M, et al. A multicentre international study of sedation for uncontrolled symptoms in terminally ill patients. Palliat Med 2000;14(4):257–265.
32. Oliver D. Opioid medication in the palliative care of motor neurone disease. Palliat Med 1998;12(2):113–115.
33. Aoki Y, Nakagawa K, Hasezawa K, et al. Significance of informed consent and truth-telling for quality of life in terminal cancer patients. Radiat Med 1997;15(2):133–135.
34. Cherny NI, Portenoy RK. Sedation in the management of refractory symptoms: guidelines for evaluation and treatment. J Palliat Care 1994;10(2):31–38.
35. Coyle N, Truog RD. Health Care Ethics Forum '94: pain management and sedation in the terminally ill. AACN Clin Issues 1994;5(3):360–365.
36. Mount B, Hamilton P. When palliative care fails to control suffering. J Pall Care 1994;10(2):24–26.
37. Rousseau P. Terminal sedation in the care of dying patients. Arch Intern Med 1996;156(16):1785–1786.
38. Miles SH, Koepp R, Weber EP. Advance end-of-life treatment planning. A research review. Arch Int Med 1996;156:1062–1068.
39. Levinsky NG. The purpose of advance medical planning—autonomy for patients or limitation of care? New Engl J Med 1996;335(10):741–743.

40. Voltz R, Akabayashi A, Reese C, Ohi G, Sass HM. End-of-life decisions and advance directives in palliative care: a cross-cultural survey of patients and health-care professionals. J Pain Symptom Manage 1998;16(3):153–162.

41. Wilson WC, Smedira NG, Fink C, McDowell JA, Luce JM. Ordering and administration of sedatives and analgesics during the withholding and withdrawal of life support from critically ill patients. JAMA 1992;267(7):949–953.

42. Kenny NP, Frager G. Refractory symptoms and terminal sedation of children: ethical issues and practical management. J Palliat Care 1996;12(3):40–45.

43. Truog RD, Berde CB, Mitchell C, Grier HE. Barbiturates in the care of the terminally ill. N Engl J Med 1992;327(23):1678–1682.

44. Haines IE, Zalcberg J, Buchanan JD. Not-for-resuscitation orders in cancer patients—principles of decision-making. Med J Aust 1990;153(4):225–229.

45. Bernat JL, Cranford RE, Kittredge FI, Rosenberg RN. Competent patients with advanced states of permanent paralysis have the right to forgo life-sustaining therapy. Neurology 1993;43:224–225.

46. Borasio GD, Voltz R. Discontinuation of mechanical ventilation in patients with amyotrophic lateral sclerosis. J Neurol 1998;245(11):717–722.

47. Cohen MH, Anderson AJ, Krasnow SH, et al. Continuous intravenous infusion of morphine for severe dyspnea. South Med J 1991;84(2):229–234.

48. Expert Working Group of the European Association for Palliative Care. Morphine in cancer pain: modes of administration. Brit Med J 1996;312:823–826.

49. McNamara P, Minton M, Twycross RG. Use of midazolam in palliative care. Pall Med 1991;5:244–249.

50. Teboul E, Chouinard G. A guide to benzodiazepine selection. Part I: pharmacological aspects. Can J Psychiatry 1990;35(8):700–710.

51. Burke AL, Diamond PL, Hulbert J, Yeatman J, Farr EA. Terminal restlessness—its management and the role of midazolam. Med J Aust 1991;155(7):485–487.

52. Stone P, Phillips C, Khullar M. Sedation in catastrophic incidents. Palliat Med 1997;11(3):253–254.

53. Mercadante S, DeConno F, Ripamonti C. Propofol in terminal care. J Pain Sympt Management 1995;10:639–642.

54. Moyle J. The use of propofol in palliative medicine. J Pain Symptom Manage 1995;10(8):643–646.

55. Sebel PS, Lowdon JD. Propofol: a new intravenous anesthetic. Anesthesiology 1989;71(2):260–277.

56. Albanese J, Martin C, Lacarelle B, Saux P, Durand A, Gouin F. Pharmacokinetics of long-term propofol infusion used for sedation in ICU patients. Anesthesiology 1990;73(2):214–217.

57. Bailie GR, Cockshott ID, Douglas EJ, Bowles BJ. Pharmacokinetics of propofol during and after long-term continuous infusion for maintenance of sedation in ICU patients. Br J Anaesth 1992;68(5):486–491.

58. Tobias JD. Propofol sedation for terminal care in a pediatric patient. Clin Pediatr (Phila) 1997;36(5):291–293.

59. Greene WR, Davis WH. Titrated intravenous barbiturates in the control of symptoms in patients with terminal cancer. South Med J 1991;84(3):332–337.

60. Craig GM. On withholding nutrition and hydration in the terminally ill: has palliative medicine gone too far? J Med Ethics 1994;20(3):139–143.

61. Stone P, Phillips C. Nutrition, dehydration and the terminally ill. J Med Ethics 1995;21(1):55.

62. Ashby M, Stoffell B. Artificial hydration and alimentation at the end of life: a reply to Craig. J Med Ethics 1995;21(3):135–140.

63. Ellershaw JE, Sutcliffe JM, Saunders CM. Dehydration and the dying patient. J Pain Sympt Management 1995;10(3):192–197.

Chapter 34

Advance Directives

Akira Akabayashi
Brian Taylor Slingsby
Raymond Voltz

NEUROLOGICAL DISORDERS AND
  ADVANCE DIRECTIVES
Neurodegenerative Diseases
Stroke
Tumors
Amyotrophic Lateral Sclerosis

Summary of Neurological Cases
A SAMPLE MODEL FOR ADVANCE CARE
  PLANNING
CULTURAL CONSIDERATIONS
SUMMARY
APPENDIX

Advance directives (ADs) are one method proposed to facilitate communication among patients, families, and health-care providers regarding the plan of care that will be considered appropriate in times of incapacity. This chapter describes the aims and benefits of AD, particularly those related to issues common to neurological diseases. Also discussed is the health-care provider's role in implementing advance care planning and the possible value of initiating discussion regarding end-of-life decisions between patient, family, and physician.

CASE HISTORY

A 66-year-old housewife was admitted to the neurology ward because of progressive weakness of her right arm that she noticed two weeks earlier. MR scan revealed a space-occupying lesion in the left temporo-parietal region consisting of central necrosis and peritumoral edema. The radiological impression of a glioblastoma multiforme was confirmed by biopsy. Because of the proximity to speech areas, the neurosurgeons advised whole-brain irradiation as first-line therapy. During irradiation, a clonic seizure of the right arm occurred with concomitant epileptic speech arrest. Anticonvulsant therapy was started, and these episodes

subsided. However, in the months following irradiation, despite high-dose dexamethasone treatment, the right hemiparesis worsened and signs of aphasia appeared. She had difficulties retrieving words, which frightened her, and at a follow-up visit an intense discussion about treatment options, prognosis, and the terminal phase took place. All her wishes regarding 'Do not resuscitate' orders, intensive care, and disease-modifying treatment were recorded. Two months later, while she was under the outpatient care of a hospice group, she suffered three generalized tonic clonic seizures and was admitted to the neurology ward. Her speech had deteriorated to such an extent that she was no longer able to communicate her preferences. However, in accordance with her AD, she was not transferred to the intensive care unit. Fortunately, using intravenous phenytoin and diazepam, her seizures were stopped on the general neurology ward. Three days later, she was transferred to the local palliative care unit, where she died peacefully three weeks later.

Discussion

This case illustrates the need, at the earliest possible time, to discuss those end-of-life decisions that are most likely to occur, depending on the underlying disease. In this case, setting up an AD was helpful for deciding about medical therapy decisions in accordance with her wishes. This act is particularly important in patients such as this one, where it is foreseeable that the ability to communicate will diminish because of the localization of the tumor.

ADs are an important means of facilitating communication among patients, families, and health-care providers regarding the plan of care desired by a patient in case of future incapacity.[1] Such directives are made while the patient remains competent, and specify the forms of medical treatment to be provided by caregivers. ADs also may designate another person to act as a proxy decision maker should the patient lose her capacity to make decisions.

The moral arguments supporting ADs in the United States are based primarily on the concept of respect for autonomy and on the patient's right to self-determination. ADs have been recommended as a means to improve communication between patients and health-care providers when making health-care decisions. Some experts believe that ADs should contain disease-specific information rather than general statements, which do not offer much assistance in most clinical situations. ADs should be seen as part of a more general plan for end-of-life decisions in which improved communication is more important than a more formal preservation of rights, achieved by simply completing a document.[1,3,4] However, whether the disease-specific ADs actually improve the patient–physician relationship has yet to be confirmed.[5]

While on the one hand, ADs are quite familiar to the palliative care patient, on the other hand, patients in clinical settings rarely express their directives regarding palliative treatment. A major difficulty of initiating an AD in the clinical setting is the inability of an individual to predict her emotions regarding future decisions. For instance, some healthy patients on religious or other grounds, may oppose receiving a blood transfusion, yet change their mind when it is a matter of life or death. In other words, it is often not feasible to predict one's final decision prior to an actual situation. Accordingly, in cases in which the future is unforeseeable, assigning a proxy decision maker can assure that one's original decisions will be followed.

The main advantage of naming a proxy is that it offers the flexibility of a trusted family member or friend who in effect takes the place of the patient in the physician–patient relationship. Although such an idea of a proxy seems ideal, many studies have documented the incongruity between a proxy's decision making and the prior wishes of the patient.[7–10] The problem seems to stem from a lack of communication and understanding of the patient's decision-making process and the values upon which it is composed. Accordingly, one solution is to have the proxy understand the patient's view on treatment through widespread discussions about end-of-life decisions, and by doing so she will be able to make correct decisions.

In the case of the 66-year-old housewife, a proxy was neither needed nor used. However, in cases in which the decision-making capacity or the patient's communication skills deteriorate, assigning a proxy is often advantageous. In instances in which the patient's family or friend plays a key role, a proxy should be discussed in order to avoid future misunderstandings between family and physician.

NEUROLOGICAL DISORDERS AND ADVANCE DIRECTIVES

There are many benefits of advance care planning in patients with neurological disease. In this section, we discuss a few neurological diseases relevant to advance care planning.

Neurodegenerative Diseases

In patients with neurodegenerative diseases (i.e. Parkinson's disease and Alzheimer's disease), it is appropriate to attend to end-of-life treatment decisions while the patient is still competent. The relatively slow progression of neurodegenerative diseases enables patient, family, and physician to discuss a disease-specific AD while decisions that lie ahead are to some extent still predictable. This advance planning avoids ambiguity concerning treatment-specific decisions. In the case of appointing a proxy, careful discussion between proxy and patient is necessary in order to facilitate adequate representation of the patient's wishes.

Stroke

While stroke is rarely foreseeable, patients with intracranial atherothrombotic disease and atherosclerosis of the internal carotid artery have a high probability of stroke. In such cases, it is recommended to discuss the possibility of an AD, including a proxy, at diagnosis.

Regardless of whether the patient decides to compose a written directive or assign a proxy, it is vital that the patient begin to discuss her directives with family and health-care providers. This will help to avoid any disagreements between family and physician in the case of a loss of decision-making capacity by the patient.

Tumors

In the case of glioblastoma multiforme and anaplastic gliomas, depending on if the tumor is a high-grade glioma (i.e. anaplastic astrocytoma, glioblastoma multiforme, anaplastic oligodendroglima, anaplastic oligostrocytoma), there exists the risk of a sudden loss of communication skills with or without consciousness, depending on the progression of the glioma. In the above-discussed case, the filing of an AD avoided any complications regarding treatment-specific decisions.

Amyotrophic Lateral Sclerosis

Patients with amyotrophic lateral sclerosis (ALS) must make a number of important and difficult treatment decisions. Although the majority of ALS patients retain cognitive faculties and mental competence throughout the course of the disease, decisions about life support for the ALS patient are ordinarily framed as issues of treatment refusal by competent patients. Accordingly, the rights of ALS patients as competent adults to refuse life support have been recognized in several court cases in the United States.[11] To avoid any disagreement between physician and patient or family, it is advantageous in advance to discuss a thorough treatment plan.

Disease symptoms such as progressive dysarthia, often leading to a total loss of the ability to communicate, or the onset of dyspnea, together with symptoms of chronic nocturnal hypoventilation, are instances where symptoms require treatment-specific decisions. With the utilization of ADs, confusion can be avoided.

The most feared symptom of ALS is dyspnea from respiratory insufficiency that alters the patient's quality of life. As soon as dyspnea develops, a proper treatment plan should be discussed. Non-invasive intermittent ventilation (NIV) via a mask is an efficient and cost-effective means of alleviating these symptoms.[12] If the patient refuses NIV, intermittent oxygen administration may be attempted. However, oxygen is inferior to NIV because of the danger of respiratory depression in chronically hypercapnic patients receiving oxygen during sleep.[13]

At this stage, it is crucial for the patient's directives to be recorded in order to avoid unwanted intubation by an emergency physician upon terminal respiratory failure. Although patients may survive for years on full 24-hour mechanical ventilation by tracheostomy, they may ultimately develop a 'locked-in' syndrome.[14] Once this happens, communication becomes difficult because of total paralysis. Some patients may wish to continue living in such a state; and others refuse further life-sustaining therapy. ADs executed at the early stage of ALS can be useful to guide the physician, but some patients change their minds about therapy as the disease progresses. Benditt et al. suggests the use of an ALS disease-specific directive as means of facilitating effective communication and adherence to the patient's wishes. [15]

Summary of Neurological Cases

There are several clinical levels of a patient's ability to communicate. In cases of dementia, Parkinson's disease, and ALS, where time is not a limiting factor, patient, family, and physician should utilize this time to discuss the issues pertaining to palliative care. The inevitable decline and foreseeable course of ALS, together with sufficient time from diagnosis to death, offer ample opportunity for physician and patient to formulate a care and treatment plan and to make end-of-life decisions upon loss of competence. In cases of neoplastic disease, the abrupt loss of communicative skills can be foreseen at the time of diagnosis; consequently, it is necessary to attend to the possibility of an AD and other advance care planning as soon as possible. Lastly, although stroke is seldom foreseen, in cases in which the risk of stoke is high, we encourage prior planning to the possible events that may lie ahead. In brief, neurological diseases and their frequency of leading to palliative care necessitate discussion concerning advance care planning.

A SAMPLE MODEL FOR ADVANCE CARE PLANNING

In the appendix, we propose a brief checklist for planning end-of-life decisions in patients with a terminal disease.[16] The proposed checklist is general and should be tailored to the patient's individual medical, social, and cultural circumstances. Depending on the patient's diagnosis and stage of disease, the issue of ventilatory support may overshadow the issue of disease-modifying treatments. From a social standpoint, each patient has her own relationships with significant others, so the role that family and friends play in advance care planning varies from individual to individual. Although later we discuss the issue of cultural differences, each patient may hold a different set of values and beliefs depending on her religious, cultural, and ethnic background.

Advance care planning is a painful issue to consider and ADs continue to be complicated because of the reality that it is human to change one's mind and that one never can know in advance how one would feel in a life or death situation not yet lived. However, the dearth of discussion regarding end-of-life decisions between patient, family, and physician is a problem that needs to be assessed. ADs should not be looked on as an end, but rather as a catalyst for the essential discussion regarding end-of-life decisions.

Despite the need for physicians to play a key role in orchestrating advance care planning, studies show that physicians tend not to raise the issue of ADs.[17] Failure to discuss ADs could be due to the belief that speaking of dying may be harmful and discouraging to patients, that the patient herself wishes not to speak of end-of-life decisions, or because of the belief that it is the patient's responsibility to bring up such issues.[11]

Patients as well are reluctant to discuss decisions regarding terminal treatment and the issues that compliment it. Patients may tend to avoid the issue of approaching death, may not want to deal with any additional paperwork, may consider ADs not an integral part in the setting of medical care, or may believe that family authority or trust in the physician makes directives unnecessary.[11] Thus, the physician's role becomes important in initiating the discussion between patient, family, and significant others, and the physician should be willing to provide advice when needed.

In short, the health-care provider's role in advance care planning needs be active, yet not to be overly accentuated. Martin et al. summarize the role as:

> The physician's role in advance care planning should be supportive and sufficiently participatory that preferences can be well understood and translated into clinical care. Physicians may raise issues, direct patients and families to appropriate resources, provide information about diagnoses and treatments tailored to their patients' individual health situations, address information needs as they arise, to help ensure that the proxy is involved in the process, and review the results of the process. Advance care planning is just like most quality clinical encounters in medicine; the physician has a key role but not all-encompassing role.[18]

CULTURAL CONSIDERATIONS

Multicultural research regarding advance care planning continues to assist health-care providers in understanding the intricacies between cultures. According to one book, where contributors from legal, medical, and philosophical disciplines described the situation in Japan, the United States, and Germany,[19] the Japanese are considered to have a traditional culture still oriented to patterns of familial loyalty with social relationships based upon status. The United States is seen to be the opposite. Germany is located between these two extremes. In the preface of the book, the accomplishment of the first phase was summarized by the editors, who stated:

> In modern societies, rich with diverse values and wishes manifest in individual expressions and convictions, there is no longer a uniform, general answer to the question of when life-supporting medical interventions should cease. The answer the physician might give if only his or her convictions mattered is not necessarily the answer for the patient, who most likely will have other religious beliefs, visions, personal expectations, hopes and fears.[19]

In the context of this diversity of values, the acceptability of ADs was assumed to be quite different in each culture or society. For example, in societies where individual autonomy is valued, well-informed adults often favor the use of medical care directives in advance.[19] This tendency towards contract-facilitated risk reduction can be seen in the writing of wills, as well as legal and non-legal contracts.

On the other hand, in some contexts there was less of a need for Ads, such as in cultures where values of prioritizing the community and family took precedence over self-determination.[19] In such an environment, there is greater reliance on filial relationships. Likewise, the patient customarily entrusts treatment-related decisions to family or the medical professional.

This cultural difference is also seen in the process of acquiring consent from the patient. According to previous cross-cultural research, signing of an AD form and appointing a proxy (durable power of attorney according to the U.S. law) is highly prevalent in the palliative care setting in the United States.[6] Needless to say, the reason for such is that palliative care is intrinsic to end-of-life decisions. Although in other cultures, such as Japan, where explicit oral consent is mostly obtained from the patient's family at time of admission to a hospice, in the United States, an explicitly written consent is signed by the patient.

Culturally independent, oral statements often serve as a first step. Yet because they may be misremembered and are occasionally burdensome to prove, patients should be encouraged to address their directives in written form; merely a note or a personal statement is adequate and will hold up legally.[2]

The United States is a nation of diverse cultures and peoples. When attending to advance care planning, the patient's individual ways of approaching life and death need to be taken into consideration. In the Los Angeles, Orange, and San Diego counties of California, where a physician is likely to treat patients of diverse cultural and ethnic backgrounds (e.g. Cambodian, Chinese, Japanese, Korean, Mexican, Thai), each individual's set of values and beliefs need to be considered in order to make the patient and her family feel most comfortable in having to face death.

Even within the same cultural background, each individual may hold a different set of values and a different opinion regarding end-of-life issues. Moreover, regardless of culture and ethnic background, each individual patient may have a unique relationship with her family and significant others.

SUMMARY

Advance directives should promote:

1. An improvement of trust-based communications between patients, families, and physicians.
2. The development of a trust-based partnership in co-operation and decision making prior to the patient's potential states of incompetence or wishlessness.
3. The relief of anxiety and the reduction of uncertainty that individuals, families, and others responsible for the patient's care might feel if they are unsure about what the patient would want or what the patient's best interests would be.
4. The alleviation of legal (and ethical) uncertainty for the physician, which often leads to over-treatment following the rules of 'defensive medicine'.
5. An advance in disease-specific care planning including neurological disorders such as ALS.[15]
6. The prevention of adverse decisions which are not in the patient's best interests.[20,21]

The aim of advance care planning is to provide better care to the patient and to avoid the misunderstandings between patient, family, and physician in the hope of making end-of-life decisions easier and more comfortable.

REFERENCES

1. Teno JM, Nelson HL, Lynn J. Advance care planning—priorities for ethical and empirical research. Hastings Cent Rep 1994;24(6):S32–S36.
2. King NMP. Making Sense of Advances Directives. Georgetown University Press, Washington D.C., 1996.
3. Miles S H, Koepp R, Weber EP. Advance end-of-life treatment planning. A research review. Arch Intern Med 1996;156:1062–1068.
4. Emanuel L. Advance directives: what have we learned so far? J Clin Ethics 1993;4:8–16.
5. Teno JM. Lessons learned and not learned from the SUPPORT project. Palliat Med 1999;13:91–93.
6. Akabayashi A, Voltz R. Advance Directives in Different Cultures. Topics in Palliative Care, Vol. 5. Oxford University Press, New York, 2001:107–122.
7. Zweibel NR, Cassel CK. Treatment choices at the end of life: a comparison of decisions by older patients and

their physician-selected proxies. Gerontologist 1989;29:615–621.

8. Meier DE, Mulvihill M, Cammer Paris BE. Substituted judgement: how accurate are proxy predictions?, Ann Intern Med 1991;115:92–98.

9. Uhlmann RF, Pearlman RA, Cain KC. Physicians' and spouses' predictions of elderly patients' resuscitation preferences, J Gerontol 1988;43:M115–121.

10. Ouslander JG, Tymchuk AJ, Rahbar B. Health care decisions among elderly long-term care residents and their potential proxies. Arch Intern Med 1989;149: 1367–1372.

11. Olick RS, Kimura R, Keilstein JT, Hayashi H, Riedl M, Siegler M. Advance care planning and the ALS patient: a cross-cultural perspective on Ads. Ann Rev Law Ethics, Band 4, 1996:531–557.

12. Brooks BR. Clinical epidemiology of amyotrophic lateral sclerosis. Neurol Clin 1996;14: 399–420.

13. Borasio GD, Voltz R. Palliative care in amyotrophic lateral sclerosis. J Neurol 1997;244 (Suppl 4):S11–S17.

14. Hayashi H, Shuuchi K, Kawada A. Amyotrophic lateral sclerosis patients living beyond respiratory failure. J Neurol Sci 1991;105:73–78.

15. Benditt JO, Smith TS, Tonelli M. Empowering the individual with ALS at the end-of-life: disease-specific advance care planning. Muscle & Nerve 2001;24: 1706–1709.

16. Voltz R, Akabayashi A, Reese C, et al. End-of-life decisions and advance directives in palliative care: a cross-cultural survey of patients and health-care professionals. J Pain Sympt Manage 1997;16(3):153–162.

17. Virmani J, Lawrence J, Schneiderman J, Kaplan RM. Relationship of advance directives to physician–patient communication. Arch Intern Med 1994;154: 909–913.

18. Martin DK, Emanuel LL, Singer PA. Planning for the end of life. Lancet 2000;356:1672–1676.

19. Sass HM, Veatch RM, Kimura R, eds. Advance Directives and Surrogate Decision Making in Health Care: United States, Germany, and Japan. Johns Hopkins University Press, Baltimore & London, 1998.

20. Emanuel LL. Appropriate use and inappropriate use of ddvance directives. J Clin Ethics 1994;5(4):357–359.

21. Kielstein R, Sass HM. Using stories to assess values and establish medical directives. Kennedy Instit Ethics J 1993;3:303–325.

APPENDIX: BRIEF CHECKLIST FOR PLANNING END-OF-LIFE DECISIONS

A. What should be discussed?

1. *Medical therapy decisions such as*
   - Disease-modifying treatments—cardiopulmonary resuscitation
   - Use of respirator—parenteral artificial nutrition
   - Enteral nutrition and hydration (e.g. through PEG)—anticoagulation
   - Antibiotics—specific emergency treatments (e.g. for pain, dyspnea, bleeding, epileptic seizure, restlessness, delirium)

2. *What is the preferred locus of care?*
   - Stay at home?
   - Admission to hospital? Which hospital? Hospice care?

3. *Who is the patient's source of support?*
   For example, family, friends, emergency phone numbers, physicians, nurses, social worker, other professionals, technical help, hospice group, proxy

3. *How is the patient coping?*
   - Is professional help in communication with relatives wanted?
   - Is spiritual help wanted?

5. *Are there personal organisatory decisions where the patient may need help?*
   For example, financial, writing a will, funeral details.

6. *Does the patient want to give an AD?*
   - Does the patient express preferences for future decisions on any issues mentioned above?
   - Does the patient want information on how to set up a written AD?

7. *Does the patient want to appoint a proxy?*
   - Is there an informal or culturally implicit appointment?
   - Does the patient want information on a formal appointment?

B. How to proceed if the patient wishes to express preferences in advance?

Any expression of preferences should be the result of an intensive and long-standing communication between patients, health-care professionals, and relatives.

1. *ADs*
   - Note orally expressed ADs in the medical record
   - Help in writing an AD:
     a) Should know patient well
     b) Patient must be fully informed about diagnosis, prognosis, options
     c) Patient must be mentally clear (statement of treating physician included)
     d) Should be as specific and individualized as possible

e) Regular (for example, monthly) revision
f) Avoid influencing the wording, but give all necessary information
g) Patient must know that AD may be changed any time
h) Witness should be present when signing

2. *Appointing a proxy*
   - Has the patient informally or (culturally) implicitly named a proxy already?
   - Help in formally appointing a proxy according to national laws
     a) Proxy must be trustworthy, fully informed, and available
     b) Try to avoid obvious conflicts of interests
     c) Regular revision and discussions
     d) Witness present when signing

Chapter 35

Refusal and Withdrawal of Treatment

James L. Bernat

INTRODUCTION
ETHICAL BASIS OF TREATMENT REFUSAL
BARRIERS TO TREATMENT REFUSAL
RESPONDING TO TREATMENT
  REFUSALS
EMPIRICAL STUDIES

REFUSAL OF HYDRATION AND
  NUTRITION
REFUSAL OF LIFE-SUSTAINING THERAPY
  IN NEUROLOGICAL PRACTICE
PRACTICAL AND LEGAL ISSUES

Refusal of medical treatment is an implicit part of the doctrine of informed consent. Competent patients and the authorized surrogate decision makers of incompetent patient have the right to refuse all forms of treatment, including life-sustaining treatment without which they will die, and also including artificial hydration and nutrition. Physicians must respect valid treatment refusals by patients and surrogates. Physicians should attempt to enhance patients' communicative and psychological capacities to maximally permit them to participate in their health decisions. Physicians who feel that patients or surrogates have made a bad decision to stop treatment can try to negotiate a time-limited trial of treatment. Patients undergoing withdrawal of life-sustaining treatment require excellent palliative care to prevent them from suffering. Studies have shown, however, that many dying patients are not receiving proper palliative care. Hospital ethics committees can help assure protection of the patient's interest in situations in which treatment conflicts arise between patients and their surrogates, and their physicians.

CASE HISTORY

A 56-year-old man with amyotrophic lateral sclerosis (ALS) had been maintained on positive-pressure home ventilation for the past three years. He had become progressively paralyzed and now was able to move only his eyes and eyelids. He had an eye-movement-directed computer communication system that permitted him to make his feelings and wishes known. His wife and two adult children were supportive of his continued home care but the expenses had become a source of difficulty. Over the course of several weeks, he had decided that the time had come to stop the ventilator. He wrote a letter to his neurologist explaining that he wished to discontinue the ventilator. His wife was ambivalent about this decision but tried to be supportive. She wondered if he was depressed and needed antidepressant treatment. He denied being depressed though did admit to being 'tired' of the ventilator and especially of his utter dependency. His neurologist engaged in a series of discussions with him and his wife over the next several weeks pursuing the reasons for his decision, his goals, his sources of pleasure and pain, and whether he might be depressed. The neurologist concluded that his decision to refuse the ventilator was rational and arranged to admit him to the hospital for ventilator withdrawal. This was accomplished with benzodiazepine sedation and intravenous morphine. He died with his family at his bedside.

INTRODUCTION

Although the provision of palliative care is not restricted categorically to dying patients, the management of the terminally ill patient comprises the most common setting for neurologists to practice palliative care. Many terminally ill patients receiving palliative care decide to refuse further life-sustaining therapy (LST) when their goals of treatment change from curative to palliative, and therefore they become concerned more about the quality of their remaining life than its quantity. Thus, the topic of withdrawal or refusal of LST is highly relevant to the subject of palliative care in neurological practice.[1]

The past three decades have witnessed a transformation in how we conceptualize the act of withholding and withdrawing LST: from being physician-centered to being patient-centered.[2] In the 1970s and 1980s, the topic was conceptualized as the physician-centered withholding or withdrawal of LST. Accordingly, physicians, ethicists, and judges strove to devise guidelines that permitted physicians to discontinue patients' LST in certain well-defined clinical circumstances. Physicians who withdrew LST from terminally ill patients were said to have committed 'passive euthanasia' when patients died as the result of their fatal underlying illnesses, because the deaths were linked causally to the withdrawal of LST.

The contemporary conceptualization is that of informed refusal of LST. Patients have the right to accept or refuse therapies offered by physicians, as described in Chapter 37 in the discussion of informed consent. When LST has been refused by a competent patient or by the legally authorized surrogate decision maker of an incompetent patient, the physician must discontinue it, except in rare circumstances discussed later. The current situation is better understood as the patient-centered refusal of LST because the patient (or surrogate), not the physician, is the locus of decision making. And when terminally ill patients refuse LST and die as a result of their underlying illnesses, it is misleading to label the physician's act to stop LST as 'passive euthanasia'. Rather, the patient's death is the outcome of the natural history of their terminal disease in the absence of LST.[3]

ETHICAL BASIS OF TREATMENT REFUSAL

The ethical basis of the right of patients to refuse LST is the basic human right of self-determination. As discussed in Chapter 37, this right originates in our consensual respect for persons and human dignity, and underlies the importance of securing patients' informed consent for treatment. Informed refusal is an intrinsic part of informed consent.

Valid refusal has the same three elements as valid consent. The patient must be given information about diagnosis, prognosis, and treatment options that a reasonable person would need to know to permit a rational decision. The patient must have the capacity to make health-care decisions ('competence') or an authorized surrogate decision maker should be approached for consent or refusal. And no physician, family member, or agency should coerce the patient, thereby assuring that the patient's consent or refusal is given freely. Patients' refusals lacking any of these elements are not valid.[4]

Informed consent and refusal are operationalized in clinical practice through the doctrine of shared decision making. The patient and physician comprise a decision-making dyad in which the physician provides essential medical information about diagnosis, prognosis, treatment options, and their expected outcomes, and then offers a treatment recommendation. The patient processes this information in the context of his/her unique personal system of values and preferences. Together they reach a mutually agreeable treatment decision that the physician then implements and the patient follows.[5]

Many dying patients lose the capacity to make treatment decisions because of the development of delirium, dementia, encephalopathy, stupor, or coma. Their right to accept or refuse therapy is not extinguished by incapacity but is transferred to a surrogate decision maker to consent or refuse on their behalf. Physicians should conduct the same consent discussion with the surrogate decision maker of an incompetent patient as with a competent patient, and they should respond to the surrogate's consent or refusal in much the same way as to that of the competent patient.

BARRIERS TO TREATMENT REFUSAL

Several barriers may impede patients from exercising their right to refuse LST, primarily because of doubt in the physician's mind that the patient's refusal is valid. Depression is one such barrier. Depression is common in terminal illness[6] and often is a factor in a terminally ill patient's decision to stop LST.[7] To the extent that concurrent depression may be altering the rationality of a dying patient's refusal of LST, physicians should consider addressing and treating a patient's concurrent depression if it is sufficiently severe.[8] Often, however, the depression may be irreversible. Some patients may hold irrational beliefs and fears regarding LST that can be dispelled by timely and compassionate counseling.[9]

Physical barriers such as paralysis and inability to communicate may complicate the logistics of decision making by dying neurological patients. For example, patients with ALS often have great difficulty communicating because of anarthria, aphonia, and ventilator dependency. Neurologists' understanding of patients' exact wishes and their degree of confidence that patients understand the medical facts they need to make health-care decisions may be improved greatly by asking occupational therapists to devise computerized communication systems. Without clear and accurate communication, physicians may lack confidence that their patients' consent or refusal is valid.[10]

Physician barriers also are important. A recent survey of neurologist members of the American Academy of Neurology showed widespread misunderstanding of the ethical, legal, and medical guidelines surrounding decisions to withhold or withdraw LST from neurological patients.[11] For example, 40% of surveyed neurologists wrongly believed that they needed to consult legal counsel before withdrawing a patient's LST and 38% incorrectly were concerned that they may be charged with a criminal offense for withdrawing LST.[11] These knowledge deficits can be overcome by improved education in end-of-life care, such as that offered in the American Medical Association's program Educating Physicians in End-of-Life Care (EPEC).[12]

Additionally, surveys of physicians have shown that they have biases in how and when they decide to respect treatment refusals by patients or surrogates. One survey found that physicians preferred to withdraw therapies:[13]

1. From organs that failed from natural, as opposed to from iatrogenic causes.
2. That had been started recently, as opposed to those that had been of long duration.
3. That would result in the patient's immediate death rather than in delayed death.
4. That would result in delayed death when in the presence of the physician's diagnostic uncertainty.

In a later study, the same investigators found that physicians were more likely to withhold or withdraw therapies related to their specialty than to other specialties.[14] The attitudes underlying these biases may be harder to change.

There are cultural differences in the practice of withholding and withdrawing LST. Two international conferences of 15 participating countries convened in Appleton, Wisconsin, United States in 1987 and 1991 attempted to formulate agreement on universal principles for withholding and withdrawing LST.[15] With only a few dissenters on relatively minor issues, the conferences were a success in formulating international guidelines. Nevertheless, some cultural differences persist, particularly in the assertions that all patients have a categorical right to refuse LST and that physicians have the duty to respect a patient's refusal of LST. The issues in medical decision making about consent and terminal care in cross-cultural setting have been reviewed.[16]

RESPONDING TO TREATMENT REFUSALS

Valid treatment refusals should be respected by physicians and implemented. Valid refusals are those made by competent patients who understand and can process the information provided by their physicians about diagnosis, prognosis, and treatment options, and who have not been coerced into a particular decision by physicians, families, or agencies. Such patients have reached a rational decision that truly represents their sincerely held personal wishes and are decisions not contaminated by psychotic depression or irrational thinking.

The troubling question arises frequently in practice of how and when physicians are justified in overruling a patient's refusal of LST. Certainly, there are very few cases in which it is ever justified for a physician to continue to treat an incipiently dying patient who has validly and explicitly refused LST. But when patients are acutely ill (but not necessarily terminally ill) and refuse LST for a potentially reversible condition early in the course of the illness, it is reasonable for physicians to proceed with caution rather than to summarily withdraw LST once a patient has refused it. I have cared for patients with Guillain–Barré syndrome or relatively minor cerebrovascular events in which the patients or their surrogates have refused LST early in the course of illness. I explained that the patients' neurological function almost certainly would improve and that it was premature to stop treatment now. But these explanations have not always been sufficient to convince them.

In cases in which the prognosis is good with treatment but the patient refuses LST, I try to negotiate a time-limited trial of therapy. I make a contract with the patient or surrogate to permit LST to continue for a specified time, pending the expected improvement. I agree that if the improvement does not occur during that time, I will honor their refusal of LST thereafter. Thus, I have had the experience both of continuing and discontinuing LST after the time-limited treatment trial depending on the patient's progress. But because of the obviously poor prognosis in dying, terminally ill patients, treatment refusals are almost always respected without physicians suggesting time-limited treatment trials.

Patients for whom LST has been withheld or withdrawn deserve ideal palliative care as discussed throughout this book. When limiting or withdrawing LST, in addition to ordering specific palliative care measures, it is essential for physicians to write specific orders clarifying those treatments that will be given and those that will not. Merely ordering 'comfort measures only' is not optimal medical practice because it unfairly thrusts upon the nursing staff the responsibility to determine which treatments count as comfort care. Our hospital palliative care service uses an overprinted, standard order page for palliative care orders that anticipates all classes of treatment and forces the responsible physician to consider in advance which therapies are appropriate in each case. Idealized examples of such order pages have been published.[17]

EMPIRICAL STUDIES

The act of patient or surrogate refusal of LST is exceedingly common. In the United States, for example, 40%–65% of intensive care unit (ICU) deaths result from withholding or withdrawing LST[18] and 74% of all ICU patients who died had at least some treatments withheld and withdrawn.[19]

Several reports have been published detailing how physicians withhold and withdraw LST from ICU patients.[20–22] But relatively few reports have focused on neurological patients. In one recent report from a neurological ICU, when brain-dead patients were excluded, 43% of dying patients were terminally extubated and their mean survival time following extubation was 7.5 hours. Morphine or fentanyl was administered to treat dyspnea in two-thirds. In a subsequent survey of surrogate decision makers, 88% stated that they were satisfied with the process of withholding and withdrawing LST.[23]

Several studies have reported the type of palliative care dying patients received during extubation. There is evidence that an awake patient is kept more comfortable if physicians rapidly dial down the ventilator settings rather than to summarily extubate the patient or to conduct prolonged terminal weaning.[24] Studies of withdrawal of LST from ICUs show that awake patients are prescribed adequate dosages of benzodiazepine drugs and opiates, and that the drugs do not appear to hasten the moment of death.[25]

Studies of termination of LST in critically ill and terminally ill children reveal results similar to those in adults. In one survey of 16 pediatric ICUs, 38% of all deaths were attributed to withdrawal of LST.[26] Two other single-institution studies disclosed that 32% and 58% of children's deaths were from withdrawing LST.[27,28] LST decisions for children, as discussed in Chapter 37, should, when possible, attempt to secure the assent of the developmentally appropriate child and should always be taken with the permission of the parents or other surrogate decision makers.

By far the largest and most comprehensive study of how physicians withdraw LST and provide palliative care to critically ill patients was the Study to Understand Prognoses and Preferences for Outcomes and Risks of Treatment (SUPPORT). SUPPORT was a four-year, two-phase study of over 9000 hospitalized, seriously ill patients in the United States, whose goals were to measure the quality of end-of-life decision making, the frequency of unnecessarily painful or prolonged deaths in the hospital, and to attempt to improve the quality of terminal care.[29]

Phase I of SUPPORT showed that there were serious shortcomings in the care of critically ill and dying patients, such as, that many patients did not receive 'Do not resuscitate' (DNR) orders until two days before death; that less than half of physicians knew their patients' cardiopulmonary resuscitation (CPR) wishes; and that half of conscious patients suffered pain before they died. Phase II of SUPPORT showed that an intervention by trained nurses to communicate to physicians the patient's up-to-date prognosis failed to influence the physicians in their treatment behaviors.[29] The SUPPORT investigators have further analyzed their data and published a number of other important articles studying various aspects of terminal care.[30–32]

The findings of SUPPORT revealed serious deficiencies in palliative and terminal care for critically ill patients in the five American hospitals studied. But the limitations of SUPPORT also must be appreciated. SUPPORT was a study not of terminally ill patients but of critically ill patients, some of whom also were terminally ill. Three-quarters of the study patients were discharged following their hospitalization and two-thirds remained alive six months later. Moreover, the determination that a critically ill patient is also terminally ill is one that can be made much more accurately in retrospect than in prospect. The typical SUPPORT patient had a critical, but not necessarily a terminal, illness that carried a 50% prognosis for living six months.[29]

The problem with the SUPPORT study was that many of the patients (40%–60%) carried an intermediate prognosis for survival. Should

such patients get purely palliative care or aggressive care? Many of these patients and their surrogates chose aggressive therapy in the hope that they would recover, and many of them did recover. Thus, there may be an explanation why many DNR orders were not written until two days before death in many cases. The hope of recovery was abandoned when it became clear that they would no longer recover.[33] Ideally, palliative care should be given along with curative care in such patients, but it was not in many SUPPORT patients.

Physicians caring for critically ill and terminally ill patients need to provide an accurate diagnosis and prognosis to permit the patient or surrogate to make the best decision of whether to continue or discontinue LST. Interestingly, in SUPPORT, the ready availability of sophisticated prognostic models had little effect on decision making. In their prognostic determinations, physicians should cite outcome studies that have been carefully performed and analyzed so the data they contain are valid. In that spirit, physicians choosing outcome studies to determine prognoses should be wary of citing studies guilty of the fallacy of the self-fulfilling prophecy.

The fallacy of the self-fulfilling prophecy refers to a study of an illness outcome that fails to control for the variable in question and therefore predicted an unnecessarily poor prognosis that falsely represented the natural history of the illness. For example, in some studies of the outcome of coma following cardiopulmonary arrest[34] and of coma after massive intracranial hemorrhage,[35] published reports include many patients whose physicians ordered cessation of LST because of their presumed poor prognoses.

But the inclusion of these cases in studies purporting to represent the natural history of the disease in question commits the fallacy of the self-fulfilling prophecy. Rather than representing the natural history of the disease in question, these studies represent the experiential history of a group of patients receiving varying levels of support. Indeed, in one study, several patients with presumably poor prognoses after massive intracranial hemorrhage, that were treated aggressively, did well.[35] The cessation of LST in the reported patients may have been ethically and medically correct but constituted poor science and contaminated the sample such that it no longer represented the natural history of treated disease.

REFUSAL OF HYDRATION AND NUTRITION

That patients are allowed to refuse LST has been accepted widely throughout the Western world. One remaining controversy concerns whether patients or surrogates can refuse artificial or oral hydration and nutrition. David Oliver considers this subject in detail in Chapter 32. The ethical issue is whether artificial or oral hydration and nutrition can be considered medical therapies that patients may refuse or whether they occupy a class of essential bodily requirements for life that physicians are obligated to continue irrespective of refusal by patient or surrogate.

Those advocating that hydration and nutrition must be continued at all times argue that, because food and fluids are essential to life in the same way oxygen is essential, it would be unethical under any circumstances for physicians to withhold or withdraw them. They point out that whereas some patients may survive without digitalis or a ventilator, no one can live without hydration or nutrition. Therefore, a physician's act to withhold or withdraw hydration and nutrition is unethical because that act would be tantamount to killing the patient.[36,37]

Those advocating that hydration and nutrition may be withdrawn or withheld cite the fact that artificial hydration and nutrition should be included in the class of therapies that patients or their surrogates are permitted to withhold or withdraw on the grounds of valid refusal. Artificial hydration and nutrition can be viewed as a medical therapy because they require the order of a physician, the action of a nurse, and medical technology to provide.[38,39] These characteristics are not applicable, however, to oral hydration and nutrition.

The principal distinction between the two viewpoints is the difference between a physician-centered perspective and a patient-centered perspective.[2] The advocates of permitting withholding and withdrawal of hydration and nutrition are patient-centered: they are concerned more with granting patients and surrogates the right to refuse

therapies than about the impact of this right on physicians who implement the refusal. Those who believe that withholding or withdrawing hydration and nutrition is morally wrong are physician-centered: they are concerned more with the complicity of physicians in the act and the moral responsibility of physicians not to participate in any act that could be construed as suicide or killing.

Patients receiving palliative care may refuse oral hydration and nutrition as well as artificial hydration and nutrition. My colleagues and I have termed this act 'patient refusal of hydration and nutrition'.[40] There now is a wealth of data on the experiences of dying patients who voluntarily stopped eating and drinking and refused supplemental enteral or parenteral hydration or nutrition. Dying patients who receive proper palliative care do not suffer when they die from the lack of hydration and nutrition.[41] Physicians have a duty to provide good palliative care during the days to weeks until they die.

REFUSAL OF LIFE-SUSTAINING THERAPY IN NEUROLOGICAL PRACTICE

To illustrate the major ethical and procedural principles discussed above, it is useful to review examples of refusal of LST in several commonly encountered neurological syndromes in which palliative care is provided to dying patients. I will briefly consider patients with: profound paralysis but retained cognition; advanced dementia; and the persistent vegetative state. These topics are discussed in further detail in Chapters 6, 8, and 12–14.

The patient with end-stage ALS exemplifies the dying patient with profound paralysis but intact cognition. Because dying ALS patients usually retain the capacity to make health-care decisions, the ethical issues surrounding their consent and refusal for LST are more straightforward than in incompetent patients. The patient should be thoroughly educated about the disease prognosis and treatment options, particularly the options to support respiration. The patient should be permitted to decide at each stage which treatment options he/she does and does not wish to have performed.[42]

Many patients dying from ALS, especially elderly patients, will permit gastrostomy tube placement and non-invasive ventilation with bilevel positive airway pressure (BiPAP) but will not permit endotracheal intubation and invasive positive-pressure ventilation. Such patients should be reassured that whichever choice they make about ventilation, the physician will support their decision. They should not be dissuaded from considering positive-pressure invasive ventilation if they wish to try it. Portable ventilators are available for home use but insurance and payment issues remain a serious concern.[43]

Dying ALS patients should be provided with proper palliative care when they decide to withhold or withdraw positive-pressure ventilation and they develop respiratory failure requiring invasive ventilation. Palliative care during dying can take place in a hospital, nursing home, or at home, depending upon the patient's wishes and logistic issues. Patients should be given adequate dosages of benzodiazepines for sedation and opiates for combating dyspnea. The comprehensive approach to palliative care in the dying ALS patient is discussed in Chapter 8.

Patients dying of advanced dementia require surrogate decision makers to consent or refuse for LST on their behalf. In the United States and many other countries, there is now a consensus that palliative care is the appropriate level of treatment for most patients with advanced Alzheimer's disease and other dementias.[44] Family members and surrogates should attempt to follow the demented patient's earlier stated wishes regarding the desirability of treatment for infections, other intercurrent illnesses, and LST. In the absence of knowing the patient's wishes, surrogates should attempt to reproduce the patient's treatment choice through a standard of substituted judgment, as discussed in Chapter 37. In the absence of knowing the patient's values and preferences, surrogates should determine what course of treatment is in the patient's best interest by balancing the burdens of treatment against its benefits.

There is strong evidence that feeding tubes do not improve the quality of life for patients with advanced dementia.[45] The American Academy of Neurology has opined that physicians have no duty to insert feeding tubes into patients with advanced dementia unless this treatment is desired by the surrogate decision maker or by advance directive from the patient.[46] There is always a duty to provide proper palliative care.

Decision making for the patient in a persistent vegetative state (PVS) is similar to that in dementia in that surrogates must consent or refuse LST on behalf of the patient. Guidelines from the American Medical Association[47] and the American Academy of Neurology[48] permit the withholding or withdrawal of LST from the PVS patient if that action follows the surrogate's valid refusal of treatment using either a substituted judgment or best interest decision-making standard. Palliative care should be provided on the chance that the patient has some capacity for suffering.

PRACTICAL AND LEGAL ISSUES

Surrogate decision making for refusal of LST creates several problems in practice, stemming primarily from the adequacy of the surrogate to make the best decision for the patient. Experienced physicians have encountered cases in which they believed that the surrogate had reached a decision that the patient would not have reached.[49] Some surrogates make decisions that satisfy their own needs rather than representing the patient's view. Conflicts of interest in family surrogate decision making are relatively common. The family member may have non-altruistic motives, such as the desire for an inheritance, that may represent an important reason for them to refuse a patient's LST.

The presence of a conflicted surrogate poses difficulty for the physician because the authority of surrogate decision making is founded on the premise that the surrogate makes the decision that is best for the patient. Some degree of conflict is inevitable and is a motivating factor even in the most loving family. Only in the presence of an overt, obvious conflict that renders the surrogate unsuitable, should the physician consider trying to replace a surrogate with a more objective person.

In the absence of a legally authorized surrogate, physicians often permit the primary family to function jointly as a surrogate. This informal appointment is reasonable because the family members can be presumed to know most about a patient's wishes and values, and care most for the patient. But sometimes, family members are divided in their opinion about what decision the patient would have made or what course of action represents the patient's best interest. Disagreement among joint surrogates creates a knotty problem: to whom should the physician listen?

I have tried to solve the problem of family disagreement by holding a joint family meeting during which we discuss the patient's diagnosis, prognosis, treatment options, and previous statements about wishes for treatment.[50] Each family member is allowed time to explain his/her viewpoint about what action is best for the patient. Usually this meeting produces consensus. But intractable disagreement sometimes persists, usually because of a pre-existing family feud in which certain members always disagree.[51] Consultation from the hospital ethics committee may be helpful to resolve such disputes. But if the dispute persists, the physician should contact the court to appoint a single, legally authorized surrogate.

The laws governing surrogate decision making vary among jurisdictions, so physicians should be knowledgeable about the relevant laws where they practice. In the United States, for example, all jurisdictions have laws permitting the appointment of durable powers of attorney for health care (also called health-care agent or health-care proxy). This agent is appointed by the patient while competent to decide on the patient's behalf once the patient becomes incompetent. The decision of this legally authorized surrogate trumps other family member conflicting opinions. Many states also have health-care proxy laws that, in the absence of a prior durable power of attorney appointment, automatically trigger the appointment of a legally authorized surrogate in the presence of patient incompetence.[52]

Hospital ethics committees can be helpful to review certain cases of refusal or withdrawal of LST. In the straightforward case of a terminally ill patient validly refusing LST, there is little to be gained by requesting such a review. But in cases in which the surrogate appears to making an incorrect decision, where there is no legally authorized surrogate, and the family members disagree, or where an uncertain prognosis renders the patient or surrogate decision questionable, a consultation

by the ethics committee may help clarify the process and protect the patient. Hospital ethics committees should not be permitted to make clinical decisions, only to facilitate correct decision making among the patient, surrogate, and physician.[53]

REFERENCES

1. Bernat JL. Ethical and legal issues in palliative care. Neurol Clin 2001;19:969–987.
2. Bernat JL. Plan ahead: how neurologists can enhance patient-centered medicine. Neurology 2001;56:144–145.
3. Bernat JL. Ethical Issues in Neurology, 2nd Ed. Butterworth–Heinemann, Boston, 2002:157–187.
4. Gert B, Culver CM, Clouser KD. Bioethics: A Return to Fundamentals. Oxford University Press, New York, 1997:131–250.
5. Brock DW. The ideal of shared decision making between physicians and patients. Kennedy Inst Ethics J 1991;1:28–47.
6. Chochinov HM, Wilson KG, Enns M, Lander S. The prevalence of depression in the terminally ill: effects of diagnostic criteria and symptom threshold judgments. Am J Psychiatry 1994;151:537–540.
7. Breitbart W, Rosenfeld B, Pessin H, et al. Depression, hopelessness, and desire for hastened death in terminally ill patients with cancer. JAMA 2000;284:2907–2911.
8. Block SD. Assessing and managing depression in the terminally ill patient. Ann Intern Med 2000;132:209–218.
9. Brock DW, Wartman SA. When competent patients make irrational choices. N Engl J Med 1990;322:1595–1599.
10. American Academy of Neurology Ethics and Humanities Subcommittee. Position statement: certain aspects of the care and management of profoundly and irreversibly paralyzed patients with retained consciousness and cognition. Neurology 1993;43:222–223.
11. Carver AC, Vickrey BG, Bernat JL, Keran C, Ringel SP, Foley KM. End of life care: a survey of U.S. neurologists' attitudes, behavior, and knowledge. Neurology 1999;53:284–293.
12. http://www.ama-assn.org/ethic/epec/
13. Christakis NA, Asch DA. Biases in how physicians choose to withdraw life support. Lancet 1993;342:642–646.
14. Christakis NA, Asch DA. Medical specialists prefer to withdraw familiar technologies when discontinuing life support. J Gen Intern Med 1995;10:491–494.
15. Stanley JM, ed. The Appleton International Conference: developing guidelines for decisions to forgo life-prolonging medical treatment. J Med Ethics 1992;18(Suppl):1–22.
16. Jecker NS, Carrese JA, Pearlman RA. Caring for patients in cross-cultural settings. Hastings Cent Rep 1995;25(1):6–14.
17. O'Toole EE, Youngner SJ, Juknialis BW, Daly B, Bartlett ET, Landefeld CS. Evaluation of a treatment

limitation policy with a specific treatment-limiting order page. Arch Intern Med 1994;154:425–432.

18. Raffin TA. Withdrawing life support: how is the decision made? JAMA 1995;273:738–739.

19. Prendergast TJ, Claessens MT, Luce JM. A national survey of end-of-life care for critically ill patients. Am J Respir Crit Care Med 1998;158:1163–1167.

20. Smedira NG, Evans BH, Grais LS, et al. Withholding and withdrawal of life support from the critically ill. N Engl J Med 1990;322:309–315.

21. Faber–Langendoen K, Bartels DM. Process of forgoing life-sustaining treatment in a university hospital: an empirical study. Crit Care Med 1992;20:570–577.

22. Prendergast TJ, Luce JM. Increasing incidence of withholding and withdrawal of life support from the critically ill. Am J Respir Crit Care Med 1997;155: 15–20.

23. Mayer SA, Kossoff SB. Withdrawal of life support in the neurological intensive care unit. Neurology 1999;52:1602–1609.

24. Gilligan T, Raffin TA. Withdrawing life support: extubation and prolonged terminal weans are inappropriate. Crit Care Med 1996;24:352–353.

25. Wilson WC, Smedira NG, Fink C, McDowell JA, Luce JM. Ordering and administration of sedatives and analgesics during the withholding and withdrawal of life support from critically ill patients. JAMA 1992;267:949–953.

26. Levetown M, Pollock MM, Cuerdon TT, Ruttimann UE, Glover JJ. Limitations and withdrawls of medical intervention in pediatric critical care. JAMA 1994;272:1271–1275.

27. Mink RB, Pollack MM. Resuscitation and withdrawal of therapy in pediatric intensive care. Pediatrics 1992;89:961–963.

28. Vernon DD, Dean JM, Timmons OD, et al. Modes of death in the pediatric intensive care unit: withdrawal and limitation of supportive care. Crit Care Med 1993;21:1798–1802.

29. SUPPORT. Principal investigators: a controlled trial to improve care for seriously ill hospitalized patients. The Study to Understand Prognoses and Preferences for Outcomes and Risks of Treatment (SUPPORT). JAMA 1995;274:1591–1598.

30. Haykim RB, Teno J, Harrell FE Jr, et al. Factors associated with do-not-resuscitate orders: patients' preferences, prognoses, and physicians' judgments. Ann Intern Med 1996;125:284–293.

31. Hamel MB, David RB, Teno J, et al. Older age, aggressiveness of care, and survival for seriously ill, hospitalized adults. Ann Intern Med 1999;131: 721–728.

32. Teno J, Lynn J, Phillips RS, et al. Do formal advance directives affect resuscitation decisions and the use of resources for seriously ill patients? J Clin Ethics 1994;5:23–30.

33. Prendergast TJ. The SUPPORT project and improving care for seriously ill patients (letter). JAMA 1996;275:1227.

34. Shewmon DA, DiGiorgio CM. Early prognosis in anoxic coma: reliability and rationale. Neurol Clin 1989;7:823–843.

35. Becker KJ, Baxter AB, Cohen WA, et al. Withdrawal of support in intracerebral hemorrhage may lead to self-fulfilling prophecies. Neurology 2001;56: 766–772.

36. Siegler M, Weisbard AJ. Against the emerging stream. Should fluids and nutritional support be discontinued? Arch Intern Med 1985;145:129–131.

37. Rosner F. Why nutrition and hydration should not be withheld from patients. Chest 1993;104:1892–1896.

38. Lynn J, Childress JF. Must patients always be given food and water? Hastings Cent Rep 1983;13(5): 17–21.

39. Steinbrook R, Lo B. Artificial feeding—solid ground, not a slippery slope. N Engl J Med 1988;318: 286–290.

40. Bernat JL, Gert B, Mogielnicki RP. Patient refusal of hydration and nutrition: an alternative to physician-assisted suicide or voluntary active euthanasia. Arch Intern Med 1993;153:2723–2728.

41. Schmitz P. The process of dying, with and without feeding and fluids by tube. Law Med Health Care 1991;19:23–26.

42. Miller RG, Rosenberg JA, Gelinas DF, et al. Practice parameter: the care of the patient with amyotrophic lateral sclerosis (an evidence-based review). Report of the Quality Standards Subcommittee of the American Academy of Neurology. Neurology 1999;52: 1311–1323.

43. Moss AH, Casey P, Stocking CB, Roos RP, Brooks BR, Siegler M. Home ventilation for amyotrophic lateral sclerosis patients: outcomes, costs, and patient, family, and physician attitudes. Neurology 1993; 43:438–443.

44. Finucane TE, Christmas C, Travis K. Tube feeding in patients with advanced dementia: a review of the evidence. JAMA 1999;282:1365–1370.

45. Gillick MR. Rethinking the role of tube feeding in patients with advanced dementia. N Engl J Med 2000;342:206–210.

46. American Academy of Neurology Ethics and Humanities Subcommittee. Ethical issues in the management of the demented patient. Neurology 1996;46:1180–1183.

47. American Medical Association Council on Scientific Affairs and Council on Ethical and Judicial Affairs. Persistent vegetative state and the decision to withdraw or withhold life support. JAMA 1990;263: 426–430.

48. American Academy of Neurology. Position of the American Academy of Neurology on certain aspects of the care and management of the persistent vegetative state patient. Neurology 1989;39:125–126.

49. Terry PB, Vettese M, Song J, et al. End-of-life decision making: when patients and surrogates disagree. J Clin Ethics 1999;10:286–293.

50. Miller DK, Coe RM, Hyers TM. Achieving consensus on withdrawing or withholding care for critically ill patients. J Gen Intern Med 1992;7:475–480.

51. Molloy DW, Clarnette RM, Braun EA, et al. Decision making in the incompetent elderly: 'the daughter from California syndrome'. J Am Geriatr Soc 1991;39: 396–399.

52. Schneiderman LJ, Arras JD. Counseling patients to counsel physicians on future care in the event of patient incompetence. Ann Intern Med 1985;102: 693–698.

53. Hafemeister TL, Hannaford PL. Resolving Disputes Over Life-Sustaining Treatment: A Health Care Provider's Guide. National Center for State Courts, Williamsburg, VA, 1996.

Chapter 36

Physician-assisted Suicide and Euthanasia

Alan Carver
Kathleen M. Foley

INTRODUCTION
STATUS OF THE LEGALIZATION OF
  PHYSICIAN-ASSISTED SUICIDE AND
  EUTHANASIA
The Netherlands
The United States
Australia
CURRENT ISSUES IN THE
  PHYSICIAN-ASSISTED SUICIDE/
  EUTHANASIA DEBATE

Physicians' Attitudes, Behaviors, and
  Knowledge
Reasons for a Patient's Request for a
  Hastened Death
DEVELOPMENT OF AN APPROACH TO
  THE DYING PATIENT
SUMMARY

Physician-assisted suicide (PAS) and euthanasia are now legal in the Netherlands and in Belgium; PAS is legal in one state, Oregon, in the United States. Although guidelines for PAS/euthanasia have been developed, they are not consistently followed. Health-care professionals' attitudes, behaviors, and knowledge influence their willingness to provide PAS/euthanasia. Such professionals lack adequate training in pain and symptom management, psychological assessment and treatment, communication skills, and ethical guidelines. Broad educational initiatives in palliative care are necessary to enable health-care professionals to care for patients who request assistance in death, providing them with competent, compassionate care.

CASE HISTORY

A 69-year-woman with widely metastatic cancer and a chest wall pain syndrome requests her physician to help her die. The patient reports poorly controlled pain, profound fatigue, and concern about being a burden to her husband. Her caregiver

husband is tearful at the time of interview as he pleads with his wife to let him care for her. A full medical and psychological evaluation following hospital admission lead to the diagnosis of epidural spinal cord compression as the cause of her chest wall radicular pain. The patient is also diagnosed as having a major depression based on her self reports, degree of hopelessness, and depressed mood. The patient is started on an aggressive pain management regimen with steroids and radiotherapy, opioids, antidepressants, and regular psychological support interventions. Her pain rapidly improves within two days and at two weeks her mood is significantly improved. When asked whether her physician should have helped her to die when she requested such help, the patient responds 'I guess not, I was depressed, but I didn't know it'.

Case Discussion

This case represents a typical example of an advanced cancer patient with pain secondary to an undiagnosed neurological complication of cancer and with depression associated with chronic pain and serious medical illness. In this patient, careful assessment and treatment of her neurological pain complaints and psychological symptoms facilitates the development of a treatment plan focused on reducing her pain and psychological symptoms and improving her quality of life. Health-care professionals must be able to appropriately diagnose and treat each symptom and develop a plan of care. Effective communication skills, coupled with knowledge and skill in diagnosing depression in a medically ill patient, require that neurologists learn these skills during residency and fellowship training. Using a stepwise approach of assessment coupled with appropriate radiologic studies and consultation with other disciplines, a combined approach of medical, neurological, psychologic care can improve the patient's symptoms.

Recent studies have demonstrated that depression in medically ill patients is responsive to antidepressant treatment and such therapy should be instituted. In this patient, pain and psychological distress were the major forces driving her request for PAS. Treatment of her pain and adequate management of her depression allowed her improved quality of life.

INTRODUCTION

This chapter will briefly review the current status of PAS and euthanasia in the Netherlands, the United States, and Australia, and discuss some specific issues in providing humane, compassionate care for dying patients and their families. For purposes of the discussion, PAS is defined as the provision of a lethal prescription by a physician to a patient for the specific purpose of ending the patient's life. Voluntary active euthanasia is defined as the administration of a lethal dose of medication to a patient for the purpose of ending the patient's life

At the current time, PAS and euthanasia are legal in two countries, the Netherlands and Belgium. PAS is legalized in one state, Oregon, in the United States. For a brief nine months, euthanasia was a legalized medical treatment in the Northern Territory of Australia. Both the Canadian and British Parliaments in the last several years have rejected challenges to their laws prohibiting PAS and euthanasia.

Several international organizations have weighed in with their opinions on the PAS/ euthanasia debate. In 1999, the Council of Europe issued recommendations on the care of the dying arguing strongly for the development of palliative care programs.[1] The Council cited the European Convention on Human Rights, Article II, which states that 'no one shall be deprived of his life intentionally'. The World Health Organization (WHO), in its monograph 'Cancer Pain Relief and Palliative Care' clearly distinguishes palliative care from PAS and euthanasia and recommends that 'member states not consider legislation allowing for physician-assisted suicide or euthanasia until they have assured for their citizens the availability of services for pain relief and palliative care'.[2] Both the WHO and the Council of Europe have conceptualized end-of-life care as a societal and public health issue.

In this debate, some have portrayed PAS and euthanasia as the compassionate response to balancing a reverence for life with the belief that death should come with dignity.[3] Others see PAS and euthanasia as a potentially cost-effective way to limit care to marginalized chronically ill patients.[4] The debate has provided the opportunity for a public discussion on the care of the seriously ill and dying. Such a discussion is critical if we are to understand patients' requests for PAS/ euthanasia and to identify existing barriers that impede seriously ill patients' access to appropriate, compassionate care. The experiences of the Netherlands, Oregon, and Australia have also informed the discussion and have demonstrated the difficulties of trying to regulate the unregulatable.[5]

STATUS OF THE LEGALIZATION OF PHYSICIAN-ASSISTED SUICIDE AND EUTHANASIA

The Netherlands

In 2001, the Dutch Parliament passed a statute that formally legalized euthanasia and PAS in the Netherlands, which had been legally sanctioned since the mid 1980s as a result of a series of case decisions. The legal sanction of PAS/euthanasia was the result of the 1984 Dutch Supreme Court decision reversing the conviction of a physician who had assisted in the death of an elderly woman, and the advocacy of the Dutch Medical Association, who defended the physician's actions. The Dutch Medical Association requested a change in the law and eventually developed a consensus on the practice of euthanasia with specific guidelines. This consensus was reached by the courts, the Dutch Medical Association, the Ministry of Justice, and the Dutch Health Council.

Two major studies, supported by the Dutch government, in 1990 and 1995, describe the Netherlands' experience with PAS and euthanasia.[6] These studies were done in part to respond to both domestic and international concerns about reports of abuse. The interpretation of these studies remains controversial, with some Dutch reviewers arguing that there is no serious problem[6] and others, including a series of international experts, identifying significant flaws in the processing, reporting, and interpretation of the data.[7,8]

The Dutch have clear guidelines for the practice of PAS and euthanasia. These include the following:

- That the request be voluntary, well-considered, and persistent
- That the patient experiences intolerable suffering that cannot be relieved
- That there is a formal consultation with a colleague
- That cases be reported

Reviews of PAS and euthanasia practices have demonstrated that these guidelines have not been consistently followed.[9] Underreporting has been a serious problem. As reported in 1990, only 18% of Dutch physicians reported their euthanasia cases to authorities as required. To encourage more reporting of cases, a simplified notification procedure was enacted. The procedure ensured that physicians would not be prosecuted if they followed the guidelines. This procedural change led to an increase in the cases reported to 41% by 1995. Yet, 59% of cases still go unreported. This number suggests a failure to fully accept and apply existing guidelines. The 1990 and 1995 surveys also showed that half of the physicians who do not report their cases wish to avoid judicial inquiry; 20% report fear of prosecution; 16% fail to fulfill requirements for accepted procedures; and 14% believe that euthanasia should be a private matter. 15%–20% of

Dutch doctors state that they will not report their cases under any circumstances.

Another guideline—that the patient have intolerable suffering that cannot be relieved—has also not been consistently followed. In 74% of cases, physicians report that such suffering was a reason for the patient's request for euthanasia, but in one quarter of the cases, fear of future suffering or fear of loss of dignity were more important. Neither of these reasons satisfy the criteria of unrelieved suffering. Formal consultations with a colleague are to take place, but this happens in only 80% of the reported cases.

What has been identified of greatest concern in the 1990 and 1995 studies is that in 0.8% of the deaths (more than 1000 cases in the Netherlands each year), physicians admitted that they actively caused death without the explicit consent of the patient. In the 1995 study, this figure is 0.7%. In both studies about one quarter of physicians stated that they had terminated the lives of patients without explicit requests from the patient to do so. It is on the basis of this data that the Dutch government has suggested that there be review panels established following a death of a patient from PAS or euthanasia to better assess the cases and scrutinize the application of the guidelines. Independent of the government reports, are a series of published case examples of how the guidelines have not been followed.[9]

Many have argued that the availability of PAS and euthanasia has in part suppressed the development and expansion of palliative care and hospice services throughout the country.[10] Dutch governmental agencies have begun to address palliative care needs and the Ministry of Health has committed funds for the development of palliative care in academic centers and palliative care units in regular nursing homes. The Netherlands, like many other countries, also has health-care professionals with little training and education in palliative care. Again, initiatives are under way to correct this situation.

The United States

In the United States there has been a century-long history of advocacy for PAS and euthanasia. At the heart of the U.S. debate has been the issue of patient autonomy and a patient's right to choose a dignified death. Americans have a right to refuse medical treatment and policies have been developed to support both withdrawal and withholding of care. A federal law, the Patient Self Determination Act, ensures a patient's right to advance directives defining how they wish to be cared for if they become incompetent and to designate a health-care proxy. Yet, the U.S. Supreme Court rejected the notion of a constitutional right to assisted suicide. In its decision it left the states free to legislate permission and prohibition of assisted suicide. It also suggested that Americans have a constitutional right to palliative care.[11]

At the present time, 38 states have laws explicitly prohibiting assisted suicide and recent attempts at PAS legislation have failed in three states—Michigan, Maine, and California. As well, courts in Florida, Colorado, and Nebraska have turned down cases requesting PAS. At the present time, Oregon is the only state that has legalized PAS. This occurred following passage of a referendum, a series of legal challenges, and then a second referendum, with the Oregon Death with Dignity Law eventually implemented in November 1997.[12] The law permits physicians to prescribe lethal medication to terminally ill patients. It differs from that of the Netherlands where euthanasia and PAS are both sanctioned. It also differs from the Netherlands in that intolerable suffering that cannot be relieved is not a basic requirement for assisted suicide in Oregon. Simply having a diagnosis of a terminal illness with a prognosis of less than six months to live is considered sufficient criteria. A patient's diagnosis and prognosis of death within six months must be confirmed by a consultant physician. Patients must submit their requests in writing 14 days following their initial oral request for assistance in death. Physicians must report the patient's death from a lethal prescription.

Although it has been strongly argued that Oregon could serve as 'a laboratory of the states', showing how assisted suicide would work, this has not occurred.[13] The Oregon Health Division (OHD) has been charged with monitoring the law and limits its reports to general epidemiologic data and information collected from physicians who have prescribed a lethal prescription. To date, the OHD has issued five reports.[14] Not all of the information that they collect is made public. The OHD has defended its limited data collection and censorship over this information as necessary to protect doctors' and patients' confidentiality. The law has no provision for an independent evaluator to study what data is available and this OHD process has prevented a fully open discussion. Again in contrast to the Netherlands, where the Dutch government has supported detailed studies, such information is currently not available from the Oregon experience.

Critics of the law have argued that the concern with physician rather than patient protection pervades the Oregon law.[15,16] Under the law, physicians are exempt from the ordinary standards of care, skill, and diligence required of Oregon physicians in other circumstances such as withdrawing life support. Instead, the physician is immunized from civil or criminal liability for actions taken in good faith in assisting a suicide, irrespective of community standards and other matters, even if the physician acts negligently. There is no enforcement mechanism in the Oregon law should physicians choose not to comply with guidelines set up by the OHD for reporting all cases in which medication for the purpose of assisted suicide has been prescribed. As noted in the Netherlands, under-reporting has been a significant problem, but the question of even ascertaining under-reporting has not been addressed by the OHD.

Of interest, the Oregon Medical Association has remained neutral in the debate about the legalization of PAS—again, in contrast to the Netherlands, where the Royal Dutch Medical Association advocated for both euthanasia and PSA. With five years of data, the OHD reports that the number of patients who have requested PSA is small. The number of prescriptions written since implementation have risen from 24 in 1998 to 58 in 2002. Sixteen patients died in 1998 and 38 in 2002. To date, 129 have died from PAS. There is a higher rate of use of PAS among patients with ALS and cancer as compared to other terminal illnesses. However, the evidence demonstrates that the numbers of requests are increasing and the numbers of prescriptions written over this period of time is also increasing.

A wide variety of non-official information sources have provided more detailed patient and physician perspectives that have suggested a more complex and controversial picture of the Oregon experience.[17] Oregon journalists have written a series of articles based on interviews with the families and physicians of patients who have been assisted in suicide.[18] Three physicians have published their personal narratives of experience with patients whom they have assisted in suicide, and have defended their role in the procedure.[19] Several surveys have captured the experience of physicians, patients, and families in end-of-life care, providing contrasting data to the OHD's reports.[20,21] Physicians who, for whatever reason, did not comply with patients' requests for suicide remain silent, with no forum in which to express their opinions.

Beyond the limits of this discussion, there are a series of assisted suicide cases that have raised serious questions about the current process. For example, although the Oregon law does require that a second physician evaluate the patient to confirm the diagnosis, prognosis, and voluntariness of choice, no provision is made for the independent selection of this consulting physician.[15] Although a psychiatric evaluation is the standard of care for suicidal patients, the Oregon law does not require it in cases of assisted suicide. Under the law, only if the physician believes that the patient might be suffering from a psychiatric or psychological disorder or find that depression is causing impaired judgment will the physician refer the patient to a licensed psychiatrist or psychologist for counseling. Depression per se is not considered sufficient reasoning for such a referral.

From a 1999 anonymous survey of Oregon physicians who received requests for PAS since the Oregon law went into effect, a picture of the inadequacy of palliative care consultations in Oregon has been noted.[20] In more than half of the 142 cases for which physicians supplied information, no palliative care intervention of any kind was provided. In less than half of the patients (68), at least one of a variety of measures referred to as substantive palliative care interventions is listed as having been suggested. In only 13% of the 142 cases was there a recommendation for a palliative care consultation. What is of particular note is that almost half of the patients for whom any interventions were made changed their minds about assisted suicide.

The OHD has also argued that economic factors do not influence the choice of PAS and that vulnerable patients are not unduly requesting PAS. Yet the data collected is insufficient to support these claims.

The legislation of PAS in Oregon has led to the development and expansion of palliative care services within the state. State studies have suggested increased referral to hospice and palliative care services, improved professional education, and heightened awareness of addressing patients' and families' complicated symptom management issues.[22]

Although several authors have called for an outside evaluation of the Oregon experience, there is little evidence to suggest that the state wishes to open this current process to outside scrutiny. Sadly, little information has been collected from patients themselves and from their families about the patients' and families' concerns for pain and symptom management, psychological support, and family support. Therefore, five years into this experience, we continue to know little about the patients and their families, their needs, and the potential of how interventions could alter patients' request for assistance in death.

Australia

In Australia, in 1995, the Rights of the Terminally Ill (ROTI) Act was passed in the Northern Territory of Australia by a vote of 13 to 12 and enacted, through passage of its regulations, in July 1996. Australia, at that time, became the first country in modern times to legalize rather than sanction euthanasia. Under the legislation, terminally ill patients who were experiencing pain, suffering, or distress to an extent deemed unacceptable, could ask their medical practitioner to help them end their lives. Consultation with a second medical practitioner in the specialty of the patient's illness was required. If the first medical practitioner did not have special qualifications in palliative care, a third consultant physician with such qualifications was required to give information to the patient on the availability of palliative care. A psychiatrist was also required to examine the patient and certify that he or she did not have a treatable or clinical depression. The Act required that a period of seven days elapse between an initial request and the patient's signing of an informed consent, witnessed by two medical practitioners. Forty-eight hours later, assistance to end life could be provided. A copy of the death certificate and relevant section of the medical record related to the illness and death in each case had to be forwarded to the coroner. The coroner was required to report to the Parliament the number of patients using the Act. In all, seven patients were euthanized by one physician—a euthanasia advocate, Dr Phillip Nitschke.[23]

One of the unintended consequences of the ROTI Act in Australia was its particular impact on the indigenous community of Aborigines who comprise nearly one quarter of the Northern Territory's population.[24] Concepts of euthanasia were unfamiliar to Aborigines; many dialects having no words for it. Assisting a person to die was considered likely to be an instrument of sorcery within their culture and traditionally regarded as morally wrong. Evidence was received, on passage of the Bill, that hospitals had become feared as places in which Aborigines could be killed without their consent. This demonstrated an unacceptable impact on the attitudes of the Aboriginal community towards health services in general.

Nine months into the law, the Federal Parliament overruled the law in the Northern Territory. In a published review of the seven patients euthanized by Dr Nitschke, Dr David Kissane pointed out that the considerable legislative effort to draft safe regulations that would protect vulnerable patients in fact failed to protect isolated, depressed, and demoralized patients.[23] Currently, both PAS and euthanasia are prohibited in Australia.

CURRENT ISSUES IN THE PHYSICIAN-ASSISTED SUICIDE/EUTHANASIA DEBATE

Physicians' Attitudes, Behaviors, and Knowledge

National and international surveys suggest that the willingness of physicians to assist patients in dying appears to be determined by numerous complex factors including their religious beliefs, personal values, medical specialty, age, practice setting, perspective on the use of financial resources, and their knowledge about palliative care principles and practices.[25]

A survey by the American Academy of Neurology of the attitudes, behaviors, and knowledge of neurologists demonstrated that there was a sizable gap between established legal, medical, and ethical guidelines for the care of the chronically ill, critically ill, and dying patients, and the beliefs and practices of neurologists.[26] For example, 29% of neurologists surveyed believed that in a patient dying of ALS, treating dyspnea with morphine sufficient to decrease ventilatory drive is the same as killing the patient; 39% think that such therapy constitutes euthanasia. Yet 72% of neurologists agree that treating dyspnea is an important part of palliative care. Although 89% agreed that withholding and withdrawing care is ethically different from assisted-suicide, 40% think they should consult legal council before stopping life-sustaining treatments, and 38% are concerned about being charged with a crime for withdrawing life-sustaining treatment. 37% think that it is illegal to give analgesics in doses that risk respiratory depression in the dying. These beliefs by neurologists are in marked contrast to a series of treatment guidelines developed by the American Academy of Neurology (AAN) emphasizing the importance of pain management and palliative care and the role of the neurologists in withholding and withdrawing care at the end-of-life.[27–33] 95% of neurologists agreed that the existence of living wills or designated health-care proxies made the decision process for the withdrawal of life-sustaining care easier, but only 31% of their patients had completed such documents.

Some neurologists stated that they would participate in PAS and voluntary euthanasia under the current U.S. legal constraints (13% and 4%), but many (44% and 28%) indicated that they would do so if the practices were legalized. In a study by Meier et al., who surveyed 3102 physicians in 10 specialties, neurologists were willing to participate in PAS and voluntary euthanasia even if illegal.[34] Neurologists in her study appeared to be more likely to participate in PAS and voluntary euthanasia than other specialty groups if it was legalized. It is not clear whether neurologists in the Meier et al. survey were making clear distinctions between good palliative care and PAS.

Neurologists do commonly receive requests for PAS. A large percentage of ALS specialists (41%) have received at least one request for PAS. This is in contrast to only 20% of general neurologists and 25% of neuro-oncologists.

Emmanuel et al. has also studied physicians' perceptions and has reported that among oncologists in the 1990s, there was a significant decline in support for euthanasia and PAS.[35] He cites the recent focus on end-of-life care, which has identified a multiplicity of interventions to improve the quality of living and dying of terminally ill patients that may have impacted on this reduction in advocacy for PAS and euthanasia. Emmanuel et al. also noted that a majority of U.S. physicians do not consider PAS or voluntary euthanasia as ethical. Moreover, U.S. physicians make clear distinctions between the practice of PAS and euthanasia, in contrast to Dutch physicians, who do not make such distinctions. It is of interest that a recent health maintenance organization in Oregon recently reported difficulty in finding physicians who would be willing to write lethal prescriptions for patients requesting PAS, suggesting perhaps a possible changing perspective of Oregon physicians in the last 4–5 years. Yet, it remains difficult to fully interpret the meaning of these surveys and how physicians' responses in such surveys relate to actual practice.

From the international perspective, there is an enormous need for studies of attitudes, behaviors, and knowledge of medical specialties and other health-care professionals in each country. Such studies can then compare such attitudes and knowledge to the existing legal, moral, and ethical guidelines in each country. Although living wills and health-care proxys are now a part of the U.S. legal system through the Patient Self-Determination Act, such legal documents are only just beginning to be widely used throughout Europe, Central Europe, Asia, and Africa. The focus on patient autonomy has been predominantly an American perspective, but clearly the rise of bioethics and the interest in patient autonomy is growing. In the United States, withholding and withdrawal of care and aggressive palliative care have been recognized by the U.S. Supreme Court as distinct from PAS and euthanasia, but in many countries these issues are currently conflated, adding further controversy to the discussions that distinguish palliative care from PAS and euthanasia.

Further complicating the variations in attitudes and behaviors among professionals, there is a profound lack of knowledge about how to provide palliative care. Three major U.S. government supported reports have indicted health-care professionals for their lack of knowledge and training in end-of-life care, and this lack of professional education and training appears to be an international issue as well.[36–38] Health-care professionals' lack of knowledge and skills in pain management, symptom control, communication skills, and ethical guidelines is the most serious challenge to developing and expanding palliative care initiatives.

Back et al., in their study of Washington State physicians whose patients requested assistance in dying, noted that physicians' lack of sophistication in assessing non-physical suffering, specifically patients' degree of existential distress, was a serious barrier to their providing care to such patients.[39] Studies emphasize that physicians struggle with their decisions to aid or not aid patients and they report feeling professionally isolated, with serious concerns, when making decisions for or against PAS.[40] These studies emphasize the need for physicians to gain competency in communicating with patients about the complex medical, social, psychological, and existential issues that occur as patients are dying.

Whether physicians are for or against PAS and euthanasia, there appears to be strong agreement that the care of the dying needs significant improvement, and there are major national and international initiatives to advance palliative care.[41]

Reasons for a Patient's Request for a Hastened Death

What the PAS/euthanasia debate has advanced is research into the domains of care for dying patients and their families, revealing the complex interaction of those who wish for hastened death and their environment, their health-care system, and their own personal beliefs. Emmanuel et al., in a detailed study of the domains of the dying process, clearly demonstrated that caregiver burden is significant in patients with a high degree of disease burden.[42] Such studies further emphasize how environmental issues play a pivotal role in patients' sense of self and, potentially, in their loss of self-respect and dignity. Lavrey et al., based on a qualitative study of 32 Canadians with HIV/AIDS, emphasized that individuals' loss of sense of self-value, from the disintegration and loss of community, has major implications for developing policies on PAS which should focus on many more issues other than the doctor/patient relationship.[43] Lavrey et al. argue that the current laws, such as exist in Oregon and the Netherlands, have not proved 'a framework to address social circumstances'.

The conceptual framework for a societal construct in the debate about PAS and euthanasia is further substantiated by people with disability, where lack of social networks for care at home often force the institutionalization of respiratory dependent or paralyzed patients.[44] Patients with ALS and neurodegenerative diseases are similarly identified because of their significant, progressive neurologic disability and need for extensive chronic care. In fact, national studies of patients with ALS show that there is marked variation in the utilization of palliative care approaches for symptom control of such as dyspnea, difficulty swallowing, drooling and ventilatory difficulties.[45] It is of interest that in Oregon, 5% of all deaths from ALS were by PAS; in the Netherlands, 20% of ALS patients chose PAS or euthanasia.[46]

As described, Ganzini and colleagues have, using an anonymous survey methodology, provided some insight into Oregon healthcare professionals' perceptions of patients requesting PAS.[21] One study reported that 46% of patients who requested PAS in Oregon, in the first two years, changed their minds after a substantive palliative care intervention was proposed or implemented. No data is available on why other patients were not offered such options. Again, from this Oregon survey data, up to 80% of patients who had prescriptions written for PAS in Oregon were receiving hospice care. Yet there is a dearth of information on the degree to which the hospice benefit meets patient and caregiver needs to reduce suffering and

caregiver burden, and why 20% of patients refused hospice services. What is now emerging in the public discussion is that it is not simply access to available palliative care therapies but the environment in which an individual lives and is cared for that can dramatically influence a patient's sense of self.

Studies have shown that patients who have requested PAS or euthanasia more commonly have chronic medical illness, with cancer, AIDS, and neurodegenerative disorders representing the most common diseases. The age of such patients is wide ranging, with most of the younger patients having a diagnosis of AIDS. The research to date suggests that the factors most commonly involved in requests for assistance are concerns about future loss of control, of being or becoming a burden to others, and fear of severe pain.[20,39]

An increasing number of studies have directly asked terminally ill patients with cancer/AIDS about their desire for death. These studies have shown that the desire for death is closely associated with depression, and that pain and lack of social supports are contributing factors.[47,48] It is now recognized that the relationship between depression and the desire to hasten death may vary among some groups of dying patients. Breitbart et al. has reported that depression and hopelessness are strongly related to interest in PAS for patients with HIV/AIDS. Emanuel et al. reported that for oncology patients and terminally ill patients, depressive symptoms were also associated with a personal interest in euthanasia and PAS.[49] Ganzini has reported that hopelessness, but not depression, was associated with ALS patients considering taking a prescription to end their life.[50]

Emanuel et al. has demonstrated that there is a relationship between the extent of caregiving needs and interest in euthanasia or PAS.[51] Such a relationship of caregiver needs was not identified by Ganzini, who was unable to show an association between burden of caring for patients and caregiver support for or opposition to a patient's request for PAS.

Emanuel et al. has argued that pain is not a major determinant of interest in or use of euthanasia or PAS.[51] Yet, in our own experience in evaluating patients in our cancer pain consultation service, fear of pain because of a previous episode of uncontrolled pain is often a driving force for patient's desire for death.[52]

From surveys of the American public, 70% report that fear of pain is a strong factor for them to consider PAS or euthanasia.[53] Future surveys need to distinguish between current pain and patients' experience with uncontrolled pain to better understand the role that pain plays in patients' request for PAS and euthanasia.

Studies have also attempted to address the interactions between uncontrolled symptoms and vulnerability to suicide in patients with cancer/AIDS. Bruera et al. has noted that patients' desire for death is independent of their physical symptoms.[54] The interactions between suicide risk and desire for death has been studied in patients with HIV/AIDS. Patients with AIDS have a high risk of suicide that is independent of physical symptoms. Among New York City residents with AIDS, the relative risk of suicide in men between the ages of 20 and 59 years was 36 times higher than the risk in men without AIDS in the same age group, and 66 times higher than the risk in the general population. Patients with AIDS who committed suicide generally did so within nine months after diagnosis; 25% had made a previous suicide attempt, 50% had reported severe depression, and 40% had seen a psychiatrist within four days before committing suicide.[55]

Suicide is the eighth leading cause of death in the United States and the incidence of suicide is higher in patients with cancer or AIDS and elderly men than in the general population. Conwell and Caine reported that depression was under-diagnosed by primary health-care physicians in a cohort of elderly patients who subsequently committed suicide; 75% of the patients had been seen by a primary care physician during the last month of life but had not received a diagnosis of depression.[56]

Studies to address the question of the effective treatment for depression on the desire for a hastened death are needed. In one report involving four patients who initially wished to hasten their death, such patients changed their mind within two weeks following treatment with psychotherapy and anti-depressants.[47] In short, there is increasing data to suggest that patients who request assistance in death experience significant psychological and existential distress that is often framed in concerns about being a burden, loss of meaning in their lives, and fear of uncontrolled symptoms.

DEVELOPMENT OF AN APPROACH TO THE DYING PATIENT

Numerous reviews have discussed the approach to the dying patient who requests assistance in death.[57–60] Cassem has described the role of the physician and several authors have written specific guidelines.[61–63] Physicians in general, and neurologists specifically, need to become acquainted with this literature and develop their own expertise in addressing the needs of patients and families as they approach death.

SUMMARY

In summary, there are serious physician-related barriers to appropriate, humane, compassionate care for the dying. These range from attitudinal and behavioral barriers to educational barriers. Physicians need to explore their own perspectives on the meaning of suffering as they develop a construct of care for the dying. They need insight into how the nature of the doctor/patient relationship influences their own decision making and impacts on that of their patients. The medical profession needs to take the lead in developing and supporting guidelines for good care of dying patients. Identifying the factors relating to physicians, patients, and the health-care system that pose as barriers to appropriate care should be the first step in any national or international dialogue on PAS/euthanasia. Such an approach can educate health-care professionals and the public on the topic of death and dying.

Death is an issue that society as a whole faces, and it requires a compassionate response, but we should not confuse compassion with competency in the care of terminally ill patients, and we should strongly advocate for improving the competency of health-care professionals as they face the challenging experience of death.

REFERENCES

1. Council of Europe. Protection of the human rights and dignity of the terminally ill and the dying. Official Gazette of the Council of Europe 1999.

2. The World Health Organization. Cancer Pain Relief and Palliative Care. Report of a WHO Expert Committee. The World Health Organization, Geneva, Switzerland, 1990.

3. Angell M. The Supreme Court and physician-assisted suicide the ultimate right. N Engl J Med 1997; 336:54–57.

4. Cohn F, Lynn J. Vulnerable people: practical rejoinders to claims in favor of assisted suicide. In: Foley K, Hendin H, eds. The Case Against Physician Assisted Suicide for the Right to Palliative Care. Johns Hopkins University Press, Baltimore, 2002:238–260.

5. Callahan D, White M. The legalization of physician-assisted suicide: creating a regulatory Potemkin village. U Richmond Law Rev 1996;3:272–278.

6. Van der Mass PJ, Van der Wal G, Haverkate I, et al. Euthanasia physician-assisted suicide, and other medical practices involving the end of life in the Netherlands 1990–1995. N Engl J Med 1996; 335:1699–1705.

7. Hendin H. Seduced by Death: Doctors, Patients, and Assisted Suicide. Norton Press, New York, 1998.

8. Hendin H, Rutenfrans C, Zylicz Z. Physician-assisted suicide and euthanasia in the Netherlands: lessons from the Dutch. JAMA 1997;277:1720–1722.

9. Hendin H. The Dutch experience. In: Foley K, Hendin H, eds. The Case Against Physician Assisted Suicide for the Right to Palliative Care. Johns Hopkins University Press, Baltimore, 2002:97–121.

10. Zylicz Z. The story behind the blank spot: hospice in Holland. Am J of Hospice and Palliative Care 1993;10:30–34.

11. Burt R. The Supreme Court speaks: not assisted suicide but a constitutional right to palliative care. N Engl J Med 1997;337:1234–1236.

12. Oregon Death with Dignity Act. Oregon Revised Statute. 1997;127:127–99.

13. Alpers A, Lo B. Physician-assisted suicide in Oregon. A bold experiment. JAMA 1995;974(6):483–487.

14. Hedberg K, Kohn M. Five years of legal physician-assisted suicide in Oregon. N Engl J Med 2003; 348:961–964.

15. Foley K, Hendin H. The Oregon Report: Don't Ask, Don't Tell. Hastings Center Report 1999;29: 37–42.

16. Foley K, Hendin H. The Oregon Experiment. In: Foley K, Hendin H, eds. The Case against Physician Assisted Suicide for the Right to Palliative Care. Johns Hopkins Press, Baltimore, 2002:144–174.

17. Hamilton NG. Oregon's culture of silence. In: Foley K, Hendin H, eds. The Case Against Physician Assisted Suicide for the Right to Palliative Care. Johns Hopkins University Press, Baltimore, 2002:175–192.

18. Kettler B. Stricken by ALS, Joan Lucas Decides to Die—Then Acts. Medford Mail Tribune, 25 June 2000.

19. Regan P. Helen. Lancet 1999;353:1265–1267.

20. Ganzini L, Nelson HD, Schmidt TA, Kraemer DF, Delorit MA, Lee MA. Physicians' experiences with the Oregon Death with Dignity Act. N Engl J Med 2000;342:557–563.

21. Ganzini L, Nelson HD, Schmidt TA, Kraemer DF, Delorit MA, Lee MA. Experiences of Oregon nurses and social workers with hospice patients who requested assistance with suicide. N Engl J Med 2002;347(8):582–588.

22. Tolle SW. Oregon assisted suicide: the silver lining. Ann Intern Med 1996;124(2):267–269.

23. Kissane DW, Street A, Nitschke P. Seven deaths in Darwin: case studies under the Rights of the Terminally Ill Act, Northern Territory, Australia. Lancet 1998;352:1097–1102.

24. Collins JJ, Brennan FT. Euthanasia and the potential adverse effects for Northern Territory Aborigines. Lancet 1997;349:1907–1908.

25. Portenoy RK, Coyle N, Kash M, et al. Determinants of the willingness to endorse assisted suicide: a survey of physicians, nurses, and social workers. Psychosomatics 1997;38:277–287.

26. Carver AC, Vickrey BG, Bernat JL, et al. 'End of life care: a survey of US neurologists' attitudes, behavior and knowledge. Neurology 1999;53:284–293.

27. Report of the Ethics and Humanities Subcommittee of the American Academy of Neurology. Position of the American Academy of Neurology on certain aspects of the care and management of the persistent vegetative state. Neurology 1989;39:125–126.

28. Report of the Ethics and Humanities Subcommittee of the American Academy of Neurology. The ethical role of neurologists in the AIDS epidemic. Neurology 1992;42:1116–1117.

29. Report of the Ethics and Humanities Subcommittee of the American Academy of Neurology. Position statement: certain aspects of the care and management of profoundly and irreversibly paralyzed patients with retained consciousness and cognition. Neurology 1993;43:222–223.

30. Report of the Ethics and Humanities Subcommittee of the American Academy of Neurology. Ethical issues in the management of the demented patient. Neurology 1996;46:1180–1183.

31. Report of the Ethics and Humanities Subcommittee of the American Academy of Neurology. Palliative care in neurology. Neurology 1996;46:870–872.

32. Report of the Ethics and Humanities Subcommittee of the American Academy of Neurology. Position statement: assisted suicide, euthanasia, and the neurologist. Neurology 1998;50:596–598.

33. Bernat JL, Goldstein ML, Viste KM. The neurologist and the dying patient. Neurology 1996;46:598–599.

34. Meier DE, Emmons CA, Wallenstein S, Quill TE, Morrison RS, Cassel CK. A national survey of physician-assisted suicide and euthanasia in the United States. N Engl J Med 1998;338:1193–1232.

35. Emanuel EJ. Euthanasia and physician assisted suicide: a review of the empirical data from the United States. Arch Intern Med 2002;162(2):142–152.

36. Field M, Cassell C, eds. Approaching Death: Improving Care at the End of Life. Division of Health Care Services, Institute of Medicine, National Academy Press,Washington DC, 1997.

37. Foley K, Gelband H, eds. Improving Palliative Care for Cancer. Institute of Medicine, National Academy Press, Washington DC, 2002.

38. Field M, Behrman RE, eds. When Children Die: Improving palliative and End-of-life Care for Children and their Families. Institute of Medicine, National Academy Press, Washington DC, 2002.

39. Back AJ, Wallace JI, Starks HF, Pearlman RA. Physician-Assisted Suicide and Euthanasia in Washington State: Patient Requests and Physician Responses. JAMA 1996;275:919–925.

40. Kohlwes RJ, Koepsell TD, Rhodes LA, Pearlman RA. Physicians' responses to patients' requests for physician-assisted suicide. Arch Intern Med 2001;161: 657–663.

41. Foley K. Advancing Palliative Care in the US. Palliative Medicine. 2003;17(2):89–91.

42. Emanuel E, Fairclough D, Slutsman J, Emanuel L. Understanding economics and other burdens of terminal illness: the experience of patients and their caregivers. Ann Intern Med 2000;132:451–458.

43. Lavery JV, Boyle J, Dickens BM, Maclean H, Singer P. Origins of the desire for euthanasia and assisted suicide in people with HIV-1 or AIDS: a qualitative sstudy. Lancet 2001;358:362–366.

44. Coleman D. Not dead yet. In: Foley K, Hendin H, eds. The Case Against Physician Assisted Suicide for the Right to Palliative Care. Johns Hopkins University Press, Baltimore, 2002:213–237.

45. Bradley WG, Anderson F, Bromberg M, et al. Current management of ALS: comparison of the ALS CARE database and the AAN practice parameter. Neurology 2001;57:500–504.

46. Veldnik JH, Wokke JH, Van Der Wal G, et al. Euthanasia and physician-assisted suicide among patient's with amyotrophic lateral sclerosis in the Netherlands. N Engl J Med 2002;346(21):1638–1644.

47. Chochinov HM, Wilson KG, Enns M, et al. Desire for death in the terminally ill. Am J Psychiatry 1995;152:1185–1191.

48. Breitbart W, Rosenfeld B, Pessin H, et al. Depression, hopelessness, and desire for hastened death in terminally ill patients with cancer. JAMA 2000;284:2907–2911.

49. Emanuel EJ. The ASCO Task Force on end of life survey. In: Foley K, Gelband H, eds. Improving Palliative Care for Cancer. National Cancer Policy Board Report. National Academy Press, Washington DC, 2001:46–47.

50. Ganzini L, Johnson WS, McFarland BH, Tolle SW, Lee MA. Atttitudes of patients with amyotrophic lateral sclerosis and their caregivers toward assisted suicide. N Engl J Med 1998;339:967–973.

51. Emanuel EJ, Fairclough DL, Slutsman J, Alpert H, Baldwin D, Emanuel LL. Assistance from family members, friends, paid caregivers and volunteers in the care of terminally ill patients. N Engl J Med 1999; 341:956–963.

52. Foley K. The relationship to pain and symptom management to patient requests for physician assisted suicide. J Pain Sympt Manage 1991;6(5):289–297.

53. Gallup Institute. Spiritual Beliefs and the Dying Process: A Report on the National Survey Conducted for the Nathan Cummings Foundation and Fetzer Institute. Gallup Institute, 1997.

54. Almazor–Suarez M, Newman C, Hanson J, et al. Attitudes of terminally ill cancer patients about euthanasia and assisted suicide: Predominance of psychosocial determinants and beliefs over symptom distress and subsequent survival. J Clin Oncol 2002;20(8):2134–2141.

55. Passik S, McDonald M, Rosenfeld B, Breitbart W. End of life issues in patients with AIDS: clinical and research considerations. J Pain and Sympt Cont 1995;3:91–111.

56. Conwell Y, Caine HD. Rational suicide and the right to die. Reality and myth. N Engl J Med 1992; 326: 1100–1103.

57. Quill TE. A physician's position on physician-assisted suicide. Bull NY Acad Med 1997;74(1): 114–118.

58. Quill TE, Meier DE, Block SD, Billings JA. The debate over physician-assisted suicide: empirical data and convergent views. Ann Intern Med 1998;128(7): 552–558.

59. Block SD. Perspectives on care at the close of life. Psychological considerations, growth and transcendence at the end of life: the art of possible. JAMA 2001;285(22):2898–2905.

60. Emanuel L. Facing requests for physician assisted suicide: toward a practical and principled skill set. JAMA 1998;280:643–647.

61. Cassem NH. The dying patient. In: Cassem NH, ed. Massachusetts General Hospital Handbook of General Hospital Psychiatry. Mosby Year Book Inc., St Louis, 1991:343.

62. Cherny NI, Coyle N, Foley KM. Guidelines in the care of the dying cancer patient. In: Cherny NI, Foley KM, eds. Hematology/Oncology Clinics of North America: Pain and Palliative Care. WB Saunders Co, Philadelphia, 1996:235–259.

63. Block SD, Billings JA. Patient requests for euthanasia and assisted suicide in terminal illness. The role of the psychiatrist. Psychosomatics 1995;36(5): 445–457.

Chapter 37

Informed Consent

James L. Bernat

INTRODUCTION
A THEORY OF INFORMED CONSENT
The Competent Patient
Shared Decision Making
The Incompetent Patient
Standards for Surrogate Decision Making

CONSENT IN MINORS
TREATMENT WITHOUT CONSENT
PRACTICAL ISSUES
CULTURAL AND LEGAL ISSUES
RESEARCH

All patients have the ethical right of informed consent and refusal that requires physicians, except in emergency treatment, to seek their permission before proceeding with medical care. This right is transferred to a legally authorized surrogate decision maker to exercise on their behalf when patients lose the capacity to make health-care decisions. Patients and surrogates require adequate information and the absence of coercion. Ideally, patients and physicians will practice shared decision making so the decision is patient-centered. Surrogates for incompetent patients should attempt to follow the explicit or implicit preferences of the patients they represent and decide in their best interest when they lack knowledge of their treatment preferences. Child patients should be included in the consent process to the extent they are capable of understanding. Consent is a process and not an event. It is a communication process that evolves over time. Consent for participation as a human research subject imposes even stricter standards of information exchange and lack of coercion than consent for treatment.

CASE HISTORY

A 62-year-old man received chemotherapy and immunotherapy in a clinical trial for the treatment of a right parietal-occipital lobe malignant glioma, following primary treatment with surgical resection

and radiation therapy. Yet, he continued to deteriorate with progressive left hemiparesis, left hemineglect, and seizures. Large dosages of three anticonvulsants sedated him and he had become cushingoid from dexamethasone. After frequent visits with his neuro-oncologist, he decided to discontinue the chemotherapy and immunotherapy and receive purely palliative treatment. His neuro-oncologist carefully explained his likely prognosis with and without the specific treatment, and together they devised a palliative treatment plan that both found acceptable. When he later became stuporous, his wife (who also was his durable power of attorney for health care) continued to consent for the palliative treatment on his behalf, and worked closely with the neuro-oncologist to agree on a treatment plan. Both the patient and his wife felt they had played an important part in treatment decisions and that the treatment at each stage respected the patient's wishes.

INTRODUCTION

The doctrine of informed consent is the ethical and legal foundation of medical practice. It acknowledges that patients possess a basic human right to provide or refuse their permission for tests and therapies suggested by physicians. That patients possess this right imparts an ethical duty (and in most parts of the world a legal duty) for physicians to obtain

383

patients' free and informed consent before proceeding with medical treatment, except in well-defined exceptional circumstances. Western common law and normative ethical principles grant all persons the rights of self-determination, privacy, and human dignity. These rights generally ban touching or causing potential bodily harm without a person's consent. Although physicians may have beneficent motives that some have argued mitigate the full need to secure patients' consent, Western society generally has required physicians to obtain patients' voluntary permission for testing and treatment.[1]

Implicit in the doctrine of informed consent is the option of informed refusal. Patients are permitted to refuse diagnostic testing or therapeutic intervention recommended by their physicians if they so choose. And specifically, all patients are permitted to refuse life-sustaining therapy if that represents their reasoned choice. The duty of physicians to respect patients' refusals of life-sustaining therapy and how palliative care is administered in that setting are discussed further in Chapter 35.

Obtaining a patient's consent for palliative care is not fundamentally different from obtaining a patient's consent for any other type of medical care. Thus most of the comments in this chapter apply equally to attempted curative medical care. In this chapter, I discuss the theory and practice of informed consent. I clarify how physicians obtain consent from a competent patient and explain how to obtain consent when patients become incompetent. I explain the concept of shared decision making and discuss the criteria and standards of surrogate decision making. I outline obtaining consent for treatment of minors and discuss emergency treatment and other exceptions to obtaining consent. I briefly touch on practical issues in obtaining and documenting consent. I end with a short discussion of legal and cultural issues in obtaining consent for palliative care.

A THEORY OF INFORMED CONSENT

A number of scholars have analyzed the doctrine of informed consent from ethical and legal perspectives to produce definitions and criteria. The most lucid of these is the analysis by Bernard Gert and Charles M. Culver.[2,3] Gert and Culver prefer the term 'valid consent' because the mere transmittal of information from physician to patient alone is inadequate for an ethically or legally sound consent. Although I agree with this formulation, for the goal of greater familiarity, here I employ the more commonly used term 'informed consent'. An analysis of informed consent should consider the criteria of obtaining informed consent in the two fundamental clinical situations: for the competent patient and the incompetent patient.

Following the usage of Gert and Culver, I employ the term 'competence' in a clinical context as a shorthand way of indicating the capacity of a patient to make health-care decisions. I specifically do not intend a legal usage that, in many jurisdictions, refers specifically to a determination of decisional capacity that can be made only in a court of law. Rather, 'competence' in my usage refers to a clinical determination of a patient's decision-making capacity made by a physician in the clinic or at the bedside. Competent patients understand that they have a decision to make, can comprehend their choices and their implications, can rationally manipulate these data to reach a clinical decision that they can consent or refuse. Physicians seek consent directly from competent patients.[2,3]

Incompetent patients, by contrast, lack the capacity to make health-care decisions. They may fail to understand the decision or its benefits and risks to them, be unable to manipulate data, or to effectively communicate their wishes. In neurological practice, the most common reasons for a patient's incompetence are dementia, delirium, or metabolic or toxic encephalopathy producing confusion, stupor, or coma. Patients with severe forms of aphasia also are incompetent because, even though their cognitive capacities may remain intact, language dysfunction impairs their ability to effectively communicate their wishes. Physicians must seek consent from the authorized surrogate decision makers of incompetent patients.

Physicians customarily make competence determinations during their interviews and examinations of patients on the basis of patients' responses to questions about their history and during more formal examinations of their mental status. Such assessments usually permit a physician to generate a firm conclusion about a patient's competence. In instances in which a patient's competence remains unclear, requesting an examination by a second physician or, where readily available, by a psychiatrist, can help resolve the competence determination. Some patients with delirium or metabolic/toxic encephalopathies have fluctuating levels of competence. This situation is particularly common in the dying patient and in the hospitalized, critically ill patient.

The Competent Patient

Two conditions make consent in the competent patient valid:
1. Physicians communicate adequate information to enable the patient to make a rational decision
2. They do not employ coercion, thereby assuring that the patient's consent is voluntary

Consents that are obtained without both of these elements are ethically invalid.[2,3]

Adequate information is that information that a reasonable person needs to know to reach a rational decision. Reasonable people need to know their diagnosis and prognosis with and without treatment. They need to know their choices and the risks, benefits, and expected outcomes of those choices. Physicians should communicate risks to the extent they are common or severe. Thus, for example, in pharmacotherapy, they should explain common but mild risks such as skin rash (0.1% risk) as well as less common but more severe risks such as dose-related pancytopenia (0.01% risk). Physicians probably do not have a duty to communicate exceedingly uncommon risks such as serious idiosyncratic reactions (0.00001% risk) because most rational people understand that freakish untoward risks are always possible and the slight chance of this event does not usually alter the patient's decision to proceed with treatment.[2,3]

Adequate information also includes the physician's reasons for the proposed tests or therapies in the context of the patient's illness. The physician's rationale for treatment is important so the patient can understand the reason to accept whatever risks are implicit in treatment by appreciating the countervailing benefits of treatment. Further, adequate information needs to be communicated in a way patients can comprehend. They should be given the opportunity to ask questions and receive answers calmly and clearly.

Lack of coercion is necessary to make the consent freely given. Coercion includes undue pressures by threats or other forces that no reasonable person could resist. It is coercive for physicians to threaten that they will not care for a patient who is unwilling to follow their exact treatment recommendations. It is not coercive for physicians to make strong treatment recommendations by factually explaining the reasons for the recommendations and citing the benefits shown in valid outcome studies. But it is coercive for physicians to exaggerate the benefits of the recommended treatment or the risks of alternative treatments or no treatment to attempt to manipulate the patient into making the 'right decision'.

Physicians may exercise a subtle form of coercion or, at least, manipulation through the framing effect. Framing refers to *how* physicians present treatment options to patients.[4] Several studies have shown that how a physician frames the decision is highly predictive of how the patient will respond. For example, the use of leading questions in framing is highly influential. Investigators testing the wishes of elderly patients to receive cardiopulmonary resuscitation (CPR) found when they framed the decision using the leading question: 'you would want us to restart your heart if it stopped, wouldn't you?' that the majority of patients answered 'yes'. But when they reframed the same question without suggesting an answer and included the statistics of CPR successes in their age group, the majority of patients declined.[5]

During an ethically acceptable consent process, it is essential that physicians frame decisions in an unbiased way. Although after objectively presenting treatment options, physicians should issue a treatment recommendation, it is wrong for physicians to unfairly influence the patient's decision by manipulating them through a biased framing of the choices. To the fullest extent possible in their discussion, physicians should clearly separate fact from opinion. This separation allows patients to understand the difference between the two and to agree upon the facts while permitting disagreement with the physician's opinion.

Shared Decision Making

Obtaining valid consent is a process not an event. It is a conversation between the patient and physician in which the physician provides information and answers the patient's questions. The process of consent takes place over time as treatment plans are developed and represents an agreement between the patient and physician on mutually shared goals and an approach to treatment. This consensual agreement approach is called shared decision making.[6]

In the shared decision-making model of consent, the physician brings to the table a technical knowledge of diseases, their diagnosis and prognosis, the available treatment options, and a knowledge of their likely outcomes with the patient's condition. The physician also brings a treatment recommendation, based on the physician's experience and judgment, that the physician believes represents the best treatment for the patient in this case. It would be wrong for a physician merely to recite a menu of options and ask the patient independently to choose one without professional guidance whatsoever.

The patient brings to the table his/her unique set of preferences and values for treatment that result from their life and health goals. Implicit in these preferences is a highly personal ranking of harms from treatment or non-treatment. For example, some patients would prefer to undergo mutilating radical surgery if doing so increased their life expectancy a statistically determined amount of time, whereas other patients would prefer to remain whole even if by doing so they lived a shorter time.

The patient interprets the data and recommendations from the physician through the filter of his/her unique values and preferences to judge the personal acceptability of each option and to choose the one that is best personally. Together, the patient and physician reach mutual agreement on the treatment plan that is then implemented and followed.

Physicians have a unique role in helping patients understand their illness and the reasons for the recommended treatment and guiding them to make the right choice.[7]

Many patients respond, 'Doctor, do whatever you feel is best for me'. There is nothing wrong with this deferral to the physician so long as it represents the patient's reasoned decision. As patients grow sicker, they often become more dependent and more often wish to defer such decisions to physicians. Voluntary deferral to a physician is not an ethical problem. Rather, the ethical problem concerns the patient who wishes to participate in treatment decisions but who is disenfranchised from doing so by a physician who fails to ask about or consider the patient's viewpoint in the decision.

The Incompetent Patient

Patients rendered incompetent by dementia, delirium, aphasia, or other conditions impairing cognitive and language capabilities lack the capacity to provide consent. But incompetent patients do not lose their right of consent. Rather, the right of consent is transferred to a surrogate (proxy) decision maker to execute on behalf of the patient. Physicians therefore must conduct exactly the same consent discussion with the surrogate of the incompetent patient as they do directly with the competent patient. Valid surrogate consent has the same elements as valid patient consent.

Surrogate decision makers can be appointed formally or informally. Many jurisdictions provide a mechanism for the appointment of a legally authorized surrogate. In the United States, for example, most states provide all citizens when competent, the opportunity to appoint another person who is vested with authority to serve as that person's legally authorized medical decision maker. The surrogate's authority is activated once the person has been rendered incompetent by illness or injury. Jurisdictions label such appointments variously as durable power of attorney for health care, health-care proxy, or health-care agent. Most jurisdictions vest this surrogate agent with the same level of medical decision-making authority as is possessed by the competent patient. Many states also have enacted health-care proxy laws that automatically appoint a legally authorized surrogate decision maker in the absence of a previously executed appointment.[8]

In many instances, however, the incompetent patient will not have previously executed a surrogate appointment and live in a jurisdiction without a health-care proxy law that would automatically appoint one. In this situation, the physician must identify an appropriate surrogate decision maker. Generally, physicians designate primary family members to this role. So long as the primary family members are in agreement with each other, this informal system works well in practice. In the face of disagreement, physicians can attempt to create consensus by diplomatic family counseling. But if this process fails and an intractable disagreement among primary family members persists, the physician should consider referral of the matter to a court of law for the formal designation of a legally authorized surrogate.

Standards for Surrogate Decision Making

Surrogate decision making for incompetent patients is difficult and stress-provoking for many surrogates because they are unsure as to the correct course of action. Good surrogates possess accurate knowledge of the health-care goals and treatment preferences of the patient they represent and the courage to uphold these goals and preferences in practice. Physicians should counsel surrogates that there are accepted ethical and legal standards for their decision making that they should attempt to employ as they execute their lonely task.[9]

The highest standard is that of expressed wishes. If the patient, when competent, had clearly expressed specific wishes about treatment in a particular situation, the surrogate should insist that this preference be followed. Following a patient's expressed wishes is the ethically most powerful standard because it permits continued respect for the autonomy and self-determination of the patient even after the patient has been rendered incompetent. But because it is uncommon for patients to have anticipated and provided guidance for the precise clinical situation that they later might develop, this standard usually cannot be applied in practice.[9]

Evidence of expressed wishes may be found in written advance directive forms such as in living will declarations or durable power of attorney appointments available in many jurisdictions. However, here too, the expressed wishes standard often cannot be applied because the terms of written directives may be too general and vague for the surrogate to apply them confidently to a particular situation. Expressed wishes also can be found in statements to families and friends made previously by the patient. Here, however, physicians should exercise caution because previous statements may not have been carefully considered judgments or may be inapplicable because they were made in a different circumstance.

In the common situation in which the patient had not previously expressed clear wishes, the standard of substituted judgment should be applied. This standard asks the surrogate to make a novel but informed decision on behalf of the patient that attempts to reproduce the precise decision the patient would have made by applying the patient's known values and preferences to the clinical situation at hand. Surrogates should understand that the decision they reach is not necessarily the one they might make for themselves. But their task is not to decide what they think is best using their own preferences or values. Executing a substituted judgment requires surrogates to attempt to reach the decision that the patient would have made using the patient's own values and preferences.[10]

Empirical studies of the accuracy of substituted judgments show that they are erroneous in approximately one-third of attempts.[11,12] Some scholars have argued that the alternatives to substituted judgment are worse and, moreover, that the standard of decision making is not as important as correctly identifying the proper person to make the decision.[13] Nevertheless, surrogates should be instructed to try to decide as the patient would decide by 'walking in the patient's shoes'. That the surrogates are asked merely to convey the wishes of the incompetent patient rather than make an independent decision lessens the potential for guilt they may feel about the decision process.

In many instances, the surrogate has no knowledge of the patient's values and preferences. This situation is common among court-appointed public guardians and surrogates of infants and young children who have never been able to express wishes. In this situation, the surrogate employs the standard of best interests. This standard asks the surrogate to balance the benefits to the patient of the proposed treatment against its harms and make an objective balance of the competing factors to determine what is in the patient's best interest. Clearly, this type of determination is ethically less powerful than the previous standards because it relies totally on the surrogate's opinion rather than trying to follow the patient's expressed wishes or what the surrogate would presume those wishes to be.[9]

Best interest determinations have been criticized because, while they purport to objectively weigh the benefits and burdens of therapy, they remain intrinsically subjective determinations that depend on the surrogate's concept of the quality of the patient's life.[13] Some surrogates assign relatively low value to life in a state of disability and may decide against providing for treatment if the patient might be disabled.[14] Surrogates using a best interest standard must exercise great caution and humility to not undervalue life of a diminished quality that the patient may be perfectly happy to continue to lead.

Irrespective of the standards used, in all instances of surrogate decision making for incompetent patients, the physician and surrogate form a decision-making dyad analogous to the shared decision-making doctrine. Effective communication between the physician and surrogate is critical. Consent in the incompetent patient remains a process of working together between the physician and surrogate for the good of the patient.

CONSENT IN MINORS

Obtaining informed consent in children and adolescents introduces additional ethical and legal complexities. In most jurisdictions, there is no legal duty to obtain the child's consent; the consent of the parents or other guardian is sufficient. Despite the fact that the child is a minor and does not enjoy the legal rights of majority, there is a growing acceptance of the ethical desirability to secure the consent of children and adolescents to the degree they can understand and participate.

In the United States, the American Academy of Pediatrics (AAP) has led the movement to extend the right of consent to children who have the capacity to participate in medical decisions. To clarify that a child or adolescent's consent is necessary but not sufficient for valid consent for their treatment, the AAP adopted and defined the term 'assent'. They argued that to achieve valid consent of children and adolescents, it is necessary to obtain the developmentally appropriate minor's assent in addition to the parents' 'permission'. The AAP chose the term 'permission' to emphasize that parental approval was insufficient without the minor's assent.[15]

The AAP states that a minor's assent for testing or treatment should include at least the following elements:

> 1) helping the patient achieve a developmentally appropriate awareness of the nature of his or her condition; 2) telling the patient what he or she can expect with tests and treatment(s); 3) making a clinical assessment of the patient's understanding of the situation and the factors influencing how he or she is responding (including whether there is appropriate pressure to accept testing or therapy); and 4) soliciting an expression of the patient's willingness to accept the proposed care. Regarding this final point, we note that no one should solicit a patient's views without intending to weigh them seriously. In situations in which the patient will have to receive medical care despite his or her objection, the patient should be told that fact and should not be deceived.[15]

Some bioethicists later warned that the child liberation views of the AAP unwisely afforded decisional latitude to children and adolescents enabling them to make bad decisions which, in the end, hurt them more than helped them.[16] Indeed, the AAP was concerned about possible conflicts between children and their parents and devoted considerable attention to advising pediatricians how to resolve such conflicts in the best interest of the minor patient. They recommended that pediatricians assess each child and adolescent individually to determine their cognitive and emotional readiness to participate in medical decisions.[15]

The legal status of consent in minors is complex. Jurisdictions have legislated varying and sometimes conflicting laws that simultaneously attempt to protect and liberate minors. For example, in the United States, most states now define the age of majority as 18 years, a change from the previous legal majority of 21 years, as a consequence of passage of the 26th amendment to the Constitution in 1971 that lowered the legal voting age to 18 years. But nearly all states also have created the category of 'emancipated minors' to acknowledge that some people under age 18 are granted the freedom to consent independently of their parents or guardians. Although the statutory definition of emancipation varies among jurisdictions, most statutes emancipate minors who are married, who have borne children, who are serving in the military, or who are financially independent from their parents. Emancipated minors have the same full legal authority to consent independently as people over the age of 18 years.[17]

Additionally, most states have designated the category of 'mature minors' to acknowledge that many adolescents between the ages of 14–18 years have achieved the cognitive and emotional capacities necessary to consent independently. In states with mature minor statutes, irrespective of their emancipation status, such mature minors are permitted to consent without direct parental involvement.[17]

Further, most states have enacted minor treatment statutes that permit adolescents over the age of 14 to consent independently for the treatment of specified conditions. Although the list of such conditions varies among jurisdictions, most statutes include the treatment of sexually transmitted diseases, birth control, pregnancy, drug abuse, and alcohol abuse. Some states enlarge the diagnosis list to include treatment for psychiatric disorders and abortion. Obviously, it is incumbent on physicians caring for children and adolescents to be aware of the relevant laws within the jurisdiction in which they practice.[17]

TREATMENT WITHOUT CONSENT

Although it is ethically and legally necessary for physicians to obtain valid consent from patients before testing or treatment, there are justified exceptions to this rule. The most common exception is during emergencies when, because of the critical time demands intrinsic to emergency treatment and the frequent unavailability of surrogates, urgently needed treatment must proceed without consent. A second, and much more rare instance, is when physicians can justify overruling patients' irrational treatment refusals.

Physicians can and should provide emergency treatment without consent in situations in which it would be harmful to delay treatment to try to obtain consent. The ethical principle of beneficence generally permits or requires urgent and needed treatment on the basis of presumed consent. In this circumstance, it is presumed that a patient would have provided consent for emergency treatment. The emergency treatment common law doctrine formalizes the concept of presumed consent but limits the treatment to generally accepted therapies in the emergency condition at issue. Experimental or unproved therapies would not be covered by the emergency treatment doctrine because, since it is not unambiguously clear that the patient would have consented to these therapies, the patient's consent cannot be presumed.[18]

A much rarer instance in which some physicians have claimed that treatment without consent is justified is when the patient has made a seriously irrational treatment refusal. Treating, in the face of an explicit refusal, on the basis that the physician knows better than the patient what is in the patient's best interest is an example of paternalism. Is such paternalism ever justified? In fact, there are exceedingly few instances in which such paternalism can be justified and essentially none in the field of palliative care.[2,3] Certainly, patients dying of terminal illnesses who refuse life-sustaining therapy usually cannot be construed to be making a seriously irrational treatment refusal when they will die within a short time anyway of their underlying illness.

There is also a legal implication of treating in the face of an explicit treatment refusal.

Such unwanted manipulation of the patient's body could be construed as battery. It is incumbent on the physician to adequately explain the basis for treatment, in the face of an explicit refusal, to attempt to justify such a paternalistic act. In the absence of a good justification, the patient who explicitly refuses consent should not be given the treatment in question.

PRACTICAL ISSUES

Numerous studies have shown that, despite physicians' acknowledgement of the need for obtaining consent and an understanding of how it should be carried out, many physicians have not integrated ideal consent behaviors into their medical practices.[19] This mismatch of theory and practice raises the question of what are the barriers to informed consent? One clear barrier is the time required for a detailed consent conversation in the context of a busy medical practice. Many physicians simply lack the time necessary to conduct detailed explanations even if they wanted to do so. Another barrier is physicians' inadvertent use of technical jargon. Some physicians use technical words that are part of their usual vocabulary that they erroneously assume patients will understand. Studies measuring patients' comprehension of medical facts discussed at a physician visit show an appallingly low level of understanding.[20] And many physicians continue to regard consent merely as a cumbersome technical requirement to obtain a signature on a consent form.

The procedural requirements for documenting consent vary among countries, institutions, and practices. In general, the more dangerous the diagnostic or therapeutic procedure, the more likely it is for a policy to require written consent. For example, in the setting of palliative care, written consent usually is not necessary for a patient to receive opiates or benzodiazepines when the physician adequately explains the choice, risks, reasons, and outcomes. But the patient who is advised to undergo a surgical procedure for pain palliation will usually be required to sign a consent form.

The signature on a consent form, however, is not the consent. It is only the formalization of a preceding conversation between the physician and patient during which the patient has made an informed decision to proceed. It is that conversation that constitutes the consent process. Risk managers in many institutions believe that a patient's signature on a consent form reduces professional liability because it formally establishes that a preceding consent discussion has taken place with the physician. However, the event of signing consent forms in some practices has been reduced to a *pro forma* exercise without an adequate preceding consent discussion. A patient's signature in such cases affords little protection to professional liability.

CULTURAL AND LEGAL ISSUES

There is a marked diversity of normative consent practices and laws throughout the world. In some cultures, the very act of a patient voluntarily consulting a physician or entering a hospital is construed as sufficient consent for testing and treatment with no attempt necessary to obtain further permission. By contrast, in the United States, the legal and ethical doctrine of consent has been formalized in innumerable hospital regulations and practice guidelines to be a fundamental and necessary step in medical care.

For example, in several cultures, it is accepted practice for physicians not to disclose to a patient the diagnosis of cancer or other serious illnesses even when they have been clearly established.[21-23] Interestingly, in most of these cultures it is acceptable to tell family members of the patient's diagnosis but the information is hidden from the patient. These practices presumably stem from a beneficent intent of family members to spare the affected person the emotional stress of discovering the existence of a serious illness. But how can a physician in these cultures obtain the patient's consent for treatment when the patient lacks the most fundamental information about his/her own diagnosis? In some of these cultures, this problem is solved because the family paternalistically provides the consent, not the patient.

Cultural variation may become an issue in cross-cultural medical treatment. For example, if a patient from a culture where disclosure of a serious diagnosis is not practiced receives medical care in a culture where patients are told their diagnoses as part of a consent process, what should physicians tell the patient? This quandary poses the conflict between respect for cultural mores and normative practices for obtaining valid consent. I have attempted to solve this conflict simply by asking the patient how much he/she wishes to know about their diagnosis and prognosis and whether I should obtain consent for treatment from him/her or from a family member on their behalf.

Similarly, laws and legal standards for consent vary among cultures and jurisdictions. Practitioners need to understand the laws within the communities in which they practice.

RESEARCH

The final area in which informed consent is relevant to the topic of palliative care is consent for participation in clinical research. The voluntary, free, and informed consent of the human research subject has been an ethical axiom for clinical research since the development of the Nuremberg Code in 1947.[24] The Code of Helsinki, drafted originally in 1964 by the World Medical Association and amended in five subsequent revisions, most recently in 2000, reiterated the requirement for voluntary consent in the Nuremberg Code and added additional ethical duties on the investigator to ensure the welfare of the human research subject at all times during the study.[25]

The ethical duties of the investigator to assure the human research subject's voluntary consent and welfare stems from the unique relationship between the investigator and the human subject. Because the goal of research is the development of generalizable knowledge, the human research subject becomes the means to accomplish that goal. In any human relationship in which a person is used solely as a means for another objective, rather than treated as an end in itself, explicit permission for that use is required from the subject, and the user of the subject incurs a special duty to protect the subject's welfare.[26]

The criteria for informed consent for research are similar to those for clinical care: the subject must be competent to consent, full information must be conveyed and understood by the human subject, and there must be an absence of coercion by people or agencies. But because the goal of research is the development of knowledge—a goal that may not be congruent with what is in the human subject's best interests—the satisfaction of each of these consent criteria is heightened in research in comparison to clinical care.

Competence to consent to service as a research subject is essential. Surrogate consent for incompetent patients to participate in research is allowable in most circumstances, but the requirements are heightened over those governing a competent patient's consent. Thus, most medical societies and commissions ruling on the criteria for surrogate consent for vulnerable patients (such as the cognitively impaired patient) to serve as research subjects require minimal risk and at least the possibility that the research can directly help the subject.[27,28] No such criteria are ordinarily required for voluntary consent by the competent human subject. The heightened criteria are designed to protect vulnerable research subjects who otherwise may be at risk of exploitation or harm because of their condition.[29]

The criterion for what counts as adequate information transmitted from the investigator to the research subject is similarly heightened. Rather than relying on the reasonable person standard of consent as is customary in clinical care, the standard in human research requires the use of detailed written material in nearly every case. The investigator must ensure that the patient understands the nature of the research and the specific role of the human subject. The written material must include an understandable, accurate, and explicit statement of the risks and potential benefits to the human subject from participating, a clause that clarifies that the subject may withdraw from the research at any time without penalty, and the name and telephone number of the responsible person to contact for any questions or problems.[26]

As is true in consent for clinical care, consent for human research participation is a process and not an event. The signature on the consent form is not the consent itself but merely a formalization of a previous consent process. Because of the technicalities of clinical research, the investigator has a special duty to answer the potential subject's questions clearly, fully, and understandably.

The criterion of absence of coercion is more stringent in research consent than in treatment consent. Coercion for research consent can be exerted in a subtle fashion that requires vigilance. It is unfortunately common in many medical centers for a patient's treating physician also to be the clinical investigator. This situation of dual agency creates a conflict of interest or at least a conflict of obligation.[30] The physician–investigator is conflicted between a duty to act in the patient's best interest and the desire to use the patient to further a research goal. That conflict consciously or subconsciously can affect how the physician–investigator frames the issue of participation in the research study to the patient–subject. Moreover, many patients will defer the decision of whether to consent to serve as research subjects to their physicians whom they trust implicitly. Or they may provide consent out of a sense of gratitude to their physician rather than from a sense of altruism.

The problem of dual agency is most troublesome, however, when it helps create and perpetuate the 'therapeutic misconception' in the patient's mind: that the true goal of the study is to help the patient's condition.[31] Despite the fact that conscientious physician–investigators attempt to explain that the patient–subject's role in the research is as an experimental subject to increase knowledge, many patients—especially those who are desperate for a possible effective treatment—continue to believe that the goal of their participation is to help their condition. The plight of 'desperate volunteers' raises the questions of implicit coercion, whereby severely ill patients may feel they have no other choice than to consent to participate in the study because, in their mind, it offers the latest and best treatment. The circumstance of dual agency adds further ethical duties to the physician–investigator to compassionately and honestly counsel the patient–subject to help dispel the therapeutic misconception.[31]

The Code of Helsinki recognizes that investigators may be conflicted in their roles and requires that an independent body approve and supervise the participation of the human subject to protect the welfare of the patient–subject.[25] In the United States this body is called the institutional review board (IRB) and in Europe and elsewhere is generally called the research ethics committee. Many of the rules of operation of these bodies have been enshrined in law. For example, United States regulations govern the operation of the IRB to require certain research conduct with respect to human subjects. In that regard, the IRB has three principal roles:[32]

1. To certify and document that the patient's full and free informed consent has been obtained
2. To demonstrate that the risks to the research subject are outweighed by the totality of potential benefits to the subject and future patients
3. To protect the privacy, confidentiality, dignity, and welfare of the human research subject

Empirical studies of the success of investigators in obtaining proper consent from human research subjects reveal discouraging results. Studies have shown that investigators spend insufficient time on the process of education of the patient in the details of the subject's participation.[33] Even when sufficient time has been spent, other studies have found that many subjects fail to understand the information in consent forms,[34] the concept of randomization,[35] or the difference between a clinical trial and ordinary therapy.[31] Thus, the theoretical requirements for an ethically acceptable consent often are not fully realized in practice.

Some research protocols pose unique difficulties for investigators to obtain consent. For example, consent for research on emergency conditions creates the same logistic difficulty in obtaining consent as in emergency medical treatment. But whereas treating physicians can employ the emergency treatment doctrine to provide patients needing emergency treatment with implied consent, no such doctrine authorizes investigators to conduct research on patients with emergency conditions. Recognizing the intractability of this problem and the benefits to society accrued in conducting emergency research, the United States Food and Drug Administration and the Department of Health and Human Services have propounded guidelines exempting human subject consent in research for emergency conditions if the research protocol qualifies and the investigators follow clearly stipulated guidelines.[36] Some of these guidelines may be relevant to certain research protocols in palliative care in which a patient–subject's consent cannot be obtained in a timely manner or at all.

REFERENCES

1. Faden R, Beauchamp TL, King NM. A History and Theory of Informed Consent. Oxford University Press, New York, 1986.
2. Culver CM, Gert B. Basic ethical concepts in neurologic practice. Semin Neurol 1984;4:1–8.
3. Gert B, Culver CM, Clouser KD. Bioethics: A Return to Fundamentals. Oxford University Press, New York, 1997:195–216.
4. Malenka DJ, Baron JA, Johansen S, et al. The framing effect of relative and absolute risk. J Gen Intern Med 1993;8:543–548.
5. Murphy DJ. Do-not-resuscitate orders: time for re-appraisal in long-term-care institutions. JAMA 1988;260:2098–2101.
6. Brock DW. The ideal of shared decision making between physicians and patients. Kennedy Inst Ethics J 1991;1:28–47.
7. Sherlock R. Reasonable men and sick human beings. Am J Med 1986;80:2–4.
8. Schneiderman LJ, Arras JD. Counseling patients to counsel physicians on future care in the event of patient incompetence. Ann Intern Med 1985;102:693–698.
9. Bernat JL. Ethical Issues in Neurology, 2nd Ed. Butterworth–Heinemann, Boston, 2002:85–88.
10. Buchanan AE, Brock DW. Deciding For Others: The Ethics of Surrogate Decision Making. Cambridge University Press, Cambridge, 1989:112–116.
11. Seckler AB, Meier DE, Mulvihill M, et al. Substituted judgment: how accurate are proxy predictions? Ann Intern Med 1991;115:92–98.
12. Sulmasy DP, Terry PB, Weisman CS, et al. The accuracy of substituted judgments in patients with terminal diagnoses. Ann Intern Med 1998;128:621–629.
13. Pearlman RA, Jonsen A. The use of quality of life considerations in medical decision-making. J Am Geriatr Soc 1985;33:344–352.
14. Uhlmann RF, Pearlman RA. Perceived quality of life and preferences for life-sustaining treatment in older adults. Arch Intern Med 1991;151:495–497.
15. American Academy of Pediatrics Committee on Bioethics. Informed consent, parental permission, and assent in pediatric practice. Pediatrics 1995;95:314–317.
16. Ross LF. Health care decision making by children. Is it in their best interest? Hastings Cent Rep 1997;27(6):41–45.
17. Holder AR. Minors' rights to consent to medical care. JAMA 1987;257:3400–3402.
18. American Academy of Neurology Ethics and Humanities Subcommittee. Consent issues in the management of cerebrovascular diseases. Neurology 1999;53:9–11.
19. Lidz CW, Meisel A, Osterweis M, Holden JL, Marx JH, Munetz MR. Barriers to informed consent. Ann Intern Med 1983;99:539–543.
20. Byrne DJ, Napier A, Cuschieri A. How informed is signed consent? Br Med J 1988;296:839–840.
21. Jecker N, Caresse J, Pearlman R. Caring for patients in cross-cultural settings. Hastings Cent Rep 1995;25(1):6–14.
22. Macklin R. Ethical relativism in a multicultural society. Kennedy Inst Ethics J 1998;8:1–22.
23. Kuczewski M, McCruden PJ. Informed consent: does it take a village? The problem of culture and truth telling. Cambridge Q Healthcare Ethics 2001;10:34–46.
24. Shuster E. Fifty years later: the significance of the Nuremberg Code. N Engl J Med 1997;337:1436–1440.
25. World Medical Association. Declaration of Helsinki: ethical principles for medical and research involving human subjects. JAMA 2000;284:3043–3045.
26. Emanuel EJ, Wendler D, Grady C. What makes clinical research ethical? JAMA 2000;283:2701–2711.
27. American College of Physicians. Cognitively impaired subjects. Ann Intern Med 1989;111:843–848.
28. National Bioethics Advisory Commission. Research Involving Persons with Mental Disorders That May Affect Decision Making Capacity. Vol 1. National Bioethics Advisory Commission, Rockville, MD, 1998.
29. Dresser R. Mentally disabled research subjects: the enduring policy issues. JAMA 1996;276:67–72.
30. Shortell SM, Waters TM, Clarke KWB, Budetti PP. Physicians as double agents: maintaining trust in an era of multiple accountabilities. JAMA 1998;280:1102–1108.
31. Appelbaum PS, Roth LH, Lidz CW, et al. False hopes and best data: consent to research and the therapeutic misconception. Hastings Cent Rep 1987;17(2):20–24.
32. American Academy of Neurology Ethics and Humanities Subcommittee. Ethical issues in clinical research in neurology: advancing knowledge and protecting human research subjects. Neurology 1998;50:592–595.
33. Lantos J. Informed consent: the whole truth for patients? Cancer 1993;72:2811–2815.
34. Lavelle–Jones C, Byrne DJ, Rice P, Cuschieri A. Factors affecting quality of informed consent. Br Med J 1993;306:885–890.
35. Snowdon C, Garcia J, Elbourne D. Making sense of randomization: responses of parents of critically ill babies to random allocation of treatment in a clinical trial. Soc Sci Med 1997;45:1337–1355.
36. Wichman A, Sandler AL. Research involving critically ill subjects in emergency circumstances: new regulations, new challenges. Neurology 1997;48:1151–1155.

PART 6
GENERAL ASPECTS

Psychological Aspects

Richard Sloan

Many neurological diagnoses are debilitating to patients, both physically and psychologically. The aim of the clinician should be to attend to both aspects, so that the patient can be helped to readjust to an acceptable quality of life with the minimum of distress. Herein lies the true art of medicine.

CASE HISTORY

During a hospital admission, Michael's neurologist had just diagnosed motor neurone disease/amyotrophic lateral sclerosis. Michael's wife had previously indicated that, if it was something serious, she didn't want him to be told. She was angry when the neurologist questioned the ethics of this, saying that she knew Michael better than he did.

Michael looked withdrawn and depressed on the ward round. Opinion amongst the staff was divided as to whether he ought to be told the bad news or not, with strong feelings being expressed on both sides. After a particularly difficult month when several of his patients on the unit had died, the neurologist felt under attack from all sides and seriously wondered why he had chosen such a stressful career in medicine.

INTRODUCTION

The diagnosis of a neurological illness and its aftermath can have profound effects on all those involved—patients, their families, and also the health-care professionals looking after them. Patients' reactions can vary from acceptance through naive ambivalence to abject horror. Dealing with the emotional reactions of patients has been highlighted as one of the most stressful areas for oncologists.[1] The same is likely to be true for progressive neurological disorders.

In cancer, there is research evidence that the patients who cope better overall are those who ask for and are given accurate information about their illness and treatment, confront their situation rather than deny it, and have a positive attitude in adversity—the 'fighting spirit'.[2] Doctors can either facilitate or unwittingly block this if they lack the necessary communication skills to detect and deal with individual patients' concerns or distress.[3] It is therefore useful for professionals to be aware of how, and how not, to respond to the various reactions they will come across.

PATIENT REACTIONS

Anxiety

Anxiety in patients or families is common and can be infectious to the professionals caring for them. It may be obvious or concealed, for instance, as anger. When recognized, it is important to openly acknowledge it. 'There seems to be something bothering you—are you able to tell me about it?' may clear the air and allow things to move on. Unaddressed anxiety may result in the consultation becoming dysfunctional or confrontational.

Much anxiety is temporary and helped by talking things through. Many patients say that the most stressful time of their disease journey is the uncertainty before the diagnosis is made and that receiving a difficult or life-threatening diagnosis was easier than previously having no diagnosis to come to terms with at all. Aware of this, clinicians can do much to reduce the psychological pain by keeping the patient as informed as possible. Many official complaints stem from patients feeling insufficiently informed. Even where there is no news as yet, it helps to acknowledge the anxiety this creates.

In other cases, simple explanations may be insufficient and the anxiety may be longer term. This may be the result of the patient's past experiences, poor social support, or ineffective coping mechanisms. Having access to specialist help is important. There is increasing evidence that short-term interventions such as cognitive therapy, as practised by clinical psychologists and others, can reduce distress to patients during difficult times.[4] This challenges negative assertions in the patient's mind such as not seeing any hope for the future, and helps them regain control of those aspects of their life they still have influence over. Anxiolytic medication may be helpful in the short term but inadvisable long-term because of the risk of physical dependence.

Anger

Strong emotions are commonly felt, if not always voiced, by neurological patients and their families. Anger may come out at various stages in the disease process—when there is a perceived delay in a diagnosis being made, the receiving of bad news, the loss of independence as the disease progresses. It can be an expression of anxiety or fear; part of the 'fight or flight' response. Health-care professionals may react in various ways to anger. If criticism is perceived, the professional may take this personally and become defensive. A confrontation may develop, even when the source of the anger was actually nothing to do with the recipient. Alternatively, professionals may avoid acknowledging the anger, because of fear of confrontation, by changing the subject or literally walking away. This can further inflame the situation, leaving the patient feeling more aggrieved.

In contrast to the business world, few clinicians or nurses receive specific training in how to deal with conflict or anger in their clients, but there are guidelines which can reduce the stress to both patients and professionals alike.

1. Allow the person to ventilate their anger. It is better to ask 'What has happened?' rather than say 'Are you angry?', as some may feel guilty about their anger and deny it.

2. Ask the patient to clarify what exactly they are angry about—it may not be what you think.

3. Empathize with them (e.g. 'I can understand that the wait for a diagnosis must have been very stressful'). Empathizing is not the same as admitting fault in yourself or another professional. It is a genuine expression of sympathy for the difficult experience the person has gone through. This can quickly defuse an escalating situation and restore trust.

4. Offer to explain the situation as you see it. This may correct misunderstandings or reveal new information which helps the patient to see things differently. If there has been a genuine error or misunderstanding on your part, patients generally appreciate and respect an apology. There is evidence that litigation is less likely if an appropriate apology is offered and medical insurance companies often encourage this. Do *not* apologize for a colleague—if you weren't there at the point of dispute, you can't be sure of what actually took place. Encourage the patient to discuss the issue with them directly or, if appropriate, offer to find out more information yourself to clarify things.

5. If the person's anger is out of control and you feel threatened or angry yourself, say that you cannot address things with them right now until things have settled down and depart.

Denial

This is a common reaction in all of us to adversity. It may present as the patient who has been told of a serious illness but who apparently hasn't taken it on board. It is a way of coping, and health-care workers must respect this. Forcing a patient to accept a difficult reality before they are ready to risks removing their main psychological support system and rejection of the messenger. In a terminal illness, many realize their fate gradually rather than straightaway and, unless the patient is initially insistent, this is probably kinder. In a few, denial may persist throughout the illness. However, as the illness progresses, especially if it has debilitating consequences, most denial will inevitably be challenged and patients will start to ask questions. It is important that they are given this opportunity in order to better adapt to their circumstances, both practically and psychologically.

Questions such as 'Is there anything more you want to ask me about your illness?' or 'How do you see things going?' allow the patient to ask for more information if they want to, or say that everything is fine if they are still coping through denial. The patient thus dictates the pace at which information is given. This is in contrast to the practice of telling every patient every detail as soon as the diagnosis is made.

The minority who choose to deny throughout the course of their disease are often the most challenging for families and professional carers. Unrealistic demands or requests may be difficult to comply with (e.g. the patient who insists on their family booking a foreign holiday for them when they are patently not safe to travel). Friction and conflict can often result. Sensitive and gentle handling of the request, with an honest discussion of the practical difficulties, is less risky than humoring the patient and facing the consequences later. Other more realistic goals can be suggested as alternatives so that the patient is not left without hope of achieving anything.

Depression

Depression is sometimes described as occurring when the gap between a person's expectations of life and reality is large. The realization that life may be reduced in quality or quantity by a neurological condition could lead to such a gap. This may occur soon after diagnosis, or later when the full implications of the illness become apparent.

There has been much debate over the difference between natural sadness as a result of a distressing diagnosis and clinical depression warranting professional intervention. The textbook features of clinical depression may help—lack of motivation, hopelessness, sleep disturbance, loss of appetite, diurnal variation in mood. However, a depressed mood lasting more than a few weeks, even in the absence of these features, may warrant a trial of antidepressant therapy. Asking the person 'Do you *feel* depressed?' is a useful screening question. Some will say not, recognizing the episode as appropriate sadness during the readjustment process.

Non-pharmacological therapies such as cognitive therapy have been shown to be just as effective as drug treatments, and in some cases more so.[4] Patients can thus be helped to modify their life goals to more achievable ones in the circumstances and thereby narrow the expectation–reality gap.

Professionals can reduce the risk of depression in several ways. There is evidence that emotional distress is more likely to occur in patients deprived of information or the opportunity to express their concerns.[5] Where this occurs, they may fantasize negatively about the outcome of their illness or feel isolated and helpless. Regularly offering to discuss any concerns counteracts this and leaves the patient feeling supported and cared for, even when the future is uncertain.

End-of-life Issues

Many patients and families, even if they know that an illness is life-threatening, often cope by 'living for today' and not worrying much about what the future holds. This makes sense, as those who can't think of anything but death and dying may be unable to make the best of what time is left.

However, there will come a time when, because of progressive weakness or other physical symptoms, difficult issues are raised in peoples' minds. It helps if professionals are prepared for the sort of questions they may be asked and how to respond.

PROGNOSIS

In relation to terminal illnesses, clinicians or nurses often have difficulty when asked 'How long?' Most people ask, not expecting a precise answer, but hoping to have some idea as to how to pace themselves or when to tackle unfinished business. It is helpful to first clarify why the person has asked. It may be because the patient needs to know when the time is right to call a son over from abroad to say their goodbyes but doesn't want to do so prematurely. A relative may need guidance as to whether it is reasonable to book a holiday and that the patient will be all right whilst they are away. This way, the question may be more directly answered, with the proviso that things can change unpredictably.

Giving a prognosis of a specific number of days, weeks, or months can be problematic. If it turns out to be an overestimate, the patient may feel resentful and deceived. Where the prediction is an underestimate, patients and their families often experience fear and trepidation as the deadline approaches, then passes. It is probably better to give a broad range of probable survival, such as 'months rather than years' or 'weeks rather than months', again with the proviso that events can prove physicians wrong.

In this context, patients and families often appreciate guidance on the indicators that suggest the disease is catching up with them. This is so that they can recognize for themselves when it is, or is not, happening. In the absence of any other reversible cause, rapidly increasing weakness and reduction of functional capacity are the most consistent indicators of approaching death.

FEAR OF DEATH

Asking 'Are you fearful for the future?' may reveal hitherto undisclosed fears about the dying process. Again, it helps to clarify exactly what the fear is for that individual. For some, it may be the assumption that pain and suffering are inevitable sooner or later. Patients with motor neurone disease/amyotrophic lateral sclerosis may have heard that they could choke to death. Without telling untruths, it should be possible to reassure patients and families that these sorts of horrific deaths are rare and, with proper access to expert symptom control, suffering can be avoided. This may be difficult for professionals who have witnessed a dreadful death and do not feel confident in dealing with a recurrence. However, early advice from palliative care specialists to discuss contingency plans in the event of distressing symptoms can pre-empt this. The 'Breathing Space Kit' was developed by the Motor Neurone Association of Great Britain specifically to provide quick and easy treatment of distressing choking or breathlessness.

Patients may gain comfort from knowing the common accounts of people who have had a 'near death experience'. Those who have been successfully resuscitated after being clinically dead after a cardiopulmonary arrest describe a pleasant, not distressing, feeling of calm and tranquility.

For others, the fear of what happens after death may be the issue. This may be helped, if the person agrees, by talking with a minister of religion.

The Concept of Hope

When faced with adversity, humans often avoid going to pieces by holding out hope for better days. In the case of serious illness, hope for a cure may persist, even where this is highly unlikely. Professionals should be wary of killing all hope—this may remove a useful coping mechanism. Nor should professionals be over-optimistic as this can jeopardize trust when reassurances turn out to be false.

The skill for the health-care professional is in helping the patient adjust their goals realistically to their situation at a pace which is acceptable to them. This may mean consoling the person who is finally realizing that they are never going to regain full functional capacity whilst giving them realistic hope that mobility can still be maintained, to a lesser degree, in a wheelchair.

For those coming to realize their mortality from a neurological disease, pledging of continuing support and comfort whatever happens is important. Saying 'I'm afraid there's nothing more we can do' may be true in terms of arresting the disease, but can be devastating to the patient who may conclude that they are condemned to a lonely, painful demise. There is *always* something that professionals can do to avoid this and maintain hope for a comfortable, peaceful death.

PROFESSIONAL GUIDELINES

Breaking Bad News

Bad news is defined as news that significantly and negatively alters a person's expectation of their future. On the diagnosis of a condition that can be easily treated, explaining this is relatively straightforward, but where the illness is difficult to treat or might result in death, the task is much more stressful and challenging.

Breaking bad news is difficult for the following reasons:
- Fear of doing it badly
- Fear of unleashing strong emotions such as anger or crying
- Fear of getting blamed for the bad news
- Fear of having failed the patient medically
- Being reminded of one's own mortality

Research shows that the majority of patients *do* want information about their illness even if the news is not good.[6] A small minority would not want to be given any negative information at any stage. The challenge is to find out what the patient's information preferences are at that particular time so that they neither feel deprived nor overwhelmed.

Many doctors still believe that communication skills for breaking bad news cannot be taught and can only be learnt on the job. However, there *are* guidelines that help make it easier for both parties.[7,8]

The factors to consider, in order, are as follows:

1. The setting
Privacy is essential, so that the patient can feel free to ask difficult questions without worrying if others are listening in. Discussing sensitive issues on the open ward is a potential breach of confidentiality. There should be no interruptions: the phone should be off the hook and bleepers handed to someone else for taking messages.

Patients often say that they would have liked to have had the option of having someone else with them when the news was broken, such as a relative or nurse. This may be helpful for picking up pieces afterwards. The patient can also check out with the other person details they may not have taken in fully the first time. When it is known that the results of investigations are likely to be through on a certain day, the patient should be asked in advance if they would like to have someone else there with them.

Some would say that these preparations suggest to the patient that the news is bound to be bad. However, it could be argued that this is good practice whether the news is good *or* bad.

2. Finding out what the patient knows or suspects
Finding out what the patient understands so far helps gauge the pace of the consultation and where the patient is starting from. Some patients may genuinely have no idea that there is anything seriously wrong; others may be terrified that they are going to die next week. 'What have you made of things so far?' is a good opening question.

3. Finding out how much more they want to know
Although the majority *will* want more information, a small minority would be devastated if told bad news at any time. 'Some people wish to know everything about their condition and others just what the doctor's treatment plan is. Which camp do you fall into?' Those who habitually cope by using denial will relate to the latter and be spared unnecessary distress.

4. Firing a warning shot
Where the patient is asking for more information, it is still important to signal that difficult news is coming before disclosing it. This lessens the blow for those still relatively unsuspecting. 'I'm afraid that the results of your investigations are not what I was hoping for.' There should then be a pause during which the doctor gauges the patient's reaction. If they look shocked, ask what is going through their mind. If in doubt as to whether to continue, ask whether they want more information or time to think about it. Where the patient says 'What do you mean, not what you were hoping for?', this is a clear request for more information and it is right to proceed.

5. Providing information in stages

It is better to give the patient small pieces of information at a time and check whether they have understood before going on to the next bit of detail—'Does this make sense to you?' or 'Do you want me to go over that again?' Launching into a monologue only to find out that the patient froze after the first sentence is a waste of time. Again, if the patient looks shocked, ask what is on their mind and check out whether they are ready to go on or not.

Where the diagnosis is inevitably fatal, this may be too much to handle straightaway. Unless they ask directly, it may be better to offer to see the patient again and find out how much more information they are ready for.

6. Acknowledging and responding to the patient's reaction to the news

When the patient looks shocked or cries, the messenger's response is crucial. Carrying on through embarrassment will appear uncaring to the patient who will be unable to take anything more in anyway. Acknowledging the distress—'This must be shocking news'—gives the patient permission not to feel embarrassed, accepting that it is natural and understandable in the circumstances.

Try to find out exactly what the source of their distress is—'Can you bear to tell me what's going through your mind right now?' This allows them to decline if it is too difficult to talk about. The reasons for the distress may seem obvious, but may be different for different people, based on previous concepts and experiences. It is an opportunity to correct misunderstandings. If the patient is expressing undue pessimism, such as thinking they are going to die next week, appropriate reassurance can be given that this is not the case.

7. Making arrangements for follow-up

It is important at the end of the consultation to make specific arrangements for the patient to be seen again and have the opportunity to clarify or ask more. Where there is no definitive medical treatment, it is tempting to tell the patient they don't need to come back again, but this can be very frightening.

Apart from offering to see them yourself, other sources of information or support should be mentioned such as disease-specific booklets, access to specialist neurological nurses, patient associations, or the patient's family physician (suitably informed). Even when there are no treatment options, this conveys to patients the feeling that they are being supported, not abandoned.

Telling Children Difficult News

Children are often subjected to collusion (see later section). The desire of parents to protect them from the difficult news that one of them has a fatal neurological illness is understandable. Yet there is strong evidence that children suffer more, both in the short and long term, if not prepared for an expected death.[9] They can be more susceptible to anxiety and depression for years afterwards and may grow up finding it difficult to make relationships with other adults, having been deceived at such an important time in their lives. Often, parents rationalize that the child is too young to understand. However, children as young as 4–5 years of age can understand the meaning and permanency of death and can sense, without being told, that something is seriously amiss within the family. When not given the opportunity to verbalize their anxieties, children often exhibit some sort of behavioral change as a symptom of their underlying unease. Excessive passivity or attention seeking may be put down to 'their age'. If the child is to be spared unnecessary added distress, such behavior is an indication for addressing the situation rather than disciplining the child.

Parents and professionals often do not know how to approach this sensitive subject and it is, therefore, often not addressed at all until after the death. In the absence of factual information, children often fantasize to fill the gap, making up reasons in their own minds for a parent's deteriorating health. They may blame themselves, concluding that it is their fault because they were naughty the other week.

In fact, children have a remarkable capacity for acceptance of difficult news and carrying on with life relatively normally provided that they are reassured that they will continue to be loved and cared for. The difficulty usually lies in the minds of the adults who fear causing more harm or becoming upset themselves. Helpful advice may be available from bereavement workers or child psychologists for parents. This may take the form of a storybook that parents can read with the child,[10] talking about the death of someone close to them, the feelings and reactions this causes in themselves and those around them. It opens up the subject so that the child can ask if there are other issues troubling them.

It is vital that health-care professionals are aware of such resources locally and can sensitively inform parents of the negative consequences of not talking honestly with children and answering their concerns.

Communication Skills

Patients consistently rate 'good communicator' as one of the essential qualities of a competent clinician.[6] Unfortunately, this is often not acknowledged by the professionals, with more emphasis placed on the technical aspects of diagnosis and disease management. The traditional medical model pays little attention to addressing each patient's personal agenda. Patients who feel they have been given inadequate information are more likely to complain. Communication is a two-way process and involves gauging and responding to the individual needs of patients rather than giving out the same information to everyone.

Unfortunately, many professionals believe they are good communicators when they are not, and that communication skills cannot be taught. They may come over to their patients as detached, cold, or arrogant. Conversely, patients who feel they have been adequately informed by a caring physician who gives them time to express their concerns experience less symptoms, both physical and psychological.[5] This does not significantly increase individual consultation time and results in greater professional job satisfaction. Like any skill, communication *can* be taught and pitfalls avoided. Those who have been trained in such skills are able to pick up and act on the verbal and non-verbal cues that patients display—so-called 'active listening'—thereby preventing misunderstandings from escalating. Bad outcomes are better tolerated by patients when their carers are seen as good providers of information.[11]

The overall conclusion must be that communication skills are good for both patient and physician well-being. As with all clinical skills, they should be expertly taught, regularly practised, and reviewed throughout a professional's career. Herein lies the challenge for medical education if mutual understanding between patients and health-care professionals is to be improved.

Coping with Collusion

Collusion is defined as a secret agreement to conspire to deceive. In health care, it usually takes the form of a relative asking the doctor not to tell the patient they have a serious illness. The colluder's motive is usually the protection of loved ones from distressing news. This instinctive action, well-meaning though it is, usually results in more distress in the long term—both for the patient, who may become isolated and anxious when getting less well, and for the colluder, as secrets become harder to maintain as the patient's health declines. If not recognized or addressed, the situation also becomes more stressful for the professionals involved. They become torn between being truthful to the patient and incurring the wrath of the colluder. It is easy for an unsuspecting professional, unaware of the collusion, to innocently disclose information and be castigated by the colluder.

Often, because of lack of training, professionals leave well alone and everyone suffers the consequences. There are, however, guidelines to prevent the situation escalating. They are based on two fundamental ethical premises:

- Patients have the right to medical information about themselves if they want it
- Patients have the right to decline medical information about themselves if they do *not* want it

The guidelines aid negotiation with the colluder so that you can find out which category the patient is in and help the colluder to understand the disadvantages of maintaining the deception. Because colluders' instinctive feelings are very strong, it is crucial to first understand and openly acknowledge why they are doing it. This prevents a confrontation developing.

GUIDELINES FOR DEALING WITH COLLUSION

1. Ascertain from the colluder why they have chosen to do it and acknowledge their reasons. If they fear the patient going to pieces, do they have any evidence from the past that this might indeed happen? Where there *is* justified concern, the clinician

should rightly be more cautious in his subsequent dialogue with the patient.

2. Find out the cost to the colluder of the collusion. Colluders may not immediately be aware of the stress on themselves or the strain on their relationship with the patient—'How have things changed between you since he got his illness?'

3. Discuss the down side to collusion—for patient and colluder. Although relatively easy to maintain at first, collusion usually becomes more and more stressful with time.

4. Negotiate with the colluder to see the patient on your own to find out how they are feeling about their situation and whether there is anything else they wish to know. Promise that you will not force information on them that they do not wish to know. However, most patients do want to know in time and, if asked, you should give honest answers. If the colluder denies access to the patient, it may be better to remain vigilant and use opportunities as they present themselves to remind the colluder of the escalating stress as it develops.

5. Interview the patient alone. If they are in denial and are not asking for any more information, allow them to maintain this coping mechanism, saying that they can always ask anything in the future if they wish to. More often, they will appreciate the opportunity to find out more, but may have been keeping quiet because of the imposed block to communication. Many patients will have come to the conclusion that their illness is a serious one (even though this has not been openly discussed) from the non-verbal clues from physicians and family. Patients often express relief when things are finally out in the open. Offer to talk with the patient and family together to share what has just been discussed.

6. Talk with patient and family together. This facilitates open communication between the family members and gets over the fear of how to break the ice.

Psychosexual Problems

Patients with progressive neurological illness often face a series of losses as their illness progresses—loss of work, mobility, independence, role as husband/parent/breadwinner: all the normal things which adults take for granted. Those around the patient will be aware of this and will wish to help compensate for those things the patient can no longer do for themselves. However, depending on the prevailing culture within families or their health-care professionals, loss of sexual function may not be acknowledged or helped. Much silent suffering can result which compounds the other losses.

For couples in a stable relationship, guilt on the part of the patient in depriving their partner of an important part of their relationship can occur. Patients who are single may fear never being attractive to a potential partner ever again. Changes in bodily appearance or image can induce self-loathing.

Professionals may feel inadequately equipped to assess or help people with sexual problems as a result of chronic illness. They may rationalize and say that it is none of their business and a private matter between the patient and their partner. By default, patients will pick up the vibes that this is not a valid area for discussion and will be unlikely to ask for help in the first place. If health-care professionals are concerned with health in its fullest meaning, this could be viewed as an abdication of responsibility. The skill, as with breaking bad news, is finding out how much the patient or their partner wants to discuss potentially sensitive issues.

Asking a question such as 'How has your illness affected your relationship with your husband/wife?' gives the patient permission to disclose as much or as little as they feel they want to. For simple issues such as concern that sexual activity may cause harm to the patient, simple reassurance may be all that is required. Couples can be encouraged to see that sexuality is not just about the sexual act and that closeness and affection are also very important and still practical. Where distress is still being experienced because of sexual dysfunction, it is important that the professionals know of local sources where a proper assessment of both physical and psychological factors can be made and practical help offered.[12]

Professional Burnout

Pressures on health-care staff have increased in recent decades. The previous 'doctor knows best' attitude is gradually being replaced by patients wanting to take an active role in discussing their diagnosis and management. With many neurological illnesses being unamenable to cure, the stresses are greater still. The cumulative effects of this can lead to so-called 'burnout' with serious dysfunction in the professional's working and private life. What are the factors that reduce the likelihood of this happening?

Research has shown that lack of a social network outside of work increases the risk of burnout in those dealing with the terminally ill.[13] So, it is important to counterbalance this with routine life-enhancing activities or hobbies.

Whilst it may not be fashionable in the macho world of medicine to share one's anxieties or perceived failures with colleagues, peer group support, either informal or formal, can counteract negative feelings and concerns.[14] Organizations that encourage this do so knowing that it ultimately results in better patient care from staff that feel respected and supported by their colleagues.

REFERENCES

1. Fallowfield LJ. Communication skills of oncologists. Forum: Trends Experi Med 1995;5(1):99–103.

2. Northouse LL. The impact of breast cancer on patients and husbands. Cancer Nurs 1989; 12: 276–284.

3. Ford S, Fallowfield LJ, Lewis S. Can oncologists detect distress in their out-patients and how satisfied are they with their performance during bad news consultations? Br J Cancer 1994;70:767–770.

4. Blackburn IM, Twaddle V. Cognitive therapy in action. Souvenir Press, London, 1996.

5. Roter DL, Hall JA, Kern DE, et al. Improving physicians' interviewing skills and reducing patients' emotional distress: a randomised clinical trial. Arch Intern Med 1995;155:1877–1884.

6. 'Patient-Centred Cancer Services?' What Patients Say. The National Cancer Alliance, Oxford, May 1996.

7. Walker G, Bradburn J, Maher J. Breaking Bad News. King's Fund Publishing, London, 1996.

8. Baile W, Buckman R. A Practical Guide to Communication Skills in Clinical Practice (CD-ROM). Medical Audio Visual Communications Inc., *dwc@mavc.com*

9. Black D. Childhood bereavement. Br Med J 1996;312:1496.

10. When Someone Special has Motor Neurone Disease. Motor Neurone Disease Association, UK, 1996. *www.mndassociation.org.*

11. Suchman AL, Roter DL, Green M, Lipkin M. Physician satisfaction with primary care office visits. Med Care 1993;31:1083–1092.

12. Association to Aid the Sexual and Personal Relationships of People with a Disability, 286 Camden Rd, London N7 OBJ.

13. Vachon, MLS. Motivation and stress experienced by staff working with the terminally ill. Death Education 1978;2:113–122.

14. Woolley H, Stein A, Forrest GC, Baum JD. Staff stress and job satisfaction at a children's hospice. Arch Dis Childhood 1989;64:114–118.

Chapter 39

Spirituality

Robert M. Taylor
Sharol L. Herr

SPIRITUALITY AND RELIGION
EMPIRIC STUDIES OF SPIRITUALITY
   AND RELIGION
SOURCES OF SPIRITUAL DISTRESS
Reflecting on the Past
Relating to the Present

Relating to the Future
SPIRITUALITY AND RELIGIOUSNESS IN
   NEUROLOGICAL DISEASE
THE NEUROLOGICAL TEAM AS
   SPIRITUAL CARE PROVIDERS
SUMMARY

Providing end-of-life care presents many challenges—some we learn about in our medical textbooks, whereas others we learn about primarily through our experience of observing, listening, and being present. Within the interdisciplinary approach to holistic care of the body, mind, and spirit in the provision of palliative care, we may witness not only the suffering and striving, but often the thriving of individuals. When we offer ourselves to others a transformation takes place allowing a breadth and depth of interaction and relationship rarely experienced in modern health care. The reaching out to others provides opportunities for awareness and growth in our usual and ordinary encounters as well. Spiritual care offers a dimension to medical care encouraging and supporting personal growth and transcendence beyond the physical experience. Opening ourselves up to these experiences will give us inspiration to continue on our course of caring.

CASE HISTORY

Sharon was just 31 when she came to the university neurology clinic complaining of severe back and left leg pain. Her medical history was otherwise unremarkable. She attributed the onset of her symptoms to an injury resulting from a fall three months previous, but her pain and weakness had progressed since then. Physical examination revealed some mild weakness of her left leg and a decreased left patellar reflex, and EMG showed evidence of fourth and fifth lumbar nerve root irritation. Sensory nerve conduction studies were normal and a MRI of the lumbar spine did not reveal any abnormality. Her pain remained severe and appeared out of proportion to any documented pathology and her poor response to adjuvant medications, but fair response to opiates led to concerns about drug abuse.

Sharon's weakness progressed slowly, eventually involving her right leg and left arm. EMGs documented more generalized denervation, but no fasciculations. Pain in the back and legs continued to be her most distressing symptom. The working diagnosis was motor neuron disease, but the lack of upper motor neuron signs suggested the possibility of a more benign syndrome.

During her three admissions to the university hospital over the next year, Sharon was not always treated well by the resident physicians. Despite her progressive symptoms, they tended to suspect her weakness was embellished. Furthermore, because her complaints of pain appeared out of proportion to her weakness and her pain could not be readily explained physiologically, drug-seeking behavior was suspected.

When Sharon's primary neurologist left the university, she followed him to his new practice.

He now admitted his patients to a large, non-profit, community hospital with an internal medicine training program. During two admissions to this hospital, she found she was treated with respect and her symptoms were taken at face value. After almost two years and several hospital stays, the diagnosis of amyotrophic lateral sclerosis (ALS) was made.

Sharon was estranged from her parents and two younger sisters after choosing a free-spirited lifestyle that conflicted with her family's values. Sharon lived several states away from her family and had not seen them in years. She lived in a small rural town with her boyfriend, who was physically disabled but able to assume primary support of Sharon. Her social history included a past history of alcohol and drug abuse.

Sharon and her family were of Jewish ancestry but not believers. As a small child she recalled having had several mystical encounters with seemingly real persons, who identified themselves as Jesus and Mary, that were very reassuring and comforting. Mary, in particular, was very nurturing. Her recollection was that, at the time, she did not perceive these figures as having any religious significance, since she believed she had never heard of Mary or Jesus before. For some time these encounters were secret to Sharon. However, one day, when her mother overheard her conversation with Mary, she chastised her severely. After that, she never saw Jesus or Mary again.

The belief system Sharon held as an adult integrated Jewish, Christian, and native American tenants and rituals. Sharon was creative and resourceful and had a way of drawing people to her. She was open and engaging and would actively seek out social and medical support. Throughout the course of her illness there were open discussions about the disease process and what would happen. Sharon strongly opposed any resuscitative measures and was confident that she would not want to be maintained on ventilatory support.

Sharon's condition progressed rapidly and after only two and a half years she presented to the emergency room with respiratory distress. After pulmonary consultation, and with encouragement from the neurologist, despite her prior reluctance, she agreed to a trial of tracheostomy and ventilatory support. Once she was stabilized on the portable ventilator she transferred to a local rehabilitation facility for teaching, prior to a planned discharge back to her apartment. However, after being in the nursing facility for three weeks, and finding life on the ventilator totally unsatisfactory, Sharon insisted on having the ventilator withdrawn. She was returned to the hospital for terminal weaning from the ventilator.

While at the rehabilitation facility Sharon had made contact with her parents and two sisters. Her mother and youngest sister had visited her during that time and her entire family came to the hospital to spend the last several days of Sharon's life with her. This was the first time that Sharon had shared a spiritual connection with her family. She spent time with her sisters, discussing art and writings. The spiritual dimension that developed was one of a connection with 'mother earth' and the 'great spirit'. Sharon and her mother were able to re-unite and bond in a way that had not happened in the past. Personal integrity and honesty were values that meant a lot to Sharon and her family, and the distance that had grown between them throughout the years seemed to fade away in the richness of Sharon's spiritual journey to her death.

As Sharon prepared for her death she engaged in many thoughtful discussions with her physicians and the hospital chaplain, with whom she had developed a relationship over the previous months. With the openness of the facility, its physicians and staff allowed Sharon the opportunity to search her soul as she proceeded on this journey. A major theme in Sharon's questioning was one of worthiness. She questioned her self-worth: 'Am I a worthy person in the universe?' 'Am I a good person?'

Identifying a legacy in her short life was also important. She had 'adopted' and mentored a young woman of whom she was very proud. The young woman was vibrant and accomplished and she felt that this would be her legacy, something well done. Broken relationships caused Sharon sadness and regret. She spent time making contact with those people, mending the torn fabric that had at one time held them close. Sharon requested contact with a rabbi and a priest in her dying. In many ways she was her own rabbi, teaching and affirming herself and her family. Sharon was a seeker, a woman trying to find her way in the world. She demonstrated great courage and inner strength. She had a confidence and faith that she was a part of something bigger, something that would live on after death. Indeed, she lives on in the hearts and minds of those who cared for her.

SPIRITUALITY AND RELIGION

Spirituality is most often defined as the desire for meaning and purpose in life.[1] Sometimes spirituality is defined also as including a sense of connectedness to others, the world as a whole, and a transcendent being or power.[2] At least in the former sense, because meaning and purpose are universal human concerns, spirituality may be considered a characteristic of all people. In the broader sense, spirituality will be important to most, if not all, people and will necessarily involve others such as family members, friends, or a religious community in the individual's experience of serious illness and dying.

Because serious illness and death raise profound questions about the ultimate meaning and purpose of life, a person's spirituality invariably plays a role in responding to and coping with the experience. If a seriously ill or dying person is religious, his or her religion will frequently serve both as an organizing principle for understanding the meaning of illness and death, as well as a support system for dealing with the situation. Furthermore, the professional carer's own spirituality or religion may influence his or her approach to terminal illness in general as well as interactions with particular dying patients. Thus it is essential that those caring for seriously ill and dying patients understand both the distinctions between spirituality and religious beliefs as well as the importance of these spheres of human experience to the patient and family or significant others.

The relationship between religion and spirituality is complex. Although historically spirituality was considered synonymous with religion, over the past few decades the meanings of the two concepts have gradually diverged. Both spirituality and religion are concerned with ultimate purposes and meanings. Religion has been defined as 'the totality of belief systems, an inner piety or disposition, an abstract system of ideas, and ritual practices'.[1] Although belief in God is an element of most religions, it is not a necessary component—the most notable exception being Buddhism. Nevertheless, religions typically provide an ordering of one's priorities and a framework for interpreting and understanding life and death. Traditionally, religion is conceived of as a communal activity with a defined history, representing a system of beliefs and practices which have served to organize the experience of its adherents and connect them to each other, the rest of

creation, and a divine or transcendent power. Thus, although religion necessarily includes spirituality, it generally is defined in a somewhat more restrictive way, emphasizing these communal and historical elements. Yet, one may speak of having a private or personal religion, in that one's spirituality may include a uniquely personal belief system incorporating one's relationship with humanity, the world, and a transcendent power, as well as personal ritual practices. A person's spirituality, therefore, may or may not include a specifically religious dimension.

Religion may serve two different, but related, functions for terminally ill patients: first, providing a core set of beliefs for understanding and interpreting important life events and, second, creating an ethical framework for medical decision making. Because religion often serves as a basis for understanding and interpreting critical life events, including illness and death, it would appear reasonable to assume that strong religious beliefs would correlate with less anxiety in the face of illness and death and increased acceptance of death. Yet research exploring the connection between religious belief and attitudes toward death have produced ambiguous results and conflicting interpretations.[1] Similarly, although religiously based ethical theories often appear to provide clear-cut guidelines for end-of-life decision making, the influence of religious values on clinical decisions is not straightforward. Certainly each of the great religions includes powerful moral imperatives and well-developed systems of ethical analysis. Yet they also may sometimes include ambiguities or controversial perspectives on difficult issues which create the possibility of uncertainty or conflict when wrenching emotional decisions are required. An example of the impact of religion on ethical decision making is the evidence from several studies that patients, physicians, and nurses who are more religious are less likely to endorse or participate in euthanasia or assisted suicide.[1] Furthermore, members of particular religious traditions, notably orthodox Judaism, Islam, and many fundamentalist Christians, are more likely than others to insist on continuing artificial hydration and nutrition for imminently dying patients.

A distinction is sometimes made between implicit meaning and found meaning; the former indicating the process by which medical information is collected and evaluated, the latter identifying the process of interpretation that permits one to comprehend the place of an event or illness in the context of one's own life. It is in this latter sense that the quest and desire for meaning are at the core of most definitions of spirituality and also in this sense that spirituality may serve as a resource for coping with terminal illness and death. The literature indicates not only that terminally ill patients report a greater spiritual orientation and outlook than either healthy persons or other hospitalized patients, but also that there is an association between spirituality and decreased psychosocial distress, as well as an enhanced sense of well-being and an increased quality of life.[1]

EMPIRIC STUDIES OF SPIRITUALITY AND RELIGION

Unfortunately, there is little data available about patients' attitudes and beliefs regarding the role of spirituality and religion in end-of-life care. In one recent study, Ehman et al.[3] surveyed 177 ambulatory patients at an academic pulmonary medicine clinic (an 83% response rate) and found that, although 83% reported a religious affiliation, only 51% reported that they considered themselves religious or very religious, whereas 13% reported that they were not religious. Yet 77% reported a belief in 'life after death' and 90% believed that prayer sometimes may influence recovery from an illness. Forty-five per cent stated that, if gravely ill, their spiritual or religious beliefs would influence their medical decisions, whereas 33% stated that their spiritual or religious beliefs would not and 22% were unsure. Asked whether, if they were gravely ill, they would want their physician to inquire as to whether they had spiritual or religious beliefs that would influence their medical decisions, 66% agreed or strongly agreed, while 9% disagreed, 7% strongly disagreed, and 18% had no opinion. Although this preference was not influenced by self-reported religiosity, 94% of those whose religious beliefs would influence their medical decisions wanted to be asked whereas, of those who did not have such beliefs, 48% would not want to be asked and 45% would

want to be asked. Only 15% of patients recalled a physician making such an inquiry. Interestingly, 13% thought that a physician should not inquire in case they might not agree with the patient's beliefs. Asked whether such an inquiry would strengthen their trust in their physician, 87% of those with beliefs that would influence their medical decisions agreed, compared to 45% of those without such beliefs.

The authors contrast their results with those obtained in three studies obtained in the early and mid 1990s, which showed only a minority of patients welcomed physician inquiry about religious or spiritual issues. These studies differed from the study of Ehman et al. in two important ways: first, the earlier studies surveyed patients in family practice clinics and, second, and probably more significantly, the earlier studies asked patients their preferences about more open-ended inquiries into their religious and spiritual beliefs. The authors speculate that patients are more likely to welcome inquiries into their religious and spiritual beliefs if these questions are framed in such a way that they indicate a legitimate medical reason for the inquiry.

Steinhauser et al.[4] surveyed seriously ill patients, recently bereaved family members, physicians, and other health-care workers, to investigate which factors each group considered the most important attributes of a good death. The questions asked included several with spiritual or religious implications. Among factors considered important by all groups (>70% agreement) that relate to spiritual or religious issues were maintaining one's dignity, having someone who will listen, saying goodbye to important people, having a nurse with whom one feels comfortable, having a physician who knows one as a whole person and with whom one can discuss fears, resolving unfinished business with family and friends, believing that one's family is prepared for one's death, and feeling prepared to die. Among those factors rated significantly more important by patients as opposed to physicians were being at peace with God (89% vs 65%), being able to help others (88% vs 44%), prayer (85% vs 55%), and feeling one's life is complete (80% vs 68%). Patients and physicians exhibited greater variation for several factors, including discussing spiritual beliefs with one's physician (important to 50% of patients and 49% of physicians), having a chance to talk about the meaning of death (58% and 66% respectively), discussing personal fears (61% and 88%), meeting with a clergy member (69% and 60%), knowing the timing of one's death (39% and 26%), and controlling the time and place of one's death (40% and 36%).

The results of this survey reinforce the importance of spiritual and religious issues for terminally ill patients and their families. However, while they indicate that physicians and other health-care workers generally understand the importance of these issues for patients, physicians may underestimate the importance to their patients of certain factors. Furthermore, these results indicate that while a majority of patients would appear to welcome discussing spiritual or religious issues with their physicians, this desire is by no means universal.

Cohen et al. recently reviewed the question of whether physicians should inquire into patient's religious and spiritual beliefs. They emphasize the need for the health-care team to be respectfully attentive to the religious and spiritual values of their patients while avoiding the implication that the care provided will be inappropriately influenced by the patient's specific religious or spiritual beliefs. They suggest that 'at a minimum' physicians should cover four areas to learn about spiritual or religious beliefs relevant to a patient's medical care:

> (1) whether the patient has religious or spiritual beliefs of general significance to him or her, (2) whether some or all of these beliefs are especially important to the patient, (3) how these beliefs might affect the patient's choices about medical care in general, and (4) how these beliefs affect the patient's treatment choices in this situation.[5]

Astrow et al. note that surveys indicate that physicians are significantly less likely than patients to express a belief in God (64% vs 95%). Yet they emphasize the importance of a broader perspective on illness, asserting that serious illness should be understood 'as both a biological fact and a spiritual challenge for all patients', encouraging health-care providers to attend to patients' religious and spiritual beliefs as an important part of providing optimal care for patients.[6]

SOURCES OF SPIRITUAL DISTRESS

When considering the patient who has advanced disease and is approaching the end of life, sources of spiritual distress can be looked at in terms of issues relating to the past, the present, and the future.[7]

Reflecting on the Past

As was noted in our case history, at the end of her life, Sharon was struggling with the issue of worthiness and a life well lived. The end of life is a time of reflection and drawing conclusions about what contribution was made in life. Worth can be evaluated in terms of relationships, accomplishments, contributions to society, work, and the legacy one has left. If in dying, the person perceives that they have not made a difference, their self-worth is devalued. Guilt can also be a source of spiritual distress when a person is dying and perceives that they will be judged or convicted by others or God for past wrongs. There may be an attempt to reconcile or remedy the wrong, to make amends, so that they may go forward peacefully to death. Reflecting on these wrongs may prompt a person to seek forgiveness or reconciliation to find peace. Acknowledging the past wrongs may be freeing in and of itself, to allow the person to find inner peace.

The past may also generate unrest and guilt for family and care givers. A sense of urgency can prompt resolution of differences and conflicts. If the guilt and shame related to the past is significant and perceived as insurmountable, the distance between the dying and others may actually become greater or at best remain strained. Guilt about failures and unfulfilled dreams can also cause spiritual distress—'If only I...' becomes a familiar lament.

Relating to the Present

In the here and now of the dying process, spiritual distress often revolves around the loss of function and roles that are familiar and comfortable and have given the individual meaning. This is disruptive for the patient and the patient's family. It is almost inevitable that when the role of the patient changes, so too do the roles of the family and/or caregiver. Physical changes begin to dictate function and dependency on others increases. Often an individual's meaning revolves around work and position and when this is disrupted personal worth is questioned. The meaning of a person's life may also be questioned when they cannot find meaning in the experience of illness and suffering. Openness to suffering having personal meaning is a difficult concept for our 21st-century culture. Victor Frankl said, 'To live is to suffer, to survive is to find meaning in the suffering.'[8]

In the experience of illness, psychological and social changes occur. These changes may include concern for maintaining standard of living, maintaining personal and professional contacts and relationships, loss of income, loss of function, and reliance on others to meet basic needs.

Relating to the Future

As we look toward dying, inevitably we must confront separation from others. Often religious beliefs provide a construct for understanding this separation and serve to offer a degree of conciliation or hope in accepting the separation. Acknowledging the separation gives an opportunity to look to the future for self and others. It allows for planning and completion of tasks that will provide for others and put 'affairs in order'. Having provided for others can allow a sense of satisfaction and completion.

SPIRITUALITY AND RELIGIOUSNESS IN NEUROLOGICAL DISEASE

The needs of patients with neurological disease will vary greatly, depending on their neurological condition, the rate of progression, their own individuality, previous experience, and family support. The challenges faced by Sharon, in the case history, highlight those faced by any person with a neurological disease. Several studies of people with amyotrophic lateral sclerosis (ALS) have considered the reactions and care of people as they face their

deterioration, and these studies may show the challenges of caring for people with advancing neurological disease.

ALS is a progressive disease, characterized by progressive weakness, but with preservation of cognitive function, leading to severe disability, inability to swallow, and respiratory failure, and invariably resulting in death, typically within three to five years of diagnosis (see Chapter 8). Although artificial hydration and nutrition (via percutaneous endoscopic gastrostomy—PEG) and respiratory support (via non-invasive assisted ventilation or tracheostomy and mechanical ventilation) are options for prolonging life, many patients refuse or discontinue these treatment options due to excessive burdens. Those who do choose them will nevertheless eventually die of complications of ALS. Because of the combination of inexorable physical deterioration and the preservation of awareness, patients with ALS are acutely conscious of their predicament and can rarely avoid making difficult life-and-death treatment decisions, creating the potential for great distress and suffering.

A recent study assessing the attitudes of patient with ALS and their caregivers toward assisted suicide[9] found that 56% of patients agreed with the statement 'Under some circumstances I would consider taking a prescription for a medicine whose sole purpose was to end my life'. Sixty-two per cent of caregivers said they would support the patient's decision for assisted suicide, and there was a 73% incidence of concordance between the patient's and caregiver's attitude toward assisted suicide. Patients who were willing to consider assisted suicide were more likely to be men, better educated, rated their quality of life lower, had a stronger sense of hopelessness, were more likely to refuse life-supporting treatment, and were more likely to have a desire to die and to have had recent thoughts of suicide. Both patients who would not consider assisted suicide and caregivers who would not support it were more likely to be religious on all measures, including church membership, frequency of religious practices, and importance of religion.

Data collected for the above study was further analyzed to evaluate patient and caregiver assessments of the patient's suffering and quality of life.[10] Twenty per cent of patients reported their suffering as 4 or greater on a 6-point Likert scale (1 = no suffering and 6 = terrible suffering). Suffering was statistically correlated with increasing pain, poorer quality of life, greater hopelessness, worsening functional status, and greater sense of being a burden to others. Psychological symptoms of depression correlated with increased suffering, but somatic symptoms of depression did not. Although the investigators found a strong correlation between self-reported suffering and poor quality of life (rated on an analogous 6-point Likert scale), they found that suffering correlated more strongly with the effects of the disease on their body and psyche, whereas quality of life was more strongly correlated with social factors. In fact, less social support was the only factor that correlated with poor quality of life but not suffering. Interestingly, there was a stronger concordance between caregiver and patient ratings of patient suffering than quality of life, suggesting that the concept of suffering may be more easily understood by others, or that suffering may elicit a greater empathic response from caregivers. However, there was no correlation between either suffering or quality of life, as reported by the patient, and religiousness or church membership.

Unfortunately, neither of the above studies attempted to assess patient or caregiver spirituality. However, taken together, these two studies suggest that, although religiousness and church membership may not alter a patient's perception of his or her suffering or quality of life, they may affect how the patient responds to the illness and the distress it causes.

A third recent study specifically investigated the impact of spirituality and religiousness on patients with ALS.[11] The investigators found an imperfect correlation between religiousness and spirituality; although those who were more religious tended to be more spiritual, those who were more spiritual but not more religious, were more likely to be female and less educated. Both religiousness and spirituality correlated with an increased sense of hope. More spiritual patients were less bothered by the possibility of not thinking after death, while more religious patients were less concerned with intellectual capacities declining with death and 'missing out on so much' after death. Correlations between treatment decisions and religiousness and spirituality included the finding that more religious patients were more likely to use Bi-Pap whereas more spiritual patients were less likely to use a PEG tube but more likely to have identified a health care proxy. Thus, the investigators concluded that both religiousness and spirituality offer a source of comfort to patients with ALS and may also affect treatment decisions.

THE NEUROLOGICAL TEAM AS SPIRITUAL CARE PROVIDERS

When the members of the team involved in the care of patients with advancing neurological disease view the person holistically and provide spiritual care, the encounter is transformed and becomes personal, whether the team member is a physician, nurse, physiotherapist, occupational therapist, speech therapist, or from another discipline. Spiritual care is an experience or encounter that can be used to comfort and allow expression. In the United States a study reported that 77% of hospitalized patients want the physician to attend to spiritual needs.[12] Although generally it is not recommended that the team members discuss religion, if there is a discovery that religious beliefs are shared and respected this can be a comfort to the patient. Spiritual care should be viewed as an experience or an encounter, not a prescription. Spiritual care can optimize expression and exploration of life and its meaning. Providing spiritual care may also bring comfort, convey respect and acceptance, and honor the patient as a unique individual. Being comfortable with providing spiritual care allows team members to explore their own spirituality and grow through the experiences of others.

The professional carer is often an agent of hope.[13] Through personal honesty and integrity they can guide individuals through painful and life-changing events and illness. They can acknowledge the significance and seriousness of an illness and at the same time honor hope and the potential of the unknown. Hopelessness has been identified as a strong predicator of adverse health outcomes and a common source of spiritual distress.

In palliative care, through developing trust and respect, the team members have the opportunity to be companions on the patient's journey with the opportunity to encourage and support the patient, especially if they have established a long-term relationship. The privilege is to be invited into such an intimate time of life experience. Serving as a facilitator for the patient to identify hopes and fears is a part of the 'companion' role and may require direct inquiry. Helping the patient identify short- and long-range goals, owing to the unpredictability of terminal and progressive illness, puts the team member in the position of spiritual mentor. Encouraging spiritual and religious practices or rituals of the patient can foster peace and comfort in palliative care.

One of the hallmarks of the palliative care model is the interdisciplinary team. There is often role blurring among the team members due to the trust that has been developed with the patient and family. The chaplain can serve as a mentor and support as team members become more comfortable with providing spiritual care themselves. Team members can be a resource to the patient and family in focusing on key areas of distress or unrest with the patient. The team should establish who will be completing a spiritual needs assessment. Several assessment tools are available in the literature. An assessment can be made of the sources of distress or worry to the patient and family by asking, 'What is your greatest concern?' A wealth of information can be obtained and help the health-care team focus on interventions that will be most meaningful to the patient.

Assessing the spiritual needs of the family can be as critical as assessing the patient's needs. Many times patients will come to a peaceful place, understanding their life is going to end. It may be very difficult for the family to come to this same comfort level for fear of being seen as abandoning the patient or giving up hope. Support to the family can facilitate the progress through grief and mourning after the patient's death. In the time of grief and bereavement the team can show their support by expressing sympathy.[14] This can be done personally, by phone, or by writing a note. Their other function in bereavement is to allow the survivors to express emotion, as listening and maintaining presence in the midst of the grief provides comfort and allows healing to begin.

A barrier to physicians and other team members providing spiritual care is differing values and beliefs. Allowing the patient the opportunity to identify his needs rather than relying on intuition or personal expectations can increase the comfort level of the professionals. Maintaining tunnel vision of clinical issues can also impede the provision of spiritual care. Choosing a spiritual care-giving mentor to confide in and provide feedback can, over time, help decrease personal discomfort with providing spiritual care. Sharing spiritual self and remaining open to a dimension beyond the physical can help the team members develop and nurture personal spirituality.

In 'Anatomy of an Illness' Norman Cousins wrote:

> Death is not the ultimate tragedy of life. The ultimate tragedy of life is depersonalization—dying in an alien and sterile area, separated from the spiritual nourishment that comes from being able to reach out to a loving hand, separated from a desire to experience the things that make life worth living, separated from hope.[15]

SUMMARY

Opportunities abound in the provision of palliative care to develop relationships and connectedness with our patients and their families. Death, like birth, stimulates an awareness of the significance of life. The awareness that a life is nearing its end often prompts reflection on one's values and beliefs. The construct of beliefs as expressed in religion and spirituality can be a source of challenge, comfort, hope, and at times distress, not only for the person who is dying, but also for their caregivers, family, and the health-care team. Helping others to confront their spiritual and religious struggles can be both difficult and rewarding. Providing holistic care requires a commitment by the palliative care team to open their hearts and minds to the core of life's meaning and the depth and wonder of the transcendent.

REFERENCES

1. Daaleman TP, VandeCreek L. Placing religion and spirituality in end-of-life care. JAMA 2000;284: 2514–2517.

2. Wolman RN. Thinking with your soul: Spiritual intelligence and why it matters. Harmony Books, New York, 2001:14–16.

3. Ehman JW, Ott BB, Short TH, Ciampa RC, Hansen–Flaschen J. Do patients want physicians to inquire about their spiritual or religious beliefs if the become gravely ill? Arch Intern Med 2000;159:1803–1806.

4. Steinhauser KE, Christakis NA, Clipp EC, McNeilly M, McIntyre L, Tulsky JA. Factors considered important at the end of life by patients, family, physicians and other care providers. JAMA 2000;284:2476–2482.

5. Cohen CB, et al. Walking a fine line: physician inquiries into patients' religious and spiritual beliefs. Hastings Center Rep 2001;31(5):29–39.

6. Astrow AB, et al. Religion, spirituality, and health care: social, ethical, and practical considerations. Am J Med 2001;110:283–287.

7. Cherney NI, Coyle N, Foley K. Guidelines in the care of the dying cancer patient. Hematology/Oncology Clinics of North America 1996;10(1):261–286.

8. Frankl VE. Man's Search for Meaning: An Introduction to Logotherapy, 4th Ed. Beacon Press, Boston, 1992.

9. Ganzini L, Johnston WS, McFarland BH, Tolle SW, Lee MA. Attitudes of patients with amyotrophic lateral sclerosis and their care givers toward assisted suicide. NEJM 1998;339:967–973.

10. Ganzini L, Johnston WS, Hoffman WF. Correlates of suffering in amyotrophic lateral sclerosis. Neurology 1999;52:1434–1439.

11. Murphy PL, Albert SM, Weber CM, Del Bene ML, Rowland LP. Impact of spirituality and religiousness on outcomes in patients with ALS. Neurology 2000;55:1581–1584.

12. Sloan RP, Bagiella E, et al. Should Physician Prescribe Religious Activities? NEJM 2000;342(25):1913–1916.

13. Warm E, Weissman D. Fast Fact and Concept No. 21; Hope and Truth Telling. September, 2000. End-of-Life Physician Education Resource Center. *www.eperc.mcw.edu.*

14. Saunderson EM, Ridsdale L. General practitioners' beliefs and attitudes about how to respond to death and bereavement: qualitative study. BMJ 1999;319:293–296.

15. Cousins N. Anatomy of an Illness as Perceived by the Patient: Reflections on Healing and Regeneration. Bantam Books, New York, 1979:133.

Chapter 40

Cultural Aspects of Care

David Oliviere
David Oliver

OVERVIEW
The Nature of Culture
Culture and Palliative Care
Components of Culture in Palliative Care
ENSURING QUALITY
Institutional Racism and Minority Groups
Consideration of Values
Role of Culture and Religion
Stereotyping and Generalization
Consideration of Our Own Attitudes
CULTURAL CARE AND PATIENT CARE
Cultural Safety

Individualized Approach to Care
Language and Communication
Personal Care
Medical Intervention—Symptom Control
    and Medication
Food Preparation and Diet
Family Involvement and Care
Religious and Spiritual Life
Needs of Refugees
ASSESSMENT AND INTERVENTION
SUMMARY

The understanding of any patient is impossible without the understanding of their culture, whether this is the wider culture of their ethnic group, nationality, or religion or the more specific culture within individual families. The place of culture in the 'total' holistic approach of palliative care should always be considered, and the issues of culture and ethnicity should be addressed in both direct and indirect patient care. These various strands and components need to be considered in the assessment and intervention with each individual patient and family, involving them closely in this assessment process. In the care of patients with neurological disease there may be specific concerns related to disability or personal care, and these issues must be considered to ensure good-quality palliative care for patients and their families.

CASE HISTORY

Gina Pantin, aged 53 years, was diagnosed with motor neuron disease some two years ago and continued to work as a psychiatric nurse for eighteen months. Her mobility was extremely poor, self-care limited, and speech slightly impaired. She was spending increasing amounts of time in bed.

The family are Black Caribbean but have been resident in this country for many years. Gina lived with her husband. Their only child lived with her own daughter, aged five, on the other side of the city.

Gina was cared for at home by her family with a package of care from the social services department. She remained in a bed in her downstairs living room. Her husband was under severe strain, just managing to maintain his own building business.

One of the major problems for Gina was her very ambivalent relationship with her daughter. She was dependent on her for care but, at the same time, was distanced from her and critical of her help.

OVERVIEW

It is impossible to understand a person without understanding his/her culture.

Within the holistic approach of palliative care, cultural aspects are integral to appreciating

415

the person and their experiences. How they interpret the world, how they behave in it, and how they perceive the value of treatment, is determined by culture. With neurological conditions particularly, patients face life in a confusing, changing world where they confront so much loss of function. Retaining the self-esteem of the patient, and leaving the inner person intact, is essential.

The Nature of Culture

Culture is a multifaceted concept. It is subtle but accounts for a person's unique outlook and identity, as culture comprises a range of features, incorporating 'institutions, language, values, religious ideals, habits of thinking, artistic expressions and patterns of social and interpersonal relationships.'[1] Helman stresses that:

> Culture is a set of guidelines (both explicit and implicit) which individuals inherit as members of a particular society and which tells them how to view the world, how to experience it emotionally and how to behave in relation to other people ...To some extent, culture can be seen as an inherited 'lens', through which individuals perceive and understand the world that they inhabit, and learn how to live within it.[2]

Culture can be experienced as a basic set of rules—some very explicit and others quite subtle—about different aspects of living, being ill, and dying. Some of these sets of 'rules' are rejected, reinforced, or amalgamated with other sets of rules over one's lifetime[3] and each patient or family displays different sets of mores, patterns of relationship, and verbal and non-verbal reactions to situations. Culture is a dynamic process and these responses are partly defined by cultural patterns learnt from babyhood; they evolve by exposure to other cultural influences.[3] Many people are mixed in their cultures and this is increasingly so as societies become pluralistic and 'inter-cultural'.

Culture and Palliative Care

Cultural and societal attitudes underlie the approach taken by professionals and the

institutions which provide health-care services. Research is increasingly demonstrating how palliative care is influenced by this and varies across countries and continents.[4]

'There are different cultural assumptions about so-called truth-telling and about the nature of autonomy'[5] as well as attitudes towards religion and spirituality, euthanasia, sedation at the end of life, and the definition of terminality.[4] An awareness of the sociocultural context in which the service is provided, from which the health-care professional comes, and the perception of the patient and family, are all essential ingredients. The understanding of these elements is part of working towards quality care for neurological patients.

The holistic model of palliative care developed in the United Kingdom at a time when society was more 'monocultural' and, in the health sector, professionals were less conscious of the cultural dimensions in patient care. Over the past few decades, communities and many countries have become more multicultural, multiethnic, and multifaith. Health-care professionals are aware of working in a 'mixed' context where colleagues and patients are from diverse cultural backgrounds

Cicely Saunders at St Christopher's Hospice developed the concepts of 'total pain' and 'total care' in the 1960s.[6] She emphasized the integration of the physical, psychological, emotional, social, and spiritual, but the concepts of 'cultural pain' and 'cultural care' were not included and yet form inherent parts of all the dimensions listed. The overall philosophy of the modern hospice and palliative care movement has always been person-centred, attending carefully to the individual needs of the patient, family, and friends. There has therefore been a developing awareness of the need to be sensitive to culture, which plays a crucial part in attempting to assess fully the needs of a patient and in providing medical intervention and care.

A health professional cannot understand the patient without appreciating his/her culture. In caring for neurological patients, issues such as dependence, disability, and death may all carry particularly prominent stigmata for some patients, families, and communities, and it is essential that these aspects are considered by all involved.

Components of Culture in Palliative Care

There are various aspects of health-care practice that relate to working with people from different cultures:

- Equality of opportunity and equity issues, including access to services and providing appropriate services for individuals from all sections of our communities
- Sensitivity to patients and families from different religions and ethnic communities
- Anti-discriminatory practice—recognizing and addressing disadvantage and oppression
- Working with the differences and diversity amongst patients and families, respecting the unique characteristics and requirements of different cultures, particularly as every family will have their own particular culture and mores

ENSURING QUALITY

Institutional Racism and Minority Groups

In founding palliative care, Cicely Saunders has said she wanted to give 'a voice for the voiceless',[7] using Archbishop Desmond Tutu's phrase. She was referring to the importance of advocating for the needs of patients and to the freedom which good pain relief and symptom control can bring. Now with the recognition of 'socially excluded' groups and the emphasis on inclusion and of 'palliative care for all', the same sentiment refers to those patients from minority cultures.

In the United Kingdom, there is a growing awareness of the element of 'institutional racism' within public services, following the Macpherson Report[8] (a report based on the enquiry into the murder of Stephen Lawrence, a young black man, where charges of institutionalized racism were made at the handling by the police involved in the murder enquiry). The report has led many organizations to question racism within their own structures. The report defines 'institutional racism' as:

> The collective failure of an organisation to provide the appropriate and professional service to

people because of their colour, culture or ethnic origin. It can be seen or detected in processes, attitudes or behaviour which amount to discrimination through unwitting prejudice, ignorance, thoughtlessness and racist stereotyping which disadvantage minority ethnic people.[8]

This can manifest itself in several ways within institutional care (in hospitals and nursing homes, hospices, and palliative care units) as well as in home care contexts. Staff attitudes, availability and access to services for black and minority peoples, and environmental conditions that primarily cater for the tastes and preferences of a majority, white population, for example, can be seen to be an imposition of the majority.

A different view of racism is expressed by the Tavistock Clinic:

> Racism and institutional inequity originate in deep-rooted unconscious processes common to all human beings to rid the personality of intolerable experience which pathologically distorts into attitudes of superiority, and hatred, both personally and socially.[9]

Indeed, research has repeatedly indicated that 'black and minority ethnic communities are particularly likely to suffer from bad health, yet many have poor access to health-care and little say in how it is delivered.'[10]

Although the research has pointed to significant inequalities in health care of minority ethnic people,[11,12] there are indications that social class accounts for some of the differences.[13] Specialists in palliative care and the needs of those from minority ethnic groups highlight that 'insensitivity, racism and lack of cultural awareness are still evident in the health services generally' and emphasize that there are various problems not only in services for these communities but also with the availability of accurate data.[14] There is growing evidence from a number of research projects of the views of culturally diverse communities towards palliative care and some of the concrete obstacles.[15]

It is important to remember that the problems exist in the world in which people from different cultures live, rather than in the person or professional who lives in it. However, a word of caution—the needs of different minority ethnic communities vary and within each group there is diversity.

Consideration of Values

The understanding of the patient and their family, community, extended network, clan, or tribe is complicated by the fact that we inevitably tend to see the world through our own cultural norms. Our own culture will color the way we assess the needs of people from other cultures. We must never assume that our culture or perspective is the norm but try to appreciate the values, norms, and attitudes of the patient and family.

In working with any individual or group, especially when there are obvious differences, we must take into account the world views that might be affecting the cultures of the professional or patient and family. There is no right or wrong view of the world, but individuals may have differing perceptions which affect the way they work. The individual has views that may be located anywhere on the continuum shown in Table 40–1, affecting how they experience the world and how they may intervene with others they meet, both socially and professionally. These concepts and values are not in themselves right or wrong states. They are largely based on eastern and western perspectives, but as we are all a mixture, it is important that we locate ourselves and our families in order to have

Table 40–1. World Views

Values	
Individuality	Groupness
Independence	Interdependence
Uniqueness	Sameness
Difference	Community
Experience	
Separate	Integrated
Concrete	Abstract
Material	Spiritual
Control over nature	At one with nature
Competition	Co-operation
Intervention	
Individual rights	Collective responsibility
Explain	Discover
Activity	Inactivity

(Based on Stjernsward J, World Health Organization, Cancer and Palliative Care Unit)[16]

an appreciation of them and their needs. The experience of pain, medical intervention, and spiritual viewpoints can all be linked to one's value system.

The above framework reinforces the need to get to know the ill person and their family rather than relying on assumption and one's own world view. We must be aware too, that some people from other cultures may be uncomfortable with a more westernized medical approach to consulting patients. Also, a knowledge of a particular culture can be a dangerous thing as we can presume certain information rather than use it to know which questions to ask.[16]

With Gina and her family, they bring a mix of values as individuals: some from their Caribbean heritage; others developed from a western viewpoint; others from a generational perspective. For example, the daughter was pregnant at 17 years old and was a single parent. She had found this acceptable but had shocked and appalled her parents. One of the major problems for Gina was her very ambivalent relationship with her daughter. She was dependent on her for care but at the same time was distanced from her and critical of her help. The differing value systems within this family accounted for some of the 'unresolved business' Gina and her family experienced. They had never come to terms with the pregnancy and all that it meant, and mother and daughter had been alienated from each other as a result.

Role of Culture and Religion

There are major differences but also overlaps between culture and religion. Every religion has its own cultural practices, conventions, and rituals; not every culture is religious. For some, religious and cultural ways of life are inextricably linked, giving meaning to body and mind. Gina belonged to a black church which offered certain support systems, communal rituals, prayer, singing, support for the dying, and bereavement traditions which drew on Christian and African conventions.

For some patients/families, even though they have not practised the religion of their childhood, their very identity, behavior, lifestyle, and celebrations are all shaped by their religious background and traditions. People can even define themselves by their religious grouping, even when their personal faith is limited or non-existent.[19] The onset of illness, dying, and death can initiate new meaning in religious practices and rituals; for others the opposite is true.

Stereotyping and Generalization

To order the world and to orient oneself within it, one has to categorize and generalize to some extent. However, when it comes to assessing and intervening with patients, this can be most unhelpful as it denies the very individuality and response to the *person* and his/her needs that we seek in palliative care. Concepts such as the uniqueness of the person and the meaning of different aspects of his/her life are part of good palliative care and we need to find the person behind the patient.

Clinical practice that 'boxes' people and categorizes them ('he's a typical...') is missing the full picture, and so often subsequent behavior is mis-interpreted through the lens of the stereotype. It is essential to recognize *where* the person is in his/her culture: there are conventionalists and fundamentalists at one end of the continuum, with liberals and reformists at the other. We need to confront prejudice and stereotypical thinking and attitudes in ourselves, our colleagues, and others.

Labels such as 'Jewish', 'Moslem', 'Catholic', 'Irish', or 'westernized' can be very limited and unhelpful. Listening and questions such as 'So tell me about what is important in your culture...religion...family' and 'If you were well enough how would you be spending your time?' can communicate genuine interest to the patient and family and a willingness to get to know them as people.

Palliative care is full of contradictions, opposites, and paradoxes, which reflect life. Working with commonality and difference is another example of holding the tension between opposing components. Whether 'South Asian' or 'South African', you need to discover the commonality and differences within the culture and where the person sits in the culture. He/she may have rejected or be apathetic to the cultural mores, practices, or rituals which the culture dictates.

In Gina's case, it would have been easy to make assumptions that it was acceptable for the family system to contain, as a matter of course, single parenthood or that the entire family was 'religious'. In fact Gina's husband did not attend the black church of which Gina was a committed member. Gina was upset and saddened by her daughter's single parenthood, despite the five years since her grand-daughter was born. Some strict mores and expectations had been transgressed.

Furthermore, generalizations that 'black people look after their own' have to be checked out and the needs of the individual family assessed. In the case of the Pantin family, there was no sizeable extended family available in this country.

Consideration of Our Own Attitudes

The reflection around one's own attitudes as well as those of colleagues, are necessary for the professionals who are concerned about the cultural aspects of care. Because of the tendency to view others' cultures through our own perspectives and to impose our own values in assessing and judging a situation, self-awareness and other colleagues' perceptions are important in correcting initial impressions and prejudices. For example, it is easy to be critical of the very ill patient who wishes to return to India to die when you are convinced that his quality of care and of life would be inferior; or of the family which speaks for their ill member, not appearing to allow them an opportunity to express a viewpoint; or of the woman patient who does all the work in the household whilst her husband and son do little to support her.

Professional values of non-judgmental attitudes, acceptance, autonomy, confidentiality, and respect can be challenged when it comes to some ethical decisions and reconciling a patient/family's differing stance. When there is a mix of views based on differing cultural traditions and patterns (e.g. the elderly Asian patient who expects her children to care for her at home whilst her daughter wishes you to support an application for residential care; the family which dictates that you do not pass confidential information to the patient regarding prognosis), the dilemmas can be magnified.

CULTURAL CARE AND PATIENT CARE

Cultural Safety

The nursing profession in New Zealand, from the late 1980s, gave birth to the concept of 'cultural safety' in order to reflect on nursing practice from the point of view of the Maori indigenous minority. The concept has been adopted by the Nursing Council of New Zealand as part of the basic curriculum for nursing training[17] and there is a growing literature on the subject.

> The effective nursing of a person/family from another culture...recognises the impact on the nurse's culture on his or her own practice. Unsafe clinical practice is any action which diminishes, demeans, or disempowers the cultural identity and wellbeing of an individual.[18]

The same basic principle can apply to all the professional disciplines that comprise the team.

Culture is subtle. Learning about death and dying rituals and about different ethnic and religious groups is desirable. However, it is more important to find the person *within* his/her cultural context and to know how to negotiate as to what he/she needs and wants.

Individualized Approach to Care

There has been much criticism of the 'checklist' or 'fact file' approach[19] in dealing with the cultural aspects of patients' care. The need to have religious and cultural requirements written down for an average or typical member of a particular group, is oversimplifying and generalizing the complex needs of people from different cultures. It avoids the individuality of the person. For example, in the area of diet, lists of the dietary needs of members of the Jewish, Moslem, or African–Caribbean communities may be interesting but do not tell us about the particular dietary needs of our patient. With Gina, in liaising with the meals service from the local social services department, it was necessary to know something of her diet but not assume her liking for Caribbean dishes.

On the other hand, common traditions, trends, and tendencies can open the way to alerting the sensitive professional as to what questions to address with the patient. By understanding that there may be specific areas that need to be addressed, a more useful conversation can be held. The essential ingredient is to be able to ask, check, and listen to the patient/family's wants and needs.[20,21]

Language and Communication

The principle that talking or counseling must be done in the language in which the person thinks, is an important one. It is, of course, impossible to really get to know the needs of the patient well when there are significant language barriers. Dependence on relatives to act as interpreters is sometimes inevitable and the quickest practical response but there may be very great difficulties in this approach. Relatives may actually reduce the communication with the professional by providing a 'filter' through which it is impossible to reach the patient and their own views and problems. If at all possible the use of a trained interpreter is important as this provides a more professional and neutral interpretation. However, experience of working with interpreters in palliative care, when emotions can be very strong and issues sensitive, can be complex and difficult. There is a need for the professional to receive training in the best use and working practices with interpreters. Interpretation is a bilingual as well as a bicultural process.[14]

Ideally, some time spent with the interpreter to prepare them for the interview, to debrief afterwards, and, for whoever oversees the work of the interpreter, to provide some training and support, makes for more positive results.

With many neurological conditions, when the patient cannot communicate verbally or effectively, the reliance on the family to interpret the patient's needs is greater. However, the professional should be aware that in many traditions there can be a reluctance to encourage disclosure of life-threatening conditions.

The use of pictures, word books, boards, and other aids is vital, and it may be necessary for a key member of staff to become particularly familiar with these tools. The basic need to check back with patients their understanding of what has been said, decided, and of terms used, cannot be emphasized enough.

Personal Care

Personal hygiene, washing and toileting, and hair and skin care are all areas where it is possible to give permission to the patient to tell you how he/she prefers procedures to be carried out. It is important to establish practices relating to personal care. The skilled clinician will be sensitive to other cultures' concern over modesty and privacy. In respecting religious and cultural practices, the need for ablutions after going to the toilet is necessary for some; fasting or facing Mecca will be necessary for others.

The gender of medical and nursing staff may be an issue for some patients and their spouses, and this needs flexibility where possible. For many, same-sex caregivers are preferred and any infringement of modesty is distressing.

Medical Intervention—Symptom Control and Medication

The expression of unhappiness in the somatization of feelings by showing discomfort in the stomach must not be confused with other signs and symptoms of pain. An awareness of how some diseases are more taboo in some cultures than others is necessary.

The tolerance of pain and other symptoms and the attitude to medication may well be intertwined with religious views of the tolerance of suffering, about remaining conscious before death, and of punishment. Therefore, there will be cultural connotations which will require exploration with the patient.

Food Preparation and Diet

Ensuring food preparation takes place in keeping with requirements of a patient's faith and culture is essential for some, optional for others. Getting to know what is important, and facilitating members of a patient's family or community to bring in or prepare the food, is an essential component in the holistic care of patients. Moreover, the need to check if the patient wishes to fast or finds the meals acceptable makes for good care. Unless dietary needs are properly met, a patient can feel very uncomfortable and unsafe.

Equally, sensitivity around methods of feeding is important. Tube feeding, for example, may have different implications for different cultures. For many the role of food is critical and the need to prolong life at all costs, desirable; for others, not. The cessation of tube feeding may have even greater significance for some communities. Consultation with religious leaders may be helpful should there be any implications for added spiritual suffering if care is seen to have inflicted additional physical suffering.

Family Involvement and Care

The roles of men and women in the particular community; the respect for older/younger members; the identification of leaders; the importance of cousins and extended family visiting the bedside, all have to be understood. Family patterns of communication, tone and level of voice, attitude, eye contact, shows of affection, and so on have to be seen in their cultural context. Furthermore, some families need to involve elders or have a community leader's/male's permission to make decisions regarding treatment, which conflict with the personal autonomy of a more western model of behavior. This can conflict, for example, over the care of a female patient where a professional may not have access to the patient and discussions are filtered through male members of the family. There is some evidence that for many minority ethnic groups, the concept of the inpatient hospice and palliative care is alien. Home care can be seen as more acceptable; the notion of a relative being sent out of the family to be looked after, taboo.

Within Gina's family, there were at least two cultural sets of expectations between the two generations, as displayed by mother's more traditional and religious approach to sex and relationships before marriage. She felt that this had been transgressed by the behavior of her daughter and her pregnancy out of marriage. This also accounted for a major communication gap and unresolved issues between mother and daughter up to and beyond the death. It affected the daughter's grief and formed much of the agenda for the bereavement work that followed.

Religious and Spiritual Life

Some patients will need to have the security and assurance of contact with a representative of their religious community. Prayers and rituals need to be respected. Conversations about pastoral matters and about finding hope and meaning in their experience of the illness, death, and bereavement are often sought through contact with religious leaders.

In Gina's case, the church members became an increasingly strong source of support to her, and her 'fundamentalist' beliefs sustained her. Opportunities to pray around her bed and other religious rituals were a great comfort to her.

Needs of Refugees

In many countries and large cities there may be refugees and those seeking asylum. They have been subject to trauma and persecution and have experienced loss on a huge scale, with suppressed memories of the events and feelings arising from them. In the crisis of a life-threatening illness, it is not uncommon for many of the emotions to be triggered and the patient/family can sometimes begin to voice earlier experiences. Whether the experience is in the recent or distant past, the emotional trauma can begin to surface in the present, in grief and guilt. It also occurs that the children of survivors begin to experience some of the emotional fallout from the older generation.[3]

ASSESSMENT AND INTERVENTION

As part of identifying the key areas of concern, the skilled clinician will be sensitive to the impact of culture on the patient's quality of care: there are specific needs and the process of getting to understand the patient's family requirements to consider. There will be areas that immediately need consideration by professionals, such as dietary requirements on religious grounds or the preference for spicy foods, the need to meet with religious leaders of the patient's faith, and the need for an interpreter.

Accurate information needs to be recorded to ensure sufficient basic data is available: names and how the patient likes to be addressed; written and spoken languages (as these might not be the same); religion; dietary requirements; details of members of the family may necessitate adequate space in notes.

To create a sense of security and trust, the clinician's sensitivity to the patient's cultural needs is essential in the *process* of caring from initial investigation, assessment, and diagnosis, through to treatment and active life-prolonging interventions, end-of-life care, death, and bereavement follow-up. All these stages are part of good supportive and palliative care and will include a mixture of information giving, treatment of symptoms, support and counseling, and the involvement of other professionals and disciplines. The ability to respond to the needs of the patient and family's uncertainty and questions will be promoted by communicating a real desire to respect the whole person, including their cultural and religious values and identity.

It is a challenge to know which questions to ask and to manage the time that is required to get to know a patient and family's more subtle needs. However, the focus on one area or question can signal to the patient/family concern and interest. They are more likely to alert the professionals if basic trust is established.

One needs to remember that each clinician works in a team; there may be other members with specific interest and time to attend more directly to the cultural and religious requirements and concerns, such as the chaplain or social worker. A clinician does not have to go it alone.

Creating an atmosphere where a professional is attentive to the lifestyle of the person sets up a 'contract' with the patient/family. Ask them if they would let you know should the care not be meeting the needs of their religion or culture, or not be carried out in the way they are used to. As professionals from another culture or even from the same, one cannot be expected to be automatically familiar with what is appropriate for the individual patient/family member.

For many patients, the crisis of illness and death highlights the traditions and rituals which offer them meaning and support. For others, there may be a rejection of cultural patterns. For good practice to be a reality, the patient has to be at the center of care, their differing needs identified and met.[22]

Care begins where difference is recognised.[23]

SUMMARY

Patients and their families will bring to the professional their problems and concerns regarding the disease and its effect on them. These problems will be in the context of their own particular culture—of their country, religion, ethnic group, or their own family. It is essential for these wider issues to be considered carefully in the assessment and care of patients and families to ensure that the care offered is both effective and acceptable to all concerned.

REFERENCES

1. Lum. Social work practice and people of color: a process and stage approach, 2nd Ed. Brooks Cole, Pacific Grove, CA, 1992.
2. Helman C. Culture, Health and Illness. Butterworth–Heinemann, Oxford, 1990.
3. Oliviere D. Cross-cultural principles of care. In: Saunders C, Sykes N. The Management of Terminal Malignant Disease. Edward Arnold, Oxford, 1993.
4. Núñez Olarte JM, Gracia Guillen D. Cultural issues and ethical dilemmas in palliative and end-of-life care in Spain. Cancer Control 2001;8(1):46–54.
5. Clark D. European palliative care in the *longue durée*. European Journal of Palliative Care 2001;8:92.
6. Clark D. Total pain: the work of Cicely Saunders and the hospice movement. American Pain Society Bulletin July/August 2000.
7. Oliviere D. A voice for the voiceless. European Journal of Palliative Care 2000;7:102–105.
8. Macpherson Report: Stephen Lawrence Enquiry. February 1999.
9. Cooper A. (Chair, Race and Equity Working Group). Race and Equity Initiatives Within the Trust. Tavistock and Portman NHS Trust (unpublished paper).
10. Cabinet Office. Involving Users. Improving the Delivery of Health Care. National Consumer Council and Service First Unit, London, 1999.
11. Department of Health. Independent Inquiry into Inequalities in Health. The Stationery Office, London, 1998.
12. Race, Health, and Social Exclusion Commission. Sick of Being Excluded. The Association of London Government, London, 2000.
13. Alexander Z. The Department of Health: Study of Black, Asian and Ethnic Minority Issues. Annex, London, 1999.
14. Firth S. Wider Horizons. The National Council for Hospice and Specialist Palliative Care Services, London, 2001.
15. Mount J, ed. Palliative Care Services for Different Ethnic Groups. National Council for Hospice and Specialist Palliative Care Services, London, 2000.
16. Oliviere D, Hargreaves R, Monroe B. Good Practices in Palliative Care: A Psychosocial Perspective. Ashgate, Aldershot, 1998:165–166.
17. Polaschek NR. Cultural safety; a new concept in nursing people of different ethnicities. J Advanced Nurs 1998;27:452–457.
18. Nursing Council of New Zealand. Guidelines for Cultural Safety in Nursing and Midwifery Education. Nursing Council of New Zealand, Wellington, 1996.
19. Gunaratnam Y. Culture is not enough. A critique of multi-culturalism in palliative care. In: Field D, Hockey J, Small N, eds. Death, Gender and Ethnicity. Routledge, London, 1997.
20. Neuberger J. Introduction. Cultural issues in palliative care. In: Doyle D, Hanks G, MacDonald N, eds. Oxford Textbook of Palliative Medicine, 2nd Ed. Oxford University Press, Oxford, 1998.
21. Neuberger J. Dying Well: A Guide to Enabling a Good Death. Hochland and Hochland, Cheshire, 1999.
22. Kagawa–Singer M, Blackhall LJ. Negotiating cross-cultural issues at the end of life. JAMA 2001;286:2993–3301.
23. Frank A. At the Will of the Body: Reflections of Illness. Houghton Mifflin, Boston, 1991.

Chapter 41

Palliative Care Education for Neurologists

Ian Maddocks

INTRODUCTION
THE CHANGING ROLE OF THE
   NEUROLOGIST
NEUROLOGY TRAINING
THE CONTENT OF PALLIATIVE CARE
   EDUCATION

Knowledge
Skills
Attitude
CONCLUSION

Although the practice of specialist neurology has changed radically over recent decades, the formal education of the neurologist has failed to keep pace with that change, with an emphasis on the mastery of new knowledge and techniques in a limited area of the discipline, which often leads to early subspecialization. There have been many calls for a greater attention to the sociocultural aspects of the patient's condition, but relatively few models to follow. Yet increasingly medicine deals with chronic conditions in which those aspects loom large in effective assessment and management. Palliative care seeks to provide a comprehensive approach to care in circumstances where any opportunity for cure has passed, with an emphasis on quality of life for the days that remain. The expertise developed in care of terminal cancer is increasingly recognised as relevant to many other advanced disease situations, including a wide range of conditions managed by neurologists. Palliative care deserves promotion as a basic component in the preparation of the specialist neurologist.

INTRODUCTION

This book was initiated by specialist physicians in palliative care and neurology who saw a need for neurologists to be better prepared for a role in the provision of palliative care to individuals with advanced and terminal neurological diseases. The Executive Board of the American Academy of Neurologists has affirmed that because many neurological diseases are progressive and incurable, optimal care requires that neurologists understand and apply the principles of palliative care, including the development of team approaches and the framing of appropriate and realistic goals for the care of dying patients.[1] The Academy also recommends palliative care as the most appropriate form of medical care for many patients with advanced dementia.[2] Some Neurology Societies, such as the American Academy of Neurology, the European Neurological Society, and the Austrian, German, and Italian Neurological Societies, have started to offer educational courses in 'Palliative care in neurology'. Concurrently, however, studies suggest that neurologists practice palliative care poorly, if at all. Neurologists in training have little exposure to suitable models of such care and faculty neurologists often seem most interested in rarities.[3]

This chapter seeks to explore how palliative care education might contribute to the preparation of the neurologist.

424

THE CHANGING ROLE OF THE NEUROLOGIST

The specialty of neurology is no different from other areas of medicine in facing an escalating growth in information, with major developments in neuroscience and increasing numbers of medical meetings and new journals. A generalist cannot know everything, and increasingly each specialty moves towards subspecialization, with neurologists 'working together in packs' so that individual practitioners can take up more limited areas of expertise.[4] Changes in the management of medicine have contributed to changes in clinical practice, with a shift away from hospitals governed by non-medical people to free-standing specialty clinics where costs can be controlled by physicians.[5] Inevitably this increases the isolation of the specialty from other disciplines.

At the same time, there has been an increase in the range of services offered, with more use by neurologists of nurse practitioners or medical assistants. This partly reflects market competition, and partly, perhaps, the recognition that patients with chronic neurological disorders have not been receiving all the neurological services they need.[6] There has been little concurrent change in neurological education, however; the emphasis remains on the application to neurological disorders of the new knowledge emanating from biomedical research, with a bias towards the quantifiable.[7] This makes it difficult to conceptualize and implement a curriculum more appropriate to the changing scene of neurology—one more balanced in its attention to quality care.

Menken has questioned whether future advances in care will follow the narrow biological model which has hitherto been seen as the triumph of modern medicine, and has called for a broader education taking fuller account of a 'biosociocultural' approach, pointing out that chronic disorders predominate in modern medicine and reflect behavior and social values.[8] He has suggested that training should focus on personal and family environment and community health, and encourages neurologists to forge links with other disciplines. Others have recommended that neurologists view continuing education as

having the goal of improving quality of care provided rather than simply increasing the knowledge base.[9] These are views are very congruent with a palliative care approach.

Traditional practice of neurology was very much focused on diagnosis: 'Where is it? What is it?' was the mantra for neurological diagnosis in my student days. Therapeutics was a less valued part of the discipline, being often ineffective in reversing established damage or degeneration. Careful history taking was followed by detailed clinical examination—eliciting subtle signs by precise attention to a well-practiced routine using eyes and ears and hands by the bedside. Little in the way of either surgical or pharmacological intervention was available to modify the course of the illness that had been brilliantly elucidated.

Newer imaging techniques of the brain and spinal cord have revolutionized the neurologists' approach to many disorders—but the need for bedside skills in diagnosis is claimed to persist:

> The nuances of neurological examination are not readily conveyed in textbooks and must be learnt at the bedside. . .[the new techniques] are no substitute for the careful neurological examination.

One of the doyens of neurology, Walshe, has noted that sophisticated diagnostic techniques call for sound clinical judgement, and are not a substitute for it.[10]

The close liaison operating between neurology and psychiatry in many centers might have been expected to bring to neurology a greater sympathy with the broader human perspectives of medicine. Merino warns that a too-narrow neuroscientific approach remains widespread, and urges neurologists to:

> understand defence mechanisms, ways of coping with adversity, motivation and family dynamics to understand fully the effects of illness and treatment on individual patients.[11]

Pain management has not been seen as a central responsibility of the neurologist and apparently remains poorly managed within the specialty. In a survey conducted in the United States, only 30% of practising neurologists felt adequately trained to diagnose and 20% to treat pain disorders. Residency program directors gave some recognition to pain management by ranking it seventh out of eight neurology subspecialties, but only 29% reported having a neurology pain specialist on the faculty.[12] Yet neurology journals give space for excellent reviews on advances in the understanding and management of pain.[13]

NEUROLOGY TRAINING

An assertion that the usual training in neurology has been too narrow, too focused on individual assessment, and little aware of broader community needs or global issues is being more widely expressed. Mencken has been a leading commentator on the changing practice of neurology, and has called for a greater role for patients and those who advocate for them in the development of education programs, suggesting that all medical students should achieve competence in public health and recognize the global health needs of human populations. He recommended clinical teaching carried out by multidisciplinary groups of teachers to help get away from the mutual reinforcement of research and specialization and a tendency for trainees to rotate through a series of narrow specialties, describing medical education as 'a moral enterprise, steeped in human and cultural values'.[14] Many palliative care physicians would share that attitude and hope that it was inherent in medical education at every level.

An effective or adequate palliative care education for the trainee neurologist ought to stem from the strongly motivating experience of care for a dying patient during undergraduate clerkship, and even a period of attachment to a hospice unit. However, much of that motivation can be diluted by the excitement of acute care and curative procedures in the senior student and junior houseman years at a busy major hospital, swayed by the applause reserved for accurate diagnosis or manual dexterity by intern or resident, and the emphasis in teaching on the fascinating rarity.

The over-full undergraduate curriculum of the modern medical school has had little room for any additions and palliative care was rarely high on the list of priorities. But increasingly, medical schools are adopting an emphasis more congruent with the biopsychosocial approach already mentioned. At the postgraduate level there are useful opportunities to study palliative care in many universities, some leading to graduate diplomas or master's awards.[15] Relatively few specialists in neurology can be expected to undertake these, but it is worth emphasizing that important contributions have been made to the practice and recognition of palliative care by individual neurologists such as Dr Kathleen Foley, who early grasped the importance of the discipline, and who advocates strongly for the neurologist as a provider of palliative care.[16,17] What will be most useful will be a change in the training of all neurologists which builds on a formative undergraduate experience and encourages a broader exposure to community practice and primary care; one which should include responsibility for the management of advanced disease and death in home and family settings.

A term as a registrar or fellow in a well-recognized palliative care unit will be most useful, particularly if it encourages the trainee to undertake the full range of responsibilities for hospital and home care, and includes day care and bereavement care programs, maintains specialist inpatient beds, and conducts education at both undergraduate and postgraduate levels. However, only a trainee with a strong motivation to learn palliative care can be expected to undertake such a term, faced with the need to encompass the burgeoning neurological literature, to seek clinical experience with leaders in this or that subspecialty of neurology, and to satisfy the demands of supervisors who lack either knowledge or interest in a discipline such as palliative care.

Further, the new discipline of palliative care remains small, and there will be relatively few opportunities for a term of attachment to a unit with an established reputation, so that the combination of few, if any, examples to follow, minimal interest or encouragement from senior practitioners, and the lack of relevant opportunities will be likely to stifle the aspirations of all but the most enthusiastic trainee neurologists who are considering a term of experience in palliative care.

THE CONTENT OF PALLIATIVE CARE EDUCATION

As in all areas of health care, a syllabus prescribed for the training of a neurologist in palliative care should address the acquisition of knowledge, skills, and attitude.

Knowledge

Relevant knowledge concerning palliative care will include patient assessment (focusing on symptom recognition and measurement) together with devising comprehensive approaches to management (including physical, psychological, and pharmacological measures) which will extend to patient and family education and organizational aspects for care delivery. New facts can be listed in a book, but there is a perspective essential to the effective delivery of palliative care which recognizes that there is no right answer; that one of the first things to learn is that the discomforts of terminal illness change often, and that what brings relief today may seem useless tomorrow.

A quotation I have found useful to share with students builds on a statement by Celibidache, the Romanian conductor—'What is written in the score is everything, except what is important'.[18]—which is modified to 'What is written in the textbook is everything except what is important'. As with the performance of music it is the *way* palliative care is delivered that matters.

A range of potential interventions and prescriptions need to be learnt, and a best choice is made on the basis of pathology, past history, personal preference, recent responses, and current distress. Awareness of facts concerned with oncology, HIV, and advanced pathologies of all kinds is most important. A knowledge of pain mechanisms and analgesic actions, a close appreciation of how to prescribe effectively those opioids that are available (the mix of analgesics varies from country to country), and familiarity with the resources of various kinds (equipment, financial assistance, home care support, volunteer support, bereavement counseling, etc.) are all most desirable.

Skills

Skills to acquire for the practice of palliative care are only partly professional; some, such as patience (a willingness to wait, listen, consider another approach) are more personal. The Australian psychiatrist, Ainslie Meares (who gave great attention to helping patients with advanced cancer), stated: 'Most of my talk was in silence, but that has been the only talk that was really worthwhile.'[19]

Skills in communication, in team working, in clinical assessment, and review of complex situations (including some which will involve family tension, conflict, or inappropriate expectations) are often more necessary than procedural skills such as paracentesis, placement of an epidural catheter for opioid delivery, or performance of a nerve block (though such procedures will sometimes bring excellent relief of discomfort, and must be included). Acquiring the skill of working in a team necessarily involves a proper awareness of the contributions to care which can be made by nurse practitioners, home support services, psychologists, physiotherapists, pastoral care workers, as well as any number of the other health specialties. The close co-operation of the neurologist, the respiratory physician, and the palliative care team in the continuing care of the patient with ALS, and the support of the involved family, is an excellent example to draw upon. But it will be important to frame that awareness with an experience of team working which has every chance of instilling a heightened respect for the different contributions which each professional brings.

Attitude

A change of attitude may be the most important key to further development of the discipline—taking an interest in the major and minor discomforts which attend advanced and terminal illness rather than in diagnosis and underlying pathology, even though those remain of major importance.

Changes in attitude are not readily effected by precept or lecture; they are acquired largely through experience. Hence the need to offer students hands-on familiarity with the care of dying persons and the support of their close family members. Desirable attitude changes include bringing to patient care a flexible and responsive compassion, building multidisciplinary teamwork, reducing the rigidity of hierarchies (e.g. helping nurses and physicians to establish common goals and mutual respect), removing opiophobia, and extending care to family members and into the bereavement period. Example is helpful, but the challenge of devising the most effective and appropriate response to real situations in concert with other dedicated companions is the most helpful way to develop new approaches to one's work. Few neurologists in training will have had exposure to such opportunities.

CONCLUSION

Palliative care has won an established place in medicine largely through its demonstration of good care for individuals with advanced cancer. Increasingly, the management methods evolved in that experience are found relevant to aged care and the support of those with advanced respiratory, cardiac, and renal disease which has moved beyond any reasonable hope of cure. Neurology is a particularly appropriate area of medicine to embrace the tenets and expertise of palliative care, being faced with many individuals whose diseases are incurable at the time of diagnosis. Ways must be found to ground palliative care within the changing world of neurological education as a basic component of what a neurologist needs to profess and practice—though how that is achieved will necessarily vary from country to country.

REFERENCES

1. Special article. Palliative care in neurology. Statement approved by the American Academy of Neurologists Executive Board. Neurology 1996;46:870–872.
2. Special article. Ethical issues in the management of the demented patient. Statement approved by the American Academy of Neurologists Executive Board. Neurology 1996;46:1180–1183.
3. Bernat JL, Goldstein ML, Viste KM. The neurologist and the dying patient. Neurology 1996; 46:589–599.
4. Kennard C. Editorial. J Neurol Neurosurg Psychiatry 1999;66:1.
5. Roberts J. Specialists in the US: what lessons? Brit Med J 1995;310:724–727.
6. Ringel SP, Vickrey BG, Rogstad TL. US neurologists: attitudes on the US health care system. Neurology 1996;47(1):279–287.
7. Ringel SP, Vickrey BG, Keran CM, Bieber J, Bradley WG. Training the future neurology workforce. Neurology 2000;54:480–484.
8. Menken M. The changing paradigm of neurologic practice and care. Implications for the undergraduate curriculum. Arch Neurol 1990;47:334–336.
9. Ringel SP, Vickrey BG. Measuring quality of care in neurology. Arch Neurol 1997;54(11):1329–1332.
10. Berger JR. On bedside teaching. Ann Int Med 1997;127(2):172.
11. Merino JG. Neurology and psychiatry—closing the great divide. Neurology 2000;55:602–603.
12. Galer BS, Keran C, Frisinger M. Pain medicine education among American neurologists: a need for improvement. Neurology 1999;52:1710–1712.
13. Foley KM. Advances in cancer pain. Arch Neurol 1999;56(4):413–417.
14. Menken M. Medical and neurological education at the millenium. Arch Neurology 2000;57(1):62–63.
15. Maddocks I. Postgraduate courses and awards in palliative care. Palliative Medicine 1992;6:269–271.
16. Foley KM. Competent care for the dying patient instead of physician-assisted suicide. N Eng J Med 1997;336:54–57.
17. Foley KM, Carver AC. Palliative care in neurology. Neurologic Clinics 2001;19(4):789–799.
18. Celibidache S. Interview. Australian Broadcasting Commission, 'World of Music', October 7, 1984.
19. Meares A. A Way of Doctoring. Hill of Content, Melbourne, 1983.

Chapter 42

So, Here's What's Happened In My Life Since Last April

Ben–Joshua Jaffee[†]

Dr Ben–Joshua Jaffee is one of the most integrated persons I know. There has never been any pretense to Ben–Joshua. He is a committed caregiver, a dedicated teacher, an academic, a friend to all who work with him. It is truly a case of 'what you see is what you get'.

The ripple effect caused among social workers by his work at the University of Washington School continues today. He was an eagerly awaited presenter at the King's College Conferences on Death and Bereavement, and an active researcher as a member of the International Work Group on Death, Dying, and Bereavement.

Dr Jaffee continues to teach us now with his acceptance of and coping with his illness, amyotrophic lateral sclerosis (ALS). His humor at his own physical problems proves once again that the human spirit is stronger than the human body.

Professor John Morgan

It's been a most difficult, challenging, and learning-filled journey that I've been on. There have been some good and beautiful experiences; many, many really hard, very unpleasant, and disappointing ones; and a few dark-night-of-the-soul transformative ones.

First, the positive ones. Last spring, Sylvia and I moved into our beautiful townhouse, with the fantastic help of loving friends and family. It *is* a lovely home, really elegant, without being ostentatious. And Sylvia's won-

[†]On December 4th, 2002, Professor Jaffee died peacefully at his home.

derful aesthetic sense and little touches have made it all the more attractive. It is so quiet and peaceful that we just enjoy sitting in the living room and feeling the silence and serenity. We have a wonderful view of Lake Washington and the Cascade Mountains, and in our east-facing bedroom we are treated to glorious sunrises. We feel blessed to be here. Our relationship has continued to deepen and to be tested, honed, challenged, and matured by having to face the cruel realities of ALS. This hasn't been an easy journey for either of us but, overall, for a three-year relationship, I think we've done remarkably well in dealing with most of those realities and in meeting most of those challenges. We've also purposely scheduled concerts, dance concerts, and operas into our lives so we could have some respite, pleasure, and enjoyment, to counterbalance the increasing harshness of the progressive nature of this disease.

And progressive it most certainly has been! Relentlessly! Even though I knew this conceptually, as is the case in most situations, it took experiencing the actuality for me to truly comprehend it. By last May, I was having such increasing difficulty eating and swallowing that there was real danger that I could aspirate food or liquid into my lungs, with resultant threat of aspiration pneumonia. So, reluctantly, I followed my doctors' advice and had a PEG feeding tube inserted into my stomach. That meant that most of my nutrition had to be taken through that tube, in the form of enriched liquid formula. I was still able to eat some regular food, only if it were blenderized and made into custard consistency, but the

429

bulk of my nourishment had to come in the formula: enough to give me the 1800 calories I needed to maintain my weight.

The problem was that all the formulas on the market contain a fair amount of sugar, in one form or another, and I've been sensitive to all sugar for years. So, it took two or three months of experimentation to find a formula with the least amount of sugar and then to figure out the rate of flow into my tube at which I could tolerate it, with only a minimal amount of sugar reaction. I take the formula by means of a pump, attached to an IV pole, which accompanies me wherever I go. I call it my Pole Star, since it plays an important role in directing where I can go and what I can do. I'm on the pump all night (thank goodness it's quite quiet!), when I take in a little more than half the formula supplement I need, leaving the remainder to be 'eaten' or 'drunk' during the day. In addition, I must also take in 700–900 cc of water each day to keep me hydrated. This I do by using a large syringe to inject the water—plus any medications—into my tube. This is another whole story: the process of tube feeding by syringe. It requires a number of different steps, each of which is essential and all of which must be taken in a specified designated sequence, in order to avoid the contents of the tube and my stomach spewing out all over the room. So, it takes a long time to do this, and requires constant attention and mindfulness to avoid accidental leakage. What an education in being present in the moment! I'm thinking of writing a piece on 'The Zen of Tube Feeding'!

I'm grateful that I also do have a back pack carrier for the pump and the feeding bag. This allows me to be mobile while I 'feed'—truly a moveable feast (though 'feast' is not quite the word I'd use to describe that vanilla flavored formula, which I can't even taste). For a couple of months, I continued taking all my vitamin and mineral supplements by mouth, until I had a severe choking episode that was bad enough for Sylvia to have to call 911 (emergency medic help). That incident put a complete stop to the oral ingestion of *any* supplements.

As my swallowing muscles became weaker, I could eat (or even taste) progressively less and less by mouth, without danger of aspirating. For the past month to six weeks, I've been eating nothing at all orally. As you can well imagine, the losses due to this development have been manifold. Besides having to give up all my favorite foods, I miss the physical sensations of chewing and of drinking and of smelling food. The important socializing rituals around food and eating are not a pleasurable and enjoyed part of my life any more: restaurant dining is out for me, and for Sylvia and me together (although she periodically goes to restaurants with friends); and shopping for food is also no longer part of my regular everyday activity. And when I do go to the co-op, which used to be really 'home' to me for so many years, I feel almost like a stranger or an alien who no longer 'belongs' there.

The bulbar palsy type of ALS that I have, first and primarily affects the entire head and throat area. Due to the degeneration and death of the lower motor neurons in the medulla, the nerves emanating from those neurons also degenerate. This, in turn deprives the muscles of the face, lips, palate, glottis, and throat of their regular stimulation and enervation, thereby causing them to weaken and to function progressively less well, and eventually, not at all.

So, my speech, which last year was beginning to be compromised but was still intelligible, has deteriorated steadily, at what to me seems to be a fairly rapid pace. Until about five or six months ago, I could make myself at least partly understood to many people who would take the time and make the effort to listen carefully. Up to that time, Sylvia was able to understand close to 90%, and then 80%, of what I was saying. However, over the past six months, she has been able to understand less and less, until she now cannot understand anything, nor can anyone else. In effect, I am no longer able to speak at all! A *major, major* loss, because throughout my life, expressing myself orally has been a central aspect of my identity, not to mention, of course, my academic career. Moreover, the same deterioration of the throat muscles that precludes me from talking, also makes it impossible for me now to sing, or even hum. And singing—to myself, to my children while putting them to sleep at night, to my partners, at synagogue services—was always an essential central source of pleasure and emotional nourishment in my life, as well as a primary means of expressing my emotions. And for the same reason, I'm unable even to chuckle or to truly laugh any more, especially that all-out, hearty, unselfconscious type of laughter that used to be so characteristic of me. Now, all that comes out is a high-pitched sort of screech that I just can't recognize as coming from me.

So, the only way I can now communicate is by writing. Thanks to Sylvia, pads of notepaper of all forms and sizes abound all over, and almost litter, our home. I also had the creative idea of using those old-time children's magic slates on which one writes, then pulls up the covering plastic sheet so that the writing disappears and the slate is blank and ready for more writing. They are very hard to find nowadays, but through the efforts of a good friend, we were able to locate a source that has them in abundance, so I'm now well supplied. This is a wonderful and highly useful 'low tech' communication tool for me to use with strangers, sales people, agency functionaries, etc. So I carry a magic slate clipped to a clipboard wherever I go outside the house, even though it is often quite awkward to carry that and the several other things I need. At first, such a 'toy' seemed totally out of place at operas, plays, and other social events. But I carry it anyway, just in case the need arises for me to 'speak' with someone.

However, by definition, the writing on the magic slate is very ephemeral; gone as soon as I lift the plastic sheet. Also, it or any kind of writing is of course useless for phone conversations. So, for months, I had to ask Sylvia or other friends to make and to answer all my phone calls. Another great loss, combined with the concomitant loss of independence and autonomy that resulted. And no one can convey the ideas and responses exactly, or sometimes even near, what I have in mind or would say. So, through my HMO (health maintenance organization) and Medicare (federal health care funding), I was able to obtain a 'LightWriter'—an electronic communication device on which I type my words and thoughts, press a key, and a synthesized voice speaks what I've written. (*Exactly* what I've written, with misspellings, skipped words, limited punctuation, etc.; all spoken out, sometimes with hilarious consequences.) This is my 'high tech' means of communication, essential on the phone, but not very helpful in social situations, where the conversation

moves so fast that I can't keep up with it as I'm writing and what I want to say is no longer relevant by the time I'm ready to 'speak' it.

A good friend, who visits me regularly, offered to write everything *he* wanted to say, just as I need to do, so he could share my experience of having to markedly slow down my communication. Also, this eliminated the former disparity in competence or sense of enablement that prevailed when I had to write everything and he could respond in speech so spontaneously, easily, freely, and rapidly. For the same reasons, Sylvia and I agreed to do the same thing. By and large, this has worked fairly well, especially when we're discussing a topic in some detail or processing an argument or misunderstanding. But it also has its important limitations and drawbacks. Perhaps the greatest one is that we can't use written communication in the dark in bed. One of my most profound losses is the loss of 'pillow talk', at night when we go to bed and in the morning before we rise. Those deeply intimate, tender, and loving exchanges, often in whispers, which were so nourishing for us, which brought us so close and which were often precursors to foreplay, are gone, no longer possible. As are gestures, which can't be readily seen in the dark and aren't capable of conveying the subtleties and nuances of inflection, pacing, and voice tone that are possible only with oral communication. And written notes, with the light on and the need for glasses, just don't cut it; not the same. A deeply felt loss for both of us. At my suggestion, we've begun looking into the possibility of our learning some sign language, so as to add more intimacy to our everyday communication, to replace some of the more 'formal' or 'cold' aspects of the written word on the page. And I know it'll take a fairly long time to master signing to the point where we can convey subtle ideas or emotions. But we'll see what happens. I'll be grateful for *any* increase in intimacy and ease of communication. (I sometimes get so tired and weary of having to write out *everything*!)

There are some major consequences of the atrophy of the lips, palate, cheeks, and swallow muscles in my type of ALS, several of which I could not have anticipated and which therefore confronted me with some painful and unwelcome surprise losses. Perhaps the principal one, which has had the most profound and far-reaching impact on my life, is that not being able to swallow means that saliva cannot be managed well and automatically, as it is in people without the disease, and as it used to be for me. I learnt that everyone generates two litres of saliva a day, but healthy people aren't aware of that because they swallow it automatically and unconsciously.

I can no longer do that. So saliva accumulates in my mouth, and not being fully swallowed, it leaks out. My lips are so weak that I cannot purse them at all. (This makes me incapable of swishing my mouth after brushing my teeth, and it also means I can no longer kiss! And in addition, loss of control over my lips means I can no longer smile. Any attempted smile results in only a grimace.) So, I can't spit out and get rid of the excess saliva except through drooling. This is a real problem when the saliva becomes so viscous that it can't leak out easily, so I can't get it out of my mouth at all. I've tried numerous medications prescribed by my neurologist to dry up the saliva and also to thin it, but thus far, none has worked. Moreover, each medication has had very unpleasant side effects which have been very hard for me to tolerate. Furthermore, the mucous, which is automatically brought up from the lungs and automatically and unconsciously swallowed by healthy people, remains all the time in the base of my throat, right above the vocal cords. There it poses the danger of aspiration because I can't either swallow it or bring it up to my mouth to expectorate it.

So, right now, perhaps the *main* difficulty I'm having to deal with is the *constant and continuous* drooling, with no let up, except while I'm asleep. (I'm not sure of the reason for this exception, but I'm very grateful for it. Otherwise I'd not be able to sleep at all and would run the risk of aspirating and drowning in my own juices.) But the minute I awaken, even before I get out of bed, the saliva starts again. It's very uncomfortable and a major nuisance, drooling all over everything, the floor, clothes, books, furniture, the computer (even as I'm typing this message)—*everything*! In addition, it causes me to cough a lot when it gets close to the tracheal opening and threatens to be aspirated. My cough response is a blessing, because it prevents aspiration, but it's very tiring.

However, I find that I've begun to be able to look at my drooling with some degree of detachment and humor, for which I'm grateful.

I see myself as a human dripping faucet that no plumber or no washer can fix. I've also concluded that, at this point in my life, even if I wanted to become one, I'd make a very poor criminal: I leave my drool prints wherever I go. I've also discovered an example of true perpetual motion: I drool on the floor, and as I'm bending over to wipe it up, I drool more in roughly the same spot. As I'm wiping that spot up, I drool still more in the same place, and on and on and on. Voila! Perpetual motion (at least until I drop with exhaustion). We've all read or heard about people who accomplish difficult tasks through the sweat of their brow. *I'm* destined to accomplish *my* difficult tasks, I've found, and indeed, any tasks, through the drool of my mouth! Really, though, my ability to joke and make puns about my drooling is really very helpful to me in getting through this aspect of the disease. In fact, it's really my salivation!

One other totally unexpected consequence of the bulbar aspect of my version of ALS seems worthy of note, because of its major impacts on very basic aspects of my body's functioning which I, like every other healthy person, took for granted and was totally unaware of. I didn't know, but abruptly and rudely learned, that it's the upper palate that normally seals off the upper section of the oral cavity from the lower section and that this makes it possible for us to develop the expulsive force necessary to blow our nose. With both my upper and lower palates very much weakened and virtually non-functional, I can no longer perform this basic and crucial function. This means that it has become very difficult, if not impossible, to keep my nasal passages clear and clean. This has become a serious matter as my tracheal airway has become more and more compromised and clogged by the constant pooling of saliva and mucous at the base of my throat. When this becomes bad, especially at night, and my nasal passages are also not clear, I've begun to feel, if only for a few seconds, the anxiety of potential asphyxiation.

A second unanticipated repercussion of the weakened palate's inability to seal off the upper from the lower section of the oral cavity and thus create an expulsive force in both the respiratory and digestive systems is that this makes it virtually impossible to 'bear down' during defecation. That becomes more than just a vexing nuisance as normal peristalsis in the intestinal tract and the colon becomes weaker due to the marked absence of roughage and bulk in the totally liquid formula and water diet I'm required to follow.

This illness, as you can see, is teaching me a great deal about anatomy and physiology that I, a massage therapist, never knew before. I doubt that even my doctors are really aware of the role of the upper palate in the two basic and essential functions I've just described to you. At least, none of them has told me about them or prepared me to anticipate them. And that Black spiritual, 'Dem Bones, Dem Bones, Dem Dry Bones' (that at least my American colleagues are very familiar with), never taught me that the palate bone is connected to the ass bone!

The final aspect of my journey with ALS that I'd like to share with you is truly a challenging and somewhat scary one. Early on in my illness, the doctors had said that, given the bulbar palsy onset of the disease, there was the *possibility* that I would not experience the atrophy and weakening of the limbs and the torso that most commonly characterize ALS. Well, that possibility did not materialize. In the past four or five months, I've experienced marked and progressive wasting of muscle and fat, first in my left hand, arm, and shoulder. In fact, my left hand and fingers have become so weak and atrophied that I can hardly hold anything even *moderately* heavy. My fingers can't bend easily, and my left arm and shoulder have lost so much muscle mass and are so weak that I can't keep them up for more than a few minutes at a time. My left little finger is constantly bent and can't really be straightened. That makes typing difficult and somewhat slower but not yet impossible, as you can see from the length of this message. My right hand is also losing muscle and strength, but being the dominant hand, it's still much stronger than the left. Nevertheless, it became so hard for me to turn on the ignition of my car with the right hand, that I had installed a remote engine start device that starts the engine at the press of two buttons on the remote. This has been a major contribution to maintaining my independence and mobility.

But speaking of buttons, I'm having much more difficulty buttoning my clothes and tying my shoes because of the progressive loss of fine motor skills with my hands. Also, I'm experiencing much greater difficulty putting on shirts and jackets by myself because my shoulders and upper arms are so much weaker.

I've lost 20 pounds in one year, mostly due to loss of muscle mass, and I see that very graphically when I look at my torso in the mirror. I'm really gaunt (but not with the wind . . . yet!). My upper back muscles must also be getting weaker because they are beginning to ache and hurt if I stand too long. Thus far, my legs appear to be functioning well, but even they are beginning to cramp a lot at night, and I've been experiencing fleeting pains in my left lower leg. So, unless this aspect of the disease either slows down or plateaus, there will be increasing limitations on my ability to function independently in various quadrants of my life, along with my inability to eat, swallow, and talk. I'm sure that that situation will present me with yet more and different losses, and with the need to grieve them.

So, I think that for me, the important and illuminating question is how have I handled all these developments during the past year. Externally and internally, how have I traveled the ALS journey from last April to now? Externally, I've followed each of the suggestions of my neurologist and other conventional doctors for managing the symptoms of this illness and trying to make it as comfortable as possible to live with those symptoms. Conventional medicine has no cure to offer for the disease, and only a single, scientifically tested drug, which was shown to extend the life of the experimental group patients on average from three to five months as compared with the control group. I took that drug and coped with its negative side effects for roughly eight months, as the symptoms got worse and worse, and finally I stopped. I'm now trying another drug that seemed to be possibly somewhat more effective in slowing the rate of the disease, but that drug has not been subjected to a randomized, double blind research study. Its side effects seem less severe for me, though it's too soon to determine whether there is *any* benefit for me. My symptoms are only increasing, as I've described above.

You may remember that in my April message I spoke of the possible miracles of alternative healing approaches and said I intended to try as many of those that seemed substantial and that came to me from people whose judgment I valued and thought was sound. I was optimistic about beating this illness in that way. Well, for over 10 months, I tried a wide range of alternative approaches, serially, so that whatever positive outcome might possibly occur, I could attribute to a given approach. I committed a substantial amount of time and funds to these efforts, and none has yielded any improvement. No miracles have occurred, and I am now much less sanguine that any will. I haven't given up totally on alternative healing methods, and recently, Sylvia and I consulted a psychic whom I have worked with many times over the past 10 years and have found to be a really authentic and clear channel. I've just begun to follow the techniques that came out of that session, and we'll see. Presently, with our not knowing how much time we have left, Sylvia wants to opt for increased quality of whatever life together we have remaining, by doing what we want and enjoying ourselves now, rather than by trying any other time-consuming alternative healing approaches with dubious outcomes. I largely agree, but I'm open to other possibilities that may emerge and that seem promising. It's my life and by nature, I'm a survivor.

It's been the way I've related to the disease internally that's been where I've struggled most, and where I've had the greatest and the hardest learning. For the first 10 months or so, periodically I'd get frustrated, angry, or very sad, and I'd cry, yell, or pound the table or the walls, or throw things as I encountered loss after loss, at what seemed to be a markedly accelerating pace. Of course, who knows better than all of us in this field that these emotions and behavioral reactions can be a 'normal', and possibly even healthy, part of the process of grieving such major and ongoing losses. But although they afforded me some transient cathartic release, somehow I always ended up feeling worse, constricted, deflated, and 'down'.

The only thing that has really enabled me to continue living through and experiencing the debilitating consequences of this illness, with at least some modicum of balance and grace, has been a basic and powerful notion, drawn from the teachings of the spiritual path I've been following the past six years. It is also contained in a couple of profound books I've read ('The Power of Now' by Eckhart Tolle,

and 'Learning to Fall: The Blessings of an Imperfect Life' by Phillip Simmons). That notion is the value and importance of being present in each moment, and of totally accepting whatever that moment brings, without wanting it to be different from what it is. That's an extraordinarily difficult space to achieve at any time. But I've found it especially daunting as I've been experiencing loss upon loss: as I've been struggling to breathe and avoid choking or possibly drowning in my own juices, with saliva and mucous clogging the upper respiratory airways; when, in the moments that I've been trying to communicate but am unable to vocalize anything but a grunt; when I can't pick up or hold a book or my clipboard in my weakening hands, or tie my shoes or button my shirt with those hands; and so on. In those moments, at first, I could reach that acceptance space for only a nanosecond at a time. Then, maybe for several seconds or possibly a minute. Now, with persistent practice, for somewhat longer periods, perhaps for as much as the better part of a day. And, I still forget or can't get there much of the time.

But when I do remember and can achieve that presence and acceptance—even for those nanoseconds—I feel a profound calmness, serenity, and even tranquility. (In those moments, I realize and actually experience, that I am much more than my body that is undergoing all that stress and turmoil. It's then that I really know, deeply, that everything is all right just as it is, and that I am, and will continue to be, all right.) Much of the time these days, I keep opening up myself to receive and experience these precious moments because I've found that for me (not necessarily for anyone else), this way of being is not simply a useful concept or an optional frill in my life. Rather, it's an absolute necessity! It's the only way I've found that I can keep going and not give up or become severely depressed in the face of the relentless march of this implacable disease toward more and more debilitating weakness, reduced functioning in all areas, and, ultimately, my end.

I've struggled, as perhaps some of you may have, with the difference between acceptance and resignation. Through my readings and my conversations with wise and spiritually grounded people, I've come up with a clear distinction that satisfies me (again, not necessarily anyone else): acceptance brings about a sense of expansion, openness, freedom of spirit, and makes one feel good and lighter; whereas resignation results in a sense of constriction, closedness, tightness of spirit, and makes one feel bad, heavier, and that one has given up. So, it's definitely acceptance that I seek and have been aiming for.

Well, dear friends and colleagues, I fear that this has been not a limited message but rather a tome. I trust I've not gone beyond the bounds of your patience, tolerance, or interest, with this very lengthy account of what's happened in my life since last you heard from me. Also, I hope that you do not feel deluged by more specifics of this disease than you ever wanted and that you'd rather not have been exposed to. It's just that it's been such a long time since I've been in contact with you. I feel so close to you—almost like family, though we really haven't spent a great deal of time together—that I felt a strong desire to share with you what life's really been like for me this past year, and how I've responded to it. This way, you now have a clear picture of where I am on my journey and how I'm doing.

Love and blessings to you all.

Index

Page numbers in *italics* indicate tables.